D0469917

MANUAL OF LABORATORY TESTS

JUNE H. CELLA, R.N., M.S.N., Ed.D.
Former Associate Professor
Department of Nursing
College of Allied Health Sciences
Thomas Jefferson University
Philadelphia, Pennsylvania

JUANITA WATSON, R.N., M.S.N.
Director of Education
Saint Agnes Medical Center
Philadelphia, Pennsylvania

Doctoral Candidate
Division of Nursing
New York University
New York, New York

F. A. DAVIS COMPANY • Philadelphia

Printed in the United States of America

Last digit indicates print number: 10 9 8 7 6 5 4

Library of Congress Cataloging-in-Publication Data

Cella, June, 1927–
 Nurse's manual of laboratory tests   /   June Cella, Juanita Watson.
   p.   cm.
 Includes bibliographies and index.
 ISBN 0-8036-1696-1
   1. Diagnosis, Laboratory—Handbooks, manuals, etc.   2. Nursing—
 Handbooks, manuals, etc.   I. Watson, Juanita, 1946–   .
 II. Title.
   [DNLM: 1. Diagnosis, Laboratory—nurses' instruction.   QY 4
 C393n]
 RB37.C43 1989
 616.07'5—dc19
 DNLM/DLC
 for Library of Congress   88-36758
                                                                           CIP

This book is dedicated to my husband, Andrew, who endured—
and endured—and endured.

JHC

This book is dedicated to my mother, Dorothy M. Watson, and to
the memory of my father, Harry A. Watson

JW

PREFACE

This book is designed to provide both students and practitioners of nursing with the information needed to care for clients undergoing laboratory tests and to use the results of the tests in planning and evaluating care. Its focus is on providing a strong, yet practical, nursing perspective. Although a number of books on laboratory studies are currently available for nurses, this text is unique in that its format provides in-depth background information and quick-reference clinical applications data in separate sections for related tests.

The Background Information sections are designed to provide the anatomic, physiologic, and pathophysiologic content necessary for a thorough understanding of the tests and their purposes. The depth of this content reflects the increasingly sophisticated knowledge base required for current nursing practice and reinforces information from supporting sciences. Since this content is presented in separate sections for groups of related tests, the reader may obtain comprehensive information that ultimately promotes in-depth understanding of the purposes of the tests and the implications of the results. The inclusion of these Background Information sections makes this book unlike many other texts on laboratory studies, which require the reader to glean background information from descriptions of individual tests and then synthesize it to achieve a more complete understanding. The Background Information sections should be especially useful for students of nursing and for practitioners who wish to increase their depth of knowledge about the tests.

The Clinical Applications Data sections provide the quick reference information frequently needed in the practice setting. For each test within the respective sections, reference values, including variations related to age and sex where applicable, are provided. In addition, the several different units of measure by which test results may be reported are included. It is recognized that reference values may vary from laboratory to laboratory. Thus, the reader is urged to consult with the laboratory performing the test to determine its usual reference ranges.

Also included in the Clinical Applications Data sections are factors that may interfere with or alter test results, as are the indications and purposes for the test. When test results have multiple or combined implications, these are included. Major contraindications and Nursing Alerts are included to provide information crucial to safe and reliable testing. Content for these sections was selected judiciously so that only information of critical importance is highlighted. Additional components of the Clinical Applications Data sections include client preparation (which is further divided into sections on client teaching and physical preparation for those tests requiring more extensive preparation), the procedure for performing the test, aftercare, and nursing observations. Where appropriate, critical observations before, during, and after the test are delineated. In contrast to the Background Information sections, most of the content in the Clinical Applications Data sections is presented in list format. Extensive cross-referencing is used to relate the Background Information and Clinical Applications Data sections.

Additional features of this manual that lend to its practical use are presentation of detailed content in tabular form where appropriate and use of appendices to describe collection of blood and urine samples, so that this information need not be repeated with every test involving these substances.

Every effort has been made to include those tests currently in use in practice settings, but to limit content on tests that are infrequently used or that are becoming outmoded. It also is recognized that new tests may have become available after the manuscript was prepared. Readers are, therefore, encouraged to keep abreast of current literature on laboratory studies and to consult with laboratories in their areas on new tests and developments in the field.

It is our belief that this book offers a new approach to providing a source of information that nurses may use in preparing clients for laboratory tests, identifying client problems, and monitoring progress toward desired goals.

JHC
JW

ACKNOWLEDGMENTS

This book would not have been possible without the help, support, and encouragement of a number of people. Special appreciation is due to the staff of the F. A. Davis Company. I am particularly indebted to Alan Sorkowitz, Nursing Developmental Editor, for his major contribution in developing the unique format of this text, for his encouragement to pursue this approach, and for always being available for help when I needed it. I would also like to acknowledge Robert Martone, Senior Nursing Editor, who encouraged me to pursue this project, and Robert H. Craven, Jr., Executive Vice President, for his support and patience as the book evolved. Special thanks also is due to Ruth De George, Nursing Department Secretary, for her invaluable assistance. Many other individuals at the F. A. Davis Company contributed to the production of this book, and I wish to extend to all of them my sincere appreciation for their expertise and dedication to the high standards necessary to producing a good book. Special recognition in this regard is due to Ann Houska and Zena Sandler Gordon, Copy Editors; Philip Ashley, Book Designer; Don B. Freggens, Jr., Artist; and Herb Powell, Director of Production.

I would also like to thank the consultants who served as reviewers of the manuscript for their thoroughness and generosity in sharing their ideas and suggestions. Your comments proved invaluable!

Throughout the process of writing this book, I received tremendous encouragement from my co-workers at Saint Agnes Medical Center. I would especially like to acknowledge the support of the staff of the Department of Continuing Education; the faculty, staff, and students of the School of Nursing; the staff of the Health Sciences Library; the staff of the Clinical Laboratory; Peggy Jones, Vice President for Nursing; Shirley Murray, Vice President for Clinical Services; and Sr. M. Clarence, O.S.F., President. God bless you all!

Special thanks also are due to several individuals who have been supportive of me over the years and who offered special encouragement when I decided to pursue writing a book. These include my sister, Ella-mae Watson Blank; my nephew, Randolph R. Blank; and my long-time friends and mentors Dorothy M. Schmeck and Dr. Dorothy A. Mereness.

Juanita Watson

In addition to the consultants and the F. A. Davis staff members whom Juanita Watson has acknowledged, I would like to thank Karen Okie and Kate Barriteau, former members of the F. A. Davis staff.

June H. Cella

CONSULTANTS

Gayle Acton, R.N., M.S.N.
Instructor
University of Texas at Austin
School of Nursing
Austin, Texas

Camille B. Bagnato, M.N., R.N.C.
Assistant Professor
University of Pittsburgh School of Nursing
University of Pittsburgh at Johnstown
Johnstown, Pennsylvania

Teresa M. Bruggeman, Ph.D., R.N.
Assistant Professor
University of Michigan
School of Nursing
Ann Arbor, Michigan

Beth M. Bukowski, R.N., M.S.N.
Nursing Quality Assurance Coordinator
Georgetown University Hospital
Department of Nursing
Washington, District of Columbia

James Bush, Ed.D., R.N.
Associate Professor
University of Washington
School of Nursing
Seattle, Washington

Bonita M. Cavanaugh, R.N., M.S.
Senior Instructor
University of Colorado Health Sciences Center
School of Nursing
Denver, Colorado

Judy C. Curtis, R.N., B.S.N.
Education Coordinator
Georgetown University Hospital
Department of Nursing
Washington, District of Columbia

Carol F. Evans, R.N., M.S.N.
Assistant Director of Continuing Education
Saint Agnes Medical Center
Philadelphia, Pennsylvania

Alice C. Geissler, R.N., CCRN
Consultant and Contract Practitioner, Critical Care
Colorado Springs, Colorado

Donna D. Ignatavicius, R.N., M.S.
Health Care Consultant
DI Associates
Easton, Maryland

Robert J. Jacobson, M.D.
Acting Chairman, Department of Medicine
Georgetown University Medical Center
Washington, District of Columbia

Mary Frances Moorhouse, R.N., C.C.P., CCRN
Consultant and Contract Practitioner, Critical Care
Colorado Springs, Colorado

Joyce Ann Sands, R.N., M.S., CCRN
Education Coordinator
Hoag Memorial Hospital
Newport Beach, California

April Hazard Vallerand, R.N., M.S.N., CCRN
Instructor
University of Florida
College of Nursing
Gainesville, Florida

CONTENTS

INDEX OF TESTS COVERED

The tests in this index are grouped according to the substance being examined and are listed alphabetically under each substance. The first number cited for each test refers to background information, and the second (in boldface type) to clinical applications data.

First number, background information; second (**bold**) number, clinical applications data.

First number, background information; second (**bold**) number, clinical applications data.

First number, background information; second (**bold**) number, clinical applications data.

First number, background information; second (**bold**) number, clinical applications data.

First number, background information; second (**bold**) number, clinical applications data.

First number, background information; second (**bold**) number, clinical applications data.

First number, background information; second (**bold**) number, clinical applications data.

1

HEMATOLOGY AND TESTS OF HEMATOPOIETIC FUNCTION

INTRODUCTION

Blood constitutes 6 to 8 percent of total body weight. Expressed as volume, women have 4.5 to 5.5 liters, men 5 to 6 liters. The principal functions of blood are the transport of oxygen, nutrients, and hormones to all tissues and the removal of metabolic wastes to the organs of excretion. Additional functions of blood are (1) regulation of temperature by transfer of heat to the skin for dissi-

1

pation by radiation and convection, (2) regulation of the pH of body fluids through the buffer systems and facilitation of excretion of acids and bases, and (3) defense against infection by transporting antibodies and other substances as needed.

Blood consists of a fluid portion, called plasma, and a solid portion that includes red blood cells (erythrocytes), white blood cells (leukocytes), and platelets (thrombocytes). Plasma comprises 45 to 60 percent of the blood volume and is composed of water (90 percent), amino acids, proteins, carbohydrates, lipids, vitamins, hormones, electrolytes, and cellular wastes.[1] Of the "solid" or cellular portion of the blood, over 99 percent consists of erythrocytes. Leukocytes and thrombocytes, although functionally essential, occupy a relatively small portion of the total blood cell mass.[2]

Erythrocytes remain within the blood throughout their normal life span of 120 days, transporting oxygen in their hemoglobin component and carrying away carbon dioxide. Leukocytes while in the blood are merely in transit, since they perform their functions in body tissue. Platelets exert their effects at the walls of blood vessels, performing no known function in the bloodstream itself.[3]

Hematology traditionally limits itself to the study of the cellular elements of the blood, their production, and the physiological derangements that affect their functions. Hematologists also are concerned with blood volume, the flow properties of blood, and the physical relationships of red cells and plasma. The numerous substances dissolved or suspended in the plasma fall within the province of other laboratory disciplines.[4]

HEMATOPOIESES

Hematopoiesis is the process of blood cell formation. In normal, healthy adults, blood cells are manufactured in the red marrow of relatively few bones, notably the sternum, ribs, vertebral bodies, pelvic bones, and proximal portions of the humerus and femur. This is in contrast to the embryo, in which blood cells are derived from the yolk sac mesenchyme. As the fetus develops, the liver, the spleen, and the marrow cavities of nearly all bones become active hematopoietic sites (Fig. 1–1). In the newborn, hematopoiesis occurs primarily in the red marrow, which is found in most bones at that stage of development. Beginning at about age 5, the red marrow is gradually replaced by yellowish fat-storage cells (yellow marrow), which are inactive in the hematopoietic process. By adulthood, blood cell production normally occurs only in those bones that retain red marrow activity.[5]

Adult reticuloendothelial cells retain the potential for hematopoiesis, although in the healthy state, reserve sites are not activated. Under conditions of hematopoietic stress in later life, the liver, the spleen, and an expanded bone marrow may resume producing blood cells.

All blood cells are believed to be derived from the "pluripotential stem cell,"[6] an immature cell that has the capability of becoming an erythrocyte, leukocyte, or thrombocyte. In the adult, stem cells in hematopoietic sites undergo a series of divisions and maturational changes to form the mature cells found in the blood (Fig. 1–2). As they achieve the "blast" stage, stem cells are committed to becoming a specific type of blood cell. This theory also explains the origin of the several types of white blood cells (neutrophils, monocytes, eosinophils, basophils, and lymphocytes). As the cells mature, they lose their ability to reproduce and cannot further divide to replace themselves. Thus, there is a need

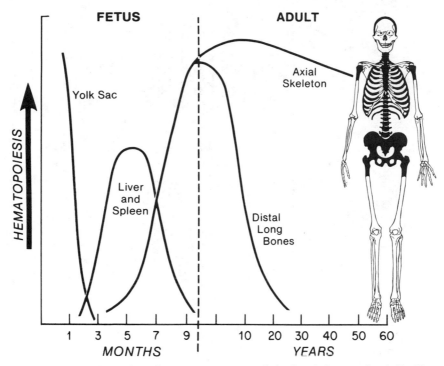

FIGURE 1-1. Location of active marrow growth in the fetus and adult. (From Hillman and Finch,[5] p 2, with permission.)

for continuous hematopoietic activity to replenish worn out or damaged blood cells.

Erythropoiesis, the production of red blood cells, and *leukopoiesis,* the production of white blood cells, are components of the hematopoietic process. Erythropoiesis maintains a population of approximately 25×10^{12} circulating red cells, or an average of 5 million erythrocytes per mm^3 of blood. The production rate is about 2 million cells per second, or 35 trillion cells per day. With maximum stimulation, this rate can be increased sixfold to eightfold, or one volume per day equivalent to the cells contained in one-half pint of whole blood.

The level of tissue oxygenation regulates the production of red blood cells; that is, erythropoiesis occurs in response to tissue hypoxia. Hypoxia does not, however, directly stimulate the bone marrow. Instead, red cell production occurs in response to *erythropoietin,* precursors of which are found primarily in the kidney and to a lesser extent in the liver. When the renal oxygen level falls, an enzyme, renal erythropoietic factor, is secreted. This enzyme reacts with a plasma protein to form erythropoietin, which subsequently stimulates the bone marrow to produce more red blood cells. Specifically, erythropoietin (1) accelerates production, differentiation, and maturation of erythrocytes; (2) reduces the time required for cells to enter the circulation, thereby increasing the number of circulating immature erythrocytes such as reticulocytes (Fig. 1–2); and (3) facilitates the incorporation of iron into red blood cells. When the number of erythrocytes produced meets the body's tissue oxygenation needs, erythro-

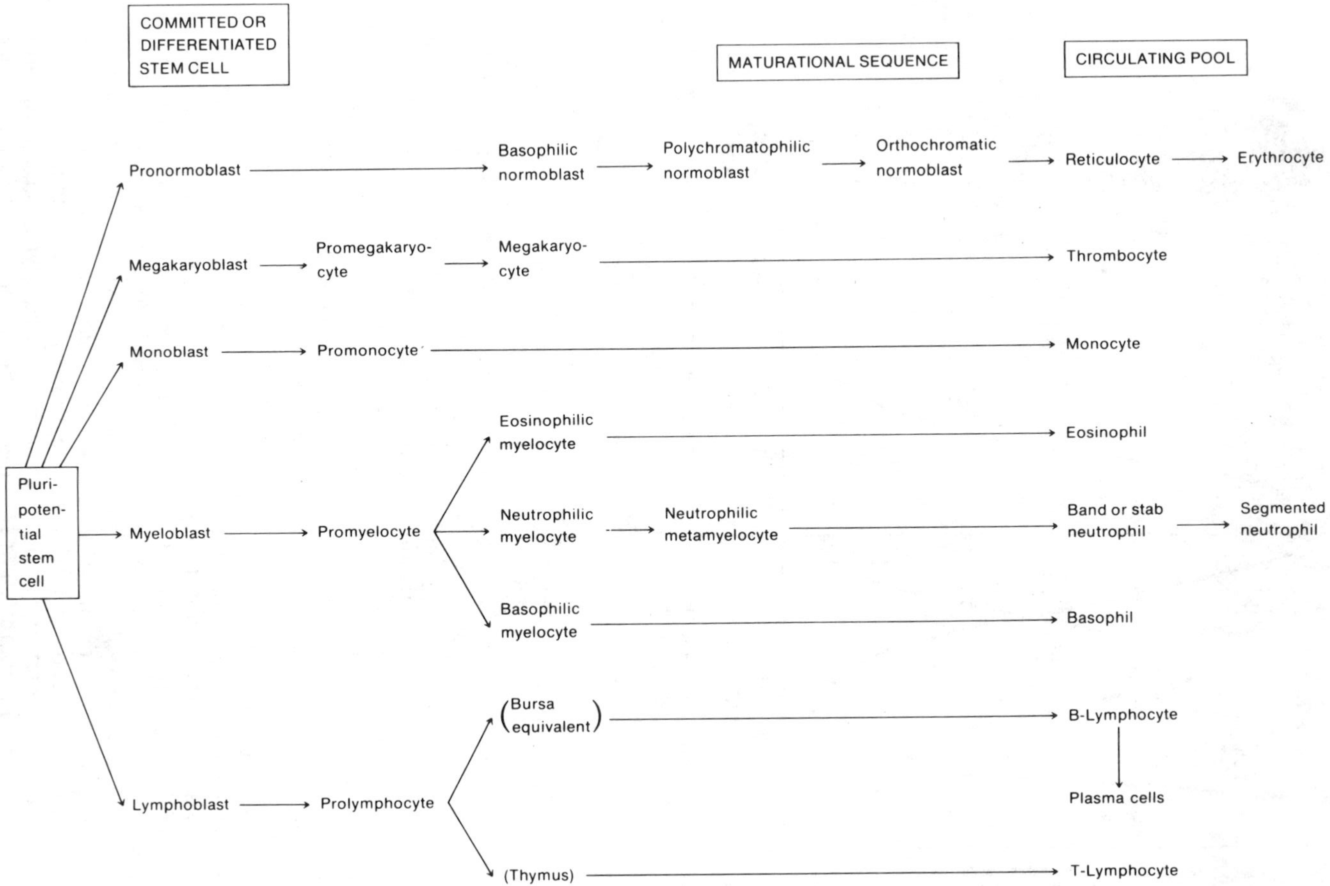

Figure 1-2. Theory of formation and maturation of blood cells (hematopoiesis). (From Price and Wilson, Pathophysiology, 3rd ed., McGraw-Hill, New York, 1986, p 181.)

TABLE 1–1. **Causes of Tissue Hypoxia That May Stimulate Erythropoietin Release**

Acute blood loss
Impaired oxygen–carbon dioxide exchange in the lungs
Low hemoglobin levels
Impaired binding of oxygen to hemoglobin
Impaired release of oxygen from hemoglobin
Excessive hemolysis of erythrocytes due to hypersplenism or hemolytic disorders of antibody, bacterial or chemical origin
Certain anemias in which abnormal red cells are produced (e.g., hereditary spherocytosis)
Compromised blood flow to the kidneys

poietin release and red cell production are reduced. Table 1–1 lists causes of tissue hypoxia that may stimulate the release of erythropoietin.

Threats to normal erythropoiesis occur (1) if sufficient amounts of erythropoietin cannot be produced, or (2) if the bone marrow is unable to respond to erythropoietic stimulation. People without kidneys or with severe impairment of renal function are unable to produce adequate amounts of renal erythropoietic factor. In these individuals, the liver is the source of erythropoietic factor. The quantity produced, however, is sufficient only to maintain a fairly stable state of severe anemia that responds minimally to hypoxemia.

Inadequate erythropoiesis may occur also if the bone marrow is depressed because of drugs, toxic chemicals, ionizing radiation, malignancies, or other disorders such as hypothyroidism. Also, in certain anemias and hemoglobinopathies, the bone marrow is unable to produce sufficient normal erythrocytes.

Other substances needed for erythropoiesis are vitamin B_{12}, folic acid, and iron. Vitamin B_{12} and folic acid are required for DNA synthesis and are needed by all cells for growth and reproduction. Because cellular reproduction occurs at such a high rate in erythropoietic tissue, formation of red blood cells is particularly affected by a deficiency of either of these substances. Iron is needed for hemoglobin synthesis and normal red cell production. In addition to dietary sources, iron from worn out or damaged red blood cells is available for reuse in erythropoiesis.[7]

Leukopoiesis, the production of white blood cells, maintains a population of 5,000 to 10,000 leukocytes per mm^3 of blood, with the capability for rapid and dramatic change in response to a variety of stimuli. No leukopoietic substance comparable to erythropoietic factor has been identified, but many factors are known to influence white cell production with a resultant excess (leukocytosis) or deficiency (leukopenia) in leukocytes.

Table 1–2 shows the causes of physiological and pathological alterations in leukopoiesis. It should be noted that white blood cell levels vary in relation to diurnal rhythms; thus, the time at which the sample is obtained may influence the results. Overall, leukocytes may increase by as many as 2,000 cells per ml from morning to evening, with a corresponding overnight decrease. Eosinophils decrease until about noon, then rise to peak between midnight and 3 A.M. This variation may be related to adrenocortical hormone levels, which peak between 4 and 8 A.M., since an increase in these hormones can cause circulating lymphocytes and eosinophils to disappear in a few hours.

TABLE 1-2. **Causes of Altered Leukopoiesis**

Causes of Leukocytosis	Causes of Leukopenia
Physiologic	*Physiologic*
Pregnancy	Diurnal rhythms
Early infancy	
Emotional stress	
Strenuous exercise	
Menstruation	
Exposure to cold	
Ultraviolet light	
Increased epinephrine secretion	
Pathologic	*Pathologic*
All types of infections	Bone marrow depression
Anemias	Toxic and antineoplastic drugs
Cushing's disease	Radiation
Erythroblastosis fetalis	Severe infection
Leukemias	Viral infections
Polycythemia vera	Myxedema
Transfusion reactions	Lupus erythematosus and other autoimmune
Inflammatory disorders	disorders
Parasitic infestations	Peptic ulcers
	Uremia
	Allergies
	Malignancies
	Metabolic disorders
	Malnutrition

EVALUATION OF HEMATOPOIESIS

Background Information

Abnormal results of studies such as a complete blood count (p. 19) and white blood count and differential (p. 41) indicate the need to determine the individual's hematopoietic function. Evaluation of hematopoiesis begins with the examination of a bone marrow sample and may subsequently require other studies. These include the reticulocyte count, serum iron, total iron-binding capacity, transferrin levels, ferritin, vitamin B_{12} and folic acid studies, and the Schilling test. All of these tests, with the exception of the Schilling test, require a sample of peripheral blood, either venous or capillary.

Although the collection of blood specimens is usually the responsibility of the laboratory technician or phlebotomist, it is often the responsibility of the nurse in emergency departments, critical care units, and community and home care settings. A detailed description of procedures for obtaining peripheral blood samples is provided in Appendix I.

BONE MARROW EXAMINATION (CLINICAL APPLICATIONS DATA, p. 11)

Bone marrow examination (aspiration, biopsy) requires removal of a small sample of bone marrow by aspiration, needle biopsy, or open surgical biopsy.

TABLE 1–3. **Causes of Alterations in Bone Marrow Cells**

Cell Type	Increased Values	Decreased Values

Reticulocytes	Compensated RBC loss
	Response to vitamin B_{12}
	  therapy
		Aplastic crisis of sickle cell
		  disease or herditary
		  spherocytosa

Neutrophils
  (total)
	Myeloid (chronic) leukemias
	Acute myeloblastic leukemia
		Aplastic anemia
		Leukemias (monocytic and
		  lymphoblastic)

Lymphocytes	Lymphatic leukemia Lymphosarcoma Lymphomas Mononucleosis Aplastic anemia	
Plasma cells	Myeloma Connective tissue disorders Infections Hypersensitivity reactions Macroglobulinemia	
Megakaryocytes	Old age Chronic myeloid leukemia Polycythemia vera Megakaryocytic myelosis Infections Idiopathic thrombocytopenia purpura Thrombocytopenia	Pernicious anemia Agranulocytosis Polycythemia vera Iron deficiency anemia

Myeloid to
  erythroid
  (M:E) ratio
	Bone marrow failure
	Myeloid leukemia
	Infections
	Leukemoid reactions
		Posthemorrhage hematopoiesis

Normoblasts	Polycythemia vera	Deficiency of folic acid or vitamin B_{12} Aplastic anemia Hemolytic anemia
Eosinophils	Bone marrow carcinoma Lymphadenoma Myeloid leukemia	

Cells normally present in hematopoietic marrow include erythrocytes and granulocytes (neutrophils, basophils, and eosinophils) in all stages of maturation, megakaryocytes (from which platelets develop), small numbers of lymphocytes, and occasional plasma cells (Fig. 1–2, p. 4). Nucleated white cells in the bone marrow normally outnumber nucleated (immature) red cells by about three to one. This is called the myeloid to erythroid (M:E) ratio.[8] Causes of increased and decreased values on bone marrow examination are presented in Table 1–3.

Since bone marrow examination involves an invasive procedure with risks of infection, trauma, and bleeding, a signed consent is required.

RETICULOCYTE COUNT (CLINICAL APPLICATIONS DATA, p. 14)

Reticulocytes are immature red blood cells. As red cell precursors mature (see Fig. 1–2, p. 4), the cell nucleus decreases in size and eventually becomes a dense structureless mass.[9] At the same time, the hemoglobin content of the cell increases. Reticulocytes are cells that have lost their nuclei but still retain fragments of mitochondria and other organelles. They also are slightly larger than mature red blood cells.[10] Red blood cells normally enter the circulation as reticulocytes and attain the mature form (erythrocytes) in 1 to 2 days.

Under the stress of anemia or hypoxia, an increased output of erythropoietin may lead to an increased number of circulating reticulocytes (see Table 1–1, p. 5). The extent of such an increase depends upon the functional integrity of the bone marrow, the severity and duration of anemia or hypoxia, the adequacy of the erythropoietin response, and the amount of available iron.[11] For example, a normal reticulocyte count in the presence of a normal hemoglobin level indicates normal marrow activity, whereas a normal reticulocyte count in the presence of a low hemoglobin level indicates an inadequate response to anemia. This may be due to defective erythropoietin production, bone marrow function, or hemoglobin formation. After blood loss or effective therapy for certain kinds of anemia, an elevated reticulocyte count (reticulocytosis) indicates that the bone marrow is normally responsive and is attempting to replace cells lost or destroyed.

Individuals with defects of red cell maturation and hemoglobin production may show a low reticulocyte count (reticulocytopenia) because the cells never mature sufficiently to enter the peripheral circulation. Pernicious anemia and thalassemia are classic causes of such ineffective erythropoiesis. A low reticulocyte count may be seen also in clients with severe iron-deficiency anemia, although to a lesser degree. It should also be noted that persons with certain chronic hemolytic diseases may experience aplastic crises in which their usually high level of reticulocytes drops abruptly, indicating that red cell production has stopped despite continuing red cell destruction.[12]

Performing a reticulocyte count involves examining a stained smear of peripheral blood for the percentage of reticulocytes in relation to the number of red blood cells present.

IRON STUDIES (CLINICAL APPLICATIONS DATA, p. 15)

Iron plays a principal role in erythropoiesis, as it is necessary for proliferation and maturation of red blood cells and for hemoglobin synthesis. Of the body's normal 4 g of iron (somewhat less in women), about 65 percent resides in hemoglobin and about 3 percent in myoglobin. A tiny but vital amount of iron is found in cellular enzymes, which catalyze the oxidation and reduction of iron. The remainder is stored in the liver, bone marrow, and spleen as ferritin or hemosiderin.[13]

Except for blood transfusions, the only way iron enters the body is orally. Normally, only about 10 percent of ingested iron is absorbed, but up to 20 percent or more can be absorbed in cases of iron-deficiency anemia. It is never possible to absorb all ingested iron, no matter how great the body's need. In addition to dietary sources, iron from worn out or damaged red blood cells is available for reuse in erythropoiesis.[14]

Serum Iron, Transferrin, and Total Iron-Binding Capacity (TIBC)

Any iron present in the serum is in transit among the alimentary tract, the bone marrow, and available iron storage forms. Iron travels in the bloodstream bound to transferrin, a protein (beta-globulin) manufactured by the liver. Unbound iron is highly toxic to the body, but there is generally much more transferrin available than is needed for iron transport. Usually, transferrin is only 30 to 35 percent saturated, with a normal range of 20 to 55 percent.

Conditions that lead to diminished protein synthesis or involve defects in iron absorption will alter the body's ability to transport iron. For example, abnormal protein homeostasis and resultant low transferrin levels are seen in chronic diseases and infections, widespread malignancy, malnutrition, and nephrotic syndrome. Serum iron levels also may be low in these disorders, and thus, the percentage saturation may remain unchanged. In contrast, if the problem is solely one of protein homeostasis, and iron stores are normal, percentage saturation will be high.

When total body iron is low, as in iron-deficiency anemia and blood loss, transferrin levels increase. Transferrin levels also increase in women in the third trimester of pregnancy and in those taking oral contraceptives. If excess transferrin is available in relation to body iron, the percentage saturation is low. Conversely, in situations of iron excess, both serum iron and percentage saturation are high. Iron excess may occur in hemachromatosis, a genetic defect of iron regulation, in lead poisoning, after multiple blood transfusions, and in severe hemolytic disorders in which iron is released from damaged red cells.[15]

Measurement of serum iron is accomplished by using a specific color reagent to quantitate iron after it is freed from transferrin. Transferrin may be measured directly through immunoelectrophoretic techniques or indirectly by exposing the serum to sufficient excess iron such that all the transferrin present can combine with the added iron. The latter result is expressed as total iron-binding capacity (TIBC). The percentage saturation is calculated by dividing the serum iron value by the TIBC value.

Ferritin

Iron is stored in the body as ferritin or hemosiderin. Many individuals who are not anemic and who can adequately synthesize hemoglobin may still have decreased iron stores. For example, menstruating women, especially those who have borne children, usually have less storage iron. In contrast, persons with disorders of excess iron storage such as hemachromatosis or hemosiderosis have extremely high serum ferritin levels.[16]

Serum ferritin levels are used to measure iron storage status and are obtained either by radioimmunoassay or enzyme-linked immunoassay. The amount of ferritin in the circulation usually is proportional to the amount of storage iron (ferritin and hemosiderin) in body tissues. It should be noted that serum ferritin levels vary according to age and sex (Fig. 1–3).

VITAMIN B$_{12}$ AND FOLIC ACID STUDIES (CLINICAL APPLICATIONS DATA, p. 16)

Vitamin B$_{12}$ (cyanocobalamin) and folic acid (pteroylmonoglutamic acid) are essential for the production and maturation of erythrocytes. Both must be present for normal DNA replication and cell division. In humans, vitamin B$_{12}$ is obtained only by eating animal proteins; hydrochloric acid (HCl) and intrinsic factor are required for absorption. Folic acid (or folate) is present in liver and in many foods of vegetable origin such as lima beans, kidney beans, and dark-green leafy vegetables. It should be noted that canning and prolonged cooking destroy folate. Normally functioning intestinal mucosa is necessary for absorption of both vitamin B$_{12}$ and folic acid.

Vitamin B$_{12}$ is normally stored in the liver in sufficient quantity to withstand 1 year of zero intake. In contrast, most of the folic acid absorbed goes directly to the tissues, with a smaller amount stored in the liver. Folate stores are adequate for only 2 to 4 months.

Vitamin B$_{12}$ deficiency is almost always associated with impaired absorption of the vitamin. Common causes include gastric surgery, decreased secretion of intrinsic factor, age-related atrophy of the gastric mucosa, surgical resection of

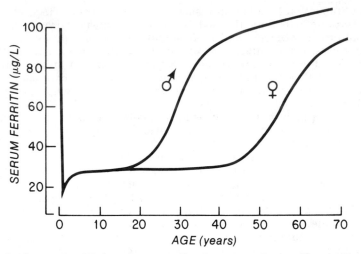

FIGURE 1-3. Serum ferritin levels according to sex and age. (From Hillman and Finch,[5] p 54, with permission.)

the ileum, and intestinal parasites or overgrowth of bacteria in the small intestine. A congenital deficiency of the plasma protein needed to transport vitamin B_{12} also may lead to deficiency despite normal dietary intake. The most common form of vitamin B_{12} deficiency in adults is pernicious anemia, a megaloblastic anemia characterized by decreased gastric production of HCl and intrinsic factor.

Folic acid deficiency also may produce a megaloblastic anemia that is indistinguishable from pernicious anemia, but the condition is usually due to deficient dietary intake, which is commonly seen in individuals with increased folate requirements (pregnancy, hemolytic anemia) whose dietary intake is poor. Folic acid deficiency also is seen in patients with certain diseases of the small intestine and liver that interfere with folic acid absorption and storage (sprue, cirrhosis).[17] Drugs that are folic acid antagonists (alcohol, anticonvulsant agents; antimalarial agents, and certain drugs used in treating leukemia) also may produce folic acid deficiency.[18] People with diseases such as chronic alcoholism, uremia, and certain malignancies commonly have folic acid deficiency.

SCHILLING TEST (CLINICAL APPLICATIONS DATA, p. 17)

The Schilling test is used to determine the cause of a vitamin B_{12} deficiency, which may be due to lack of intrinsic factor or malabsorption in the ileum. Absorption of vitamin B_{12} requires that it be bound to intrinsic factor, a glycoprotein secreted by the gastric mucosa. Pernicious anemia, the most common and severe form of vitamin B_{12} deficiency, involves a deficiency of intrinsic factor, which reduces absorption of vitamin B_{12} in the ileum. Intestinal malabsorption syndromes also may cause vitamin B_{12} deficiency.

The test involves administration of a capsule of vitamin B_{12} labeled with a radioactive substance. Oral administration of the labeled vitamin B_{12} is used to determine gastrointestinal absorption of the vitamin. An injection of nonradioactive vitamin B_{12} also is given, to enhance saturation of binding sites, intestinal absorption, and renal excretion of the radioactive B_{12}. A 24-hour urine specimen is then collected.

When absorption is normal, vitamin B_{12} in excess of body needs is excreted by the kidneys. If absorption is impaired, vitamin B_{12} either does not appear in the urine or is found only in limited amounts; the unabsorbed B_{12} is excreted in the stool. Test results are expressed as the percentage of radiolabeled vitamin B_{12} excreted in the urine in relation to the amount given.

If less than 5 to 15 percent of the radioactive vitamin B_{12} is excreted, a two-stage test is indicated. In this test, an oral dose of intrinsic factor is given in addition to the labeled and unlabeled doses of the vitamin. If subsequent excretion of vitamin B_{12} reaches normal levels, pernicious anemia is confirmed; if not, malabsorption syndrome is present.[19]

Clinical Applications Data

BONE MARROW EXAMINATION (BACKGROUND INFORMATION, p. 6)
Reference Values

Cell Type (%)	Adults	Infants	Children
Undifferentiated	0–1.0	—	—
Reticulocytes	0.5–2.5	—	—
Neutrophils (total)	56.5	32.4	57.1
Myeloblasts	0.3–5.0	0.62	1.2
Promyelocytes	1.4–8 0	0.76	1.4
Myelocytes	4.2–15.0	2.5	18.4
Neutrophilic	5.0–19.0	—	—
Eosinophilic	0.5–3.0	—	—
Basophilic	0–0.5	—	—
Bands (stabs)	13.0–34.0	14.1	0
Lymphocytes	14.0–16.0	49.0	16.0
Monocytes	0.3–6.0	—	—
Plasma cells	0.3–3.9	0.02	0.4
Megakaryocytes	0.1–3.0	0.05	0.1
M:E ratio	2.3–3.5:1	4.4:1	2.9:1
Pronormoblasts	0.2–1.3	0.1	0.5
Normoblasts	25.6	8.0	23.1
Basophilic	1.4–4.0	0.34	1.7
Polychromatophilic	6.0–29.0	6.9	18.2
Orthochromic	1.0–4.6	0.54	2.7
Eosinophils	0.5–3.0	2.6	3.6
Basophils	0–0.2	0.07	0.06

There may be differences in normal values among individuals and in values obtained by different laboratory techniques.

Indications/Purposes for Bone Marrow Examination

- Evaluation of abnormal results of complete blood count (e.g., anemia), or of white blood cell count with differential (e.g., increased numbers of leukocyte precursors), or of both tests
- Monitoring effects of exposure to bone marrow depressants
- Monitoring bone marrow response to antineoplastic or radiation therapy for malignancies

■ Evaluation of hepatomegaly (enlarged liver) or splenomegaly (enlarged spleen)

■ Identification of bone marrow hyperplasia or hypoplasia, although the study may not indicate the cause of the quantitative abnormality

■ Determination of marrow differential (proportion of the various types of cells present in the marrow) and the myeloid to erythroid (M:E) ratio

■ Diagnosis of various disorders associated with abnormal hematopoiesis
 □ Multiple myeloma
 □ Most leukemias, both acute and chronic
 □ Disseminated infections (granulomatous, bacterial, fungal)
 □ Lipid or glycogen storage diseases
 □ Hypoplastic anemia (which may be due to chronic infection, hypothyroidism, chronic renal failure, advanced liver disease, and a number of "idiopathic" conditions)
 □ Erythropoietic hyperplasia (which may be caused by iron deficiency, thalassemias, hemoglobinopathies, disorders of folate and vitamin B_{12} metabolism, hypersplenism, G-6-PD deficiency, hereditary spherocytosis, and antibody-mediated bacterial or chemical hemolysis)
 □ Lupus erythematosus
 □ Porphyria erythropoietica
 □ Parasitic infestations
 □ Amyloidosis
 □ Polycythemia vera
 □ Aplastic anemia (which may be due to drug toxicity, idiopathic marrow failure, or infection)

Contraindications

■ Known coagulation defects, although the test may be done anyway if the importance of the information to be obtained outweighs the risks involved in performing the test

Client Preparation

Client Teaching. Explain to the client:

■ the purpose of the study

■ that it will be done at the bedside by a physician and requires about 20 minutes

■ the general procedure, including the sensations to be expected (momentary pain as the skin is injected with local anesthetic and again as the needle penetrates the periosteum, the "pulling" sensation as the specimen is withdrawn)

■ that discomfort will be minimized with local anesthetics or systemic analgesics

■ that the site may remain tender for several weeks

For children, provide equipment and a doll with which to role-play a simulated procedure.

For all clients, encourage questions and verbalization of concerns about the procedure appropriate to the client's age and mental status.

Ensure that a signed consent has been obtained.

Physical Preparation

■ Take and record vital signs

■ Provide a hospital gown if necessary to provide access to the biopsy site or to

prevent soiling of the client's clothes with the solution used for skin preparation
■ Administer premedication prescribed for pain or anxiety.

The Procedure

The client is assisted to the desired position depending on the site to be used. In young children, the most frequently chosen site is the proximal tibia; vertebral bodies T10 through L4 are preferred in older children. In adults, the sternum or iliac crests are the preferred sites.

The prone or side-lying position is used if the spinous processes are the sites to be used. (These sites are preferred if more than one specimen is to be obtained.) The client may also be sitting, supported by a pillow on an over-bed table for this site. The side-lying position is used if the iliac crest or tibia is the site. For sternal punctures, the supine position is used.

The skin is prepared with an antiseptic solution, draped, and anesthetized, preferably with procaine, as it is painless when injected. Asepsis must be meticulous to prevent systemic infection.

For aspiration, a large needle with stylet is advanced into the marrow cavity. Penetration of the periosteum is painful. The stylet is removed and a syringe is attached to the needle. An aliquot of 0.5 ml of marrow is withdrawn. At this time, the discomfort is a "pulling" sensation rather than pain. The needle is removed and pressure applied to the site. The aspirate is immediately smeared on slides and, when dry, sprayed with a fixative.

For needle biopsy, the local anesthetic is introduced deeply enough to include the periosteum. A special cutting biopsy needle is introduced through a small skin incision and bored into the marrow cavity. A core needle is introduced through the cutting needle and a plug of marrow is removed. The needles are withdrawn and the specimen placed in a preservative solution. Pressure is applied to the site for 5 to 10 minutes and a dressing applied.

Aftercare

The client is assisted to lie on the biopsied side, if the iliac crest was entered, or supine, if the vertebral bodies were used, to maintain pressure on the site for 10 to 15 minutes. For sternal punctures, the supine position or other position of comfort may be used. Bedrest is recommended for at least 30 minutes following the procedure. An ice bag may be applied to the puncture site to alleviate discomfort and prevent bleeding. Analgesics also may be administered to alleviate discomfort.

Nursing Observations

Pretest

■ Assess the client's understanding of explanations provided
■ Assess the client's degree of anxiety about the procedure
■ Take and record vital signs and compare with the client's usual baseline values

During the Test

■ Remain with the client, noting responses to the procedure

Post-test

■ Take and record vital signs and compare with pretest reading
■ Assess the puncture site every 10 to 15 minutes for bleeding

■ Assess the degree of discomfort after the effects of the local anesthetic wear off

RETICULOCYTE COUNT (BACKGROUND INFORMATION, p. 7)

Reference Values

Adults: 0.5 to 2.0% of red blood cells; may be higher in pregnant females

Neonates: 3.2% of red blood cells, declining to 0.5% by 2 months of age

Indications/Purposes for Reticulocyte Count

■ Evaluation of the adequacy of bone marrow response to stressors such as anemia or hypoxia
  - □ A normal response is indicated by an increase in the reticulocyte count
  - □ Failure of the reticulocyte count to increase may indicate depressed bone marrow functioning, defective erythropoietin production, and/or defective hemoglobin production
■ Evaluation of anemia of unknown etiology to determine the type of anemia
  - □ Elevated reticulocyte counts are found in hemolytic anemias and sickle cell disease
  - □ Decreased counts are seen in pernicious anemia, thalassemia, aplastic anemia, and severe iron-deficiency anemia
■ Monitoring response to therapy for anemia
  - □ In iron-deficiency anemia, therapeutic administration of iron should produce reticulocytosis within 3 days and the count should remain elevated until normal hemoglobin levels are achieved
  - □ Vitamin B_{12} therapy for pernicious anemia should cause a prompt, continuing reticulocytosis
■ Monitoring physiologic response to blood loss
  - □ Following a single hemorrhagic episode, reticulocytosis should begin in 24 to 48 hours and peak in 4 to 7 days
  - □ Persistent reticulocytosis or a second rise in the count indicates continuing blood loss
■ Confirmation of aplastic crisis in clients with known aplastic anemia as evidenced by a drop in the usually high level of reticulocytes, indicating that red cell production has stopped despite continuing red cell destruction

Client Preparation

Client preparation is the same as that for any study involving the collection of a peripheral blood sample (see Appendix I).

The Procedure

If the client is an adult, a venipuncture is performed and the sample is collected in a lavender-topped tube. A capillary sample may be obtained in infants and children, as well as in adults for whom venipuncture may not be feasible.

Aftercare and Nursing Observations

Care and assessment following the procedure are the same as for any study involving the collection of a peripheral blood sample (see Appendix I).

IRON STUDIES (BACKGROUND INFORMATION, p. 8)

Reference Values

Normal values for serum iron, transferrin, total iron-binding capacity (TIBC), and ferritin are shown below. Note that values vary according to age and sex. There also is a diurnal variation in serum iron levels, with highest levels occurring in the morning and lowest levels in the evening. This variation is unaffected by meals, except in iron-deficient individuals.[20]

Serum Iron	
Newborn	350 to 500 µg/dl
Children	40 to 200 µg/dl
Adults	
Men	60 to 170 µg/dl
Women	50 to 130 µg/dl
Elderly	40 to 80 µg/dl
Transferrin	
Newborn	60 to 170 mg/dl
Adult	250 to 450 mg/dl
% Saturation (of Transferrin)	
Newborn	65% saturation
Adult	20 to 55% saturation
TIBC	
Children	100 to 350 µg/dl
Adults	300 to 360 µg/dl
Elderly	200 to 310 µg/dl
Ferritin	
Children	20 to 40 µg/dl
Adults	
Men	50 to 200 µg/dl (average 100 µg/dl)
Women (menstruating)	12 to 100 µg/dl (average 30 µg/dl)

Indications/Purposes for Iron Studies

■ Anemia of unknown etiology to determine cause and type of anemia
  □ Decreased serum iron with increased transferrin levels is seen in iron-deficiency anemia and blood loss
  □ Decreased serum iron and decreased transferrin levels may be seen in disorders that involve diminished protein synthesis or defects in iron absorption (e.g., chronic diseases, infections, widespread malignancy, malabsorption syndromes, malnutrition, nephrotic syndrome); percentage saturation of transferrin may be normal if serum iron and transferrin levels are proportionately decreased; if the problem is solely one of protein homeostasis (with normal iron stores), percentage saturation will be high
■ Support for diagnosing hemachromatosis or other disorders of iron metabolism and storage
  □ Serum iron and ferritin levels may be elevated in hemachromatosis and hemosiderosis; percentage saturation of transferrin is elevated, whereas TIBC is decreased
■ Monitoring hematologic responses during pregnancy, when serum iron is usually decreased, transferrin levels are increased (in the third trimester), percentage saturation is low, TIBC may be increased, and ferritin may be

decreased (*note:* transferrin levels may be increased in women taking oral contraceptives, while ferritin levels may be decreased in women who are menstruating or who have borne children)

Client Preparation

Client preparation is the same as that for any study involving the collection of a peripheral blood sample (see Appendix I). Blood for serum iron and TIBC should be drawn in the morning, in the fasting state, and 24 hours or more after discontinuing iron-containing medications.[21]

The Procedure

A venipuncture is performed and the sample collected in a red-topped tube. A capillary sample may be obtained in infants and children, as well as in adults for whom venipuncture may not be feasible.

Aftercare and Nursing Observations

Care and assessment following the procedure are the same as for any study involving the collection of a peripheral blood sample (see Appendix I). Food, fluids, and medications withheld prior to the test should be resumed after the sample is obtained.

VITAMIN B₁₂ AND FOLIC ACID STUDIES (BACKGROUND INFORMATION, p. 9)

Vitamin B_{12}	Serum	200 to 900 pg/ml
Folic acid	Serum	7 to 9 µg/ml
	Red cells	165 to 600 µg/dl

Indications/Purposes for Vitamin B₁₂ and Folic Acid Studies

■ Determination of the cause of megaloblastic anemia
  □ Diagnosis of pernicious anemia, a megaloblastic anemia characterized by vitamin B_{12} deficiency
  □ Diagnosis of megaloblastic anemia due to deficient folic acid intake or increased folate requirements (e.g., in pregnancy and hemolytic anemias), or both, as indicated by decreased serum levels of folic acid
■ Monitoring response to disorders that may lead to vitamin B_{12} deficiency (e.g., gastric surgery, age-related atrophy of the gastric mucosa, surgical resection of the ileum, intestinal parasites, overgrowth of intestinal bacteria)
■ Monitoring response to disorders that may lead to folate deficiency (e.g., disease of the small intestine, sprue, cirrhosis, chronic alcoholism, uremia, some malignancies)
■ Monitoring effects of drugs that are folic acid antagonists (e.g., alcohol, anticonvulsants, antimalarials, and certain drugs used to treat leukemia)
■ Monitoring effects of prolonged parenteral nutrition

Client Preparation

Client preparation is the same as that for any study involving the collection of a peripheral blood sample (see Appendix I). Samples should be drawn after the client has fasted for 8 hours and before injections of vitamin B_{12} have been given. Alcohol also should be avoided for 24 hours prior to the test.

The Procedure

A venipuncture is performed and the sample collected in a red-topped tube. A capillary sample may be obtained in infants and children, as well as in adults for whom venipuncture may not be feasible.

Aftercare and Nursing Observations

Care and assessment following the procedure are the same as for any study involving the collection of a peripheral blood sample (see Appendix I). Foods and drugs withheld prior to the test may be resumed after the sample is obtained.

SCHILLING TEST (BACKGROUND INFORMATION, p. 10)

Reference Values

Normally, individuals excrete from 15 to 40 percent of a 0.5 μg dose of radioactive vitamin B_{12} and from 5 to 40 percent of a 1.0 μg dose.

Clients with impaired absorption excrete less than 7 percent of the smaller dose and from 0 to 3 percent of the larger dose.

Interfering Factors

- Recent radiodiagnostic tests with residual radioactive material in the body
- Incomplete collection of the timed urine sample
- Administration of laxatives prior to the test, as they may impair intestinal absorption of vitamin B_{12}

Indications/Purposes for the Schilling Test

- Identification of deficiency in vitamin B_{12} absorption (one-stage test)
- Determination of the cause of vitamin B_{12} deficiency by differentiating between pernicious anemia and gastrointestinal malabsorption problems
  - ☐ In pernicious anemia, urinary excretion of vitamin B_{12} approaches normal levels when intrinsic factor is administered as part of the study (two-stage test)
  - ☐ In gastrointestinal malabsorption problems, urinary excretion of vitamin B_{12} is decreased

---

Nursing Alert

In clients with severe renal disease, the urine collection time may need to be prolonged to 48 to 72 hours. The normal percentage of labeled vitamin B_{12} will eventually be excreted, however, as long as the client does not have impaired vitamin B_{12} absorption.

Client Preparation

Client Teaching. Explain to the client:

- that although this is a urine test, its purpose is to determine the cause of anemia
- that fasting is required for at least 8 hours prior to the test
- that laxatives should be avoided for 24 to 48 hours prior to the test, so that there is adequate absorption of the vitamin B_{12} administered by mouth
- that the nurse should be notified if diarrhea occurs prior to the test
- that a capsule of radioactive vitamin B_{12} will be given orally and that 1 to 2 hours later an intramuscular injection of vitamin B_{12} (not radioactive) will be administered
- the importance of saving all urine for 24 hours and of avoiding contamination of the urine by feces or toilet tissue
- the time the urine collection begins and ends
- that a special container for the urine will be provided

Assure the client that the amount of radiation received via the radioactive vitamin B_{12} is so small that it is harmless

Encourage questions and verbalization of concerns about the test

Physical Preparation

- Ensure to the extent possible that the client fasts for at least 8 hours and does not drink water for 1 hour prior to the test
- Ensure to the extent possible that laxatives are withheld for 24 to 48 hours prior to the test
- Provide the client with an appropriate urine collection device (e.g., urinal for a male client; urine specimen container that is inserted under the seat of a commode or toilet for a female client)
- Provide a 24-hour urine collection container

The Procedure

One-Stage Test

The client voids and the urine is discarded. If the client has recently had radionuclide studies, a sample of the urine to be discarded may be sent to the laboratory for radioactivity determination.

A capsule containing 0.5 to 1.0 μg of cobalt 57–labeled vitamin B_{12} is given orally. One to 2 hours later (depending on the laboratory's preference), an intramuscular dose of 1000 μg unlabeled vitamin B_{12} is administered.

Food and fluids are resumed after the intramuscular dose of the vitamin is given.

All urine is collected for 24 hours in a container without preservatives (48 to 72 hours for clients with severe renal disease) and is sent to the laboratory for analysis (see Appendix II).

Two-Stage Test

The client voids and the urine is discarded. If the test is done on the day following a one-stage test, a specimen from the first morning voiding should be checked by the laboratory for persistent radioactivity.

A capsule containing 0.5 to 1.0 μg of cobalt 57–labeled vitamin B_{12} is given orally. The client may then eat breakfast.

A 60 μg dose of intrinsic factor is administered orally. One to 2 hours later, an intramuscular dose of 1000 μg unlabeled vitamin B_{12} is administered.

All urine is collected for 24 hours in a container without preservatives (48 to 72 hours for clients with severe renal disease) and is sent to the laboratory for analysis (see Appendix II).

Aftercare

There is no specific aftercare. Food and fluids withheld prior to the test are resumed after administration of either unlabeled vitamin B_{12} or intrinsic factor, depending on whether a one- or a two-stage test was performed.

Nursing Observations

Pretest

- Assess the client's understanding of the explanations provided
- Assess the client's ability to follow instructions for the procedure, especially those pertaining to the 24-hour urine collection
- Assess the client's degree of anxiety about receiving a radioactive substance
- Ascertain if the client has had any recent radiodiagnostic tests that may affect results of the Schilling test
- Assess the client's bowel elimination patterns, as diarrhea due to laxatives or enteritis may alter test results by impairing absorption of vitamin B_{12}

During the Test

- Note the amount of each voiding and report diminishing amounts
- Observe the client for compliance with the urine collection and assist as necessary

Post-Test

- Assess the client to ensure that normal dietary intake has resumed

---
COMPLETE BLOOD COUNT (CBC)

Background Information

A complete blood count (CBC) includes (1) enumeration of the cellular elements of the blood, (2) evaluation of red cell indices, and (3) determination of cell morphology by means of stained smears. Counting is performed by automated electronic devices capable of rapid analysis of blood samples with a measurement error of less than 2 percent.[22]

Reference values for the CBC vary across the life cycle and between the sexes. In the neonate, when oxygen demand is high, the number of erythrocytes also is high. As demand decreases, destruction of the excess cells results in decreased erythrocyte, hemoglobin, and hematocrit levels. During childhood, red cell levels again rise, although hemoglobin levels may decrease slightly.

In prepubertal children, the normal erythrocyte and hemoglobin levels are the same for males and females. During puberty, however, values for males rise, while values for females decrease. In males, these higher values persist to age 40 or 50, decline slowly to age 70, and then decrease rapidly thereafter. In females, the drop in hemoglobin and hematocrit that begins with puberty reverses at about age 50, but never rises to prepubertal levels or to that of males of the same age.

The difference between adult males and females is due partly to menstrual blood loss in women and partly to the effects of androgens in men. Castration of adult men usually causes hemoglobin and hematocrit to decline to levels near

TABLE 1–4. Reference Values for Complete Blood Count

CBC Component	Newborn	1 Month	6 Months	1–10 Years	Adult Male	Adult Female
Red blood cells (RBC)	4.8–7.1 million/mm³	4.1–6.4 million/mm³	3.8–5.5 million/mm³	4.5–4.8 million/mm³	4.6–6.2 million/mm³	4.2–5.4 million/mm³
Hematocrit	44–64%	35–49%	30–40%	35–41%	40–54%	38–47%
Hemoglobin	14–24 g/dl	11–20 g/dl	10–15 g/dl	11–16 g/dl	13.5–18 g/dl	12–16 g/dl
Red cell indices						
MCV*	96–108 μm³	82–91 μm³	—	—	80–94 μm³	81–99 μm³
MCH†	32–34 pg	27–31 pg	—	—		27–31 pg
MCHC‡	32–33%	32–36%	—	—		32–36%
Stained red cell examination	Normochromic and normocytic for all age groups and both sexes (see p. 26)					
White blood cells (WBC)	9,000–30,000/mm³	6,000–18,000/mm³	6,000–16,000/mm³	5,000–13,000/mm³	5,000–10,000/mm³	
Differential WBC						
Neutrophils	45% or less by 1 wk	40% or less by 4 wk	32%	60% after age 2 yr	54–75% (3,000–7,500/mm³)	
Bands	—	—	—	—	3–8% (150–700/mm³)	
Eosinophils	—	—	—	0–3%	1–4% (50–400/mm³)	
Basophils	—	—	—	1–3%	0–1% (25–100/mm³)	
Monocytes	—	—	—	4–9%	2–8% (100–500/mm³)	
Lymphocytes	41% or more by 1 wk	56% by 4 wk	61%	59% after age 2 yr	25–40% (1,500–4,500/mm³)	
T-lymphocytes	—	—	—	—	60–80% of lymphocytes	
B-lymphocytes	—	—	—	—	10–20% of lymphocytes	
Platelets	140,000–300,000/mm³	150,000–390,000/mm³	200,000–473,000/mm³	150,000–450,000/mm³	150,000–450,000/mm³	

* Mean corpuscular volume.
† Mean corpuscular hemoglobin.
‡ Mean corpuscular hemoglobin concentration.

Table 1-5. Drugs That May Cause Blood Dyscrasias

Generic Name or Class	Trade Names
Acetaminophen and acetaminophen compounds	Arthralgen, Bancap, Capital, Coastalgesic, Colrex, Comtrex, Co-Tylenol, Darvocet-N, Datril, Dialog, Dolene, Duadacin, Duradyne, Esgic, Excedrin, Gaysal, Liquiprin, Metrogesic, Midrin, Nebs, Neopap Supprettes, Nyquil, Ornex, Panadol, Parafon Forte, Pavadon, Percogesic, Phrenilin, Sedapap, Sinarest, Sinutab, Sunril, Supac, Tempra, Tussagesic, Tylenol, Valadol, Vanquish, Wygesic
Acetophenazine maleate	Tindal
Aminosalicylic acid	PAS, Parasal, Teebacin
Amphotericin B	Fungizone, Mysteclin F
Antineoplastic agents	
Arsenicals	
Carbamazepine	Tegretol
Chloramphenicol	Chloromycetin
Chloroquine	Aralen
Ethosuximide (methsuximide, phensuximide)	Zarontin
Furazolidone	Furoxone
Halperidol	Haldol
Hydantoin derivatives	
Ethotoin	Peganone
Mephenytoin	Mesantoin
Phenytoin	Dilantin, Dantoin, Diphenylan
Hydralazine	Apresoline, Apresazide, Bolazine, Ser-Ap-Es, Serpasil-Apresoline
Hydroxychloroquine sulfate	Plaquenil
Indomethacin	Indocin
Isoniazid	INH, Nydrazid, Rifamate
MAO inhibitors	Eutonyl, Nardil, Parnate
Mefenamic acid	Ponstel
Mepacrine	Atabrine
Mephenoxalone	Trepidone
Mercurial diuretics	Thiomerin
Metaxalone	Skelaxin
Methaqualone	Quaalude, Sopor
Methyldopa	Aldoclor, Aldomet, Aldoril
Nitrites	
Nitrofurantoin	Cyantin, Furadantin, Macrodantin
Novobiocin	Albamycin
Oleandomycin	Matromycin
Oxyphenbutazone	Oxalid, Tandearil
Paramethadione	Paradione
Trimethadione	Tridione
Penacillamine	Cuprimine, Depen
Penicillins	
Phenacemide	Phenurone
Phenobarbital	
Phenylbutazone	Azolid, Butazolidin, Sterazolidin
Phytonadione	AquaMEPHYTON, Konakion
Primaquine	
Primidone	Mysoline
Pyrazolone derivatives	Butazolidin, Tandearil, Oxalid
Pyrimethamine	Daraprim

TABLE 1-5—*Continued*

Generic Name or Class	Trade Names
Rifampin	Rifadin, Rifamate, Rimactane, Rimactazid
Radioisotopes	
Spectinomycin	Trobicin
Sulfonamides	
Mafenide	Sulfamylon cream
Phthalylsulfathiazole	Sulfathalidine
Sulfabenzamide	Sultrin vaginal cream
Sulfacetamide	Bleph, Cetamide ointment, Sulamyd, Optosulfex, Sultrin vaginal cream
Sulfachlorpyridazine	Sonilyn
Sulfacytine	Renoquid
Sulfadiazine	Silvadene
Sulfameter	Sulla
Sulfamethizole	Thiosulfil forte
Sulfamethoxazole	Azo Gantanol, Bactrim, Gantanol, Septra
Sulfamethoxy pyridazine	Midicel
Sulfanilamide	AVC vaginal cream, Vagitrol suppositories
Sulfasalazine	Azulfidine, Sulcolon
Sulfathiazole	Sultrin vaginal cream, Triple Sulfa cream
Sulfinpyrazone	Anturane
Sulfisoxazole	Azo-Gantrisin, Gantrisin, SK-Soxazole, Sulfizin, Sulfizole, Vagilia vaginal cream
Sulfones	Sulfoxone, DDS, Avlosulfon, dapsone
Sulfonylureas	
Tolbutamide	Orinase
Chlorpropamide	Diabinese
Acetohexamide	Dymelor
Tolazamide	Tolinase
Tetracyclines	Achromycin
Chlortetracycline	Aureomycin
Demechlocycline	Declomycin
Doxycycline	Doxychel, Doxy-C, Vibramycin, Vibratabs
Meclocycline	Meclan
Methacycline	Rondomycin
Minocycline	Minocin
Oxytetracycline	Oxlopar, Terramycin, Tetramine
Thiazide diuretics (rare hematologic side effects)	Diuril, Ademol, Saluron, ExNa, Enduron, Naturetin, Naqua, Renese
Thiocyanates	
Tripelennamine	Pyribenzamine, PBZ
Troleandomycin	Cyclamycin, TAO capsules and suspension
Valproic acid	Valproate
Vitamin A	Aquasol A, Alphalin

those of adult females. It should be noted that there is a decline in erythrocytes for both sexes in old age.[23]

More detailed discussions of the red blood cell and white blood cell components of the CBC are included in succeeding sections of this chapter. Platelets are discussed in Chapter 2.

Clinical Applications Data

Reference Values

The components of the CBC and their reference values across the life cycle are shown in Table 1–4.

Indications/Purposes for a Complete Blood Count

Because the CBC provides a great deal of information about the overall health of the individual, it is an essential component of a complete physical examination, especially when performed upon admission to a health care facility or prior to surgery. Other indications for a CBC are listed below.

- Suspected hematologic disorder, neoplasm, or immunologic abnormality
- History of hereditary hematologic abnormality
- Suspected infection (local or systemic, acute or chronic)
- Monitoring effects of physical or emotional stress
- Monitoring desired responses to drug therapy and undesired reactions to drugs that may cause blood dyscrasias (Table 1–5)
- Monitoring progression of nonhematologic disorders such as chronic obstructive pulmonary disease, malabsorption syndromes, malignancies, and renal disease

Client Preparation

Client preparation is the same as that for any study involving the collection of a peripheral blood sample (see Appendix I).

The Procedure

A venipuncture is performed and the sample collected in a lavender-topped tube. A capillary sample may be obtained in infants and children, as well as in adults for whom venipuncture may not be feasible.

Aftercare and Nursing Observations

Care and assessment following the procedure are the same as for any study involving the collection of a peripheral blood sample (see Appendix I).

ERYTHROCYTE STUDIES

Background Information

The mature red blood cell (erythrocyte) is a biconcave disk with an average life span of 120 days. Because it lacks a nucleus and mitochondria, it is unable to synthesize protein and its limited metabolism is barely enough to sustain it. Erythrocytes function primarily as containers for hemoglobin. As such, they transport oxygen from the lungs to all body cells and transfer carbon dioxide from the cells to the organs of excretion. The red blood cell is resilient and capable of extreme changes in shape. It is admirably designed to survive its many trips through the circulation.[24]

Old, damaged, and abnormal erythrocytes are removed mainly by the spleen and also by the liver and red bone marrow. The iron is returned to plasma transferrin (see p. 8) and is transported back to the erythroid marrow or stored within the liver and spleen as ferritin and hemosiderin (see p. 9). The bilirubin component of hemoglobin is carried by plasma albumin to the liver, where it is conjugated and excreted into the bile. Most of this conjugated bilirubin is ultimately excreted in the stool, although some appears in the urine or is returned to bile.

The hematologist determines the numbers, structure, color, size, and shape of erythrocytes; the types and amount of hemoglobin they contain; their fragility; and whether they contain abnormal components.

ERYTHROCYTE COUNT (CLINICAL APPLICATIONS DATA, p. 33)

The erythrocyte count, a component of the complete blood count (CBC), is the determination of the number of red blood cells (RBCs) per mm^3. In international units, this is expressed as the number of RBCs per liter of blood. The test is less significant itself than in computing hemoglobin, hematocrit, and red cell indices.

Many factors influence the level of circulating erythrocytes. Decreased numbers are seen in disorders involving impaired erythropoiesis (see p. 3), excessive blood cell destruction (e.g., hemolytic anemia), and blood loss, and in chronic inflammatory diseases. A relative decrease also may be seen in situations in which there is increased body fluid in the presence of a normal number of RBCs (e.g., pregnancy). Increases in the erythrocyte count are most commonly seen in polycythemia vera, chronic pulmonary disease with hypoxia and secondary polycythemia, and dehydration with hemoconcentration. Excessive exercise, anxiety, and pain also produce higher erythrocyte counts. Many drugs may cause a decrease in circulating RBCs (Table 1–5), while a few drugs such as methyldopa and gentamicin may cause an increase.[25]

HEMATOCRIT (CLINICAL APPLICATIONS DATA, p. 34)

Blood consists of a fluid portion (plasma) and a solid portion that includes red blood cells, white blood cells, and platelets. More than 99 percent of the total blood cell mass is composed of red blood cells. The hematocrit (packed red cell volume) measures the proportion of red blood cells in a volume of whole blood and is expressed as a percentage.

Several methods may be used to perform the test. In the classic method, anticoagulated venous blood is pipetted into a tube 100 mm long and then centrifuged for 30 minutes so that the plasma and blood cells separate. The volumes of packed red cells and plasma are read directly from the millimeter marks along the side of the tube. In the micro method, venous or capillary blood is used to fill a small capillary tube, which is then centrifuged for 4 to 5 minutes. The proportions of plasma and red cells are determined by means of a calibrated reading device. Both techniques allow visual estimation of the volume of white cells and platelets.[26]

With the newer, automated methods of cell counting, the hematocrit is calculated indirectly as the product of the red cell count and mean cell volume (MCV). Although generally quite accurate, certain clinical situations may cause errors in interpreting the hematocrit. Abnormalities in red cell size and extremely elevated white blood cell counts may produce false hematocrit values. Elevated blood glucose and sodium may produce elevated hematocrits because of the resultant swelling of the erythrocyte.[27]

Normally, the hematocrit parallels the erythrocyte count. Thus, factors influencing the erythrocyte count also will affect the results of the hematocrit (see p. 24).

HEMOGLOBIN (CLINICAL APPLICATIONS DATA, p. 35)

Hemoglobin is the main intracellular protein of the red blood cell. Its primary function is to transport oxygen to the cells and remove carbon dioxide from them for excretion by the lungs. The hemoglobin molecule consists of two main components, heme and globin. Heme is composed of the red pigment, porphyrin, and iron, which is capable of combining loosely with oxygen. Globin is a protein that consists of nearly 600 amino acids organized into four polypeptide chains. Each chain of globin is associated with a heme group.

Each red blood cell contains approximately 250 million molecules of hemoglobin, with some erythrocytes containing more hemoglobin than others. The oxygen binding-carrying-releasing capacity of hemoglobin depends on the ability of the globin chains to shift position normally during the oxygenation-deoxygenation process. Structurally abnormal chains that are unable to shift normally have decreased oxygen-carrying ability. This decreased oxygen transport capacity is characteristic of anemia.

Hemoglobin also functions as a buffer in the maintenance of acid-base balance. During transport, carbon dioxide (CO_2) reacts with water (H_2O) to form carbonic acid (H_2CO_3). This reaction is speeded by carbonic anhydrase, an enzyme contained in red blood cells. The carbonic acid rapidly dissociates to form hydrogen ions (H^+) and bicarbonate ions (HCO_3^-). The hydrogen ions combine with the hemoglobin molecule, thus preventing a build-up of hydrogen ions in the blood. The bicarbonate ions diffuse into the plasma and play a role in the bicarbonate buffer system. As bicarbonate ions enter the bloodstream, chloride ions (Cl^-) are repelled and move back into the erythrocyte. This "chloride shift" maintains the electrical balance between red blood cells and plasma.[28]

Hemoglobin determinations are of greatest use in the evaluation of anemia, as the oxygen-carrying capacity of the blood is directly related to the hemoglobin level, rather than to the number of erythrocytes. In order to interpret results accurately, the hemoglobin level must be determined in combination with the hematocrit level (see p. 24). Normally, hemoglobin and hematocrit levels parallel each other and are commonly used together to express the degree of anemia. The combined values also are useful in evaluating situations involving blood loss and related treatment. The hematocrit is normally three times the hemoglobin level (i.e., hematocrit = 3 × hemoglobin). If erythrocytes are abnormal in shape or size, or if hemoglobin manufacture is defective, the relationship between hemoglobin and hematocrit is disproportionate.[29,30]

RED CELL INDICES (CLINICAL APPLICATIONS DATA, p. 36)

Red cell indices are calculated mean values that reflect the size, weight, and hemoglobin content of individual erythrocytes. They consist of the mean corpuscular volume (MCV), the mean corpuscular hemoglobin (MCH), and the mean corpuscular hemoglobin concentration (MCHC). MCV indicates the *volume* of the hemoglobin in each red blood cell; MCH is the *weight* of the hemoglobin in each red blood cell; MCHC is the *proportion* of hemoglobin contained in each red blood cell. MCHC is a valuable indicator of hemoglobin deficiency and of the oxygen-carrying capacity of the individual erythrocyte. A cell of abnormal size, abnormal shape, or both, may contain an inadequate proportion of hemoglobin.

Red cell indices are used mainly in identifying and classifying types of ane-

TABLE 1-6. **Classification of Anemias**

Anemia	Examples of Causes	MCV (μm^3)	MCH (pg)	MCHC (%)
Normocytic, normochromic	Sepsis, hemorrhage, hemolysis, drug-induced aplastic anemia, radiation, hereditary spherocytosis	82-92	25-30	32-36
Microcytic, normochromic	Renal disease, infection, liver disease, malignancies	<80	20-25	27
Microcytic, hypochromic	Iron deficiency, lead poisoning, thalassemia, rheumatoid arthritis	50-80	12-25	25-30
Macrocytic, normochromic	Vitamin B_{12} and folic acid deficiency, some drugs, pernicious anemia	95-150	30-50	32-36

mias. Anemias are generally classified according to red cell size and hemoglobin content. *Cell size* is indicated by the terms normocytic, microcytic, and macrocytic. *Hemoglobin content* is indicated by the terms normochromic, hypochromic, and hyperchromic. Table 1-6 shows anemias classified according to these terms and in relation to the results of red cell indices.

In order to calculate the red cell indices, the results of an erythrocyte count, hematocrit, and hemoglobin are necessary. Thus, factors that may influence these three determinations (e.g., abnormalities of red cell size or extremely elevated white cell counts) may also result in misleading red cell indices. For this reason, a stained blood smear may be used to compare appearance with calculated values and to determine the etiology of identified abnormalities.

STAINED RED CELL EXAMINATION (CLINICAL APPLICATIONS DATA, p. 37)

The stained red cell examination (red cell morphology) involves examination of red blood cells under a microscope. It is usually done to compare the actual appearance of the cells with the calculated values for red cell indices. Cells are examined for abnormalities in color, size, shape, and contents. The test is performed by spreading a drop of fresh anticoagulated blood on a glass slide. The addition of stain to the specimen is used to enhance red cell characteristics.

As with red cell indices, red cell color is described as normochromic, hypochromic, or hyperchromic, indicating respectively normal, reduced, or elevated amounts of hemoglobin. Cell size may be described as normocytic, microcytic, or macrocytic, depending on whether cell size is normal, small, or abnormally large, respectively. Cell shape is described using terms such as poikilocyte, anisocyte, leptocyte, and spherocyte (Table 1-7). The cells are examined also for inclusions or abnormal cell contents; for example, Heinz bodies, Howell-Jolly bodies, Cabot's rings, and siderotic granules (Table 1-8).

HEMOGLOBIN ELECTROPHORESIS (CLINICAL APPLICATIONS DATA, p. 37)

The hemoglobin molecule consists of four polypeptide globin chains and four heme components containing iron and the red pigment porphyrin. Hemoglobin formation is genetically determined, and the types of globin chains normally formed are termed alpha (α), beta (β), gamma (γ), and delta (δ). Combi-

TABLE 1–7. **Red Blood Cell Abnormalities Seen on Stained Smear**

Descriptive Term	Observation	Significance
Macrocytosis	Cell diameter >8 μm MCV >95 μm³	Megaloblastic anemias Severe liver disease Hypothyroidism
Microcytosis	Cell diameter <6 μm MCV <80 μm³ MCHC <27	Iron deficiency anemia Thalassemias Anemia of chronic disease
Hypochromia	Increased zone of central pallor	Diminished hemoglobin content
Hyperchromia	Microcytic, hyperchromic cells Increased bone marrow stores of iron	Chronic inflammation Defect in ability to utilize iron for Hgb synthesis
Polychromatophilia	Presence of red cells not fully hemoglobinized	Reticulocytosis
Poikilocytosis	Variability of cell shape	Sickle cell disease Microangiopathic hemolysis Leukemias Extramedullary hematopoiesis Marrow stress of any cause
Anisocytosis	Variability of cell size	Reticulocytosis Transfusing normal blood into microcytic or macrocytic cell population
Leptocytosis	Hypochromic cells with small central zone of hemoglobin ("target cells")	Thalassemias Obstructive jaundice
Spherocytosis	Cells with no central pallor, loss of biconcave shape MCHC high	Loss of membrane relative to cell volume Hereditary spherocytosis Accelerated red blood cell destruction by reticuloendothelial system
Schistocytosis	Presence of cell fragments in circulation	Increased intravascular mechanical trauma Microangiopathic hemolysis
Acanthocytosis	Irregularly spiculated surface	Irreversibly abnormal membrane lipid content Liver disease Abetalipoproteinemia
Echinocytosis	Regularly spiculated cell surface	Reversible abnormalities of membrane lipids High plasma free fatty acids Bile acid abnormalities Effects of barbiturates, salicylates, and so on
Stomatocytosis	Elongated, slitlike zone of central pallor	Hereditary defect in membrane sodium metabolism Severe liver disease
Elliptocytosis	Oval cells	Hereditary anomaly, usually harmless

Adapted from Widmann, FK: Clinical Interpretation of Laboratory Tests, ed 9. FA Davis, Philadelphia, 1983, p 22.

TABLE 1–8. **Types of Abnormal Red Cell Inclusions and Their Causes**

Type (Composition)	Causes of Inclusions

Heinz bodies (denatured hemoglobin)	Alpha-thalassemia
	G-6-PD deficiency
	Hemolytic anemias
	Methemoglobinemia
	Splenectomy
	Drugs:
	   Analgesics
	   Antimalarials
	   Antipyretics
	   Furacin
	   Furadantin
	   Phenolhydrazine
	   Sulfonamides
	   Tolbutamide
	   Vitamin K (large doses)

Basophilic stippling (residual cytoplasmic RNA)	Anemia due to liver disease Lead poisoning Thalassemia
Howell-Jolly bodies (fragments of residual DNA)	Splenectomy Intense or abnormal red cell production resulting from hemolysis or inefficient erythropoiesis
Cabot's rings (composition unknown)	Same as for Howell-Jolly bodies
Siderotic granules (iron-containing granules)	Abnormal iron metabolism Abnormal hemoglobin manufacture

nations of these chains form various types of hemoglobin. Disorders of synthesis and production of globin chains result in the formation of abnormal hemoglobins.

Hemoglobin electrophoresis is a technique for identifying the types of hemoglobin present and for determining the percentage of each type. Exposed to an electrical current, the several types of hemoglobins migrate toward the positive pole at different rates. The patterns created are compared with standard patterns.

At birth, most red cells contain fetal hemoglobin (Hgb F), which is made up of two alpha chains and two gamma chains. Within a few months, through sequential suppression and activation of individual genes, fetal hemoglobin largely disappears and is replaced by adult hemoglobin (Hgb A). Hemoglobin A, composed of two alpha chains and two beta chains, comprises more than 95 percent of hemoglobin in adults. A minor type of hemoglobin, Hgb A_2, which consists of two alpha chains and two delta chains, also is found in small amounts (2 to 3 percent) in adults. Traces of Hgb F persist throughout life (Fig. 1–4).[31]

More than 150 genetic abnormalities in the hemoglobin molecule have been identified. These are termed thalassemias and hemoglobinopathies. Thalassemias are genetic disorders in globin chain synthesis that result in decreased production rates of alpha or beta globin chains. Hemoglobinopathies refer to disorders involving abnormal amino acid sequence in the globin chains.

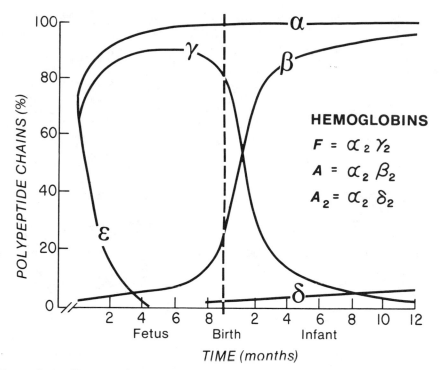

FIGURE 1-4. Changes in hemoglobin with development. (From Hillman and Finch,[5] p 9, with permission.)

In alpha thalassemia, for example, there is decreased production of alpha chains and Hgb A. The oversupply of beta chains results in the formation of hemoglobin H, which consists of four beta chains (Fig. 1–5). Complete absence of alpha chain production (homozygous thalassemia A) is incompatible with life and generally results in stillbirth during the second trimester of pregnancy. The cord blood of such fetuses shows high levels of hemoglobin Barts, a type of hemoglobin that evolves from unpaired gamma chains. Hemoglobin Barts has such a high affinity for oxygen itself that it releases none to the tissues.

In beta thalassemia minor, there is a decrease in beta chain production and, therefore, a reduction in the amount of Hgb A formed. In beta thalassemia major, all beta chain production is lost and no Hgb A is formed. The alpha chains are then used to form Hgb F and Hgb A_2.

Among the most common hemoglobin abnormalities are the sickle cell disorders, in which there is a double beta gene defect that results in the production of hemoglobin S. In Hgb S, the amino acid valene is substituted for glutamine at a critical position on the globin chain. This causes the beta chains to "lock" when deoxygenated, deforming the erythrocyte into the sickled shape. Repeated sickling damages red cell membranes and shortens the cells' life span. The abnormally shaped cells pass more sluggishly through the circulation, leading to impaired tissue oxygenation.

The gene for Hgb S is most prevalent in black populations and may be present as either sickle cell trait (having one recessive gene for Hgb S) or sickle cell disease (having both recessive genes for Hgb S). The Sickledex test, a screening test for sickle cell disorders, detects sickled erythrocytes under conditions of

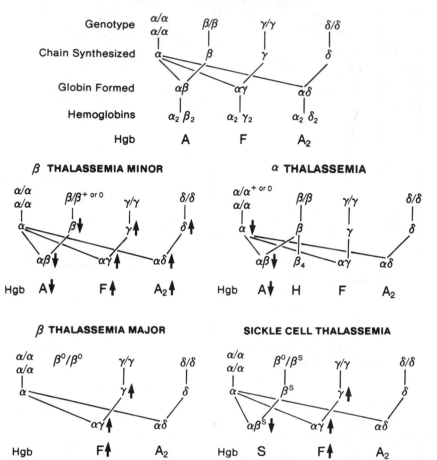

FIGURE 1-5. Formation of normal and abnormal hemoglobins. (From Hillman and Finch,[5] p 74, with permission.)

oxygen lack. Hemoglobin electrophoresis is necessary, however, to differentiate sickle cell trait (20 to 40 percent Hgb S) from sickle cell disease (70 percent Hgb S).

There are many other types of abnormal hemoglobins due to defects in globin chain synthesis. Hemoglobin C, for example, has an abnormal amino acid substitution on the beta chain and may lead to a form of mild hemolytic anemia. Other examples of abnormal hemoglobins due to rearrangement or substitution of the amino acids on the globin chains include hemoglobin E and hemoglobin Lepore (beta chain abnormalities) and hemoglobin Constant Spring (alpha chain abnormality).[32]

It should be noted that other disorders involving hemoglobin pertain to the oxygen-combining ability of the heme portion of the molecule. Examples of types of hemoglobin associated with such disorders are methemoglobin (Hgb M) and carboxyhemoglobin. Hgb M is formed when the iron contained in the heme portion of the hemoglobin molecule is oxidized to a ferric instead of a ferrous form, thus impairing its oxygen-combining ability. Methemoglobinemia may be hereditary or acquired. The acquired form may be caused by excessive radiation or by the toxic effects of chemicals and drugs (e.g., nitrates, phenacetin, lidocaine). It should be noted that Hgb F is more easily converted to Hgb M than is Hgb A.

Carboxyhemoglobin results when hemoglobin is exposed to carbon monoxide. Although this type of hemoglobin is most commonly seen in individuals with excessive exposure to automobile exhaust fumes, it may also occur in heavy smokers.[33] Tests other than hemoglobin electrophoresis are used to determine the presence of methemoglobin and carboxyhemoglobin.

OSMOTIC FRAGILITY (CLINICAL APPLICATIONS DATA, p. 38)

The osmotic fragility test determines the ability of the red cell membrane to resist rupturing in a hypotonic saline solution. Normal disk-shaped cells can imbibe water and swell significantly before membrane capacity is exceeded, but spherocytes (red cells that lack the normal biconcave shape) and cells with damaged membranes burst in saline solutions only slightly less concentrated than normal saline. Conversely, in thalassemia, sickle cell disease, and other disorders, red cells are more than normally resistant to osmotic damage (Table 1–9).

The test is performed by exposing red cells to increasingly dilute saline solutions. The percentage of the solution at which the red cells swell and rupture is then noted.

RED CELL ENZYMES (CLINICAL APPLICATIONS DATA, p. 39)

In order to maintain normal shape and flexibility as well as to combine with and release oxygen, red cells must generate energy. The needed energy is produced almost exclusively through the breakdown of glucose, a process that is catalyzed by a number of enzymes. Deficiencies of these enzymes are associated with hemolytic anemia. Two of the most common deficiencies, both hereditary, involve the red cell enzymes glucose-6-phosphate dehydrogenase and pyruvate kinase.

TABLE 1–9. Causes of Altered Erythrocyte Osmotic Fragility

Decreased Fragility	Increased Fragility
Iron-deficiency anemias	Hereditary spherocytosis
Hereditary anemias (sickle cell, hemoglobin C, thalassemias)	Hemolytic anemias
	Autoimmune anemias
	Burns
Liver diseases	Toxins (bacterial, chemical)
Polycythemia vera	Hypotonic infusions
Splenectomy	Transfusion with incompatible blood
Obstructive jaundice	Mechanical trauma to RBCs (prosthetic heart valves, disseminated intravascular clotting, parasites)
	Enzyme deficiencies (PK, G-6-PD)

Glucose-6-Phosphate Dehydrogenase

Glucose-6-phosphate dehydrogenase (G-6-PD) is an enzyme pivotal in generating the reduced form of nicotinamide adenine dinucleotide phosphate (NADPH) through the pentose pathway in glucose metabolism. Over 100 structural and functional variants of the normal G-6-PD molecule (called type B) have been identified, most of which are clinically insignificant. One variant form (called type A) does, however, produce clinical disease. The type A variant is caused by a sex-linked genetic defect. The abnormal gene is carried by females and is transmitted to males who inherit the disorder.

Persons with the type A enzyme (15 percent of American blacks) experience no difficulty until challenged by an oxidative stressor, which induces rapid intravascular hemolysis of susceptible cells. Among these stressors are systemic infections, septicemia, metabolic acidosis, and exposure to oxidant drugs (aspirin, Benemid, Chloromycetin, Furadantin, Orinase, phenacetin, quinine, quinidine, sulfonamides, primaquine, and thiazide diuretics).

A Mediterranean variant also may occur, especially in individuals of Greek and Italian extraction, and in some small, inbred Jewish populations. This variant has severely reduced enzymatic activity and leads to more severe hemolytic episodes, which are triggered by a greater variety of stimuli and are less likely to be self-limited than in persons with the type A variant. In addition to the oxidative stressors just listed, ingestion of fava beans is known to precipitate hemolytic events in individuals with Mediterranean type G-6-PD deficiency.[34]

Pyruvate Kinase

Pyruvate kinase (PK) functions in the formation of pyruvate and adenosine diphosphate (ADP) in glycolysis. The pyruvate thus formed is subsequently converted to lactate. Red cells that lack PK have a low affinity for oxygen. Episodes of hemolysis in individuals lacking this enzyme are severe and chronic, and are exacerbated by stressors such as infection.

The inherited form of this disorder is transmitted as an autosomal recessive trait; both parents must carry the abnormal gene in order for the child to be affected. The acquired form of PK deficiency is usually due to either drug ingestion or metabolic liver disease.

ERYTHROCYTE SEDIMENTATION RATE (ESR, SED RATE) (CLINICAL APPLICATIONS DATA, p. 40)

The erythrocyte sedimentation rate (ESR, sed rate) measures the rate at which red blood cells in anticoagulated blood settle to the bottom of a calibrated tube. In normal blood, relatively little settling occurs because the gravitational pull on the red cells is almost balanced by the upward force exerted by the plasma. If plasma is extremely viscous or if cholesterol levels are very high, the upward trend may virtually neutralize the downward pull on the red cells. In contrast, anything that encourages red cells to aggregate or stick together will increase the rate of settling. Inflammatory and necrotic processes, for example, cause an alteration in blood proteins that results in clumping together of red cells owing to surface attraction. These clumps of red cells are called *rouleaux*. If the proportion of globin to albumin increases, or if fibrinogen levels are especially high, rouleaux formation is enhanced and the sedimentation rate increases.[35]

An elevated ESR usually indicates the presence of an inflammatory or necrotic process. Additional tests are needed to determine the underlying cause. Results of the ESR may be used to monitor the response to treatment for various

TABLE 1–10. Causes of Altered Erythrocyte Sedimentation Rates

Increased Rate	Decreased Rate
Pregnancy (uterine and ectopic)	Polycythemia vera
Toxemia of pregnancy	Congestive heart failure
Collagen disorders (immune disorders of connective tissue)	Sickle cell, Hgb C disease
	Degenerative joint disease
Inflammatory disorders	Cryoglobulinemia
Infections	Drug toxicity (salicylates, quinine derivatives,
Acute myocardial infarction	adrenal corticosteroids)
Most malignancies	
Drugs (oral contraceptives, dextran, penicillamine, methyldopa, procainamide, theophylline, vitamin A)	
Severe anemias	
Myeloproliferative disorders	
Renal disease (nephritis)	
Hepatic cirrhosis	
Thyroid disorders	
Acute heavy metallic poisoning	

inflammatory disorders (e.g., rheumatoid arthritis, lupus erythematosus). The test also may help to document the presence of organic disease when other physical findings are noncontributory. Specific causes of altered ESRs are presented in Table 1–10.

Clinical Applications Data

ERYTHROCYTE COUNT (BACKGROUND INFORMATION, p. 24)
Reference Values

Newborn	4.8–7.1 million/mm^3
1 month	4.1–6.4 million/mm^3
6 months	3.8–5.5 million/mm^3
1–10 years	4.5–4.8 million/mm^3
Adult	
Male	4.6–6.2 million/mm^3
Female	4.2–5.4 million/mm^3

Interfering Factors

- Excessive exercise, anxiety, pain, and dehydration may lead to false elevations
- Hemodilution in the presence of a normal number of RBCs may lead to false decreases (e.g., excessive administration of intravenous fluids, normal pregnancy)

■ Many drugs may cause a decrease in circulating RBCs (see Table 1–5, p. 21)
■ Drugs such as methyldopa and gentamicin may cause an elevated erythrocyte count

Indications/Purposes for an Erythrocyte Count:

■ Routine screening as part of a complete blood count (CBC) (see p. 19)
■ Suspected hematologic disorder involving red blood cell destruction (e.g., hemolytic anemia)
■ Monitoring effects of acute or chronic blood loss
■ Monitoring response to drug therapy that may alter the erythrocyte count (see Table 1–5, p. 21)
■ Monitoring clients with disorders associated with elevated erythrocyte counts (e.g., polycythemia vera, chronic obstructive pulmonary disease)
■ Monitoring clients with disorders associated with decreased erythrocyte counts (e.g., malabsorption syndromes, malnutrition, liver disease, renal disease, hypothyroidism, adrenal dysfunction, bone marrow failure)

Client Preparation

Client preparation is the same as that for any study involving the collection of a peripheral blood sample (see Appendix I).

The Procedure

A venipuncture is performed and the sample collected in a lavender-topped tube. A capillary sample may be obtained in infants and children, as well as in adults for whom venipuncture may not be feasible.

Aftercare and Nursing Observations

Care and assessment following the procedure are the same as for any study involving the collection of a peripheral blood sample (see Appendix I).

HEMATOCRIT (BACKGROUND INFORMATION, p. 24)
Reference Values

Newborn	44–64%
1 month	35–49%
6 months	30–40%
1–10 years	35–41%
Adult	
Male	40–54%
Female	38–47%

Note that values vary across the life cycle and between the sexes (see p. 19).

Interfering Factors

■ Abnormalities in red blood cell size and extremely elevated white blood cell counts may alter hematocrit values
■ Elevated blood glucose and sodium may produce elevated hematocrits because of swelling of the erythrocyte

■ Factors that alter the erythrocyte count such as hemodilution and dehydration also will influence the hematocrit (see p. 33)

Indications/Purposes for Hematocrit

■ Routine screening as part of a complete blood count (CBC) (see p. 19)
■ Along with a hemoglobin (i.e., an "H and H"), to monitor blood loss and response to blood replacement
■ Along with a hemoglobin, to evaluate known or suspected anemia and related treatment
■ Along with a hemoglobin, to monitor hematologic status during pregnancy
■ Monitoring responses to fluid imbalances or to therapy for fluid imbalances
  □ A decreased hematocrit may indicate hemodilution
  □ An increased hematocrit may indicate dehydration

Client Preparation

Client preparation is the same as that for any study involving the collection of a peripheral blood sample (see Appendix I).

The Procedure

The volume of the sample needed depends on the method used to determine the hematocrit. With the exception of the classic method of hematocrit determination, a capillary sample is usually sufficient to perform the test. If a venipuncture is performed, the sample is collected in a lavender-topped tube.

Aftercare and Nursing Observations

Care and assessment following the procedure are the same as for any study involving the collection of a peripheral blood sample (see Appendix I).

HEMOGLOBIN (BACKGROUND INFORMATION, p. 25)

Reference Values

Newborn	14–24 g/dl
1 month	11–20 g/dl
6 months	10–15 g/dl
1–10 years	11–16 g/dl
Adult	
Male	13.5–18 g/dl
Female	12–16 g/dl

Ratio of hemoglobin to hematocrit = 3:1

Interfering Factors

■ Factors that alter the erythrocyte count may also influence hemoglobin levels (see p. 33)

Indications/Purposes for Hemoglobin Determination

■ Routine screening as part of a complete blood count (CBC) (see p. 19)
■ Along with a hematocrit (i.e., an "H and H"), to evaluate known or suspected anemia and related treatment

■ Along with a hematocrit, to monitor blood loss and response to blood replacement
■ Along with a hematocrit, to monitor hematologic status during pregnancy

Client Preparation

Client preparation is the same as that for any study involving the collection of a peripheral blood sample (see Appendix I).

The Procedure

A venipuncture is performed and the sample collected in a lavender-topped tube. A capillary sample may be obtained in infants and children, as well as in adults for whom venipuncture may not be feasible.

Aftercare and Nursing Observations

Care and assessment following the procedure are the same as for any study involving the collection of a peripheral blood sample (see Appendix I).

RED CELL INDICES (BACKGROUND INFORMATION, p. 25)

Reference Values

Normal values for red cell indices are shown in Table 1–4 (p. 20) in relation to the complete blood count and also are repeated below for adults. Values in newborn infants are slightly different, but adult levels are achieved within approximately 1 month of age.

	Men	**Women**
MCV	80–94 μm^3	81–99 μm^3
MCH	27–31 pg	27–31 pg
MCHC	32–36%	32–36%

Interfering Factors

■ Because red cell indices are calculated from the results of the erythrocyte count, hemoglobin, and hematocrit, factors that influence the latter three tests also will influence red cell indices (e.g., abnormalities of red cell size, extremely elevated white blood cell counts)

Indications/Purposes for Red Cell Indices

■ Routine screening as part of a complete blood count (CBC) (see p. 19)
■ Identification and classification of anemias (see Table 1–6, p. 26)

Client Preparation

Client preparation is the same as that for any study involving the collection of a peripheral blood sample (see Appendix I).

The Procedure

A venipuncture is performed and the sample collected in a lavender-topped tube. A capillary sample may be obtained in infants and children, as well as in adults for whom venipuncture may not be feasible.

Aftercare and Nursing Observations

Care and assessment following the procedure are the same as for any study involving the collection of a peripheral blood sample (see Appendix I).

STAINED RED CELL EXAMINATION (BACKGROUND INFORMATION, p. 26)
Reference Values

In a normal smear, all cells are uniform in color, size, and shape and are free of abnormal contents. A normal red cell may be described as a normochromic, normocytic cell.

Indications/Purposes for a Stained Red Cell Examination

- Abnormal calculated values for red cell indices
- Evaluation of anemia and related disorders involving red blood cells (see Tables 1–6, p. 26; 1–7, p. 27; and 1–8, p. 28)

Client Preparation

Client preparation is the same as that for any study involving the collection of a peripheral blood sample (see Appendix I).

The Procedure

A venipuncture is performed and the sample collected in a lavender-topped tube. A capillary sample may be obtained in infants and children, as well as in adults for whom venipuncture may not be feasible.

Aftercare and Nursing Observations

Care and assessment following the procedure are the same as for any study involving the collection of a peripheral blood sample (see Appendix I).

HEMOGLOBIN ELECTROPHORESIS (BACKGROUND INFORMATION, p. 26)
Reference Values

The normal values for hemoglobin electrophoresis shown below are for adults. In newborn infants, 60 to 90 percent of hemoglobin may consist of Hgb F. This amount decreases to 10 to 20 percent by 6 months of age and to 2 to 4 percent by 1 year. Abnormal forms of hemoglobin (e.g., Hgb S, Hgb H) are not normally present.

Hgb A	95–97%
Hgb A_2	2–3%
Hgb F	1–2%

Indications/Purposes for Hemoglobin Electrophoresis

- Suspected thalassemia, especially in individuals with positive family histories for the disorder
- Differentiation among the types of thalassemias

■ Evaluation of a positive Sickledex test (see p. 29) to differentiate sickle cell trait (20 to 40 percent Hgb S) from sickle cell disease (70 percent Hgb S)
■ Evaluation of hemolytic anemia of unknown etiology
■ Diagnosis of Hgb C anemia
■ Identification of the numerous types of abnormal hemoglobins, most of which do not produce clinical disease

Client Preparation

Client preparation is the same as that for any study involving the collection of a peripheral blood sample (see Appendix I).

The Procedure

A venipuncture is performed and the sample collected in a lavender-topped tube. A capillary sample may be obtained in infants and children, as well as in adults for whom venipuncture may not be feasible.

Aftercare and Nursing Observations

Care and assessment following the procedure are the same as for any study involving the collecting of a peripheral blood sample (see Appendix I).

OSMOTIC FRAGILITY (BACKGROUND INFORMATION, p. 31)

Reference Values

Normal erythrocytes will rupture in saline solutions of 0.30 to 0.45 percent. Red cell rupture in solutions of greater than 0.50 percent saline indicates increased fragility. Lack of red cell rupture in solutions of less than 0.30 percent saline indicates decreased red cell fragility.

Indications/Purposes for Osmotic Fragility

■ Confirmation of disorders that alter red cell fragility, including hereditary anemias (see Table 1–9, p. 31)
■ Evaluation of the extent of extrinsic damage to red cells from burns, inadvertent instillation of hypotonic intravenous fluids, microorganisms, and excessive exercise

Client Preparation

Client preparation is the same as that for any study involving the collection of a peripheral blood sample (see Appendix I).

The Procedure

A venipuncture is performed and the sample collected in a green-topped tube. A capillary sample may be obtained in infants and children, as well as in adults for whom a venipuncture may not be feasible.

Aftercare and Nursing Observations

Care and assessment following the procedure are the same as for any study involving the collection of a peripheral blood sample (see Appendix I).

RED CELL ENZYMES (BACKGROUND INFORMATION, p. 31)
Reference Values

G-6-PD	4.3–11.8 IU/g Hgb
	125–281 U/dl PRBCs
	251–511 U/10^6 cells
	1,211–2,111 IU/ml PRBCs
PK	2.0–8.8 U/g Hgb
	0.3–0.91 mg/dl

Interfering Factors

■ Young red blood cells have higher enzyme levels than do older ones; thus, if the tests are performed within 10 days of a hemolytic episode (when the body is actively replacing lost cells through increased erythropoiesis) or after a recent blood transfusion, the results may be falsely normal

Indications/Purposes for Red Cell Enzymes

■ Hemolytic anemia of uncertain etiology, especially when it occurs in infancy or early childhood
■ Suspected G-6-PD or PK deficiency, especially in individuals with positive family histories or when jaundice occurs in response to stressors, oxidant drugs, or foods such as fava beans

Client Preparation

Client preparation is the same as that for any study involving the collection of a peripheral blood sample (see Appendix I).

The Procedure

A venipuncture is performed and the sample collected in a lavender-topped tube. A capillary sample may be collected in infants and children, as well as in adults for whom venipuncture may not be feasible.

Aftercare and Nursing Observations

Care and assessment following the procedure are the same as for any study involving the collection of a peripheral blood sample (see Appendix I).

ERYTHROCYTE SEDIMENTATION RATE (ESR, SED RATE) (BACKGROUND INFORMATION, p. 32)
Reference Values

Normal values for the erythrocyte sedimentation rate (ESR) are shown below. Note that several laboratory methods may be used to determine the ESR. Values will vary according to the method used.

	Wintrobe (mm/hr)	Westergren (mm/hr)	Cutler (mm/hr)
Men			0–8
< age 50 years	0–7	0–15	
> age 50 years	5–7	0–20	
Women			0–10
< age 50 years	0–15	0–20	
> age 50 years	25–30	0–30	

	Landau Micro Method	Smith Micro Method
Children		
Newborn–2 years	1–6	0–1 (newborn)
4–14 years	1–9	3–13

Interfering Factors

■ Delays in performing the test after the sample is collected may retard the ESR and cause abnormally low results; the test should be performed within 3 hours of collecting the sample

Indications/Purposes for Erythrocyte Sedimentation Rate

■ Suspected organic disease when symptoms are vague and clinical findings uncertain
■ Identification of the presence of an inflammatory or necrotic process
■ Monitoring response to treatment for various inflammatory disorders (e.g., rheumatoid arthritis, lupus erythematosus)
■ Support for diagnosing disorders associated with altered ESRs (see Table 1–10, p. 33)

Client Preparation

Client preparation is the same as that for any study involving the collection of a peripheral blood sample (see Appendix I).

The Procedure

A venipuncture is performed and the sample collected in a lavender-topped tube. A capillary sample may be obtained in infants and children, as well as in adults for whom venipuncture may not be feasible.

The sample should be transported promptly to the laboratory, as the test must be performed within 3 hours of collecting the sample. Delays may retard the ESR and cause abnormally low results.

Aftercare and Nursing Observations

Care and assessment following the procedure are the same as for any study involving the collection of a peripheral blood sample (see Appendix I).

LEUKOCYTE STUDIES

Background Information

Leukocytes (white blood cells, WBCs) constitute the body's primary defense against "foreignness." That is, leukocytes protect the body from foreign organisms, substances, and tissues. The main types of leukocytes are neutrophils, monocytes, eosinophils, basophils, and lymphocytes. All of these cells are produced in the bone marrow. Lymphocytes may be produced in other sites in addition to the bone marrow. Each of these types of leukocytes has different functions, and each behaves as a related but different system.[36]

Neutrophils and monocytes, the most mobile and active phagocytic leukocytes, are capable of breaking down various proteins and lipids such as those in bacterial cell membranes. The function of eosinophils is uncertain, although they are believed to detoxify foreign proteins that enter the body through the lungs or intestinal tract. The function of basophils also is not clearly understood, but the cells themselves are known to contain heparin, histamine, and serotonin. Basophils are believed to cause increased blood flow to injured tissues, while preventing excessive intravascular clotting. Lymphocytes play an important role in immunity and may be divided into two main categories, B-lymphocytes and T-lymphocytes. B-lymphocytes are responsible for humoral immunity and antibody production. It is B-lymphocytes that ultimately develop into the antibody-producing plasma cells (see Fig. 1–2, p. 4). T-lymphocytes are responsible for cellular immunity and interact directly with the antigen.[37,38] Lymphocytes and related studies are discussed in greater detail in Chapter 3.

It should be noted that leukocytes perform their functions outside of the vascular bed. Thus, white cells are merely in transit while in the blood. Because of the many leukocyte functions, alterations in the number and types of cells may be indicative of numerous pathophysiological problems.

WHITE BLOOD CELL COUNT (WBC) (CLINICAL APPLICATIONS DATA, p. 45)

The white blood cell count (WBC) determines the number of leukocytes per mm^3 of whole blood. The counting is performed very rapidly by electronic devices. The WBC may be performed as part of a complete blood count (CBC), alone or with differential white cell count. An elevated WBC is termed *leukocytosis;* a decreased count, *leukopenia.* In addition to the normal physiological variations in white count, many pathological problems may result in an abnormal WBC (see Table 1–2, p. 6).

In general, leukocytosis is seen in infection, inflammation, leukemia, and parasitic infestations. Leukopenia is seen in bone marrow depression, severe infection, viral infections, autoimmune diseases, malignancies, and malnutrition. It should be noted that an alteration in total white cell count indicates the degree of response to a pathological process but is not specifically diagnostic for any one disorder. A more complete evaluation is obtained through the differential white blood cell count.

DIFFERENTIAL WHITE BLOOD CELL COUNT (CLINICAL APPLICATIONS DATA, p. 46)

The differential white blood cell count indicates the percentage of each type of leukocyte present per mm^3 of whole blood. If necessary for further evaluation

TABLE 1-11. **Causes of Altered WBC Differential by Cell Type**

Cell Type	Increased Levels	Decreased Levels
Neutrophils	Stress (allergies, exercise, childbirth, surgery) Extremes of temperature Acute hemorrhage or hemolysis Infectious diseases Inflammatory disorders (rheumatic fever, gout, rheumatoid arthritis, drug reactions, vasculitis, myositis) Tissue necrosis (burns, crushing injuries, abscesses, malignancies) Metabolic disorders (uremia, eclampsia, diabetic ketoacidosis, thyroid crisis, Cushing's syndrome) Drugs (epinephrine, histamine, lithium, heavy metals, heparin, digitalis, ACTH) Toxins and venoms (turpentine, benzene) Leukemia (myelocytic)	Bone marrow depression (viruses, toxic chemicals, overwhelming infection, Felty's syndrome, Gaucher's disease, myelofibrosis, hypersplenism, pernicious anemia, radiation) Anorexia nervosa, starvation, malnutrition Malignancies Folic acid deficiency Vitamin B_{12} deficiency Acromegaly Addison's disease Thyrotoxicosis Anaphylaxis Disseminated lupus erythematosus Drugs (alcohol, Pyramidon, Butazolidin, phenacetin, penicillin, chloramphenicol, streptomycin, Dilantin, Mesantoin, Phenurone, PBZ, aminophylline, quinine, chlorpromazine, barbiturates, dinitrophenols, sulfonamides, antineoplastics)
Bands (immature neutrophils)	Infections Antineoplastic drugs Any condition that causes neutrophilia	None, as bands should be absent or present only in small numbers
Basophils	Leukemia Hodgkin's disease Polycythemia vera Ulcerative colitis Nephrosis Chronic hypersensitivity states	None, as normal value is 0-1%
Eosinophils	Sickle cell disease Asthma Chorea Hypersensitivity reactions Parasitic infestations Autoimmune diseases Addison's disease Malignancies Sarcoidosis Chronic inflammatory diseases and dermatoses Leprosy Hodgkin's disease Polycythemias Ulcerative colitis	Disseminated lupus erythematosus Acromegaly Elevated steroid levels Stress Infectious mononucleosis Hypersplenism Cushing's syndrome Congestive heart failure Hyperplastic anemia Hormones (ACTH, thyroxine, epinephrine)

TABLE 1-11—*Continued*

Cell Type	Increased Levels	Decreased Levels

Monocytes	Autoallergies
	Pernicious anemia
	Splenectomy
	Infections (bacterial, viral,
	  mycotic, rickettsial,
	  amoebiasis)
	Cirrhosis
	Collagen diseases
	Ulcerative colitis
	Regional enteritis
	Gaucher's disease
	Hodgkin's disease
	Lymphomas
	Carcinomas
	Monocytic leukemia
	Radiation
	Polycythemia vera
	Sarcoidosis
	Weil's disease
	Systemic lupus erythematosus
	Hemolytic anemias
	Thrombocytopenia purpura
		Not characteristic of specific
		  disorders

Lymphocytes	Infections (bacterial, viral)
	Lymphosarcoma
	Ulcerative colitis
	Bantis' disease
	Felty's syndrome
	Myeloma
	Lymphomas
	Addison's disease
	Thyrotoxicosis
	Malnutrition
	Rickets
	Waldenström's
	  macroglobulinemia
	Lymphocytic leukemia
		Immune deficiency diseases
		Hodgkin's disease
		Rheumatic fever
		Aplastic anemia
		Bone marrow failure
		Gaucher's disease
		Hemolytic disease of the
		  newborn
		Hypersplenism
		Thrombocytopenia purpura
		Transfusion reaction
		Massive transfusions
		Pernicious anemia
		Septicemia
		Pneumonia
		Burns
		Radiation
		Toxic chemicals (benzene,
		  bismuth, DDT)
		Antineoplastic agents
		Adrenal corticosteroids (high
		  doses)

of results, the percentage for each cell type can be multiplied by the total white blood cell count to obtain the absolute number of each cell type present.

Causes of alterations in the differential white cell count according to type of leukocyte are presented in Table 1–11. In general, elevated neutrophil counts are associated with infectious, inflammatory, and necrotic processes. An increase in immature neutrophils (i.e., bands, stabs) indicates the body's

TABLE 1–12. **Causes of Alterations in White Blood Cell Enzymes**

Enzyme	Causes of Alterations	
	Elevated levels	*Decreased levels*
Leukocyte alkaline phosphatase (LAP)	Chronic myelocytic leukemia	Acute myelocytic leukemia
	Polycythemia vera	Acute monocytic leukemia
	Myelofibrosis	Chronic granulocytic
	Leukemoid reactions	leukemia
	Oral contraceptives	Anemias (aplastic,
	Pregnancy	pernicious)
	ACTH excess	Thrombocytopenia
	Cushing's syndrome	Infectious mononucleosis
	Down's syndrome	Paroxysmal nocturnal
	Multiple myeloma	hemoglobinuria
	Lymphomas	Hereditary
		hypophosphatasia
		Collagen diseases
	Positive	*Negative*
Periodic acid–Schiff (PAS) stain	Acute granulocytic leukemia	Early granulocyte
	Acute lymphoblastic	precursors
	leukemia	Normal erythrocyte
	Erythroleukemia	precursors
	Amyloidosis	Mature RBCs
	Thalassemia	
	Lymphomas	
	Severe iron-deficiency	
	anemia	

attempt to produce more neutrophils in response to the pathological process. An increase in bands is sometimes referred to as a "shift to the left." This terminology derives from the traditional headings used on laboratory slips to report WBC differential results:

Bands   Neutrophils   Eosinophils   Basophils   Monocytes   Lymphocytes

In contrast, the meaning of a "shift to the right" is less well defined. This may refer to an increase in neutrophils or other granulocytes, or to an increase in lymphocytes or monocytes.

Increases in eosinophils are most commonly seen in allergic responses and parasitic infections, whereas increases in basophils may be seen in leukemias, Hodgkin's disease, and polycythemia vera. Elevations in monocyte levels are most commonly seen in chronic inflammatory and infectious processes, and during recovery from acute infections. Increased lymphocytes also may be seen in chronic inflammatory and infectious processes, as well as in lymphomas and lymphocytic leukemias.

WHITE BLOOD CELL ENZYMES (CLINICAL APPLICATIONS DATA, p. 47)

White blood cells in peripheral blood samples retain enzymatic activity and can alter substrates added in the laboratory. The presence of enzymatic activity is useful in studying cells that are so morphologically abnormal on stained smear that it is difficult to determine from which cell line they originated (see Fig. 1–2, p. 4). The two most common white cell enzyme tests are the test for leukocyte alkaline phosphatase (LAP), an enzyme found in neutrophils, and the periodic acid–Schiff stain, which tests for enzymes found in granulocytes and erythrocytes. Both tests are used to diagnose hematologic disorders, especially leukemias. Specific causes of alterations in white cell enzymes are presented in Table 1–12. Additional details of each test are briefly discussed subsequently.

Leukocyte Alkaline Phosphatase (LAP)

Leukocyte alkaline phosphatase (LAP) is an enzyme found in neutrophils. This enzyme is completely independent of serum alkaline phosphatase, which reflects osteoblastic activity and hepatic function. The LAP content of neutrophils increases as the cells mature; therefore, the LAP study is useful in assessing cellular maturation and in evaluating departures from normal differentiation.

The LAP study is used to distinguish among various hematologic disorders. For example, LAP increases in polycythemia vera, myelofibrosis, and leukemoid reactions to infections, but decreases in chronic granulocytic leukemia. As all of these conditions have increased numbers of immature circulating neutrophils, LAP scores can be helpful in differentiating among them.

Periodic Acid–Schiff (PAS) Stain

In the periodic acid–Schiff (PAS) stain, compounds that can be oxidized to aldehydes are localized by brilliant fuschia staining. Many elements in many tissues are PAS-positive, but in blood cells the PAS-positive material of diagnostic importance is cytoplasmic glycogen. Early granulocyte precursors and normal erythrocyte precursors are PAS-negative. Mature red cells remain PAS-negative, but granulocytes acquire increasing PAS positivity as they mature.[39]

Clinical Applications Data

WHITE BLOOD CELL COUNT (BACKGROUND INFORMATION, p. 41)
Reference Values

The normal range of white blood cells for adults is 5,000 to 10,000. Variations in the white blood cell count across the life cycle are shown in Table 1–4 (p. 20). Abnormal results may be classified by degree of severity as indicated below.

	Elevations	Decreases
Slight	11,000–20,000	3,000–4,500
Moderate	20,000–30,000	1,500–3,000
Severe	>50,000	<1,500

Indications/Purposes for a White Blood Cell Count

- Routine screening as part of a complete blood count (CBC) (see p. 19)
- Suspected inflammatory or infectious process (see Table 1–2, p. 6)
- Suspected leukemia, autoimmune disorder, or allergy
- Suspected bone marrow depression
- Monitoring response to stress, malnutrition, and therapy for infectious or malignant processes

Client Preparation

Client preparation is the same as that for any study involving the collection of a peripheral blood sample (see Appendix I).

The Procedure

A venipuncture is performed and the sample collected in a lavender-topped tube. A capillary sample may be obtained in infants and children, as well as in adults for whom venipuncture may not be feasible.

Because of the normal diurnal variation of WBC levels, it is important to note the time the sample was obtained (see p. 5).

Aftercare and Nursing Observations

Care and assessment following the procedure are the same as for any study involving the collection of a peripheral blood sample (see Appendix I).

DIFFERENTIAL WHITE BLOOD CELL COUNT (BACKGROUND INFORMATION, p. 41)

Reference Values

The normal percentage of each white cell type in adults is shown below. Variations across the life cycle are listed in Table 1–4 (p. 20).

Bands	3–8%
Neutrophils	54–75%
Eosinophils	1–4%
Basophils	0–1%
Monocytes	2–8%
Lymphocytes	25–40%

Indications/Purposes for Differential White Blood Cell Count

■ Routine screening as part of a complete blood count (CBC) (see p. 19)
■ Abnormal total white cell count to determine the source of the elevation
■ Confirmation of the presence of various disorders associated with increases and decreases in the several types of white blood cells (see Table 1–11, p. 42)
■ Monitoring response to treatment for acute infections, with a therapeutic response indicated by a decreasing number of bands and a stabilizing number of neutrophils
■ Monitoring physiologic responses to antineoplastic therapy

Client Preparation

Client preparation is the same as that for any study involving the collection of a peripheral blood sample (see Appendix I).

The Procedure

A venipuncture is performed and the sample collected in a lavender-topped tube. A capillary sample may be obtained in infants and children, as well as in adults for whom venipuncture may not be feasible.

Aftercare and Nursing Observations

Care and assessment following the procedure are the same as for any study involving the collection of a peripheral blood sample (see Appendix I).

WHITE BLOOD CELL ENZYMES (BACKGROUND INFORMATION, p. 44)
Reference Values

Leukocyte alkaline phosphatase (LAP)	13–130 units
Periodic acid–Schiff (PAS) stain	Granulocytes—positive
	Agranulocytes—negative
	Granulocyte precursors—negative
	Erythrocytes—negative
	Erythrocyte precursors—negative

Indications/Purposes for White Blood Cell Enzymes

■ Identification of morphologically abnormal white blood cells on stained smear
■ Suspected leukemia or other hematologic disorders (see Table 1–12, p. 44)

Client Preparation

Client preparation is the same as that for any study involving the collection of a peripheral blood sample (see Appendix I).

The Procedure

A capillary sample is generally preferred for these tests. The sample is spread on a slide, fixed, and stained.

Aftercare and Nursing Observations

Care and assessment following the procedure are the same as for any study involving the collection of a peripheral bood sample (see Appendix I).

REFERENCES

1. Hole, JW: Human Anatomy and Physiology, ed 4. Wm C Brown, Dubuque, IA, 1987, p 614.
2. Widmann, FK: Clinical Interpretation of Laboratory Tests, ed 9. FA Davis, Philadelphia, 1983, p 3.
3. *Ibid.*
4. *Ibid.*
5. Hillman, RS and Finch, CA: Red Cell Manual, ed 5. FA Davis, Philadelphia, 1985, pp 1–2.
6. Price, S and Wilson, L: Pathophysiology, ed 3. McGraw-Hill, New York, 1986, p 180.
7. Hole, *op cit*, p 619.
8. Widmann, *op cit*, p. 5.
9. Hillman and Finch, *op cit*, pp 4–5.
10. Widmann, *op cit*, p 8.
11. Hillman and Finch, *op cit*, p 5.

12. Widmann, *op cit*, p 9.
13. *Ibid*, p 11.
14. *Ibid*.
15. *Ibid*, pp 11–12, 265–266.
16. *Ibid*, p 266.
17. Hillman and Finch, *op cit*, pp 78–82.
18. Fischbach, F: A Manual of Laboratory Diagnostic Tests, ed 3. JB Lippincott, Philadelphia, 1988, p 71.
19. Widmann, *op cit*, p 15.
20. Hillman and Finch, *op cit*, p 52.
21. Widmann, *op cit*, p 12.
22. Hillman and Finch, *op cit*, p 35.
23. Widmann, *op cit*, p 19.
24. Hillman and Finch, *op cit*, p 10.
25. Fischbach, *op cit*, p 38.
26. Widmann, *op cit*, pp 17–18.
27. Hillman and Finch, *op cit*, p 36.
28. Hole, *op cit*, p 603.
29. Hillman and Finch, *op cit*, p 36.
30. Widmann, *op cit*, pp 18–19.
31. Hillman and Finch, *op cit*, p 9.
32. *Ibid*, pp 73–75.
33. Fischbach, *op cit*, pp 63–66.
34. Widmann, *op cit*, pp 40–41.
35. *Ibid*, pp 33–34.
36. Boggs, DR and Winkelstein, A: White Cell Manual, ed 4. FA Davis, Philadelphia, 1983, p 1.
37. Hole, *op cit*, pp 625–627.
38. Boggs and Winkelstein, *op cit*, pp 63–65.
39. Widmann, *op cit*, pp 44–46.

BIBLIOGRAPHY

Beare, PG, Rahr, VA, and Ronshausen, CA: Nursing Implications of Diagnostic Tests, ed 2. JB Lippincott, Philadelphia, 1985.

Bio-Science Handbook, ed 12. Bio-Science Laboratories, Van Nuys, CA, 1979.

Byrne, CJ, Saxton, DF, Pelikan, PK, and Nugent, PM: Laboratory Tests: Implications for Nursing Care, ed 2. Addison-Wesley, Menlo Park, CA, 1986.

Frohlich, ED: Pathophysiology: Altered Regulatory Mechanisms in Disease, ed 3. JB Lippincott, Philadelphia, 1983.

Garza, D and Becan-McBride, K: Phlebotomy Handbook. Appleton-Century-Crofts, Norwalk, CT, 1984.

Groer, MW and Shekleton, ME: Basic Pathophysiology: A Conceptual Approach, ed 2. CV Mosby, St Louis, 1983.

Jensen, MD and Bobak, IM: Maternity and Gynecologic Care: The Nurse and the Family, ed 3. CV Mosby, St Louis, 1985.

Kee, JL: Laboratory and Diagnostic Tests with Nursing Implications, ed 2. Appleton & Lange, Norwalk, CT, 1987.

Luckman, J and Sorenson, KC: Medical-Surgical Nursing: A Psychophysiologic Approach, ed 3. WB Saunders, Philadelphia, 1987.

Malseed, R: Pharmacology: Drug Therapy and Nursing Considerations. JB Lippincott, Philadelphia, 1985.

Mathewson, MK: Pharmacotherapeutics: A Nursing Process Approach. FA Davis, Philadelphia, 1986.

Nurse's Reference Library: Diagnostics, ed 2. Springhouse Corporation, Springhouse, PA, 1986.

Pagana, KD and Pagana, TJ: Diagnostic Testing and Nursing Implications: A Case Study Approach, ed 2. CV Mosby, St Louis, 1986.

Porth, C: Pathophysiology: Concepts of Altered Health States, ed 2. JB Lippincott, Philadelphia, 1986.

Selkurt, EE: Basic Physiology for the Health Sciences, ed 2. Little, Brown & Co, Boston, 1982.

Tilkian, SM, Conover, MB, and Tilkian, AG: Clinical Implications of Laboratory Tests, ed 4. CV Mosby, St Louis, 1987.

Wallach, J: Interpretation of Diagnostic Tests: A Handbook Synopsis of Laboratory Medicine, ed 4. Little, Brown & Co, Boston, 1986.

Widmann, FK: Pathobiology: How Disease Happens. Little, Brown & Co, Boston, 1978.

Williams, SR. Nutrition and Diet Therapy, ed 4. CV Mosby, St Louis, 1981.

2

HEMOSTASIS AND TESTS OF HEMOSTATIC FUNCTION

─────────────────────── **INTRODUCTION** ───────────────────────

Hemostasis is the collective term for all the mechanisms the body uses to protect itself from blood loss. In other words, failure of hemostasis leads to hemorrhage. Hemostatic mechanisms are organized into three categories: (1) vascular activity; (2) platelet function; and (3) coagulation.

50

Vascular Activity

Vascular activity consists of constriction of muscles within the walls of the blood vessels in response to vascular damage. This vasoconstriction narrows the path through which the blood flows and may sometimes entirely halt blood flow. The vascular phase of hemostasis affects only arterioles and their dependent capillaries; large vessels cannot constrict sufficiently to prevent blood loss. Even in small vessels, vasoconstriction provides only the briefest sort of hemostasis.

Platelet Function

Platelets serve two main functions: (1) to protect intact blood vessels from endothelial damage provoked by countless microtraumas of day-to-day existence; and (2) to initiate repair when blood vessel walls are damaged through the formation of platelet plugs.

When overt trauma or microtrauma damages blood vessels, platelets adhere to the altered surface. Adherence requires the presence of ionized calcium (coagulation factor IV), fibrinogen (coagulation factor I), and a protein associated with coagulation factor VIII, called von Willebrand's factor (VWF). The process of adherence involves reversible changes in platelet shape and, usually, the release of adenosine diphosphate (ADP), adenosine triphosphate (ATP), calcium, and serotonin. With a strong enough stimulus, the next phase of platelet activity, platelet aggregation, occurs and results in the formation of a loose plug in the damaged endothelium. The platelet plug aids in controlling bleeding until a blood clot has had time to form.[1,2]

Platelets generate prostaglandins that ultimately promote platelet adherence, while the endothelial cells lining the blood vessels produce a different prostaglandin that inhibits platelet aggregation. Ingestion of aspirin inhibits the actions of the prostaglandins released by platelets, an effect that may persist for many days after a person takes even a small amount of aspirin. Aspirin also may affect the actions of the prostaglandins produced by endothelial cells, but not to the extent that it affects platelet prostaglandins.[3] Thus, the net effect of aspirin is to inhibit hemostasis.

Thrombin, which is generated by the coagulation sequence (see further on), independently promotes release of substances from the platelets. Release of platelet factor 3 enhances coagulation mechanisms, thereby increasing thrombin generation. Platelet factor 4, also released by platelets, reinforces the interactions between coagulation and platelet aggregation by neutralizing the naturally generated anticoagulant, endogenous heparin.[4]

Coagulation

Coagulation is a complex process whereby plasma proteins interact to form a stable fibrin gel.[5] The fibrin strands thus formed create a meshwork that cements blood components together, a process known as syneresis. Ultimately, a blood clot is formed.[6,7] Normal coagulation depends on the presence of all clotting factors and follows specific sequences known as pathways or cascades.

At least 30 substances are believed to be involved in the clotting process. Those that are most significant are shown in Table 2–1. Note that clotting factors are now designated by Roman numerals. The "a" indicates an activated clotting factor.[8] There is no factor VI, as that number was originally assigned to what is now known to be activated factor V.[9]

TABLE 2–1. Clotting Factors

I	Fibrinogen
Ia	Fibrin
II	Prothrombin
IIa	Thrombin
III	Thromboplastin, tissue thromboplastin
IV	Calcium, ionized calcium
V	Accelerator globulin (AcG), proaccelerin, labile factor
VII	Proconvertin, autoprothrombin I, serum prothrombin conversion accelerator (SPCA)
VIIa	Convertin
VIII	Antihemophilic factor (AHF), antihemophiliac globulin (AHG)
IX	Christmas factor, antihemophilic factor B, plasma thromboplastin component (PTC), autoprothrombin II
X	Stuart factor, Stuart-Prower factor, autoprothrombin III
XI	Plasma thromboplastin antecedent (PTA)
XII	Hageman factor
XIII	Fibrin-stabilizing factor

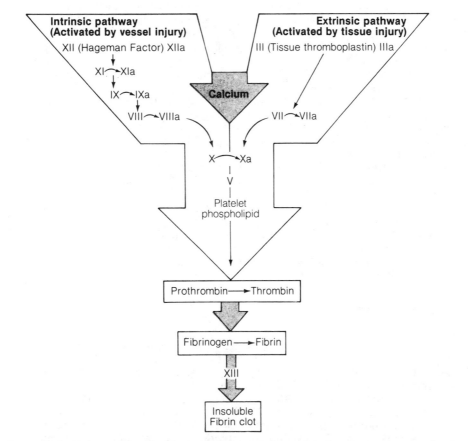

FIGURE 2–1. Schematic diagram of the intrinsic, extrinsic, and common final coagulation pathways. (From Porth,[6] p 169, with permission.)

Each of the clotting factors is involved at a specific step in the coagulation process, with one clotting factor leading to activation of the next factor in the sequence. Three major clotting sequences have been identified: (1) the intrinsic pathway, (2) the extrinsic pathway, and (3) the common final pathway.

The intrinsic pathway is activated when blood comes in contact with the injured vessel wall; the extrinsic pathway is activated when blood is exposed to damaged tissues. Both pathways are needed for normal hemostasis, and both lead to the common final pathway.[10] A schematic representation of the intrinsic, extrinsic, and common pathways is shown in Figure 2–1.

The common final pathway is initiated with the activation of factor X. Factors X and V, along with platelet phospholipid and calcium, combine to form prothrombin activator, which converts prothrombin to thrombin. Thrombin subsequently converts fibrinogen to fibrin gel. Thrombin also enhances platelet release reactions, augments the activation of factors V and VIII, and activates factor XIII.[11] Stable (insoluble) fibrin is formed in the presence of activated factor XIII.

Calcium plays an important role throughout the coagulation process. It is necessary for the activation of factors VII, IX, X, and XI; for the conversion of prothrombin (factor II) to thrombin; and for the formation of fibin. Hypocalcemia usually does not cause bleeding difficulties, however, because cardiac arrest occurs before levels are low enough to precipitate abnormal hemostasis. Citrate, oxalate, and ethylenediaminotetracetic acid (EDTA) are anticoagulants because they bind calcium and prevent it from participating in the clotting process. Any one of these substances may be added to the vacuum tubes used to collect peripheral blood samples when an uncoagulated specimen is needed (see Appendix I, Table A–1).[12]

Antagonists to Hemostasis

Both platelet activation and coagulation are self-perpetuating processes that could potentially continue until an injured vessel is completely occluded. Coagulation inhibitors are present to prevent excessive clotting and to dissolve the clot as tissue repair occurs.

Maintaining adequate blood flow aids in diluting and removing clotting factors and in dispersing aggregated platelets. Partially activated coagulation factors are carried to the liver and reticuloendothelial system where they are degraded.[13] There are also two specific anticoagulation mechanisms that help to prevent excessive clotting: (1) the fibrinolytic system, and (2) the antithrombin system.

In the fibrinolytic system, fibrin strands are broken down into progressively smaller fragments by a proteolytic enzyme, *plasmin.* Although plasmin does not circulate in active form, its precursor, *plasminogen,* does. Plasminogen is converted into plasmin by several plasminogen activators, among them factor XII, urokinase, and streptokinase. Once activated, plasmin digests fibrin and splits fibrinogen into peptide fragments (fibrin split products) and degrades factors V, VIII, and XIII. In addition, the fibrin split products interfere with platelet aggregation, reduce prothrombin, and interfere with conversion of soluble fibrin to insoluble fibrin. It should be noted that plasma also contains agents that neutralize plasmin itself. Among these are antiplasmin and alpha$_1$-antitrypsin. A balance between proplasmin and antiplasmin substances aids in maintaining normal coagulation.[14]

The antithrombin system protects the body from excessive clotting by neutralizing the clotting capability of thrombin.[15] Although various substances inhibit thrombin, the most important one is antithrombin III (AT III), a substance that abolishes the activity of thrombin (activated factor II), activated factors X, XI, and XII, and plasmin. Another name for AT III is heparin cofactor. Heparin augments by approximately 100 times the affinity of AT III and the activated clotting factors upon which it acts. A deficiency of AT III, which can be congenital or acquired, makes the individual prone to excessive clotting. Platelet factor 4, which is released when platelets are broken down, inhibits AT III activity.[16]

PLATELET STUDIES

Background Information

Circulating platelets (thrombocytes) are anuclear, cytoplasmic disks that bud off from megakaryocytes, large multinucleated cells found in the bone marrow[17,18] (see Fig. 1–2, p. 52). Platelets survive in the circulation for about 10 days.

Regulation of platelet production is ascribed to *thrombopoietin* by analogy to erythropoietin (see pp. 3 and 5 in Chapter 1), although no single substance has been specifically identified. With pronounced hemostatic stress or marrow stimulation, platelet production can increase seven to eight times normal. Newly generated platelets are larger and have greater hemostatic capacity than mature circulating platelets.[19]

Two thirds of the total number of platelets are in the systemic circulation, while the remaining third exists as a pool of platelets in the spleen. The pool exchanges freely with the general circulation.[20] The spleen also aids in removing old or damaged platelets from the circulation. In disorders involving exaggerated splenic activity (hypersplenism), 90 percent of the body's platelets may be trapped in the enlarged spleen, and the client is predisposed to excessive bleeding. Hypersplenism is seen in certain acute infections (e.g., infectious mononucleosis, miliary tuberculosis), connective tissue diseases (e.g., rheumatoid arthritis, lupus erythematosus), myeloproliferative diseases (e.g., leukemias, lymphomas, hemolytic anemias), and chronic liver diseases (e.g., cirrhosis).[21]

The functions of platelets are discussed in the introduction to this chapter. In general, individuals with too few platelets, or with platelets that function poorly, experience numerous, pinpoint-sized hemorrhages (petechiae) and multiple small, superficial bruises (ecchymoses). Frequently, there is generalized oozing from mucosal surfaces and from venipuncture sites or other small, localized injuries. Large, deep hematomas and bleeding into joints are not characteristic of platelet deficiency (thrombocytopenia).[22]

Platelet studies involve evaluating the number and function of circulating platelets. Platelet numbers are assessed by the platelet count (see further on). Studies of platelet function include bleeding time, platelet aggregation, platelet survival time, clot retraction, and the capillary fragility (tourniquet) test. It should be noted that disorders of platelet function (thrombopathies) are less common than disorders of platelet number. An overview of the causes of altered platelet function is provided in Table 2–2.

PLATELET COUNT (CLINICAL APPLICATIONS DATA, p. 59)

Platelets may be counted manually or with electronic counting devices. Although larger numbers of platelets are capable of being examined with elec-

TABLE 2–2. **Overview of Causes of Altered Platelet Function**

Increased Function	Decreased Function
Trauma	Severe liver disease
Surgery	Uremia
Fractures	Myeloproliferative disorders
Strenuous exercise	Dysproteinemias
Pregnancy	Glanzmann's disease (thrombasthenia)
	Bernard-Soulier syndrome (hereditary giant platelet syndrome)
	Idiopathic thrombocytopenia purpura
	Infectious mononucleosis
	von Willebrand's disease
	Drugs such as:
	Aspirin and other antiflammatory agents
	Antihistamines
	Antidepressants
	Alcohol
	Methylxanthines

tronic counting, the procedure is subject to error if (1) the white blood count (WBC) is greater than 10,000 per mm^3, (2) there is severe red cell fragmentation, (3) the diluting fluid contains extraneous particles, (4) the plasma sample settles too long during processing, or (5) platelets adhere to one another.

Causes of increased numbers of platelets (thrombocytosis, thrombocythemia) and decreased numbers of platelets (thrombocytopenia) are presented in Table 2–3.

BLEEDING TIME (CLINICAL APPLICATIONS DATA, p. 60)

One of the best indicators of platelet deficiency is prolonged bleeding after a controlled, superficial injury; that is, capillaries subjected to a small, clean incision bleed until the defect is plugged by aggregating platelets (see p. 51). When platelets are inadequate in number, or if their function is impaired, bleeding time is prolonged.

If the platelet count falls below 10,000 per mm^3, bleeding time is prolonged. Prolonged bleeding time with a platelet count of greater than 100,000 per mm^3 indicates platelet dysfunction. Bleeding time is prolonged in von Willebrand's disease, an inherited deficiency of von Willebrand's factor, a protein associated with clotting factor VIII that is necessary for normal platelet adherence. Aspirin ingestion also prevents platelet aggregation and may prolong bleeding time for as long as 5 days after a single 300 mg dose.[23] Other causes of prolonged bleeding times are listed in Table 2–4.

PLATELET AGGREGATION TEST (CLINICAL APPLICATIONS DATA, p. 62)

Platelet aggregation can be measured by bringing platelet-rich plasma into contact with known inducers of platelet aggregation. Most inducers, such as collagen, epinephrine, and thrombin, act through the effects of ADP, which is released by the platelets themselves (see p. 51). Adding exogenous ADP causes platelet aggregation directly. Ristocetin, an antibiotic, may also be used for this test.[24]

TABLE 2–3. Causes of Altered Platelet Levels

Increased Levels (Thrombocytosis)	Decreased Levels (Thrombocytopenia)	
	Decreased Production	*Increased Destruction*
Leukemias (chronic)	Vitamin B/folic acid deficiencies	Idiopathic thrombocytopenia purpura
Polycythemia vera	Radiation	Splenomegaly due to liver disease
Anemias (posthemorrhagic and iron-deficiency)	Viral infections	
Splenectomy		Lymphomas
Tuberculosis and other acute infections	Leukemias (acute)	Hemolytic anemias
Hemorrhage	Histiocytosis	Rocky Mountain spotted fever
Carcinomatosis	Bone marrow malignancies	Sarcoidosis
Trauma	Fanconi's syndrome	Meningococcemia
Surgery	Wiskott-Aldrich syndrome	Antibody/HLA antigen reactions
Chronic heart disease		
Cirrhosis	Uremia	Hemolytic disease of the newborn
Chronic pancreatitis	Drugs such as	Congenital infections (CMV, herpes, syphilis, toxoplasmosis)
Childbirth	Chlorothiazides	
Drugs such as:	Alcohol	Disseminated intravascular coagulation (DIC)
Epinephrine	Chloramphenicol	Immune complex formation
	Anticonvulsants	Chronic cor pulmonale
	Isoniazid	Miliary tuberculosis
	Carbamates	Burns
	Pyrazolones	Drugs such as:
	Sulfonamides	Quinine
	Sulfonylureas	Digitoxin
	Streptomycin	Heparin
	Anticancer drugs	Aspirin
		Thiazides
		Quinidine
		Gold salts
		DDT
		Benzenes

Platelet aggregation is quantitated by determining whether platelet-rich plasma becomes clear as evenly suspended platelets aggregate and fall to the bottom of a test tube. Normally, platelet aggregates should be visible in less than 5 minutes.

Platelet aggregation in response to specific inducing agents is diagnostic for specific disorders. Aspirin, other anti-inflammatory agents, and many phenothiazines markedly inhibit the aggregating effect of collagen and epinephrine but do not interfere with the direct action of added ADP. Individuals with uremia, severe liver disease, or advanced alcohol-related conditions often develop platelet dysfunction. These conditions depress the release-inducing effects of

TABLE 2-4. Causes of Prolonged Bleeding Time

Drugs	Diseases
Aspirin and other salicylates (OTC cold remedies, analgesics)	von Willebrand's disease
	Hypersplenism
Alcohol	Glanzmann's disease (thrombasthenia)
Anticoagulants	Leukemias
Chlorothiazides	Aplastic anemia
High molecular weight dextran	Connective tissue diseases
Mithramycin	Disseminated intravascular coagulation (DIC)
Streptokinase	Hypothyroidism
Sulfonamides	Hepatic cirrhosis
Thiazide diuretics	Malignancies such as Hodgkin's disease and multiple myeloma
	Measles
	Mumps
	Scurvy
	Bernard-Soulier syndrome (hereditary giant platelet syndrome)

collagen and epinephrine and of directly added ADP. Myeloproliferative disorders and dysproteinemias may cause similar results.

Individuals with von Willebrand's disease have platelets that respond normally to epinephrine, collagen, and ADP. Without von Willebrand's factor in their plasma, however, their platelets will not be aggregated by ristocetin.[25]

Other disorders that may impair platelet aggregation include Glanzmann's disease (thrombasthenia), Bernard-Soulier syndrome (hereditary giant platelet syndrome), idiopathic thrombocytopenia purpura, and infectious mononucleosis. Drugs that interfere with platelet aggregation are listed in Table 2-5.

PLATELET SURVIVAL TEST (CLINICAL APPLICATIONS DATA, p. 63)

The platelet survival test measures the survival time of circulating platelets. This is accomplished by labeling the individual's platelets with radioactive chromium and then measuring the daily count of "tagged" platelets for 10 days.

TABLE 2-5. Drugs That Impair Platelet Aggregation

Antihistamines
Salicylates
Sulfinpyrazone
Phenylbutazone
Phenothiazines
Tricyclic antidepressants
Anti-inflammatory drugs, both steroids and nonsteroidal types
Dipyridamole
Caffeine
Aminophylline

Because the procedure involves injection of a radioactive substance, a signed consent may be required.

Platelets have a normal life span of about 10 days. If platelet survival time is decreased, there will generally be a proportional decrease in the platelet count. Within a few days of continuing platelet destruction, platelet production may increase two to eight times normal. If the production rate does not compensate for the increased rate of destruction, thrombocytopenia will persist.

Many diseases may result in increased platelet destruction. The most common cause is systemic activation of the coagulation cascade, also known as disseminated intravascular coagulation (DIC) or consumptive coagulopathy. Conditions commonly associated with DIC are shock, severe crush and burn injuries, surgical trauma, tissue infarction, overwhelming sepsis, and obstetrical complications such as abruptio placenta. Abnormal platelet consumption also is seen in disorders involving vascular injury such as thrombotic thrombocytopenia purpura, hemolytic-uremia syndrome, and vasculitis, and occasionally with intravascular prosthetic devices.

Disorders involving the immune system also may cause excessive platelet destruction. The most common of these is autoimmune (idiopathic) thrombocytopenia purpura, an acute self-limited or chronic disorder in which platelet survival is extremely short and is usually measured in minutes to hours. Other causes of immune-mediated platelet destruction include chronic lymphocytic leukemia, lymphomas, systemic lupus erythematosus, and isoimmune neonatal thrombocytopenia.

Drug sensitivity reactions may produce increased platelet destruction owing to immune mechanisms. Those drugs most frequently associated with thrombocytopenia are quinine, quinidine, sulfonamide derivatives, gold salts, and possibly heparin. It should be noted that thrombocytopenia due to gold salt administration may occur months after the drug is administered.

Other causes of decreased platelet survival time include post-transfusion purpura (a life-threatening disorder that may occur 1 to 2 weeks after a blood transfusion and is most common in women who have been pregnant), hemolytic anemia, alcoholic liver disease with splenomegaly, severe protein deficiency, spider bites, rubella, and use of extracorporeal circulation during various surgical procedures (see Table 2–3, p. 56).[26]

CLOT RETRACTION TEST (CLINICAL APPLICATIONS DATA, p. 65)

When blood collected in a test tube first clots, the entire column of blood solidifies. As time passes, the clot diminishes in size. Serum (the fluid remaining after blood coagulates) is expressed, and only the red cells remain in the shrunken fibrin clot. Because platelets are necessary for this process to occur, the speed and extent of clot retraction roughly reflects the adequacy of platelet function. Individuals with thrombocytopenia or platelet dysfunction, for example, have samples with scant serum and a soft, plump, poorly demarcated clot.

The results of the clot retraction test should be evaluated in relation to other hematologic, platelet, and coagulation studies. If the client has a low hematocrit, for example, the clot is small and the volume of serum is great. In contrast, individuals with polycythemia or hemoconcentration have poor clot retraction because the numerous red blood cells contained in the clot separate the fibrin strands and interfere with normal retraction.

If fibrinogen levels are low, the initial clot is so fragile that the fibrin strands rupture and red cells spill into serum when retraction begins. If there is excessive fibrinolysis, as often happens with reduced fibrinogen levels, the incubated tube may contain only cells and fibrin with no fibrin clot at all. Low fibrinogen levels and excessive fibrinolysis are seen in DIC.[27]

The clot retraction test also can be modified to demonstrate the inhibitory

---
TABLE 2–6. Causes of Positive Rumple-Leeds Capillary Fragility Test

---

Strongly positive (grade 4)	Glanzmann's disease (thrombasthenia)
	Idiopathic thrombocytopenia purpura (ITP)
	Scurvy
	Thrombocytopenia due to acute infectious disease (measles, influenza, scarlet fever)
	Aplastic anemia
	Leukemia
	Chronic renal disease
Moderately positive (grade 3)	Hepatic cirrhosis
Slightly positive (grade 2)	Decreased estrogen levels
	Dysproteinemia
	Polycythemia vera
	Allergic and senile purpuras
	Deficiency of vitamin K, factor VII, fibrinogen, or prothrombin
	von Willebrand's disease

---

effect of antiplatelet antibodies, especially those associated with drugs. Clot retraction is abolished if more than 90 percent of platelet activity is neutralized. Serum suspected of containing antibodies can be added to normal blood to see if retraction is inhibited.[28]

RUMPLE-LEEDS CAPILLARY FRAGILITY TEST (TOURNIQUET TEST) (CLINICAL APPLICATIONS DATA, p. 65)

The capillary fragility test indicates the ability of capillaries to resist rupturing under pressure. Excessive capillary fragility may be due to either abnormalities of capillary walls or thrombocytopenia. The causes of positive test results are listed in Table 2–6.

The test is performed by applying a blood pressure cuff inflated to 100 mm Hg to the client's arm for 5 minutes. The number of petechiae resulting in a circumscribed area are then counted.

This test is unnecessary in the presence of obvious petechiae or large ecchymoses. It also should not be performed on clients known to have or suspected of having disseminated intravascular coagulation (DIC).

Clinical Applications Data

PLATELET COUNT (BACKGROUND INFORMATION, p. 54)
Reference Values

150,000 to 450,000/mm^3 (average = 250,000/mm^3)

Values vary slightly across the life cycle, with lower platelet counts seen in newborns (see Table 1–4, p. 20).

Interfering Factors

■ Altered test results may occur if:
  ☐ the white blood cell count is greater than 100,000 per mm^3
  ☐ there is severe red blood cell fragmentation
  ☐ the fluid used to dilute the sample contains extraneous particles

☐ the plasma sample settles too long during processing
☐ platelets adhere to one another
☐ the client is receiving drugs that alter platelet functions and numbers (see Tables 2–2, p. 55, and 2–3, p. 56)
■ Traumatic venipunctures may lead to erroneous results due to activation of the coagulation sequence
■ Excessive agitation of the sample may cause the platelets to clump together and adhere to the walls of the test tube, thus altering test results

Indications/Purposes for Platelet Count

■ Family history of bleeding disorder
■ Signs of abnormal bleeding such as epistaxis, easy bruising, bleeding gums, hematuria, and menorrhagia
■ Determination of effects of diseases and drugs known to alter platelet levels (see Table 2–3, p. 56)
■ Identification of individuals who may be prone to bleeding during surgical, obstetrical, dental, or invasive diagnostic procedures, as indicated by a platelet count of approximately 50,000 to 100,000 per mm^3
■ Identification of individuals who may be prone to spontaneous bleeding, as indicated by a platelet count of less than 15,000 to 20,000 per mm^3
■ Differentiation between decreased platelet production and decreased platelet function
  ☐ Platelet dysfunction is defined as a long bleeding time (see p. 55) with a platelet count of greater than 100,000 per mm^3 [29]

Client Preparation

Client preparation is the same as that for any study involving the collection of a peripheral blood sample (see Appendix I).

The Procedure

A venipuncture is performed and the sample collected in a lavender-topped tube. A capillary sample may be obtained in infants and children, as well as in adults for whom venipuncture may not be feasible.

Aftercare and Nursing Observations

Care and assessment following the procedure are essentially the same as for any study involving the collection of a peripheral blood sample. Because the client may have a platelet deficiency, digital pressure should be maintained directly on the puncture site for 3 to 5 minutes after the needle is withdrawn. The site also should be inspected after the procedure for excessive bruising.

BLEEDING TIME (BACKGROUND INFORMATION, p. 55)

Reference Values

Values vary according to the method used to perform the test (see section on procedure).

Method	Normal Values
Duke	1 to 3 minutes
Ivy	3 to 6 minutes
Template	3 to 6 minutes

When the platelet count is low, bleeding time may be calculated from platelet numbers using the formula shown below. The result should be evaluated in relation to the normal values for the Ivy and template methods.

$$\text{Bleeding time} = 30.5 - \frac{\text{Platelet count/mm}^3}{3850}$$

The calculated value also may be compared with the actual results of bleeding time obtained by the Ivy and template methods. An actual bleeding time longer than the calculated result suggests defective platelet function in addition to reduced numbers. It is also possible to detect above-normal hemostatic capacity in cases in which active young platelets compose the entire population of circulating platelets, since young platelets have enhanced hemostatic capabilities.[30] This phenomenon may be seen in disorders involving increased platelet destruction (see Table 2–3, p. 56).

Interfering Factors

■ Ingestion of aspirin and aspirin-containing medications within 5 days of the test may prolong the bleeding time. Other drugs that may prolong bleeding time are listed in Table 2–4 (p. 57).

Indications/Purposes for Bleeding Time

■ Family history of bleeding disorders, especially von Willebrand's disease (tests of platelet adhesiveness and levels of factor VIII also are necessary to confirm the diagnosis of von Willebrand's disease)
■ Signs of abnormal bleeding such as epistaxis, easy bruising, bleeding gums, hematuria, and menorrhagia
■ Thrombocytopenia as indicated by platelet count
■ Identification of individuals who may be prone to bleeding during surgical, obstetrical, dental, or invasive diagnostic procedures
■ Determination of platelet dysfunction as indicated by a prolonged bleeding time with a platelet count of greater than 100,000 per mm^3
■ Determination of effects of diseases and drugs known to affect bleeding time (see Table 2–4, p. 57)

Client Preparation

Client Teaching. Explain to the client:

■ the purpose of the test
■ that it will be done by a laboratory technician and requires approximately 15 minutes
■ the procedure, including the momentary discomfort to be expected when the skin is incised

Encourage questions and verbalization of concerns about the procedure appropriate to the client's age and mental status.

Physical Preparation

Aspirin and aspirin-containing medications should be withheld for at least 5 days prior to the test. Other drugs that may prolong bleeding time (see Table 2–4, p. 57) also should be withheld.

The Procedure

The test may be performed using the Duke, Ivy, or template method. All three methods involve piercing the skin and observing the duration of bleeding time from the puncture site. Welling blood must be removed, but gently so as not to disrupt the fragile platelet plug. After the skin is pierced, oozing blood is removed at 15-second intervals by touching filter paper to the drop of blood without touching the wound itself. As platelets accumulate, bleeding slows and the oozing drop of blood gets smaller. The end point occurs when there is no fluid blood left to produce a spot on the filter paper.[31] The test is timed with a stop watch.

For all methods, the site to be used is cleansed with antiseptic and allowed to dry. In the Duke method, the ear lobe is incised 3 mm deep with a sterile lancet. For the Ivy and template methods, the volar surface of the forearm is used. A blood pressure cuff is applied above the elbow and inflated to 40 mm Hg; the pressure is maintained throughout the test. In the Ivy method, two incisions 3 mm deep are made freehand with sterile lancets. In the template method, two incisions, each 1 mm deep and 9 mm long, are made with a standardized template. The advantage of the template method is the ability to achieve a reproducible, precise incision every time.

The elapsed time at the point when bleeding ceases is recorded. In the event that bleeding persists beyond 10 minutes, the test is discontinued and a pressure dressing is applied to the puncture site(s).

Aftercare

When the test is completed, a sterile dressing or Bandaid is applied to the site. For persistent bleeding, ice may be applied to the site in addition to the pressure dressing.

Nursing Observations

Pretest

- Assess the client's level of anxiety about the procedure
- Assess the client's understanding of explanations provided
- Inquire about recent use of drugs that may alter test results (see Table 2–4, p. 57), especially aspirin, aspirin-containing medications, and anticoagulants

During the Test

- If feasible, remain with the individual during the test, noting responses to the procedure

Post-Test

- Observe the puncture site(s) every 5 minutes for bleeding. Clients with clotting factor disorders may rebleed after initial bleeding has stopped. This may occur approximately 20 to 30 minutes after the initial procedure
- Check the puncture site(s) at least twice daily for infection or failure to heal
- For Ivy and template methods, assess for excessive bruising at the blood pressure cuff application site

PLATELET AGGREGATION TEST (BACKGROUND INFORMATION, p. 55)

Reference Values

Platelet aggregates should be visible in less than 5 minutes.

Interfering Factors

- Ingestion of aspirin and other drugs known to interfere with platelet aggregation within 5 to 7 days of the test (see Table 2–5, p. 57)

■ Delay in processing the sample or excessive agitation of the sample may alter test results

Indications/Purposes for Platelet Aggregation Test

■ Suspected von Willebrand's disease or other inherited platelet disorder
■ Evaluation of platelet aggregation in clients with disorders known to cause alterations (e.g., uremia, severe liver disease, myeloproliferative disorders, dysproteinemias)
■ Therapy with drugs known to alter platelet aggregation (see Table 2–5, p. 57)

Client Preparation

Client preparation is essentially the same as that for any study involving the collection of a peripheral blood sample (see Appendix I). It is generally recommended that the person abstain from food for 8 hours prior to the test and, if possible, from drugs that may impair platelet aggregation for 5 to 7 days prior to the test.

The Procedure

A venipuncture is performed and the sample collected in a light blue-topped tube.

Aftercare and Nursing Observations

Care and assessment following the procedure are essentially the same as for any study involving the collection of a peripheral blood sample. Because the client may have a platelet deficiency, digital pressure should be maintained directly on the puncture site for 3 to 5 minutes after the needle is withdrawn. The site also should be inspected after the procedure for excessive bruising.

PLATELET SURVIVAL TEST (BACKGROUND INFORMATION, p. 57)

Reference Values

In normal, healthy individuals, platelets labeled with radioactive chromium will disappear in about 10 days, the normal survival time for platelets. The daily counts are plotted on a graph. A normal steady-state will yield a linear disappearance pattern (Fig. 2–2). The normal platelet turnover rate is about 35,000 per mm³ platelets per day.[32]

Platelet turnover may be calculated from the platelet count divided by the platelet survival time with a correction for the number of platelets normally pooled in the spleen (usually about one third of all platelets). In normal states, platelet turnover also measures the delivery of viable platelets from the marrow to the circulation and is used as a measure of effective thrombocytopoiesis.[33]

Interfering Factors

■ Therapy with drugs known to alter platelet survival (e.g., quinine, quinidine, sulfonamide derivatives, gold salts, and possibly heparin), unless the test is being performed to evaluate such drug effects

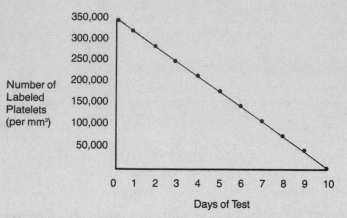

FIGURE 2–2. Normal platelet survival. (Adapted from Thompson, and Harker,[17] p 18.)

Indications/Purposes for Platelet Survival Test

- Evaluation of thrombocytopenia of unknown etiology
- Monitoring the effects of therapy with drugs known to alter platelet survival (see Interfering Factors and Table 2–3, p. 56)
- Evaluation of the effects of known or suspected disorders associated with excessive platelet destruction (see Table 2–3, p. 56)
- Unexplained purpura occurring after blood transfusions, spider bites, and extracorporeal circulation for surgical procedures
- Splenomegaly (enlarged spleen) of unknown etiology

Client Preparation

In general, client preparation is the same as that for any study involving the collection of peripheral blood samples (see Appendix I). The individual is informed that a radioactive substance will be injected intravenously but that the amount of radiation received is so small that it is harmless. A signed consent may be required.

The need for daily venipuncture for 10 days should be emphasized. For non-hospitalized individuals, arrangements may need to be made for daily transportation to the laboratory or for obtaining the samples in the home setting.

The Procedure

A venipuncture is performed and a 7 ml sample is obtained in a lavender-topped tube, to which an isotope (^{51}Cr) is added. An alternative approach is to tag donor platelets with the isotope. The tagged platelets are then injected intravenously into the client. Venous samples are collected at 1- and 2-hour intervals after the tagged platelets are infused.

Daily venous or capillary samples are obtained for 10 days and are analyzed for the number of tagged platelets.

Aftercare and Nursing Observations

Care and assessment following the procedure are essentially the same as for any study involving the collection of peripheral blood samples (see Appendix

I). Since the patient may have platelet deficiency or dysfunction, digital pressure should be maintained directly on the puncture site for 3 to 5 minutes after each venipuncture. The sites should also be inspected for excessive bruising.

CLOT RETRACTION TEST (BACKGROUND INFORMATION, p. 58)

Reference Values

A normal clot, gently separated from the side of the test tube and incubated at 37°C (98.6°F), shrinks to about half of its original size within an hour. The result is a firm, cylindrical fibrin clot that contains all the red blood cells and is sharply demarcated from the clear serum.

Interfering Factors

■ Rough handling of the sample alters clot formation.

Indications/Purposes for Clot Retraction Test

■ Evaluation of the adequacy of platelet function
■ Evaluation of thrombocytopenia of unknown etiology
■ Suspected antiplatelet antibodies due to immune disorders or drug-antibody reactions
■ Suspected abnormalities of fibrinogen or fibrinolytic activity
■ Monitoring response to conditions that predispose to DIC

Client Preparation

Client preparation is the same as that for any study involving the collection of a peripheral blood sample (see Appendix I).

The Procedure

A venipuncture is performed and approximately 5 ml of blood is collected in a red-topped tube. The sample is sent promptly to the laboratory.

Aftercare and Nursing Observations

Care and assessment following the procedure are essentially the same as for any study involving the collection of a peripheral blood sample. Because the client may have platelet dysfunction or deficiency, digital pressure should be maintained directly on the puncture site for 3 to 5 minutes after the needle is withdrawn. The site also should be inspected after the procedure for excessive bruising.

RUMPLE-LEEDS CAPILLARY FRAGILITY TEST (TOURNIQUET TEST) (BACKGROUND INFORMATION, p. 59)

Reference Values

Less than 10 petechiae (excluding those which may have been present prior to the test) in a 2-inch circle is considered normal. Results also may be reported

Grade	Number of Petechiae in 2″ Circle
1	0–10 (normal or negative result)
2	10–20
3	20–50
4	50

according to the scale shown below, with grade 1 indicating a normal or negative result. Causes of positive results are listed in Table 2–6, p. 59.

Interfering Factors

■ Repetition of the test on the same extremity within 1 week will yield inaccurate results

Indications/Purposes for Rumple-Leeds Capillary Fragility Test (Tourniquet Test)

■ History of "easy bruising" or production of petechiae by the application of a tourniquet for venipuncutre
■ Verification of increased capillary fragility, although the test itself is not specific for any particular bleeding disorder (see Table 2–6, p. 59)

Client Preparation

Client Teaching. Explain to the client:

■ the purpose of the test
■ the procedure, including the degree of discomfort to be expected from the inflated blood pressure cuff
Encourage questions and verbalization of concerns about the procedure.

Physical Preparation

■ Inspect the client's forearms and select a site that is as free as possible of petechiae
■ Measure an area 2 inches in diameter; the site may be circled lightly with a felt-tipped marker if necessary for reference
■ If petechiae are present in the site to be measured, note and record the number

The Procedure

A blood pressure cuff is applied to the arm and inflated to 100 mm Hg. The pressure is maintained for 5 minutes. The blood pressure cuff is then removed and the petechiae counted and the number recorded.

Aftercare and Nursing Observations

There is no specific aftercare. If the arm feels "tense" or "full," it may be elevated for a few minutes to hasten venous drainage. Nursing observations consist primarily of noting the presence or absence of petechiae pretest and posttest.

--- **COAGULATION STUDIES** ---

Background Information

Coagulation studies are performed to evaluate the components and pathways of the coagulation sequence (see pp. 51 to 53). Innumerable tests have been devised to diagnose inherited, acquired, and iatrogenic deficiencies of coagulation. Some of these require specialized techniques or rare reagents available only in laboratories that perform many such tests. Other tests are less precisely diagnostic but more available and more readily applicable to immediate clinical situations. The tests included here are widely available.

Screening tests of hemostatic function include the platelet count, bleeding time, prothrombin time (PT), and partial thromboplastin time (PTT). When a "coagulation profile" or "coagulagram" is ordered, it includes the four screening tests plus clotting time and activated partial thromboplastin time (aPTT).

PROTHROMBIN TIME (PT, PRO TIME) (CLINICAL APPLICATIONS DATA, p. 72)

The prothrombin time (PT, pro time) is used to evaluate the extrinsic pathway of the coagulation sequence. It represents the time required for a firm fibrin clot to form after tissue thromboplastin (coagulation factor III) and calcium are added to the sample. These added substances directly activate factor X, the key factor in all three coagulation pathways (see Fig. 2–1, p. 52). Neither platelets nor the factors involved in the intrinsic pathway are necessary for the clot to form.

To give a normal PT result, plasma must have at least 100 mg per dl of fibrinogen (normal: 150 to 400 mg per dl) and adequate levels of factors X, VII, V, and II (prothrombin). Since the test bypasses the clotting factors of the intrinsic pathway, the PT cannot detect the two most common congenital coagulation disorders: (1) deficiency of factor VIII (hemophilia A or "classic" hemophilia), and (2) deficiency of factor IX (hemophilia B, or Christmas disease). Also, thrombocytopenia will not prolong the PT.

Congenital deficiencies of the factors necessary for a normal PT are very rare. Acquired coagulation disorders that prolong the PT are, however, quite common. Among these are liver disease and ingestion of coumarin anticoagulants.

Prothrombin is a vitamin K–dependent protein produced by the liver. Thus, any disorder that impairs the liver's ability to use vitamin K or form proteins (e.g., the various types of cirrhosis) will prolong the PT. Anticoagulants of the coumarin family act by inhibiting hepatic synthesis of the vitamin K–dependent factors II, VII, IX, and X. Drugs that enhance the anticoagulant effects of coumarin (e.g., salicylates, steroids, quinidine, alcohol) may prolong the PT even more. In contrast, barbiturates and oral contraceptives antagonize the effects of coumarin.[34]

PARTIAL THROMBOPLASTIN TIME (PTT)/ACTIVATED PARTIAL THROMBOPLASTIN TIME (aPTT) (CLINICAL APPLICATIONS DATA, p. 73)

The partial thromboplastin time (PTT) is used to evaluate the intrinsic and common pathways of the coagulation sequence. It represents the time required for a firm fibrin clot to form after phospholipid reagents similar to thromboplastin reagent are added to the specimen. Because coagulation factor VII is not required for the PTT, the test bypasses the extrinsic pathway (see Fig. 2–1, p. 52).

To give a normal PTT result, factors XII, XI, IX, VIII, X, V, II (prothrombin), and I (fibrinogen) must be present in the plasma. The PTT is more sensitive than the prothrombin time (PT) in detecting minor deficiencies of clotting factors, as factor levels below 30 percent of normal will prolong the PTT.

The activated partial thromboplastin time (aPTT) is essentially the same as the PTT but is faster and more reliably reproducible. In this test, the thromboplastin reagent may be kaolin, celite, or ellagic acid, all of which more rapidly activate factor XII.

This test is used most often to monitor the effects of heparin therapy, as the PTT changes in relation to the heparin level. The PTT also may be used to detect deficiencies in clotting factors, especially those associated with the two most common congenital coagulation disorders: (1) hemophilia A or "classic hemophilia" (deficiency of factor VIII); and (2) hemophilia B or Christmas disease (deficiency of factor IX).

It is possible to infer which factors are deficient by comparing the results of the PTT with those of the PT. A prolonged PTT with a normal PT points to a deficiency of factors XII, XI, IX, and VIII and to von Willebrand's disease. In contrast, a normal PTT with a prolonged PT occurs only in factor VII deficiency.[35]

In addition to heparin therapy and coagulation factor deficiencies, the following also will prolong the PTT: circulating products of fibrin and fibrinogen degradation, polycythemia, severe liver disease, vitamin K deficiency, disseminated intravascular coagulation (DIC), and established therapy with coumarin anticoagulants.

WHOLE BLOOD CLOTTING TIME (COAGULATION TIME, CT; LEE-WHITE COAGULATION TIME) (CLINICAL APPLICATIONS DATA, p. 74)

Whole blood clotting time, also known as coagulation time (CT) or Lee-White coagulation time, is the oldest but least accurate of the coagulation tests. It measures how long it takes blood to clot in a test tube. Because the sensitivity of the test is low, coagulation problems of mild to moderate severity will not be apparent. Heparin prolongs clotting time; therefore, the test was once used to monitor heparin therapy. Partial thromboplastin time (PTT/aPTT) is currently used to evaluate such therapy.

THROMBIN CLOTTING TIME (TCT, PLASMA THROMBIN TIME) (CLINICAL APPLICATIONS DATA, p. 75)

The thrombin clotting time (TCT, plasma thrombin time) is used to evaluate the common final pathway of the coagulation sequence. Preformed thrombin (coagulation factor IIa), usually of bovine origin, can be added to the blood sample to convert fibrinogen (factor I) directly to a fibrin clot. Because the test bypasses the intrinsic and extrinsic pathways, deficiencies in either one do not affect the TCT (see Fig. 2–1, p. 52).

Thrombin-induced clotting is very rapid, and the test result can be standardized to any desired normal value (usually 10 to 15 seconds). The TCT is prolonged if fibrinogen levels are below 100 mg per dl (normal: 150 to 400 mg per dl), if the fibrinogen present is functioning abnormally, or if fibrinogen inhibitors (e.g., streptokinase, urokinase) are present (see p. XX). In all these conditions, the prothrombin time (PT) and partial thromboplastin time (PTT) also are prolonged.[36]

PROTHROMBIN CONSUMPTION TIME (PCT, SERUM PROTHROMBIN TIME)
(CLINICAL APPLICATIONS DATA, p. 75)

The prothrombin consumption time (PCT, serum prothrombin time) measures utilization of prothrombin when a blood clot forms. Normally, the formation of a clot "consumes" prothrombin by converting it to thrombin. Individuals with deficiencies in platelets, platelet factor 3, or the factors involved in the intrinsic coagulation pathway (see pp. 51 to 53, and Fig. 2-1, p. 52) are not able to convert as much prothrombin to thrombin. In such cases, excess prothrombin remains in the serum after the clot is formed, thus shortening the PCT. The PCT also may be shortened in persons receiving anticoagulant therapy or who have disseminated intravascular coagulation (DIC), hypoprothrombinemia, and cirrhosis.

Abnormal PCT results must be evaluated in relation to coagulation studies such as prothrombin time (PT), partial thromboplastin time (PTT), and factor assays, to differentiate platelet factor deficiencies from clotting factor deficiencies.

FACTOR ASSAYS (CLINICAL APPLICATIONS DATA, p. 76)

If the prothrombin time (PT) or partial thromboplastin time (PTT/aPTT) is abnormal but the nature of the factor deficiency unknown, specific coagulation factors may be measured. Factor assays require specialized techniques not available in many laboratories. Factor assays are used to discriminate among mild, moderate, and severe deficiencies and to follow the course of acquired factor inhibitors. States associated with particular factor deficiencies are presented in Table 2-7.

Factors of the extrinsic (II, V, VII, X) and intrinsic (VIII, IX, XI, XII) coagulation pathways are usually measured separately. The factor XIII assay is a separate test in which a blood clot is observed for 24 hours. Clot dissolution within this time indicates severe factor XIII deficiency. The test for fibrinogen (factor I) is discussed further on.

PLASMA FIBRINOGEN (CLINICAL APPLICATIONS DATA, p. 77)

In the common final pathway, fibrinogen (factor I) is converted to fibrin by thrombin (see Fig. 2-1, p. 52). Plasma fibrinogen studies are based on the fact that, in normal healthy individuals, the serum should contain no residual fibrinogen after clotting has occurred.

Three different techniques may be used to perform the test: (1) standard assay (classical procedure); (2) immunologic technique; and (3) heat-precipitation tests. In the standard assay, thrombin is added to the blood sample to induce clotting. Since fibrinogen is a plasma protein, the amount of protein in the resulting clot is measured. The quantity of precursor fibrinogen present is then extrapolated from this value. In the immunological technique, the degree of reactivity between the plasma sample and antifibrinogen antibodies is measured. The assumption underlying this method is that any plasma constituent that reacts with antifibrinogen antibodies is, indeed, fibrinogen. Heat-precipitation tests are based on a similar assumption that all the material responsive to the precipitation technique is really fibrinogen.[37]

Decreased values are seen primarily in clients with DIC. In this disorder, the plasma contains little or no clottable fibrinogen, but there is usually a variable amount of heat-precipitable or immunologically reactive material. Congenital fibrinogen deficiency is rare. Individuals with this disorder have low values on all tests for fibrinogen. In congenital and acquired dysfibrinogenemias,

TABLE 2-7. States Associated With Coagulation Factor Deficiencies

Factor	Synonym(s)	States Associated with Deficiency	
		Congenital	*Acquired*
Extrinsic Pathway			
II	Prothrombin	Hypoprothrombinemia	Vitamin K deficiency Liver disease
V	Accelerator globulin (AcG), Proaccelerin, Labile factor	Parahemophilia	Liver disease Acute leukemia Surgery
VII	Proconvertin, autoprothrombin I, serum prothrombin conversion accelerator (SPCA)	Factor VII deficiency	Liver disease Vitamin K deficiency Antibiotic therapy
X	Stuart factor, Stuart-Prower factor, autoprothrombin III	Stuart factor deficiency	Liver disease Vitamin K deficiency Anticoagulants Normal pregnancy Disseminated intravascular coagulation (DIC) Hemorrhagic disease of the newborn
Intrinsic Pathway			
VIII*	Antihemophilic factor (AHF), antihemophilic globulin (AHG)	Hemophilia A (classic hemophilia) von Willebrand's disease	Disseminated intravascular coagulation (DIC) Fibrinolysis
IX	Christmas factor, antihemophilic factor B, plasma thromboplastin component (PTC), autoprothrombin II	Hemophilia B (Christmas disease)	Liver disease Vitamin K deficiency Anticoagulants Nephrotic syndrome
XI	Plasma thromboplastin antecedent (PTA)	Factor XI deficiency	Liver disease Vitamin K deficiency Anticoagulants Congenital heart disease
XII	Hageman factor	Hageman trait	Normal pregnancy Nephrotic syndrome
Common Pathway			
XIII	Fibrin-stabilizing factor	Factor XIII deficiency	Liver disease Lead poisoning Multiple myeloma Agammaglobulinemia Elevated fibrinogen levels Postoperatively

*Factor VIII is increased in normal pregnancy (as is factor X) and in states of inflammation and other physiological stress.

fibrinogen-like molecules are found in the plasma, but coagulation is absent, delayed, or peculiar.[38]

Other disorders associated with low fibrinogen levels include severe liver disease and cancer of the prostate, lung, or pancreas.

Elevated fibrinogen levels are seen in immune disorders of connective tissue; inflammatory disorders such as glomerulonephritis; late pregnancy; oral contraceptive use; and cancer of the breast, stomach, or kidney. Hyperfibrinogenemia alone, however, does not necessarily predispose the client to thrombosis unless other factors (e.g., hemoconcentration, thrombocytosis, atherosclerotic disease) are present.[39]

Erroneous results may occur in individuals who have received transfusions of whole blood, plasma, or fractions within 4 weeks prior to the test.

FIBRIN SPLIT PRODUCTS (FSP) (CLINICAL APPLICATIONS DATA, p. 78)

After a fibrin clot has formed, the fibrinolytic system acts to prevent excessive clotting (see p. 53). In this system, plasmin digests fibrin. Fibrinogen also may be degraded if there is a disproportion among plasmin, fibrin, and fibrinogen. The substances that result from this degradation—fibrin split products (FSP) or fibrinogen degradation products (FDP)—interfere with normal coagulation and with formation of the hemostatic platelet plug.

Normally, FSPs are removed from the circulation by the liver and reticuloendothelial system. In situations such as widespread bleeding or DIC, however, FSPs are found in the serum.

Tests for FSP are performed on serum using immunological techniques. Since FSPs do not coagulate, they remain in the serum after fibrinogen is removed through clot formation. Antifibrinogen antibodies are added to the serum to detect the presence of FSPs. Because normal serum contains neither FSPs nor fibrinogen, there should be nothing present to react with the antibodies. If a reaction occurs, FSPs are present.[40]

Elevated levels are seen in DIC, liver disease, various obstetrical complications (e.g., pre-eclampsia, abruptio placenta, intrauterine fetal death), congenital heart disease, leukemia, thermal injury, thromboembolic states, renal disease, transplant rejection, and after cardiothoracic surgery.

Administration of heparin, fibrinolytic drugs such as streptokinase and urokinase, and large doses of barbiturates may also produce elevated FSP levels.

EUGLOBULIN LYSIS TIME (CLINICAL APPLICATIONS DATA, p. 79)

The euglobulin lysis time is used to document excessive fibrinolytic activity (see p. 53). Euglobulins are proteins that precipitate from acidified dilute plasma; these include fibrinogen, plasminogen, and plasminogen activator, but very little antiplasmin activity. In euglobulins prepared from normal blood, the initial clot dissolves in 2 to 6 hours. With excessive fibrinolytic activity, a clot will form if thrombin is added to the sample. The appearance of the clot is abnormal from the start, however, and lysis of the clot occurs within a few minutes to approximately 1 hour.[41]

Shortened euglobin lysis times are seen in fibrinolytic therapy with streptokinase or urokinase, prostatic cancer, severe liver disease, extensive vascular trauma or surgery, and shock.

The euglobulin lysis time may be abnormally short in individuals with normal fibrinolytic activity but reduced fibrinogen, because of the reduced amount of fibrin available to be lysed.[42]

Clinical Applications Data

PROTHROMBIN TIME (PT, PRO TIME) (BACKGROUND INFORMATION, p. 67)
Reference Values

Males	9.6–11.8 seconds
Females	9.5–11.3 seconds

Because values may vary according to the source of the substances added to the sample and the type of laboratory equipment used, the result usually is evaluated in relation to a "control" sample obtained from an individual with normal hemostatic function.

Test results are sometimes given as "percent" of normal activity, comparing the client's results against a curve that shows the normal clotting rate of diluted plasma. The normal value in this case is 100 percent; however, the method itself is thought to be inaccurate, as dilution affects the clotting process.

Interfering Factors

■ Numerous drugs may alter the PT results, including:
  □ drugs that prolong the PT, such as coumarin derivatives, quinidine, quinine, thyroid hormones, ACTH, steroids, alcohol, phenytoin, indomethacin, and salicylates
  □ drugs that may shorten the PT, such as barbiturates (especially chloral hydrate), oral contraceptives, and vitamin K
■ Traumatic venipuncture may lead to erroneous results owing to activation of the coagulation sequence
■ Excessive agitation of the sample may erroneously prolong the PT
■ A fibrinogen level of less than 100 mg per dl (normal: 150 to 400 mg per dl) may prolong the PT

Indications/Purposes for Prothrombin Time

■ Signs of abnormal bleeding such as epistaxis, easy bruising, bleeding gums, hematuria, and menorrhagia
■ Identification of individuals who may be prone to bleeding during surgical, obstetrical, dental, or invasive diagnostic procedures
■ Evaluation of response to anticoagulant therapy with coumarin derivatives and determination of dosage required to achieve therapeutic results
■ Differentiation of clotting factor deficiencies of V, VII, and X, which will prolong the PT, from congenital coagulation disorders such as hemophilia A (factor VIII) and hemophilia B (factor IX), which will not alter the PT
■ Monitoring the effects on hemostasis of conditions such as liver disease, protein deficiency, and fat malabsorption

Client Preparation

In general, client preparation is the same as that for any study involving the collection of a peripheral blood sample (see Appendix I). As many drugs may affect the PT result, all medications taken by the client should be noted. If the individual is receiving anticoagulant therapy, the time and amount of the last dose should be noted.

The Procedure

A venipuncture is performed and the sample collected in a light blue–topped tube. Traumatic venipunctures and excessive agitation of the sample should be avoided.

Aftercare and Nursing Observations

Care and assessment following the procedure are essentially the same as for any study involving the collection of a peripheral blood sample. Because the client may have a coagulation deficiency, digital pressure should be maintained directly on the puncture site for 3 to 5 minutes after the needle is withdrawn. The site also should be inspected after the procedure for excessive bruising.

PARTIAL THROMBOPLASTIN TIME (PTT)/ACTIVATED PARTIAL THROMBOPLASTIN TIME (aPTT) (BACKGROUND INFORMATION, p. 67)

Reference Values

PTT	30–45 seconds
aPTT	35–45 seconds (values may vary among laboratories)

Interfering Factors

- Heparin and established therapy with coumarin derivatives will alter the PTT
- Traumatic venipunctures may lead to erroneous results due to activation of the coagulation sequence
- Excessive agitation of the sample may prolong the PTT

Indications/Purposes for PTT/aPTT

- Signs of abnormal bleeding such as epistaxis, easy bruising, bleeding gums, hematuria, and menorrhagia
- Identification of individuals who may be prone to bleeding during surgical, obstetrical, dental, or invasive diagnostic procedures
- Evaluation of responses to anticoagulant therapy with heparin and/or established therapy with coumarin derivatives, and determination of dosage required to achieve therapeutic results
- Detection of congenital deficiencies in clotting factors such as hemophilia A (factor VIII) and hemophilia B (factor IX), which alter the PTT
- Monitoring the effects on hemostasis of conditions such as liver disease, protein deficiency, and fat malabsorption

Client Preparation

In general, client preparation is the same as that for any study involving the collection of a peripheral blood sample (see Appendix I). If the individual is receiving anticoagulant therapy, the time and amount of the last dose should be noted.

The Procedure

A venipuncture is performed and the sample collected in a light blue–topped tube. Traumatic venipunctures and excessive agitation of the sample should be avoided.

Aftercare and Nursing Observations

Care and assessment following the procedure are essentially the same as for any study involving the collection of a peripheral blood sample. As the client may have a coagulation deficiency, digital pressure should be maintained directly on the puncture site for 3 to 5 minutes after the needle is withdrawn. The site also should be inspected after the procedure for excessive bruising.

WHOLE BLOOD CLOTTING TIME (COAGULATION TIME, CT; LEE-WHITE COAGULATION TIME) (BACKGROUND INFORMATION, p. 68)

Reference Values

4 to 8 minutes

Because this test is relatively insensitive and difficult to standardize, a normal result does not rule out a coagulation defect.

Interfering Factors

■ Heparin prolongs the whole blood clotting time
■ Traumatic venipuncture may lead to erroneous results

Indications/Purposes for Whole Blood Clotting Time

■ Evaluation of response to heparin therapy
  ☐ Adequate anticoagulation is indicated by a clotting time of about 20 minutes
■ Signs of abnormal bleeding such as epistaxis, easy bruising, bleeding gums, hematuria, and menorrhagia
■ Suspected congenital coagulation defect that involves the intrinsic coagulation pathway (e.g., deficiencies of factors VIII, IX, XI, and XII)

Client Preparation

In general, client preparation is the same as that for any study involving the collection of a peripheral blood sample (see Appendix I). If the individual is receiving heparin anticoagulant therapy, the time and amount of the last dose should be noted.

The Procedure

A venipuncture is performed and 3 ml of blood collected in a syringe and then discarded. A new syringe, glass or plastic, is attached to the venipuncture needle, and an additional 3 ml of blood is withdrawn. Traumatic venipunctures and excessive movement of the needle in the vein must be avoided if accurate results are to be obtained.

As the second sample is withdrawn, timing is begun with a stopwatch. The sample is immediately and gently transferred into three glass tubes (1 ml in each). The test tubes are placed in a water bath at 37°C and are tilted gently every 30 seconds until a firm clot has formed in each tube.

Timing is completed when all tubes contain firm clots, and the interval is recorded as the clotting time.

Aftercare and Nursing Observations

Care and assessment following the procedure are essentially the same as for any study involving the collection of a peripheral blood sample. Because the client may have a coagulation deficiency, digital pressure should be maintained directly on the puncture site for 3 to 5 minutes after the needle is withdrawn. The site should be inspected after the procedure for excessive bleeding.

THROMBIN CLOTTING TIME (TCT, PLASMA THROMBIN TIME) (BACKGROUND INFORMATION, p. 68)

Reference Values

10 to 15 seconds (values vary among laboratories)

Interfering Factors

■ A fibrinogen level of less than 100 mg per dl (normal: 150 to 400 mg per dl) will prolong the TCT
■ Abnormally functioning fibrinogen will prolong the TCT
■ Fibrinogen inhibitors such as streptokinase and urokinase will prolong the TCT
■ Traumatic venipunctures and excessive agitation of the sample may alter results

Indications/Purposes for Thrombin Clotting Time

■ Confirmation of suspected disseminated intravascular coagulation (DIC) as indicated by a prolonged TCT
■ Detection of hypofibrinogenemia or defective fibrinogen
■ Monitoring the effects of heparin or fibrinolytic therapy (e.g., with streptokinase)

Client Preparation

In general, client preparation is the same as that for any study involving the collection of a peripheral blood sample (see Appendix I). Current medications taken by the client should be noted. If the individual is receiving anticoagulant therapy, the time and amount of the last dose should be noted.

The Procedure

A venipuncture is performed and the sample collected in a light blue–topped tube. Traumatic venipunctures and excessive agitation of the sample should be avoided.

Aftercare and Nursing Observations

Care and assessment following the procedure are essentially the same as for any study involving the collection of a peripheral blood sample. As the client may have a coagulation deficiency, digital pressure should be maintained directly on the puncture site for 3 to 5 minutes after the needle is withdrawn. The site also should be inspected after the procedure for excessive bruising.

PROTHROMBIN CONSUMPTION TIME (PCT, SERUM PROTHROMBIN TIME) (BACKGROUND INFORMATION, p. 69)

Reference Values

15 to 20 seconds with more than 80 percent of the prothrombin consumed

Interfering Factors

■ Traumatic venipunctures and excessive agitation of the sample may alter test results
■ Therapy with anticoagulants may shorten the PCT

Indications/Purposes for Prothrombin Consumption Time

■ Suspected deficiency of platelet factor 3 or of the clotting factors involved in the intrinsic coagulation pathway (i.e., factors VIII, IX, XI, and XII), as indicated by a shortened PCT
■ Suspected DIC, as indicated by a shortened PCT
■ Monitoring the effects on hemostasis of conditions such as liver disease and protein deficiency

Client Preparation

In general, client preparation is the same as that for any study involving the collection of a peripheral blood sample (see Appendix I). If the patient is receiving anticoagulant therapy, the time and amount of the last dose should be noted.

The Procedure

A venipuncture is performed and the sample collected in a red-topped tube. As with other coagulation studies, traumatic venipunctures and excessive agitation of the sample should be avoided.

Aftercare and Nursing Observations

Care and assessment following the procedure are essentially the same as for any study involving the collection of a peripheral blood sample. Because the client may have a coagulation deficiency, digital pressure should be maintained directly on the puncture site for 3 to 5 minutes after the needle is withdrawn. The site also should be inspected after the procedure for excessive bruising.

Factor Assays (Background Information, p. 69)
Reference Values

	Extrinsic Pathway
Factor II	70–130 mg/100 ml
Factor V	70–130 mg/100 ml
Factor VII	70–150 mg/100 ml
Factor X	70–130 mg/100 ml
	Intrinsic Pathway
Factor VIII	50–200 mg/100 ml
Factor IX	70–130 mg/100 ml
Factor XI	70–130 mg/100 ml
Factor XII	30–225 mg/100 ml
	Common Pathway
Factor XIII	Dissolution of a formed clot within 24 hr

Normal values vary among laboratories.

Interfering Factors

■ Therapy with anticoagulants and other drugs known to alter hemostasis
■ Traumatic venipunctures and excessive agitation of the sample may alter test results

Indications/Purposes for Factor Assays

■ Prolonged PT or PTT of unknown etiology
  ☐ If the PT is prolonged but the PTT is normal, factors of the extrinsic pathway are evaluated (i.e., factors, II, V, VII, and X)
  ☐ If the PTT is prolonged but the PT is normal, factors of the intrinsic pathway are evaluated (i.e., factors VIII, IX, XI, XII)
■ Monitoring the effects of disorders and drugs known to lead to deficiencies in clotting factors (see Table 2–7, p. 70)

Client Preparation

Client preparation is the same as that for any study involving the collection of a peripheral blood sample (see Appendix I). Current medications taken by the client should be noted. If the individual is receiving anticoagulant therapy, the time and amount of the last dose should be noted.

The Procedure

For assays of the factors involved in the intrinsic and extrinsic coagulation pathways, a venipuncture is performed and the sample collected in a light blue–topped tube. For factor XIII assays, the sample is collected in a red-topped tube. As with other coagulation studies, traumatic venipunctures and excessive agitation of the sample should be avoided. The samples should be sent to the laboratory immediately.

Aftercare and Nursing Observations

Care and assessment following the procedure are essentially the same as for any study involving the collection of a peripheral blood sample. Because the client may have a coagulation deficiency, digital pressure should be maintained directly on the puncture site for 3 to 5 minutes after the needle is withdrawn. The site also should be inspected after the procedure for excessive bruising.

Plasma Fibrinogen (Background Information, p. 69)

Reference Values

150–450 mg/dl

Interfering Factors

■ Transfusions of whole blood, plasma, or fractions within 4 weeks prior to the test may lead to erroneous results
■ Traumatic venipuncture and excessive agitation of the sample may alter test results

Indications/Purposes for Plasma Fibrinogen

■ Confirmation of suspected disseminated intravascular coagulation (DIC), as indicated by decreased fibrinogen levels

■ Evaluation of congenital or acquired dysfibrinogenemias
■ Monitoring hemostasis in disorders associated with low fibrinogen levels (e.g., severe liver diseases, and cancer of the prostate, lung, or pancreas)
■ Detection of elevated fibrinogen levels, which may predispose to excessive thrombosis in various situations (e.g., immune disorders of connective tissue; glomerulonephritis; oral contraceptive use; cancer of the breast, stomach, or kidney)

Client Preparation

Client preparation is the same as that for any study involving the collection of a peripheral blood sample (see Appendix I). Current medications taken by the client should be noted, especially anticoagulants and oral contraceptives.

The Procedure

A venipuncture is performed and the sample collected in a light blue–topped tube. As with other coagulation studies, traumatic venipunctures and excessive agitation of the sample should be avoided. The sample should be sent to the laboratory immediately.

Aftercare and Nursing Observations

Care and assessment following the procedure are essentially the same as for any study involving the collection of a peripheral blood sample. Because the client may have a coagulation deficiency, digital pressure should be maintained directly on the puncture site for 3 to 5 minutes after the needle is withdrawn. The site also should be inspected after the procedure for excessive bruising.

FIBRIN SPLIT PRODUCTS (FSP) (BACKGROUND INFORMATION, p. 71)

Reference Values

Less than 5 μ per ml

Interfering Factors

■ Heparin, fibrinolytic drugs such as streptokinase and urokinase, and large doses of barbiturates may produce elevated levels of FSP
■ Traumatic venipunctures and excessive agitation of the sample may alter test results

Indications/Purposes for Fibrin Split Products

■ Confirmation of suspected disseminated intravascular coagulation (DIC), as indicated by elevated FSP levels
■ Evaluation of response to therapy with fibrinolytic drugs
■ Monitoring the effects on hemostasis of trauma, extensive surgery, obstetrical complications, and disorders such as liver disease

Client Preparation

Client preparation is the same as that for any study involving the collection of a peripheral blood sample (see Appendix I). Current medications taken by the client should be noted, especially heparin and fibrinolytic drugs.

The Procedure

A venipuncture is performed and the sample collected in a red-topped tube or in a special tube provided for the FSP test by the laboratory. As with other coagulation studies, traumatic venipunctures and excessive agitation of the sample should be avoided. The sample should be sent to the laboratory promptly.

Aftercare and Nursing Observations

Care and assessment following the procedure are essentially the same as for any study involving the collection of a peripheral blood sample. As the client may have a coagulation deficiency, digital pressure should be maintained directly on the puncture site for 3 to 5 minutes after the needle is withdrawn. The site also should be inspected after the procedure for excessive bruising.

EUGLOBULIN LYSIS TIME (BACKGROUND INFORMATION, p. 71)

Reference Values

Lysis in 2 to 6 hours

Interfering Factors

- Decreased fibrinogen levels may lead to falsely shortened lysis time because of the reduced amount of fibrin to be lysed
- Traumatic venipunctures and excessive agitation of the sample may alter results

Indications/Purposes for Euglobulin Lysis Time

- Suspected abnormal fibrinolytic activity as indicated by lysis of the clot within about 1 hour
- Differentiation of primary fibrinolysis from disseminated intravascular coagulation (DIC), which usually presents with a normal euglobulin lysis time
- Monitoring the effects of fibrinolytic therapy on normal coagulation

Client Preparation

Client preparation is the same as that for any study involving the collection of a peripheral blood sample (see Appendix I). It should be noted whether the client is receiving fibrinolytic therapy.

The Procedure

A venipuncture is performed and the sample collected in a light blue–topped tube. As with other coagulation studies, traumatic venipuncture and excessive agitation of the sample should be avoided. The sample should be sent to the laboratory promptly.

Aftercare and Nursing Observations

Care and assessment following the procedure are essentially the same as for any study involving the collection of a peripheral blood sample. Because the client may have a coagulation deficiency, digital pressure should be maintained directly on the puncture site for 3 to 5 minutes after the needle is withdrawn. The site also should be inspected after the procedure for excessive bruising.

REFERENCES

1. Widmann, FK: Clinical Interpretation of Laboratory Tests, ed 9. FA Davis, Philadelphia, 1983, pp 116–118.
2. Langfitt, DE: Critical Care: Certification Preparation and Review. Robert J Brady Co, Bowie, MD, 1984, pp 395–396.
3. Widmann, *op cit*, p 117.
4. *Ibid.*
5. *Ibid.*
6. Porth, C: Pathophysiology: Concepts of Altered Health States, ed 2. JB Lippincott, Philadelphia, 1986, p 168.
7. Langfitt, *op cit*, p 411.
8. *Ibid*, pp 410–411.
9. Porth, *op cit*, p 169.
10. *Ibid*, p 121.
11. Widmann, *op cit*, p 119.
12. *Ibid*, p 121.
13. *Ibid*, p 124.
14. *Ibid*, pp 124–125.
15. Langfitt, *op cit*, p 413.
16. Widmann, *op cit*, p 125.
17. Thompson AR and Harker, LA: Manual of Hemostasis and Thrombosis, ed 3. FA Davis, Philadelphia, 1983, p 9.
18. Widmann, *op cit*, p 116.
19. *Ibid.*
20. Thompson and Harker, *op cit*, p 18.
21. Professional Guide to Diseases, ed 2. Springhouse Corporation, Springhouse, PA, 1987, pp 1026–1027.
22. Widmann, *op cit*, p 126.
23. *Ibid.*
24. *Ibid*, pp 129–130.
25. *Ibid*, p 130.
26. Thompson and Harker, *op cit*, pp 73–79.
27. Widmann, *op cit*, p 129.
28. *Ibid*, pp 128–129
29. Thompson and Harker, *op cit*, p 61.
30. Widmann, *op cit*, p 127.
31. *Ibid*, p 126.
32. Thompson and Harker, *op cit*, p 19.
33. *Ibid.*
34. Widmann, *op cit*, pp 132–135.
35. *Ibid*, pp 134–136.
36. *Ibid*, p 138.
37. *Ibid*, pp 138–139.
38. *Ibid*, p 139.
39. Thompson and Harker, *op cit*, p 142.
40. *Ibid*, pp 139–140.
41. *Ibid*, pp 140–141.
42. Widmann, *op cit*, p 141.

BIBLIOGRAPHY

Beare, PG, Rahr, VA, and Ronshausen, CA: Nursing Implications of Diagnostic Tests, ed 2. JB Lippincott, Philadelphia, 1985.
Bio-Science Handbook, ed 12. Bio-Science Laboratories, Van Nuys, CA, 1977.
Braunstein, J: Outlines of Pathology. CV Mosby, St Louis, 1982.

Byrne, CJ, Saxton, DF, Pelikan, PK, and Nugent, PM: Laboratory Tests: Implications for Nursing Care, ed 2. Addison-Wesley, Menlo Park, CA, 1986.

Fischbach, FT: A Manual of Laboratory Diagnostic Tests, ed 3. JB Lippincott, Philadelphia, 1988.

Frohlich, ED: Pathophysiology: Altered Regulatory Mechanisms in Disease, ed 3. JB Lippincott, Philadelphia, 1983.

Guyton, AC: Textbook of Medical Physiology, ed 7. WB Saunders, Philadelphia, 1986.

Harvey, AM, Johns, RJ, Owens, AH, and Ross, RS: The Principles and Practice of Medicine, ed 21. Appleton-Century-Crofts, New York, 1984.

Jensen, MD and Bobak, IM: Maternity and Gynecologic Care: The Nurse and the Family, ed 3. CV Mosby, St Louis, 1985.

Kee, JL: Laboratory and Diagnostic Tests With Nursing Implications, ed 2. Appleton & Lange, Norwalk, CT, 1987.

Luckmann, J and Sorensen, KC: Medical-Surgical Nursing: A Psychophysiologic Approach, ed 3. WB Saunders, Philadelphia, 1987.

Michaels, D: Diagnostic Procedures: The Patient and The Health Care Team. John Wiley and Sons, New York, 1983.

Pagana, KD and Pagana TJ: Diagnostic Testing and Nursing Implications: A Case Study. Ed 2. CV Mosby, St Louis, 1986.

Pagana KD and Pagana TJ: Pocket Nurse Guide to Laboratory and Diagnostic Tests. CV Mosby, St Louis, 1986.

Schmidt, RM and Margolin, S: Harper's Handbook of Therapeutic Pharmacology. Harper and Row, Philadelphia, 1981.

Tilkian, SM, Conover, MB, and Tilkian, AG: Clinical Implications of Laboratory Tests, ed 4. CV Mosby, St Louis, 1987.

Wallach, J: Interpretation of Diagnostic Tests: A Handbook Synopsis of Laboratory Medicine, ed 4. Little, Brown and Co, Boston, 1986.

IMMUNOLOGY AND IMMUNOLOGIC TESTING

INTRODUCTION

The immune system protects the body from invasion by foreign elements ranging from microorganisms and pollens to transplanted organs and subtly altered autologous proteins. An antigen is any substance that elicits an immune response in an immunocompetent host to whom that substance is foreign.

The cells responsible for immune reactivity are lymphocytes and macrophages. The primary function of the lymphocytes is to react with antigens and thus initiate immune responses. There are two main categories of immune response: (1) the cell-mediated response, produced by locally active T-lymphocytes present at the same time and place as the specific antigen; and (2) the humoral response, the manufacture by B-lymphocytes of antibody proteins that enter body fluids for widespread distribution throughout the body.

The immune system also removes damaged or wornout cells and destroys abnormal cells as they develop in the body. The cells responsible for these functions are the macrophages, which engulf particulate debris (phagocytosis) and also secrete a vast array of enzymes, enzyme inhibitors, oxidizing agents, chemotactic agents, bioactive lipids (prostaglandins and related substances), complement components, and products that stimulate or inhibit multiplication of other cells. These phagocytic and secretory activities help mediate responses to immune stimulation. Macrophages also are critically important in the induction of immunity. Only after macrophages process antigen and present it to lymphocytes can immunologic reactivity develop.[1]

Laboratory tests can demonstrate with remarkable sensitivity many of the body's immune activities. In general, quantification of cellular components, presence and activities of antibodies and antigens, and the measurement of biologically active secretions constitute the laboratory tests of immune functions.

TESTS OF LYMPHOCYTE FUNCTIONS

Background Information

Lymphocytes, the second most numerous of the several types of white cells in the peripheral blood (see Table 1–4, p. 20), are essential components of the immune system. Diseases affecting lymphocytes frequently manifest as an inability to protect the individual against environmental pathogens (immune deficiency disorders) or as the development of immune reactions to the individual's own cells.[2]

The lymphocytes in the circulation represent only a small fraction of the total body pool of these cells. The majority are located in the spleen, lymph nodes, and other organized lymphatic tissues. The lymphocytes in the blood are able to enter and leave the circulation freely. Thus, there is continuous movement of cells from one area or compartment to another. Despite this process, the number of lymphocytes in the blood and tissues is kept quite constant. Lymphocytes have been divided into two major categories based on their immunologic activity: T-lymphocytes and B-lymphocytes. There also is a third group of lymphocytes that lack the characteristics of either T- or B-cells; these are called null cells.[3]

T-lymphocytes are primarily responsible for cell-mediated immunity, which requires direct cell contact between the antigen and the lymphocyte. This immune reaction occurs at the local site and generally develops slowly. Examples of cell-mediated immune responses include reactions against intracellular pathogens such as bacteria, viruses, fungi, and protozoa; positive tuberculin skin test results; contact dermatitis; transplant rejection (acute and chronic reactions); and tumor immunity.

As with other blood cells, T-lymphocytes develop from stem cells (see Fig. 1–2, p. 4) and then migrate to the thymus where they proliferate and mature.

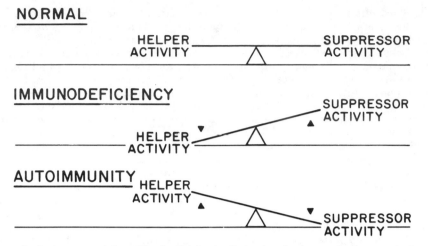

FIGURE 3–1. In normal, healthy individuals, there is a balance between helper and suppressor activities. Many immunodeficiency syndromes appear to be caused by a disturbance of this balance such that a state of unresponsiveness is created. This could result from either a lack of helper activity or an excess of suppressor activity. Conversely, autoimmunity, which results from aberrant responses directed at the host's own antigens, could result from abnormal immunoregulation from either excessive helper or reduced suppressor activities. (From Boggs and Winkelstein,[2] p 71, with permission.)

Thymopoiesis is, however, an ineffective process and many T-lymphocytes die either within the thymus or shortly after leaving it. Only a small portion of the T-lymphocytes reach the peripheral tissues as mature T-cells, capable of effecting cell-mediated immunity.[4]

It should be noted that the thymus functions primarily during fetal life. The peripheral T-lymphoid system is fully developed at birth and normally does not require a constant input of new cells for maintenance after birth. Thus, it is possible to surgically remove the thymus (e.g., as is done to treat myasthenia gravis) without impairing the individual's cell-mediated immune system. In contrast, failure of the thymus to develop during fetal life leads to a severe defect in cellular immunity (DiGeorge's syndrome), usually resulting in death during infancy as a consequence of repeated infections.[5]

Two subsets of T-lymphocytes have been identified: helper T-cells and suppressor T-cells. Helper T-cells promote the proliferation of T-lymphocytes, stimulate B-lymphocyte reactivity and activate macrophages, thereby increasing their bactericidal and cytotoxic functions. Suppressor T-cells limit the magnitude of the immune response. In normal individuals, there is a balance between helper and suppressor activities. Many immune diseases are associated with deficiencies or excesses of the T-lymphocyte subtypes (Fig. 3–1).[6]

The B-lymphocytes are responsible for humoral immunity through the production of circulating antibodies. Examples of humoral immunity include elimination of encapsulated bacteria, neutralization of soluble toxins, protection against viruses, transplant rejection (hyperacute reaction), and possible tumor immunity. Pathological alterations in antibody production are responsible for disorders such as autoimmune hemolytic anemia, immune thrombocytopenia, allergic responses, some forms of glomerulonephritis and vasculitis, and transfusion reactions.[7]

B-lymphocyte precursors are found in the fetal liver and bone marrow; how-

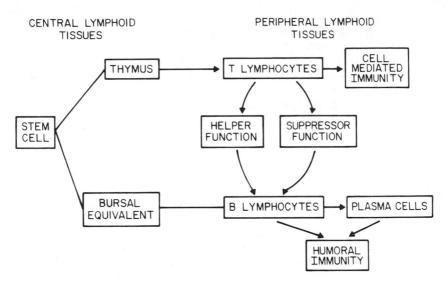

CENTRAL LYMPHOID
TISSUES

PERIPHERAL LYMPHOID
TISSUES

FIGURE 3–2. The relationships between the T-lymphocyte and B-lymphocyte systems. (From Boggs and Winkelstein,[2] p 64, with permission.)

ever, the maturation of the B-lymphoid system is less well defined than that of T-cells. In birds, the stem cells mature into B-cells in the bursa of Fabricius. No organ equivalent of this has been found in humans, although the bone marrow and fetal liver are thought to be the most likely sites.[8]

Actual production of antibodies (immunoglobulins) occurs in plasma cells, the most differentiated form of B-lymphocyte. All B-lymphocytes have immunoglobulins (Ig) on their surfaces. These serve as receptors for specific antibodies. Five classes of immunoglobulins are currently identified (IgG, IgM, IgA, IgD, and IgE). Immune activation requires interaction not only of surface Ig with the specific antigen, but also of the B-lymphocytes with helper T-cells. The activated B-lymphocytes undergo transformation into immunoblasts that replicate and then differentiate into either plasma cells, which produce antibodies, or memory cells ("small lymphocytes"), which retain the ability to recognize the antigen. Similar memory cells have been found in the T-lymphocyte system.[9]

The relationships between the T-lymphocyte and B-lymphocyte systems are diagrammed in Figure 3–2. In both cellular and humoral immune responses, initial exposure to specific antigens initiates the primary immune response. Depending upon the nature and quantity of the antigen, it may take days, weeks, or months for the cells to recognize and respond to the antigen. Subsequent exposure to the same antigen, however, elicits the secondary (anamnestic) response much more rapidly than the primary response.[10]

Tests of lymphocyte functions include T- and B-lymphocyte assays, immunoblast transformation tests, and immunoglobulin assays.

T- AND B-LYMPHOCYTE ASSAYS (CLINICAL APPLICATIONS DATA, p. 91)

T- and B-lymphocyte assays are used to diagnose a number of immunological disorders (Tables 3–1 and 3–2). A variety of methods are employed. The most common way to assess T-cell activity is to measure the individual's response to delayed hypersensitivity skin tests. This involves intradermal injection of minute amounts of several antigens to which the individual has previously been sensitized (e.g., tuberculin, mumps, Candida). Erythema and indur-

TABLE 3–1. **Causes of Altered Levels of T- and B-Lymphocytes**

Increased Levels	Decreased Levels
T-Lymphocytes	
Acute lymphocytic leukemia	DiGeorge's syndrome
Multiple myeloma	Chronic lymphocytic leukemia
Infectious mononucleosis	Acquired immunodeficiency syndrome
Grave's disease	(AIDS)
	Hodgkin's disease
	Nezelof's syndrome
	Wiskott-Aldrich syndrome
	Waldenström's macroglobulinemia
	Severe combined immunodeficiency
	(SCID)
	Long-term therapy with immunosupressive
	drugs
B-Lymphocytes	
Chronic lymphocytic leukemia	Acute lymphocytic leukemia
Multiple myeloma	X-linked agammaglobulinemia
DiGeorge's syndrome	SCID
Waldenström's macroglobulinemia	
Acute lupus erythematosus	

ation should occur at the site within 24 to 48 hours. Absence of response is termed anergy, and thus, the test is frequently called an anergy panel. Anergy to skin tests reflects either a temporary or a permanent failure of cell-mediated immunity.[11]

Other measures of T- and B-lymphocytes involve determining the number of cell types present. T-lymphocytes are recognized by their ability to form rosettes with sheep erythrocytes (i.e., the sheep red cells surround the T-lym-

TABLE 3–2. **Disorders Associated with Abnormal T-Cell Subsets**

Immune Deficiency Diseases (Helper and/or Suppressor Activity)
Common variable hypogammaglobulinemia
Acute viral infections (infectious mononucleosis, cytomegalic inclusion disease)
Chronic graft-versus-host disease
Multiple myeloma
Chronic lymphocytic leukemia
Primary biliary cirrhosis
Sarcoidosis
Immunosuppressive drugs (azathioprine, corticosteroids, cyclosporin A)
Acquired immunodeficiency syndrome (AIDS)
Autoimmunity (Helper and/or Suppressor Activity)
Connective tissue diseases (systemic lupus erythematosus)
Acute graft-versus-host disease
Autoimmune hemolytic anemia
Multiple sclerosis
Myasthenia gravis
Inflammatory bowel diseases
Atopic eczema

Adapted from Boggs and Winkelstein,[2] p 72.

phocyte). Although the sheep erythrocytes adhere to the cell membrane of the T-lymphocytes, they will react to neither B-lymphocytes nor null cells.[12]

T-lymphocytes and their subsets also may be distinguished by their ability to react with various monoclonal antibodies. Monoclonal antibodies constitute a single species of immunoglobulins with specificity for a single antigen and are produced by immunizing mice with specific antigens. The most commonly used monoclonal antibodies to T-lymphocytes are designated T3, T4, and T8. T3 is a pan-T-cell antibody that reacts with a determinant present on all mature peripheral T-lymphocytes and can, therefore, be used to enumerate the total number of T-cells present. T4 antibodies identify helper T-cells, while T8 antibodies identify suppressor T-cells.[13]

Other monoclonal antibodies include T10, T9, and T6. T10 and T9 antibodies react with very immature T-lymphocytes (thymocytes) that are found in the thymus gland but not in the peripheral circulation. T10 antigen also is seen in mature thymocytes that are localized primarily in the medullary regions of the thymus. T6 antibodies also react with certain immature thymocytes. As T-lymphocytes mature, reactivity to T6 antibodies is lost. Tests involving reactivity to immature T-lymphocytes are useful in diagnosing T-cell leukemias and lymphomas.[14]

B-lymphocytes are detected by immunofluorescent techniques. This is accomplished by mixing lymphocyte suspensions with heterologous antisera to immunoglobulins that have been labeled with a dye such as fluorescein. The antisera combine with B-lymphocytes and when the suspension is examined by fluorescent microscopy, only B-lymphocytes appear.[15]

T- and B-lymphocytes can be differentiated by electron microscopy, as T-cells are smooth and B-cells have surface projections. This technique is not, however, available in many laboratories.

IMMUNOBLAST TRANSFORMATION TESTS (CLINICAL APPLICATIONS DATA, p. 93)

When responding to a specific antigen, mature lymphocytes undergo a series of morphological and biochemical changes that enable them to become actively proliferating cells (immunoblasts). The lymphocytes enlarge, synthesize new nucleic acids and proteins, and undergo a series of mitoses. This proliferative expansion increases the pool of antigen-responsive cells (Fig. 3–3).[16] Immunoblast transformation tests evaluate the capability of lymphocytes to change to proliferative cells and, thus, to respond normally to antigenic challenge.

Several methods of performing immunoblast transformation tests may be used. Nonimmune transformation tests involve exposing a sample of the client's lymphocytes to mitogens, agents that cause normally responsive lymphocytes to become immunoblasts independent of any antigenic effect. Effective mitogens include plant extracts such as phytohemagglutinin (PHA), concanavalin A (con A), and pokeweed mitogen. PHA and con A stimulate primarily T-lymphocytes; pokeweed stimulates both T- and B-lymphocytes, although the effect on B-lymphocytes is greater. Approximately 72 hours after the lymphocytes have been incubated with the mitogens, radiolabeled thymidine is added and is then incorporated into the deoxyribonucleic acid (DNA) of the proliferating cells. The rate of uptake of radioactive thymidine indicates the extent of lymphocyte proliferation.[17]

After immune capability has been established, antigen-specific transformation tests can demonstrate whether the person's T-cells have encountered specific antigens. That is, an individual's cell-mediated immunities can be documented by observing how T-cells respond to a battery of known antigens (e.g., soluble viral or bacterial antigens, tissue antigens of human white cells from organ donors).

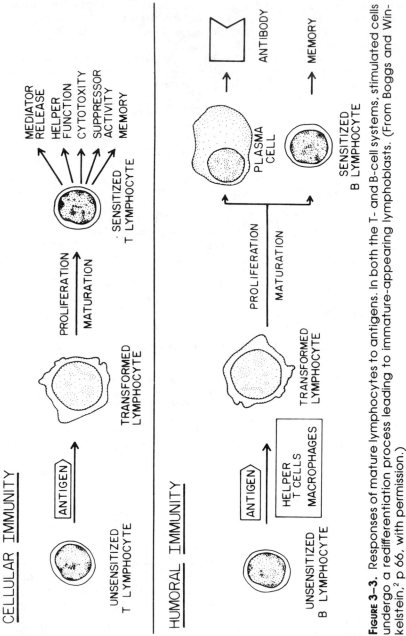

CELLULAR IMMUNITY

UNSENSITIZED T LYMPHOCYTE → ANTIGEN → TRANSFORMED LYMPHOCYTE → PROLIFERATION MATURATION → SENSITIZED T LYMPHOCYTE

MEDIATOR RELEASE
HELPER FUNCTION
CYTOTOXITY
SUPPRESSOR ACTIVITY
MEMORY

HUMORAL IMMUNITY

UNSENSITIZED B LYMPHOCYTE → ANTIGEN / HELPER T CELLS MACROPHAGES → TRANSFORMED LYMPHOCYTE → PROLIFERATION MATURATION → PLASMA CELL → ANTIBODY

SENSITIZED B LYMPHOCYTE → MEMORY

Figure 3–3. Responses of mature lymphocytes to antigens. In both the T- and B-cell systems, stimulated cells undergo a redifferentiation process leading to immature-appearing lymphoblasts. (From Boggs and Winkelstein,[2] p 66, with permission.)

TABLE 3-3. Immunoglobulins

Class	Locations	Functions	Causes of Altered Levels	
			Increased	Decreased
IgG	Plasma Interstitial fluid Placenta	Produces antibodies against bacteria, viruses, and toxins Protects neonate Activates the complement system Is a major factor in secondary (anamnestic) response	Infections—all types, acute and chronic Starvation Liver disease Rheumatic fever Sarcoidosis IgG myeloma	Lymphocytic leukemia Agammaglobulinemia Amyloidosis Toxemia of pregnancy
IgA	Respiratory tract Gastrointestinal tract Genitourinary tract Tears Saliva Milk, colostrum Exocrine secretions	Protects mucous membranes from viruses and bacteria Includes antitoxins, antibacterial agglutinins, antinuclear antibodies, and allergic reagins Activates complement through the alternative pathway	Autoimmune diseases Chronic infections Liver disease Wiskott-Aldrich syndrome IgA myeloma	Lymphocytic leukemia Agammaglobulinemia Malignancies Hereditary ataxia telangiectasia Hypogammaglobulinemia Malabsorption syndromes
IgM	—	Primary responder to antigens Produces antibody against rheumatoid factors, gram-negative organisms, and the ABO blood group Activates the complement system	Lymphosarcoma Brucellosis, actinomycosis Trypanosomiasis Relapsing fever Malaria Infectious mononucleosis Rubella virus in newborn Waldenström's macroglobulinemia Chronic infections IgD myelomas	Lymphocytic leukemia Agammaglobulinemia Amyloidosis IgG and IgA myeloma Dysgammaglobulinemia
IgD	Serum Cord blood	Unknown		—
IgE	Serum Interstitial fluid	Allergic reactions Anaphylaxis Protects against parasitic worm infestations	Atopic skin disorders Hay fever Asthma Anaphylaxis IgE myeloma	Congenital agammaglobulinemia

The mixed lymphocyte culture (MLC) technique is widely used in testing prior to organ transplantation. This test is based on the fact that cultured lymphocytes can recognize and respond to foreign antigens that have not previously sensitized the host. Immunologically responsive lymphocytes cultured together with cells possessing unfamiliar or unknown surface antigens will gradually develop sensitivity; after a lag period of 48 to 72 hours, the responding cells undergo immunoblast transformation if the stimulating cells possess antigens different from those of the host.[18]

IMMUNOGLOBULIN ASSAYS (CLINICAL APPLICATIONS DATA, p. 94)

Immunoglobulins are serum antibodies produced by the plasma cells of the B-lymphocytes. Immunoglobulins (Ig) have been subdivided into the five classes, IgG, IgA, IgM, IgD, and IgE; their functions are listed in Table 3–3. IgG, IgA, and IgM have been further divided into subclasses (e.g., IgG_1, IgG_2, IgG_3, and IgG_4).

Four techniques may be used to assess immunoglobulins: (1) serum protein electrophoresis, (2) immunoelectrophoresis, (3) radial immunodiffusion, and (4) radioimmunoassay. Serum protein electrophoresis, although not specific to the immunoglobulins, may indicate the presence of immunological disorders such that additional testing may not be needed. Electrophoresis separates the serum proteins into albumin and globulin components, with the latter being further broken down into alpha₁, alpha₂, beta, and gamma fractions. Most of the gamma fraction derives from IgG molecules, whereas IgM contributes to the beta portion.[19]

Three types of alterations in immunoglobulins can be identified by serum protein electrophoresis: (1) hypogammaglobulinemia, a reduction in the total

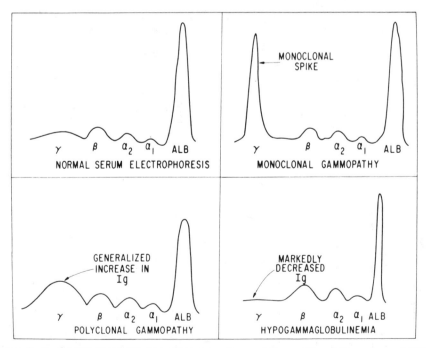

FIGURE 3–4. Serum protein electrophoretic patterns. (From Boggs and Winkelstein,[2] p 84, with permission.)

TABLE 3-4. Conditions Causing Excessive Globulin Levels

Monoclonal Gammopathies

Usually found	Multiple myeloma; Waldenström's macroglobulinemia; heavy chain disease; essential cryoglobulinemia
Sometimes found	Chronic lymphocytic leukemia; lymphomas; "benign" monoclonal gammopathy; age > 80
Rarely found	Amyloidosis; autoimmune disorders; chronic active hepatitis; biliary cirrhosis

Polyclonal Gammopathies

Usually found	Advanced cirrhosis; chronic active hepatitis; biliary cirrhosis; sarcoidosis; narcotics addiction; systemic lupus erythematosus; congenital infections; many parasitic diseases
Sometimes found	Chronic infections; infectious mononucleosis; pulmonary hypersensitivity diseases; rheumatoid arthritis; amyloidosis; scleroderma
Rarely found	Down's syndrome; berylliosis; immunoglobulin A disorders

From Widmann,[1] p 186, with permission.

quantity of immunoglobulins; (2) monoclonal gammopathy, excessive amounts of single immunoglobulins or proteins related to immunoglobulins (seen in multiple myeloma and macroglobulinemia); and (3) polyclonal gammopathy, excessive amounts of several different immunoglobulins (seen in many infections and diffuse inflammatory conditions).[20,21] Examples of these serum protein electrophoretic patterns are diagrammed in Figure 3-4. Additional examples of disorders associated with monoclonal and polyclonal gammopathies are listed in Table 3-4.

Immunoelectrophoresis is not a quantitative technique, but it provides such detailed separation of the individual immunoglobulins that modest deficiencies are readily detected. Radial immunodiffusion allows measurement of the quantity of individual immunoglobulins to concentrations as low as 10 to 20 mg per dl. Radioimmunoassay provides better results when immunoglobulin levels are below 20 mg per dl. Serum IgD and IgE are normally well below this level, as are immunoglobulin levels in most body fluids other than serum.

Clinical Applications Data

T- AND B-LYMPHOCYTE ASSAYS (BACKGROUND INFORMATION, p. 85)
Reference Values

T-lymphocytes	60 to 80% of circulating lymphocytes*
B-lymphocytes	10 to 20% of circulating lymphocytes
Null cells	5 to 20% of circulating lymphocytes
Helper T-lymphocytes	50 to 65% of circulating T-lymphocytes
Suppressor T-lymphocytes	20 to 35% of circulating T-lymphocytes
Ratio of helper to suppressor T-lymphocytes 2:1	

*A decreased lymphocyte count (lymphopenia) usually indicates a decrease in the number of circulating T-lymphocytes.

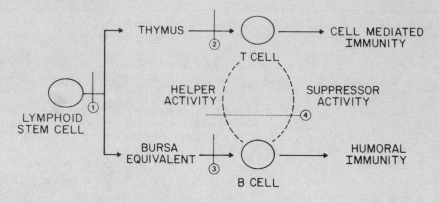

① SEVERE COMBINED IMMUNODEFICIENCY DISEASE (SCID)

② DI GEORGE SYNDROME

③ X-LINKED AGAMMAGLOBULINEMIA

④ COMMON VARIABLE HYPOGAMMAGLOBULINEMIA (CVH)

FIGURE 3–5. Several immunodeficiency diseases can be viewed as cellular blocks in the normal maturation of lymphocytes. (From Boggs and Winkelstein,[2] p 87, with permission.)

Indications/Purposes for T- and B-Lymphocyte Assays

■ Diagnosis of disorders associated with abnormal levels of T- and B-lymphocytes (see Table 3–1, p. 86)

■ Diagnosis of disorders associated with abnormal T-cell subtypes (see Table 3–2, p. 86)

■ Support for diagnosing acquired immunodeficiency syndrome (AIDS), as indicated by decreased helper T-cells, normal or increased suppressor T-cells, and a decreased ratio of helper to suppressor T-cells

■ Diagnosis of severe combined immunodeficiency (SCID), an inherited disorder characterized by failure of the stem cell to differentiate into T- and B-lymphocytes (Fig. 3–5)

■ Diagnosis of DiGeorge's syndrome characterized by failure of the thymus (and parathyroids) to develop with a resulting decrease in T-lymphocytes (Fig. 3–5)

■ Diagnosis of X-linked agammaglobulinemia characterized by severe B-lymphocyte deficiency (Fig. 3–5)

■ Diagnosis of common variable hypogammaglobulinemia (CVH) characterized by absent, decreased, or defective B-cells and most commonly due to either lack of helper T-lymphocytes or abnormal suppressor T-cells (Fig. 3–5)

Client Preparation

Client preparation is the same as that for any study involving the collection of a peripheral blood sample (see Appendix I).

The Procedure

A venipuncture is performed and the sample collected in a green-topped tube or other type of blood collection tube, depending on laboratory preference.

Aftercare and Nursing Observations

Care and assessment following the procedure are the same as for any study involving the collection of a peripheral blood sample. Since the client may be immunosuppressed, the site should be observed for signs of infection.

IMMUNOBLAST TRANSFORMATION TESTS (BACKGROUND INFORMATION, p. 87)

Reference Values

Nonimmune transformation tests	A stimulation index of greater than 10 indicates immunocompetence
Antigen-specific transformation tests	A stimulation index of greater than 3 indicates prior exposure to the antigen
Mixed lymphocyte culture	Nonresponsiveness indicates good histocompatibility

Interfering Factors

■ Radioisotope studies performed within 1 week of the test may alter test results
■ Pregnancy or oral contraceptive use may lead to a decreased response to phytohemagglutinin (PHA) in nonimmune transformation tests (see p. 93)

Indications/Purposes for Immunoblast Transformation Tests

■ Support for diagnosing immunodeficiency disorders as indicated by a decreased response to nonimmune transformation tests
■ Identification of microorganisms to which the individual was previously exposed as indicated by an increased response to antigen-specific transformation tests
■ Support for identifying compatible organ donors and recipients as indicated by nonresponsiveness on mixed lymphocyte culture

Client Preparation

Client preparation is the same as that for any study involving the collection of a peripheral blood sample (see Appendix I). All clients should be interviewed to determine whether they have undergone any radioisotope tests within the past week, or, if female, whether she is pregnant or using oral contraceptives.

The Procedure

A venipuncture is performed and the sample collected in a green-topped tube or other type of blood collection tube, depending on laboratory preference. The sample should be transported to the laboratory promptly.

Aftercare and Nursing Observations

Care and assessment following the procedure are the same as for any study involving the collection of a peripheral blood sample. As the client may be immunosuppressed, the site should be observed for signs of infection.

IMMUNOGLOBULIN ASSAYS (BACKGROUND INFORMATION, p. 90)

Reference Values

Serum Protein Electrophoresis

Constituent	Percentage of Total Protein
Albumin	52–68
Globulin	32–48
alpha$_1$-globulin	2.4–5.3
alpha$_2$-globulin	6.6–13.5
beta-globulin	8.5–14.5
gamma-globulin	10.7–21.0

Immunoglobulins

	IgG (mg/dl)	IgA (mg/dl)	IgM (mg/dl)	IgD (mg/dl)	IgE (mg/dl)
Neonate	650–1250	0–12	5–30	—	—
6 mo	200–1100	10–90	10–80	—	—
1 yr	300–1400	20–150	20–100	—	—
6 yr	550–1500	50–175	22–100	—	—
12 yr	660–1450	50–200	30–120	—	—
16 yr	700–1050	70–225	35–75	—	—
Adult	800–1800	100–400	55–150	0.5–3	0.01–0.04
Percentage of total immunoglobulins in adult	75–80%	15%	10%	0.2%	0.0002%

Interfering Factors

■ Immunizations within 6 months prior to the test may alter test results
■ Transfusions of either whole blood or fractions within 2 months may alter test results

Indications/Purposes for Immunoglobulin Assays

■ Suspected immunodeficiency, either congenital or acquired
■ Suspected immunoproliferative disorders such as multiple myeloma or Waldenström's macroglobulinemia
■ Suspected autoimmune disorder
■ Suspected malignancy involving the lymphoreticular system
■ Monitoring effects of chemotherapy or radiation therapy, or both, which may suppress the immune system
■ Identification of hypogammaglobulinemia, monoclonal gammopathy, and polyclonal gammopathy by serum protein electrophoresis (see Figure 3–4, p. 90, and Table 3–4, p. 91)
■ Support for diagnosing a variety of disorders associated with altered immunoglobulin levels (see Table 3–3, p. 89)

Client Preparation

Client preparation is the same as that for any study involving the collection of a peripheral blood sample (see Appendix I). Intake of food and fluid is usually not restricted, although some laboratories do require food restriction. The client should be interviewed to determine if he or she has received immunizations within 6 months prior to the test or transfusions of whole blood or fractions within 2 months prior to the test.

The Procedure

A venipuncture is performed and the sample collected in a red-topped tube or other type of blood collection tube, depending on laboratory preference. The sample should be transported to the laboratory promptly.

Aftercare and Nursing Observations

Care and assessment following the procedure are the same as for any study involving the collection of a peripheral blood sample. Because the client may be immunosuppressed, the site should be observed for signs of infection.

TESTS OF THE COMPLEMENT SYSTEM

Background Information

Complement is a system of protein molecules, the sequential interactions of which produce biological effects on surface membranes, on cellular behavior, and on the interactions of other proteins. Each of the proteins of the complement system is inactive by itself. Activation occurs through a cascade-like sequence after contact with substances such as IgG or IgM antigen-antibody complexes, aggregated IgA, certain naturally occurring polysaccharides and lipopolysaccharides, activation products of the coagulation system, and bacterial endotoxins. Activation of the complement system results in an inflammatory response that destroys or damages cells.

Complement proteins are identified by letters and numbers and are listed here in order of activation in the "classical pathway" of the complement cascade: $C1_q$, $C1_r$, $C1_s$, C4, C2, C3, and then C5 through C9. The "alternate pathway" bypasses C1, C4, and C2 activation and begins directly with C3. The key step in the alternate pathway is activation of properdin, a serum protein without biological effects in its inactive form. Contact with aggregated IgA, with bacterial endotoxins, or with complex molecules such as dextran, agar, and zymosan alters properdin and initiates the sequence at C3.[22]

Complete activation to C9 leads to membrane disruption and irreversible cell damage. Along the way to complete activation, the following activities occur: C2 releases a low-molecular weight peptide with kinin activity; activation of products of C3 and C5 affect mast cells, smooth muscle, and leukocytes to produce an anaphylactic effect; other elements of C3 and C5 bind to cell membranes and render them more susceptible to phagocytosis, a process called opsonization; fragments of C3 and C4 cause immune adherence, in which complement-coated particles bind to cells whose surface membranes have complement receptors; activated C3 and C4 also are capable of virus neutralization; C3 and C5 exert chemotactic activity on neutrophils; and the C5 to C9 complex influences the procoagulant activity of platelets. Conversely, procoagulant factor XII can initiate C1 activation, while plasmin (the substance that dissolves fibrin) and thrombin (which converts fibrinogen to fibrin) can cleave C3 into its active form.[23]

Numerous methods are used to evaluate the complement system. In general, increased concentrations are seen in acute inflammatory conditions, while decreased levels are seen in generalized immune disorders, since complement is consumed in the course of many antigen-antibody reactions and in certain chronic inflammatory conditions.

SERUM COMPLEMENT ASSAYS (CLINICAL APPLICATIONS DATA, p. 97)

Radioimmunoassay and immunodiffusion techniques have made it possible to quantify each of the complement components. For clinical purposes, however, only total complement, C3, and C4 are measured. Total complement is measured by exposing a sample of human serum to sheep red cells coated with complement-requiring antibody. Results are expressed as CH_{50} units, reflecting the dilution at which adequate complement exists to lyse one half of the test cells. C3 and C4 levels are measured individually by radial immunodiffusion. These latter tests take 24 to 36 hours to complete and results are easily affected by improper handling of the specimen.[24]

The causes of alterations in C3 and C4 levels are presented in Table 3–5.

TABLE 3–5. Causes of Alterations in C3 and C4 Levels

Component	Increased Levels	Decreased Levels
C3	Acute rheumatic fever Rheumatoid arthritis Early SLE* Most cancers	Advanced SLE Glomerulonephritis Renal transplant rejection Chronic active hepatitis Cirrhosis Multiple sclerosis Anemias Gram-negative septicemia Subacute bacterial endocarditis Inborn C3 deficiency Serum sickness Immune complex disease

C4	Rheumatoid
	  spondylitis
	Juvenile rheumatoid
	  arthritis
	Most cancers
		SLE
		Lupus nephritis
		Acute poststreptococcal glomerulonephritis
		Chronic active hepatitis
		Cirrhosis
		Subacute bacterial endocarditis
		Inborn C4 deficiency
		Serum sickness
		Immune complex disease

*SLE = Systemic lupus erythematosus.

IMMUNE COMPLEX ASSAYS (CLINICAL APPLICATIONS DATA, p. 98)

Immune complexes are combinations of antigen and antibody which are capable of activating the complement cascade. While the activated agent is directed against the immune complex, tissues which are "innocent bystanders" may also be severely damaged, especially when immune complexes are produced too rapidly for adequate clearance by the body. Immune complexes are commonly present in autoimmune disorders and also are found in immune hypersensitivities which do not involve autoimmunity.

Clinical Applications Data

SERUM COMPLEMENT ASSAYS (BACKGROUND INFORMATION, p. 96)
Reference Values

Total Complement (CH_{50})		40 to 90 units/ml
C3	Males	80 to 180 mg/dl
	Females	76 to 120 mg/dl
C4	Males	15 to 60 mg/dl
	Females	15 to 52 mg/dl

Values for total complement, C3, and C4, may vary according to laboratory methods and the reference range established by the laboratory performing the test.

Interfering Factors

■ Failure to transport the sample to the laboratory immediately may alter test results, as complement deteriorates rapidly at room temperature
■ Hemolysis of the sample may alter test results

Indications/Purposes for Serum Complement Assays

■ Suspected acute inflammatory disorder as generally indicated by elevated total complement levels
■ Suspected immune and/or infectious disorder (e.g., acute glomerulonephritis, systemic lupus erythematosus [SLE], rheumatoid arthritis, hepatitis, subacute bacterial endocarditis, gram-negative sepsis) as indicated by decreased total complement levels
■ Support for diagnosing hereditary deficiencies of complement components as indicated by decreased levels of total complement and/or of specific components such as C3 and C4 (Table 3–5)
■ Support for diagnosing cancer, especially that of the breast, lung, digestive system, cervix, ovary, and bladder, as indicated by increased levels of C3 and C4 (Table 3–5)
■ Monitoring the progression of malignant disease as indicated by declining complement levels as the disease progresses
■ Support for diagnosing a variety of immune and inflammatory disorders as indicated by altered C3 and C4 levels (Table 3–5)

■ Monitoring progress following various immune and inflammatory disorders as indicated by levels approaching or within the reference ranges

Client Preparation

Client Preparation is the same as that for any study involving the collection of a peripheral blood sample (see Appendix I).

The Procedure

A venipuncture is performed and the sample collected in a red-topped tube or other type of blood collection tube, depending on laboratory preference. The sample must be handled gently to avoid hemolysis and must be transported to the laboratory immediately.

Aftercare and Nursing Observations

Care and assessment following the procedure are the same as for any study involving the collection of a peripheral blood sample.

IMMUNE COMPLEX ASSAYS (BACKGROUND INFORMATION, p. 97)

Reference Values

Immune complexes are not normally found in the serum.

Interfering Factors

■ Rough handling of the sample and failure to transport the sample promptly to the laboratory may cause deterioration of any immune complexes present

Indications/Purposes for Immune Complex Assays

■ Suspected immune disorders such as systemic lupus erythematosus, scleroderma, dermatomyositis, polymyositis, glomerulonephritis, and rheumatic fever as indicated by the presence of immune complexes
■ Monitoring the effects of therapy for various immune disorders
■ Suspected serum sickness or allergic reactions to drugs as indicated by the presence of immune complexes

Client Preparation

Client preparation is the same as that for any study involving the collection of a peripheral blood sample (see Appendix I).

The Procedure

A venipuncture is performed and the sample collected in a red-topped tube or other type of blood collection tube, depending on laboratory preference. The sample must be handled gently and transported to the laboratory promptly.

Aftercare and Nursing Observations

Care and assessment following the procedure are the same as for any study involving the collection of a peripheral blood sample.

RADIOALLERGOSORBENT TEST FOR IgE (RAST)

Background Information

IgE antibodies are responsible for hypersensitivity reactions described as atopic (allergic) or anaphylactic. Examples of IgE-mediated diseases include hay fever, asthma, certain types of eczema, and idiosyncratic, potentially fatal reactions to insect venoms, penicillin, and other drugs or chemicals.

Almost all of the body's active IgE is bound to tissue cells, with only small amounts in the blood. Thus, IgE antibodies cannot circulate in search of antigen, but must wait for antigens to appear in their area. Once this happens, the interaction of IgE antibodies with specific antigens causes mast cells (tissue basophils) to release histamine and other substances that promote vascular permeability.[25]

The radioallergosorbent test (RAST) for IgE measures the quantity of IgE antibodies in the serum after exposure to specific antigens selected on the basis of the person's history. RAST has replaced skin tests and provocation procedures, which were inconvenient, painful, and hazardous to the client.

Clinical Applications Data

Reference Values

If the client is not allergic to the antigen, IgE antibody is not detected. A positive test result in relation to a specific antigen is more than 400 percent of control. Results of the test may vary depending on the reference serum used for the control.

Interfering Factors

■ Radioisotope tests within 1 week prior to the test may alter results

Indications/Purposes for Radioallergosorbent Test for IgE (RAST)

■ Onset of asthma, hay fever, dermatitis
■ Systemic reaction to insect venom, drugs, or chemicals
■ Identification of the specific antigen(s) to which the client reacts
■ Monitoring response to desensitization procedures

Client Preparation

Client preparation is the same as that for any study involving the collection of a peripheral blood sample (see Appendix I). All clients should be interviewed to determine if they have undergone any radioisotope tests within the past week.

The Procedure

A venipuncture is performed and the sample collected in a red-topped tube or other type of blood collection tube, depending on laboratory preference. The

Table 3–6. Summary of Autoantibody-related Disorders and Tests Used in Diagnosis

Antibody	Incidence		
	Present in 90% or More of Cases	Present in 50–90% of Cases	Present in < 50% of Cases
C-reactive protein (CRP)	Rheumatic fever Rheumatoid arthritis Acute bacterial infections Viral hepatitis	Active tuberculosis Gout Advanced cancers Leprosy Cirrhosis Burns Peritonitis	Multiple sclerosis Guillain-Barré syndrome Scarlet fever Varicella Surgery Intrauterine contraceptive devices
Rheumatoid factor (RF)	Rheumatoid arthritis	Early rheumatoid arthritis Systemic lupus erythematosus (SLE) Scleroderma Dermatomyositis	Advanced age Juvenile rheumatoid arthritis (20%) Infectious diseases Healthy adults (<5%)
Antinuclear antibodies (ANA	SLE	Sjögren's syndrome Scleroderma	Burns Asbestosis

Test			
Anti-DNA	Active SLE	Drug-induced SLE-like syndrome Chronic active hepatitis Heart disease, with long-term procainamide therapy	Juvenile chronic polyarthritis Rheumatoid arthritis Rheumatic fever Myasthenia gravis Advanced age Dermatomyositis Polyarteritis nodosa Primary biliary cirrhosis
	SLE in remission		Juvenile rheumatoid arthritis Progressive systemic sclerosis Drug-induced SLE-like syndrome Uveitis
Cold agglutinins	Atypical pneumonia Influenza Pulmonary embolus	Viral infections Infectious mononucleosis Lymphoreticular malignancy	Congenital syphilis Malaria Anemia Cirrhosis
LE cell preparation Cryoglobulins	SLE Raynaud's syndrome Cryoglobulinemia	— —	— —

allergy panel desired should be indicated on the laboratory request form. Each panel usually consists of six antigens.

Aftercare and Nursing Observations

Care and assessment following the procedure are the same as for any study involving the collection of a peripheral blood sample.

AUTOANTIBODY TESTS

Background Information

Antibodies directed against "self" components are believed to be responsible for the pathogenesis of many diseases. Some of these show wide-spread systemic involvement (Table 3–6), whereas others are confined to a specific organ system (Table 3–7).

Clinical Applications Data

Reference Values

C-reactive protein (CRP)	Negative to trace
Antinuclear antibodies (ANA)	Negative
Rheumatoid factor (RF)	Negative (<1:20)
Anti-DNA antibodies	<1 µg/ml
Antimitochondrial antibodies	Negative
Antiskin antibodies	Negative
Antiadrenal cortex antibodies	Negative
Antithyroglobulin, antithyroid microsome antibodies	<1:100
Anti–smooth muscle antibodies	Negative
Antiparietal cell, anti-intrinsic factor antibodies	Negative
Anti–striated muscle antibodies	Negative
Antimyocardial antibodies	Negative
Lupus erythematosus cell test (LE Prep)	Negative
Cold agglutinins	<1:16
Cryoglobulins	Negative
Antiglobulin tests (Coombs' tests)*	
Direct	Negative
Indirect	Negative

*See also Chapter 4.

Interfering Factors

■ Many drugs may cause false-positive results in certain autoantibody tests (Table 3–8)

Indications/Purposes for Autoantibody Tests

■ Signs and symptoms of the disorder for which each test is pathognomonic or for which the test provides confirming data (see Tables 3–6 and 3–7)
■ Monitoring response to treatment for autoimmune disorders

TABLE 3–7. Cell and Tissue-Specific Antibodies

Antibody Target Cell/Tissue	Diseases for Which the Test Is Usually Diagnostic	Other Diseases in Which This Antibody May Also Be Present
Skeletal muscle	Myasthenia gravis	
Cardiac muscle	Myocardial infarction	Acute rheumatic fever
Smooth muscle	Chronic active hepatitis	Biliary cirrhosis Viral hepatitis Infectious mononucleosis SLE (10%)
Mitochondria	Primary biliary cirrhosis Drug-induced jaundice	Chronic active hepatitis Viral hepatitis SLE (20%)
Skin	Pemphigus	—
Altered IgG	Rheumatoid arthritis	—
Adrenal cells	Addison's disease	—
Intrinsic factor, parietal cells	Pernicious anemia	SLE (5%)
Long-acting thyroid stimulator	Grave's disease Hashimoto's thyroiditis	—
Long-acting thyroid microsomes	Primary myxedema Juvenile lymphocytic thyroiditis Grave's disease	SLE (5%) Pernicious anemia (25%) Allergies Healthy adults
Thyroglobulin	Hashimoto's thyroiditis Primary myxedema Grave's disease	Pernicious anemia Allergies Healthy adults (5–10%)
Salivary ducts	Sjögren's syndrome	Rheumatoid arthritis
Red blood cell membrane	Autoimmune hemolytic anemia	Transfusion reaction
Platelet cell membrane	Idiopathic thrombocytopenia purpura	—
Basement membranes of lungs, renal glomeruli	Goodpasture's syndrome Glomerulonephritis	—

SLE = Systemic lupus erythematosus.

TABLE 3–8. Drugs That May Cause False-Positive Reactions in Autoantibody Tests*

Antibiotics	Para-aminosalicylic acid
Anti-DNA	Penicillin
Chlorpromazine	Phenylbutazone
Clofibrate	Phenytoin
Ethosuximide	Procainamide
Griseofulvin	Prophylthiouracil
Hydralazine	Quinidine
Isoniazid	Radioactive diagnostics
Mephenytoin	Streptomycin
Methyldopa	Sulfonamides
Methysergide	Tetracyclines
Oral contraceptives	Trimethadione

*The drugs listed here may cause false-positive reactions in the following tests: antinuclear antibodies, LE prep, and antiglobulin (Coombs') tests.

Client Preparation

Client preparation is the same as that for any study involving the collection of a peripheral blood sample (see Appendix I). Medications that the client is currently taking should be noted, as many drugs may interfere with test results. Food and fluids are not restricted, except for the cryoglobulin test which requires a 4-hour fast from food.

The Procedure

The procedure is the same for all autoantibody tests, except cryoglobulins. A venipuncture is performed and the sample collected in a red-topped tube. For cryoglobulins, the sample is collected in a prewarmed, red-topped tube. The sample must be handled gently to avoid hemolysis and sent promptly to the laboratory.

Aftercare and Nursing Observations

Care and assessment following the procedure are the same as for any study involving the collection of a peripheral blood sample. Food withheld prior to the test should be resumed.

IMMUNOLOGIC TESTS IN MICROBIOLOGY

Background Information

Exposure to bacteria, fungi, viruses, and parasites induces production of antibodies that may be identifiable only during acute disease or that may remain identifiable for many years. Exposure may be through immunization, from previous infection so minimal that it passes unrecognized, or from current symptomatic or prepathogenic infection.

The concentrations of antibody are referred to as the titer, and their predictable patterns are useful in diagnosing the disease and monitoring its course.

FUNGAL ANTIBODY TESTS (CLINICAL APPLICATIONS DATA, p. 107)

Most pathogenic fungi elicit antibodies in immunocompetent hosts. Tests for fungal antibodies employ complement fixation, immunodiffusion, and agglutination techniques. Table 3–9 indicates the fungal infections for which tests are available and causes of alterations in test results.

ANTISTREPTOCOCCAL ANTIBODY TESTS (CLINICAL APPLICATIONS DATA, p. 108)

Group A beta-hemolytic streptococci characteristically produce a variety of extracellular products capable of stimulating antibody production. Such antibodies do not act on the bacteria and have no protective effect, but their existence indicates recent presence of active streptococci. Antibody is most reliably produced in response to streptolysin O, and the test for this antibody is termed an antistreptolysin O (ASO) titer. Antibodies in response to hyaluronidase, streptokinase, deoxyribonuclease B, and nicotinamide also may be produced, with respective designations of AH, anti-SK, ADN-B, and anti-NADase. When

TABLE 3–9. **Immunologic Tests in Microbiology**

Organism	Tests Available	Causes of Alterations
Fungi		
Histoplasma capsulatum	CF, I	Prior exposure to organism or cross-reactive agent; recent skin test
Blastomyces dermatitidis	CF, I	Blastomycosis
Coccidioides immitis	CF, I	Acute or chronic infection; repeated skin testing with coccidiodin
Aspergillus furnigatus	CF, I	Pulmonary aspergillosis; aspergillosis allergy
Cryptococcus neoformans	A	Test demonstrates antigen, not antibodies, in infection
Sporotrichum schenckii	A	Deep tissue infection
Protozoa		
Toxoplasma gondii	IFA	Acute or chronic toxoplasmosis
Mycoplasma		
Mycoplasma pneumoniae	CF, CA	Primary atypical pneumonia

A = Agglutination; CA = Cold agglutinins; CF = Complement fixation; I = Immunodiffusion; IFA = Indirect fluorescent antibody tests.

ASO titers are low, tests for these latter antibodies may be performed to substantiate the diagnosis, as these are more sensitive tests.

Elevated antistreptococcal antibody titers may occur in healthy carriers of beta-hemolytic streptococci. Elevated levels are seen also in those with rheumatic fever, glomerulonephritis, bacterial endocarditis, scarlet fever, otitis media, and streptococcal pharyngitis.

FEBRILE AGGLUTINATION TESTS (CLINICAL APPLICATIONS DATA, p. 109)

When the suspected infecting organism is difficult or dangerous to culture, serologic (i.e., antigen-antibody) diagnosis is made by means of agglutination tests using antigens that react with the individual's antibodies. Diseases that may be diagnosed using these tests, along with the type of febrile agglutination test used, are listed in Table 3–10.

VIRAL ANTIBODY TESTS (CLINICAL APPLICATIONS DATA, p. 110)

Because viral cultures may not be available or may be disproportionately expensive in relation to the potential benefit (i.e., effective antiviral treatment is not available for most organisms), viral antibody tests are used to determine exposure to and infection with certain viruses (Table 3–11).

As a number of tests may be performed, requests for viral antibody tests must include enough clinical information to permit selecting the appropriate study. A request for "viral studies" is virtually meaningless.

HETEROPHILE ANTIBODY TESTS (CLINICAL APPLICATIONS DATA, p. 110)

Diagnosis of infectious mononucleosis, caused by Epstein-Barr virus (EBV), depends on serologic (i.e., antigen-antibody) confirmation of clinical manifes-

TABLE 3–10. **Febrile Agglutination Tests**

Diseases	Test
Rickettsial Infections Rocky Mountain spotted fever; typhus (murine, scrub, epidemic, and recrudescent)	Weil-Felix reaction (*Proteus* antigen test)
Salmonella Infections Typhoid and paratyphoid fevers	Widal's test (O and H antigen tests)
Brucella Infections Cattle, hog, goat (hosts may transmit infections to humans)	*Brucella* agglutination test (slide agglutination test)
Tularemia Rabbit fever and deer fly fever	Tularemia agglutination test (tube dilution test)

TABLE 3–11. **Tests for Viral Diseases**

Virus/Disease	Appropriate Serologic Tests
Respiratory syndromes Influenza Parainfluenza	CF, HI
Adenoviruses	CF, HI, NT
Chlamydia Respiratory syncytial virus	CF, IFA
Arbovirus Colorado tick fever Yellow fever	CF, HI, NT
Meningoencephalitis	Antibodies to echo, herpes, polio, and coxsackie viruses by neutralization tests
Herpes viruses Herpes simplex* Varicella zoster Cytomegalovirus*	Fluorescein-tagged antibodies in cells
Epstein-Barr virus	Heterophile antibody (Monotest), agglutination test, IFA
Rubella* Mumps Measles	IgM titers, CF, HI
Infectious hepatitis	IgM titers, IgG titers, hepatitis A virus antibodies (HAV-Ab), CF, RIA
Serum hepatitis	Antibodies to hepatitis B virus surface antigen (HBsAg) (HBsAb)
Cytomegalic inclusion disease	CF, HI
Acquired immunodeficiency syndrome (AIDS)	Human immunodeficiency virus (HIV) antibodies, Western blot (WB), IFA

Note: In the TORCH test, antibodies to *Toxoplasma gondii* (see Table 3–9), rubella virus, cytomegalovirus, and herpes virus are measured.

CF = Complement fixation; HI = Hemagglutination inhibition; IFA = Immunofluorescent antibody; NT = Neutralization test; RIA = Radioimmunoassay.

tations. The hallmark of EBV infection is the heterophil antibody, also called the Paul-Bunnel antibody, an IgM that agglutinates sheep or horse red cells.

Forssman antibody, which may be present in the serum of normal persons as well as in that of individuals with serum sickness, also agglutinates with sheep erythrocytes. The Davidsohn differential absorption test may be used to distinguish between the Paul-Bunnel antibody and the Forssman antibody.

Currently, more rapid and sensitive tests are available that use horse red cells in a single-step agglutination test.[26] These tests (e.g., Monospot, Mono-screen, Monocheck, and Monostion) are used as screening tests for infectious mononucleosis and are gradually replacing the more traditional techniques.

Clinical Applications Data

FUNGAL ANTIBODY TESTS (BACKGROUND INFORMATION, p. 104)

Reference Values

Organism	Complement Fixation Titers	Immuno-diffusion Test	Agglutination	Other Tests
Fungi				
Histoplasma capsulatum	<1:8	Negative	—	—
Blastomyces dermatitidis	<1:8	Negative	—	—
Coccidioides immitis	<1:2	Negative	—	—
Aspergillus fumigatus	<1:8	Negative	—	—
Cryptococcus neoformans	—	—	Negative	—
Sporotrichum schenckii	—	—	1:40	—
Protozoa				
Toxoplasma gondii	—	—	—	Indirect fluorescent antibody (IFA) tests <1:16
Mycoplasma				
Mycoplasma pneumoniae	<1:256	—	Cold agglutinins <1:16	—

Interfering Factors

■ Recent fungal skin tests may alter results
■ Obtaining the sample near fungal skin lesions may contaminate the specimen and alter test results

Indications/Purposes for Fungal Antibody Tests

■ Suspected infection with the fungus for which the test is performed
■ Persistent pulmonary symptoms after pneumonia
■ Acute meningitis of unknown etiology
■ Identification of the state of infection by rising or falling titers

■ Confirmation of previous exposure to the fungus despite absence of clinical signs of illness

Client Preparation

Client preparation is the same as that for any study involving the collection of a peripheral blood sample (see Appendix I). The client should be interviewed to determine if he or she has undergone any recent fungal skin tests that may alter test results.

The Procedure

A venipuncture is performed and the sample collected in a red-topped tube. Venipuncture should not be performed on or near any fungal skin lesions. The sample must be handled gently and transported promptly to the laboratory.

Aftercare and Nursing Observations

Care and assessment following the procedure are the same as for any study involving the collection of a peripheral blood sample.

ANTISTREPTOCOCCAL ANTIBODY TESTS (BACKGROUND INFORMATION, p. 104)

Reference Values

Antistreptolysin O (ASO) titer	
Preschool children	<85 Todd units/ml
School-age children	<170 Todd units/ml
Adults	<85 Todd units/ml
Anti–deoxyribonuclease B (ADN-B) titer	
Preschool children	<60 Todd units/ml
School-age children	<170 Todd units/ml
Adults	<85 Todd units/ml
Antihyaluronidase (AH) titer	<128 Todd units/ml
Antistreptokinase (Anti-SK) titer	<128 Todd units/ml

Interfering Factors

■ Therapy with antibiotics and adrenal corticosteroids may result in falsely decreased levels
■ Elevated blood beta-lipoproteins may result in falsely elevated levels

Indications/Purposes for Antistreptococcal Antibody Tests

■ Suspected streptococcal infection, to confirm the diagnosis
■ Detecting and monitoring response to therapy for poststreptococcal illnesses such as rheumatic fever and glomerulonephritis
■ Differentiation of rheumatic fever from rheumatoid arthritis, with the former indicated by elevated levels

Client Preparation

Client preparation is the same as that for any study involving the collection of a peripheral blood sample (see Appendix I). Medications that the client is currently taking or has recently taken should be noted, as therapy with antibiotics and adrenal corticosteroids may alter test results.

The Procedure

A venipuncture is performed and the sample collected in a red-topped tube. A capillary sample may be obtained in infants and children, as well as in adults for whom a venipuncture may not be feasible. The sample must be handled gently and sent promptly to the laboratory.

Aftercare and Nursing Observations

Care and assessment following the procedure are the same as for any study involving the collection of a peripheral blood sample.

FEBRILE AGGLUTINATION TESTS (BACKGROUND INFORMATION, p. 105)
Reference Values

Weil-Felix reaction (*Proteus* antigen test)	<1:80
Widal's test (O and H antigen tests)	<1:160
Brucella agglutination test (slide agglutination test)	<1:80
Tularemia agglutination test (tube dilution test)	<1:40

Interfering Factors

■ Vaccination, chronic exposure to infected animals, and cross-reactions with other antibodies may result in falsely elevated titers
■ Individuals who are immunosuppressed or receiving antibiotic therapy may have false-negative results

Indications/Purposes for Febrile Agglutination Tests

■ Determination of possible cause of fever of unknown origin (FUO)
■ Suspected typhus, Rocky Mountain spotted fever, or other disorder for which selected tests are specific
■ Suspected "carrier" state for typhoid
■ Positive blood or stool culture for *Salmonella*

Client Preparation

Client preparation is the same as that for any study involving the collection of a peripheral blood sample (see Appendix I). A thorough history should be obtained in order to identify possible sources of false-positive or -negative results.

The Procedure

A venipuncture is performed and the sample collected in a red-topped tube. The sample must be handled gently to avoid hemolysis and transported immediately to the laboratory.

Aftercare and Nursing Objectives

Care and assessment following the procedure are the same as for any study involving the collection of a peripheral blood sample.

VIRAL ANTIBODY TESTS (BACKGROUND INFORMATION, p. 105)

Reference Values

In general, lack of exposure to the virus yields a negative test result. Reference values vary with the type of viral antibody test. The laboratory performing the test should be consulted.

Indications/Purposes for Viral Antibody Tests

■ Suspected acquired immunodeficiency syndrome (AIDS) or exposure to human immunodeficiency virus (HIV)
■ Retrospective confirmation of viral infection
■ Determination of immunity to rubella in women of childbearing age
■ Confirmation of exposure to rubella in early pregnancy
■ Suspected herpes encephalitis
■ Determination of immunity to chickenpox in children with leukemia, as this infection may be fatal in such children
■ Identification of asymptomatic carriers of cytomegalovirus (CMV)
■ Monitoring the course of prolonged viral disease

■ Monitoring mothers and neonates for exposure to viral infections that may cause congenital disease in the newborn infant (usually done by the TORCH test—see Table 3–11, p. 106)

Client Preparation

Client preparation is the same as that for any study involving the collection of a peripheral blood sample (see Appendix I).

The Procedure

A venipuncture is performed and the sample collected in a red-topped tube. The sample must be handled gently to avoid hemolysis, and transported promptly to the laboratory.

Aftercare and Nursing Observations

Care and assessment following the procedure are the same as for any study involving the collection of a peripheral blood sample. Women of childbearing age with low rubella titers should be appropriately immunized.

HETEROPHILE ANTIBODY TESTS (BACKGROUND INFORMATION, p. 105)

Reference Values

Negative, or a titer of less than 1:56

Interfering Factors

■ False-positive results may occur in the presence of narcotic addiction, serum sickness, lymphomas, hepatitis, leukemia, cancer of the pancreas, and phenytoin therapy

Indications/Purposes for Heterophile Antibody Tests

■ Suspected infectious mononucleosis (of individuals with Epstein-Barr virus [EBV] infectious mononucleosis, 95 percent will have a positive result, 86 percent in the first week of illness)

Client Preparation

Client preparation is the same as that for any study involving the collection of a peripheral blood sample (see Appendix I). A thorough history should be obtained in order to identify possible sources of false-positive results.

The Procedure

A venipuncture is performed and the sample collected in a red-topped tube. For screening tests, the directions accompanying the test kit are followed. For traditional tests, the sample should be sent to the laboratory promptly.

Aftercare and Nursing Observations

Care and assessment following the procedure are the same as for any study involving the collection of a peripheral blood sample.

TESTS FOR SYPHILIS

Background Information

Infection with *Treponema pallidum* provides two distinct categories of antibodies: (1) reagin (a nonspecific antibacterial antibody); and (2) antitreponemal antibody. Reagin tests, by their nature nonspecific, include the Wassermann and Reiter complement fixation tests, now seldom used. Reagin tests currently used for screening are the venereal disease research laboratory (VDRL) and rapid plasma reagin (RPR) flocculation tests. Because reagin screening tests often yield false-positive reactions (Table 3–12), positive test results are confirmed by means of treponemal antibody tests. The best of these is the fluorescent treponemal antibody test (FTA-ABS) with absorbed serum.[27]

FLUORESCENT TREPONEMAL ANTIBODY TEST (FTA-ABS) (CLINICAL APPLICATIONS DATA, p. 112)

In this test, a sample of the client's serum is layered onto a slide fixed with *Treponema pallidum* organisms. If antibody is present, it will attach to the organisms and can subsequently be demonstrated by its reaction with fluorescein-labeled antiblobulin serum.

The fluorescent treponemal antibody test (FTA-ABS) rarey gives false-positive results, except sporadically in clients with systemic lupus erythematosus (SLE); the pattern of fluorescence may have an atypical beaded appearance in these cases. Elderly individuals and clients with immune complex diseases (see p. 97) occasionally also have false-positive results.[28]

TABLE 3–12. Causes of False-Positive Reactions to Reagin Tests

Transiently Positive	Persistently Positive
Occurring in > 10% of clients with the following:	
Infectious mononucleosis	Systemic lupus erythematosus
Malaria	Rheumatoid arthritis
Brucellosis	Illicit drug use
Typhus	Hepatitis
Lymphogranuloma venereum	Leprosy
Subacute bacterial endocarditis	Malaria
	Advanced age
	Nonsyphilitic treponemal disease (pints, yaws, bejel)
Occurring rarely in clients with the following:	
Hepatitis	Tuberculosis
Measles	Scleroderma
Chickenpox	
Mycoplasma pneumonia	
After smallpox vaccination	

VENEREAL DISEASE RESEARCH LABORATORY (VDRL) AND RAPID PLASMA REAGIN (RPR) TESTS (CLINICAL APPLICATIONS DATA, p. 113)

The venereal disease research laboratory (VDRL) and rapid plasma reagin (RPR) tests are flocculation tests for reagin and are used in screening for syphilis. The VDRL test uses heat-inactivated serum and can be done on slides or in tubes. The RPR test uses unheated serum or plasma, which is added to a reagent-treated plasma card. Automated procedures have been adapted for multichannel analyzers.[29]

It is noted that these tests are not specific for antibodies to *Treponema pallidum*, and many factors, including laboratory procedures, may cause false-positive results (Table 3–12).

Clinical Applications Data

FLUORESCENT TREPONEMAL ANTIBODY TEST (FTA-ABS) (BACKGROUND INFORMATION, p. 111)

Reference Values

Negative

Interfering Factors

■ False-positive results may occasionally occur in elderly individuals and in clients with systemic lupus erythematosus or other immune complex diseases

Indications/Purposes for Fluorescent Treponemal Antibody Test

■ Confirmation of the presence of treponemal antibodies in the serum (*note:* the test also may be applied to cerebrospinal fluid [CSF] to diagnose tertiary syphilis)

■ Verification of syphilis as the cause of positive VDRL and RPR test results (see p. 112)

Client Preparation

Client preparation is the same as that for any study involving the collection of a peripheral blood sample (see Appendix I). The person's history should be reviewed for possible sources of false-positive results.

The Procedure

A venipuncture is performed and the sample collected in a red-topped tube. The sample must be handled gently to avoid hemolysis, and transported promptly to the laboratory.

Aftercare and Nursing Observations

Care and assessment following the procedure are the same as for any study involving the collection of a peripheral blood sample.

VENEREAL DISEASE RESEARCH LABORATORY (VDRL) AND RAPID PLASMA REAGIN (RPR) TESTS (BACKGROUND INFORMATION, p. 112)

Reference Values

Results are reported qualitatively as strongly reactive, reactive, weakly reactive, or negative. A degree of quantification is possible by diluting the serum and reporting the highest titer that remains positive. Positive results must be further evaluated either by repeat testing or with tests specific for antitreponemal antibodies.[30]

Interfering Factors

■ Many factors, including laboratory procedures, may cause false-positive results (see Table 3–12, p. 112)

Indications/Purposes for VDLR and RPR Tests

■ Routine screening for possible syphilis
■ Known or suspected exposure to syphilis, including congenital syphilis
■ Verification of an antigen-antibody reaction to reagin, although a positive result is not necessarily diagnostic for syphilis
■ Monitoring response to treatment for syphilis, with effective treatment indicated by decreasing titers

Client Preparation

Client preparation is the same as that for any study involving the collection of a peripheral blood sample (see Appendix I). A thorough history should be obtained in order to identify possible causes of false-positive results (see Table 3–12, p. 112). It is recommended that alcohol ingestion be avoided for 24 hours prior to the test.

The Procedure

A venipuncture is performed and the sample collected in a red-topped tube. The sample must be handled gently to avoid hemolysis and transported promptly to the laboratory.

For neonates, a sample of cord blood may be obtained at delivery. Subsequent samples of venous blood from the infant may be required if the mother's titer is lower than that of the infant, indicating active syphilis in the infant despite successful treatment of the mother.

Aftercare and Nursing Observations

Care and assessment following the procedure are the same as for any study involving the collection of a peripheral blood sample.

IMMUNOLOGIC TESTS RELATED TO CANCER

Background Information

Certain globulins and antigens are commonly found in early fetal life, but their presence in excessive amounts in adults is abnormal. Measurement of these substances in humans has been used most recently in the diagnosis and treatment of cancer.

SERUM ALPHA-FETOPROTEIN (AFP) (CLINICAL APPLICATIONS DATA, p. 115)

During the first 10 weeks of life, the major serum protein is not albumin, but alpha-fetoprotein (AFP). Fetal liver synthesizes huge quantities of AFP until about the 32nd week of gestation. Thereafter, synthesis declines until at 1 year of age the serum normally contains no more than 30 ng per ml.

Resting liver cells (hepatocytes) normally manufacture very little AFP, but rapidly multiplying hepatocytes resume synthesis of large amounts.[31] Thus, the test's greatest usefulness is in monitoring for recurrence of hepatic carcinoma or metastatic lesions involving the liver. In such instances, AFP levels may be thousands of times normal (e.g., 10,000 to 100,000 ng per ml, when the normal value is less than 30 ng per ml). Successful treatment of hepatocellular carcinoma results in an immediate drop in AFP levels, while recurrence of hepatic carcinoma will cause AFP levels to rise 1 to 6 months before the client becomes symptomatic. It should be noted that 30 to 50 percent of Americans with liver cancer do not have elevated AFP levels. More consistent elevations are seen in those Asian and African populations with a very high incidence of hepatocellular carcinoma.[32]

Determination of serum AFP levels also may be used in diagnosing hepatoblastoma, embryonal gonadal teratoblastoma, and ataxia-telangiectasia (hereditary progressive ataxia associated with oculocutaneous telangiectasis). Elevated levels (e.g., 500 ng per ml) also may be seen in individuals with cirrhosis or chronic active hepatitis, and in those recovering from viral or toxic hepatitis.

Measurement of AFP levels in maternal blood and amniotic fluid is used to detect certain fetal abnormalities, especially neural tube defects such as anencephaly, spina bifida, and myelomeningocele (see Chapter 10 and Table 10–1, p. 400). Routine prenatal screening includes determination of the mother's serum AFP level at 13 to 16 weeks of pregnancy. If maternal blood levels are elevated on two samples obtained 1 week apart, an ultrasound may be performed and AFP levels in amniotic fluid may be analyzed. Other possible causes of elevated AFP levels during pregnancy include multiple pregnancy and fetal demise.

TABLE 3–13. Causes of Alterations in CEA Levels

Cause of Alteration	Percentage With CEA Levels (ng/ml)			
	<2.5	2.6–5	5.1–10	>10
Nonsmokers	97	3	0	0
Smokers	81	15	3	1
Ex-Smokers	93	5	1	1
Carcinomas				
Colorectal	28	23	14	34
Pulmonary	24	25	25	25
Gastric	39	32	10	19
Pancreatic	9	31	26	35
Breast	53	21	13	14
Head/Neck	48	32	14	5
Other	53	27	12	9
Leukemias	63	25	8	5
Lymphoma	65	24	11	0
Sarcoma	68	26	5	0
Benign tumors	82	12	6	1
Benign breast disease	85	11	4	0
Pulmonary emphysema	43	37	16	4
Alcoholic cirrhosis	29	44	24	2
Ulcerative colitis	69	18	8	5
Regional ileitis	60	27	11	2
Gastric ulcer	55	29	15	1
Colorectal polyps	81	14	3	1
Diverticulitis	73	20	5	2

CARCINOEMBRYONIC ANTIGEN (CEA) (CLINICAL APPLICATIONS DATA, p. 116)

Carcinoembryonic antigen (CEA) is a glycoprotein normally produced only during early fetal life and during rapid multiplication of epithelial cells, especially those of the digestive system. Elevations of CEA occur with many cancers, primary and recurrent, as well as with a number of nonmalignant diseases and in smokers (Table 3–13). Although the test is not diagnostic for any specific disease, it is used primarily when various types of carcinomas are suspected.

CEA levels are used also to evaluate response to cancer therapy. If therapy is effective, CEA levels should approach normal within 4 to 6 weeks of treatment. The test also may be used to monitor clients for recurrence of carcinoma, which may produce elevated CEA levels several months before symptoms appear.

Clinical Applications Data

SERUM ALPHA-FETOPROTEIN (AFP) (BACKGROUND INFORMATION, p. 114)
Reference Values

Neonate	600,000 ng/ml
1 year old to adult	<30 ng/ml

Indications/Purposes for Serum Alpha-Fetoprotein (AFP)

■ Monitoring for hepatic carcinoma or metastatic lesions involving the liver, as indicated by highly elevated levels (e.g., 10,000 to 100,000 ng per ml)
■ Monitoring response to treatment for hepatic carcinoma, with successful treatment indicated by an immediate drop in levels
■ Monitoring for recurrence of hepatic carcinoma, with elevated levels occurring 1 to 6 months before the client becomes symptomatic
■ Suspected hepatitis or cirrhosis as indicated by slightly to moderately elevated levels (e.g., 500 ng per ml)
■ Routine prenatal screening for fetal neural tube defects and other disorders, as indicated by elevated levels
■ Suspected intrauterine fetal death, as indicated by elevated levels
■ Support for diagnosing embryonal gonadal teratoblastoma, hepatoblastoma, and ataxia-telangiectasia

Client Preparation

For serum studies, client preparation is the same as that for any study involving the collection of a peripheral blood sample (see Appendix I). For amniotic fluid studies, the client is prepared for amniocentesis, as described in Chapter 10.

The Procedure

For serum studies, a venipuncture is performed and the sample collected in a red-topped tube. The sample must be handled gently to avoid hemolysis, and transported promptly to the laboratory. For amniotic fluid studies, amniocentesis is performed (see Chapter 10).

Aftercare and Nursing Observations

Care and assessment following the procedures are the same as for any study involving collection of a peripheral blood sample or amniocentesis (see Chapter 10).

CARCINOEMBRYONIC ANTIGEN (CEA) (BACKGROUND INFORMATION, p. 115)

Reference Values

Less than 2.5 ng per ml

Interfering Factors

■ Levels may be elevated in smokers who do not have malignancies

Indications/Purposes for Carcinoembryonic Antigen (CEA)

■ Monitoring clients with inflammatory intestinal disorders with a high risk of malignancy
■ Suspected carcinoma of the colon, pancreas, or lung, as these cancers produce the highest CEA levels
■ Monitoring CEA response to therapy for cancer, with effective treatment indicated by normal levels within 4 to 6 weeks
■ Monitoring for recurrence of carcinoma, with elevated levels occurring several months before the client becomes symptomatic

■ Suspected leukemia, gammopathy, or other disorder associated with elevated CEA levels (see Table 3–13, p. 115)

Client Preparation

Client preparation is the same as that for any study involving the collection of a peripheral blood sample (see Appendix I).

The Procedure

A venipuncture is performed and the sample collected in a red-topped tube. The sample must be handled gently to avoid hemolysis, and transported promptly to the laboratory.

Aftercare and Nursing Observations

Care and assessment following the procedure are the same as for any study involving collection of a peripheral blood sample.

REFERENCES

1. Widmann, FK: Clinical Interpretation of Laboratory Tests, ed 9. FA Davis, Philadelphia, 1983, pp 167–168.
2. Boggs, DR and Winkelstein, A: White Cell Manual, ed 4. FA Davis, Philadelphia, 1983, p 61.
3. *Ibid*, pp 61–62.
4. *Ibid*, p 63.
5. *Ibid*, pp 63–64.
6. *Ibid*, pp 68–71.
7. *Ibid*, p 74.
8. Widmann, *op cit*, p 169.
9. *Ibid*.
10. *Ibid*.
11. Boggs and Winkelstein, *op cit*, p 69.
12. *Ibid*.
13. *Ibid*, pp 69–73.
14. *Ibid*, pp 72–73.
15. *Ibid*, p 74.
16. *Ibid*, p 65.
17. Widmann, *op cit*, pp 179–180.
18. *Ibid*, p 180.
19. *Ibid*, pp 181–182.
20. *Ibid*, pp 181–184.
21. Boggs and Winkelstein, *op cit*, pp 83–84.
22. Widmann, *op cit*, p 176.
23. *Ibid*, pp 175–176.
24. *Ibid*, pp 184–185.
25. *Ibid*, p 173.
26. *Ibid*, pp 379–381.
27. *Ibid*, pp 387–392.
28. *Ibid*, p 391.
29. *Ibid*, p 390.
30. *Ibid*.
31. *Ibid*, p 325.
32. *Ibid*.

BIBLIOGRAPHY

Beare, PG, Rahr, VA, and Ronshausen, CA: Nursing Implications of Diagnostic Tests, ed 2. JB Lippincott, Philadelphia, 1985.

Bio-Science Handbook, ed 12. Bio-Science Laboratories, Van Nuys, CA, 1977.

Byrne, CJ, Saxton, DF, Pelikan, PK, and Nugent, PM: Laboratory Tests: Implications for Nursing Care, ed 2. Addison-Wesley, Menlo Park, CA, 1986.

Fischbach, FT: A Manual of Laboratory Diagnostic Tests, ed 3. JB Lippincott, Philadelphia, 1988.

Kee, JL: Laboratory and Diagnostic Tests with Nursing Implications, ed 2. Appleton & Lange, Norwalk, CT, 1987.

Luckmann, J and Sorensen, KC: Medical-Surgical Nursing: A Psychophysiologic Approach, ed 3. WB Saunders, Philadelphia, 1987.

Mathewson, MK: Pharmacotherapeutics: A Nursing Process Approach. FA Davis, Philadelphia, 1986.

Michaels, D: Diagnostic Procedures: The Patient and the Health Care Team. John Wiley & Sons, New York, 1983.

Nurse's Reference Library: Diagnostics, ed 2. Springhouse Corporation, Springhouse, PA, 1986.

Pagana, KD and Pagana, TJ: Diagnostic Testing and Nursing Implications: A Case Study Approach, ed 2. CV Mosby, St Louis, 1986.

Price, SA and Wilson, LM: Pathophysiology: Clinical Concepts of Disease Processes, ed 3. McGraw-Hill, New York, 1986.

Spencer, RT, Nichols, LW, Lipkin, GB, Waterhouse, HP, West, FM, and Bankert, EG: Clinical Pharmacology and Nursing Management, ed 2. JB Lippincott, Philadelphia, 1986.

Tilkian, SM, Conover, MB, and Tilkian, AG: Clinical Implications of Laboratory Tests, ed 4. CV Mosby, St Louis, 1987.

Wallach, J: Interpretation of Diagnostic Tests, ed 4. Little, Brown & Co, Boston, 1986.

Widmann, FK: Pathobiology: How Diseases Happen. Little, Brown & Co, Boston, 1978.

4

IMMUNO-HEMATOLOGY AND BLOOD BANKING

TESTS COVERED

First number, background information; second number, clinical applications data

INTRODUCTION

Immunohematology is the study of the antigens present on blood cell membranes and the antibodies stimulated by their presence. For red cells, more than 300 antigenic configurations have been discovered and classified. A specific biological role has been identified for only a few of these (e.g., ABO and Rh typing for blood transfusions). One commonality is that blood cell antigens are inherited, and the genes that determine them follow the laws of Mendelian genetics.[1] Thus, many of the numerous blood cell antigens that have been identified to date have their greatest usefulness in genetic studies.

The focus of this chapter is on tests of blood cell antigens and related antibodies that are used in determining the compatibility of blood and blood products for transfusions.

ABO BLOOD TYPING

Background Information

The ABO blood group system was discovered in 1901 by Landsteiner, while the theory for inheritance of ABO blood groups was first proposed by Bernstein in 1924. The first blood groups described by Landsteiner were A, B, and O, with the blood group indicating the presence or absence of a specific antigen on the red cell membrane. In 1902, Landsteiner's associates, Sturle and von Descatello, discovered the fourth ABO blood group, AB.[2]

The major antigens in the ABO system are A and B. An individual with A antigens has type A blood; an individual with B antigens has type B blood. A person with both A and B antigens has type AB blood, and one having neither A nor B antigens has type O blood. The genes that determine presence or absence of A or B antigens reside on chromosome number 9.[3]

Immunologically competent individuals older than 6 months of age have serum antibodies that react with the A and B antigens absent from their own red cells (Table 4–1). Thus, a person with type A blood has anti-B antibodies, while one with type B blood has anti-A antibodies. Individuals with type AB blood have neither of these antibodies, while those with type O blood have both. These antibodies are not inherited, but develop after exposure to environmental antigens that are chemically similar to red cell antigens (e.g., pollens and bacteria). Individuals do not, however, develop antibodies to their own red cell antigens.[4,5]

Anti-A and anti-B antibodies are strong agglutinins and cause rapid, complement-mediated destruction (see Chapter 3, p. 95) of any incompatible cells encountered. Although most of the anti-A and anti-B activity resides in the IgM class of immunoglobulins (see Chapter 3, p. 90), some activity rests with IgG. Anti-A and anti-B antibodies of the IgG class coat the red cells without immediately affecting their viability and can readily cross the placenta, resulting in hemolytic disease of the newborn. Persons with type O blood frequently have more IgG anti-A and anti-B than do individuals with type A or B blood. Thus, ABO hemolytic disease of the newborn affects infants of type O mothers almost exclusively.[6]

When blood transfusions are required, the client is normally given blood of his or her same type to prevent adverse antigen-antibody reactions. In emergency situations, however, some individuals may be given blood of other ABO types. For example, since type O blood has neither A nor B antigens, it may be

TABLE 4–1. Antigens and Antibodies in ABO Blood Groups

Blood Group	Antigens on Red Cells	Antibodies in Serum	Whites	Blacks	American Indians	Orientals
A	A	Anti-B	40	27	16	28
B	B	Anti-A	11	20	4	27
O	Neither	Anti-A Anti-B	45	49	79	40
AB	A and B	Neither	4	4	<1	5

Frequency (%) in US Populations spans the last four columns.

From Widmann,[1] p 199, with permission.

given to individuals with types A, B, and AB blood. Thus, a person with type O blood is called a *universal donor*. Since type O blood does have anti-A and anti-B antibodies, however, it should be administered slowly when given to non-O individuals. Further, because persons with type O blood have both anti-A and anti-B antibodies, they can receive only type O blood.

The situation is reversed for those with type AB blood. Since these individuals lack anti-A and anti-B antibodies, they may receive transfusions of types A, B, and O blood in emergencies when type AB blood is not available. Thus, a person with type AB blood is called a *universal recipient*.

ABO blood typing is an agglutination test in which the client's red cells are mixed with anti-A and anti-B sera, a process known as *forward grouping*. The procedure is then reversed and the person's serum is mixed with known type A and type B cells (i.e., *reverse grouping*). When a transfusion is to be administered, cross-matching blood from the donor and the recipient is performed along with typing. Cross-matching detects antibodies in the sera of the donor and the recipient, which may lead to a transfusion reaction due to red cell destruction (see p. 125).

Clinical Applications Data

Reference Values

The normal distribution of the four ABO blood groups in the United States is shown in Table 4–1 (p. 120). Discrepancies in the results of forward and reverse grouping may occur in infants, the elderly, and those who are immunosuppressed or who have a variety of immunological disorders.[7]

Indications/Purposes for ABO Typing

■ Identification of the client's ABO blood type, especially prior to surgery or other procedures in which blood loss is a threat and/or for which replacement may be needed
■ Identification of donor ABO blood type for stored blood
■ Determination of ABO compatibility of donor's and recipient's bloods
■ Identification of maternal and infant ABO blood types, to predict potential hemolytic disease of the newborn

Client Preparation

Client preparation is the same as that for any study involving the collection of a peripheral blood sample (see Appendix I). Immunosuppressive drugs taken by the client or presence of immunological disorder should be noted.

The Procedure

A venipuncture is performed and the sample collected in a red-topped tube or other type of blood collection tube, depending on laboratory preference. The sample must be handled gently to avoid hemolysis, and sent promptly to the laboratory.

Although correct client identification is important for all laboratory and diagnostic procedures, it is crucial when blood is collected for ABO typing. One of the most common sources of error in ABO typing is incorrect identification of the client and the specimens obtained.[8]

Aftercare and Nursing Observations

Care and assessment following the procedure are the same as for any study involving the collection of a peripheral blood sample. The client should be informed of his or her blood type and the information should be recorded on a card or other document (e.g., driver's license) that the client would normally carry in the event of an emergency requiring a blood transfusion.

Rh TYPING

Background Information

After the ABO system, the Rh system is the group of red cell antigens with the greatest importance.[9] The existence of this system was first reported in 1940 by Landsteiner and Weiner. The antigen was called the Rh factor, because it was produced by immunizing guinea pigs and rabbits with red cells of rhesus monkeys. The researchers found that the serum from the immunized animals not only agglutinated rhesus monkey red cells but also the red cells of approximately 85 percent of humans. Thus, human red cells could be classified into two new blood types. Rh-positive and Rh-negative. This discovery was a great breakthrough in explaining transfusion reactions to blood that had been tested for ABO compatibility, as well as in explaining hemolytic disease of the newborn not due to ABO incompatibility between mother and fetus.[10]

It is now known that the Rh system includes many different antigens. The major antigen is termed Rh_o or D. Persons whose red cells possess D are called Rh-positive; those who lack D are called Rh-negative, no matter what other Rh antigens are present. This is because the D antigen is more likely to provoke an antibody response than any other red cell antigen, including those of the ABO system. The other major antigens of the Rh system are C, E, c, and e.[11] It should also be noted that among blacks, there are many quantitative and qualitative variants of the Rh antigens that do not always fit into the generally accepted classifications.[12]

Rh-negative individuals may produce anti-D antibodies if exposed to Rh-positive cells through either blood transfusions or pregnancy. While 50 to 70 percent of Rh-negative individuals will develop antibodies if transfused with Rh-positive blood, only 20 percent of Rh-negative mothers develop anti-D antibodies after carrying an Rh-positive fetus. This difference is due to the greater number of cells involved in a blood transfusion than in pregnancy.

When Rh antibodies develop, they are predominantly IgG. Thus, they coat the red cells and set them up for destruction in the reticuloendothelial system. The antibodies seldom activate the complement system (see Chapter 3, p. 95). Anti-D antibodies readily cross the placenta from mother to fetus and are the most common cause of severe hemolytic disease of the newborn. Immunosuppressive therapy (e.g., with Rhogam) successfully prevents antibody formation when given to an unimmunized Rh-negative mother just after delivery or abortion of an Rh-positive fetus.[13]

Rh typing involves an agglutination test in which the client's red cells are mixed with serum containing anti-D antibodies. Agglutination indicates that the D antigen is present, and the person is termed Rh-positive.

Clinical Applications Data

Reference Values

The D antigen is present on the red cells of 85 percent of whites and a higher percentage of blacks, American Indians, and Asians.

Indications/Purposes for Rh Typing

■ Identification of the client's Rh type, especially prior to surgery or other procedures in which blood loss is a threat and/or for which replacement may be needed
■ Identification of donor Rh type for stored blood
■ Determination of Rh compatibility of donor's and recipient's bloods
■ Identification of maternal and infant Rh types, to predict potential hemolytic disease of the newborn
■ Determination of anti-D antibody titer after sensitization by pregnancy with an Rh-positive fetus
■ Determination of the need for immunosuppressive therapy (e.g., with Rhogam) when an Rh-negative woman has delivered or aborted an Rh-positive fetus

Client Preparation

Client preparation is the same as that for any study involving the collection of a peripheral blood sample (see Appendix I).

The Procedure

A venipuncture is performed and the sample collected in a red-topped tube or other type of blood collection tube, depending on laboratory preference. The sample must be handled gently to avoid hemolysis, and sent promptly to the laboratory.

As with ABO typing, correct client and sample identification is crucial in avoiding erroneous results.

Aftercare and Nursing Observations

Care and assessment following the procedure are the same as that for any study involving the collection of a peripheral blood sample. As with ABO typing, the client should be informed of his or her Rh type. Women of childbearing age who are Rh-negative should be informed of the need for follow-up should pregnancy occur.

ANTIGLOBULIN TESTS (COOMBS' TESTS)

Background Information

Antiglobulin (Coombs') tests are used to detect nonagglutinating antibodies or complement molecules on red cell surfaces. They are employed most commonly in immunohematology laboratories and blood banks for routine cross-matching, antibody screening tests and preliminary investigations of hemolytic anemias.[14,15]

The tests are based on the principle that immunoglobulins (i.e., antibodies) act as antigens when injected into a nonhuman host. This principle was originally published by Moreschi in 1908, but his findings drew little notice. In 1945, Coombs independently rediscovered the principle when he prepared anti-human serum by injecting human serum into rabbits. The rabbit antibody produced against the human globulin was then collected and purified. This anti-human globulin (AHG) was used to demonstrate incomplete human antibodies that were adsorbed to red cells and did not cause visually apparent agglutination unless Coombs' rabbit serum was used. The two applications of the test currently used are (1) the direct antiglobulin test (direct Coombs) and (2) the indirect antiglobulin test (indirect Coombs).[16]

DIRECT ANTIGLOBULIN TEST (DAT, DIRECT COOMBS) (CLINICAL APPLICATIONS DATA, p. 125)

It is never normal for circulating red cells to be coated with antibody. The direct antiglobulin test (DAT, direct Coombs) is used to detect abnormal in vivo coating of red cells with antibody globulin (IgG), or complement, or both.

When this test is performed, the red cells are taken directly from the sample, washed with saline (to remove residual globulins left in the client's serum surrounding the red cells, but not actually attached to them), and mixed with antihuman globulin (AHG). If the AHG causes agglutination of the client's red cells, specific antiglobulins may be used to determine if the red cells are coated with IgG, complement, or both.

The most common cause of a positive DAT is autoimmune hemolytic anemia in which affected individuals have antibodies against their own red cells. Other causes of positive results include hemolytic disease of the newborn, transfusion of incompatible blood, and red cell sensitizing reactions due to drugs. In the latter, the red cells may be coated with the drug or with immune complexes composed of drugs and antibodies that activate the complement system.[17,18] Drugs associated with such reactions are listed in Table 4–2. Positive DAT results may also be seen in individuals with mycoplasma pneumonia, leukemias, lymphomas, infectious mononucleosis, lupus erythematosus and other immune disorders of connective tissue, and in metastatic carcinoma.

TABLE 4–2. **Drugs That May Cause Positive Results in Direct Antiglobulin Tests**

Aldomet	Penicillin
Alkeran	Pronestyl
Apresoline	Quinidine
Dilantin	Rifampin
Isoniazid	Streptomycin
Keflin	Sulfonamides
Levodopa	Tetracycline
Loridine	Thorazine

Indirect Antiglobulin Test (IAT, Indirect Coombs, Antibody Screening Test) (Clinical Applications data, p. 126)

The indirect antiglobulin test (IAT, indirect Coombs, antibody screening test) is used primarily to screen blood samples for unexpected circulating antibodies that may be reactive against transfused red blood cells.

In this test, the client's serum serves as the source of antibody, and the red cells to be transfused as the antigen. The test is performed by incubating the serum and red cells in the laboratory (in vitro) to allow any antibodies present every opportunity to attach to the red cells. The cells are then washed with saline to remove any unattached serum globulins, and antihuman globulin (AHG) is added. If the client's serum contains an antibody that reacts with and attaches to the donor red cells, the AHG will cause the antibody-coated cells to agglutinate.

If there is no agglutination after addition of AHG, it means that no antigen-antibody reaction has occurred. The serum may contain an antibody, but the red cells against which it is tested do not have the relevant antigen. Thus, the reaction is negative.[19]

Applications of the IAT include compatibility testing (cross-matching), antibody screening, testing for the weak Rh variant antigen D^u, and determining antibody titers in Rh-negative women sensitized by an Rh-positive fetus. In certain of these methods, the client's serum is exposed to specific red cell antigens, thus allowing for demonstration of specific antibodies if present. Antibody titers are determined by testing various dilutions of the client's serum against red cells known to possess the corresponding antigen.[20,21]

Clinical Applications Data

Direct Antiglobulin Test (DAT, Direct Coombs') (Background Information, p. 124)

Reference Values

Negative (no agglutination)

Interfering Factors

■ Many drugs may cause positive reactions (Table 4–2)

Indications/Purposes for Direct Antiglobulin Test

■ Suspected hemolytic anemia or hemolytic disease of the newborn as indicated by a positive reaction
■ Suspected transfusion reaction as indicated by a positive result
■ Suspected drug sensitivity reaction as indicated by a positive result

Client Preparation

For samples collected by venipuncture, client preparation is the same as that for any study involving the collection of a peripheral blood sample (see Appendix I). Drugs currently taken by the client should be noted.

If the test is to be performed on the newborn, the parent(s) should be informed that a sample of umbilical cord blood will be obtained at delivery and will not result in blood loss to the infant.

The Procedure

A venipuncture is performed and the sample collected in a red-topped tube or other type of blood collection tube, depending on laboratory preference. For cord blood, the sample is collected in a red- or lavender-topped tube (depending on the laboratory) from the maternal segment of the cord after it has been cut and before the placenta has been delivered.

Aftercare and Nursing Observations

For venipunctures, care and assessment following the procedure are the same as for any study involving the collection of a peripheral blood sample. No specific care is necessary following collection of a cord blood sample.

INDIRECT ANTIGLOBULIN TEST (IAT, INDIRECT COOMBS, ANTIBODY SCREENING TEST) (BACKGROUND INFORMATION, p. 125)

Reference Values

Negative (no agglutination)

Interfering Factors

■ Recent administration of dextran, whole blood or fractions, or intravenous contrast media may result in a false-positive reaction

Indications/Purposes for Indirect Antiglobulin Test

■ Antibody screening and cross-matching prior to blood transfusions, especially to detect antibodies whose presence may not be elicited by other methods such as ABO and Rh typing
■ Determination of antibody titers in Rh-negative women sensitized by an Rh-positive fetus (see p. 125)
■ Testing for the weak Rh variant antigen D^u
■ Detection of other antibodies in maternal blood that may be potentially harmful to the fetus

Client Preparation

Client preparation is the same as that for any study involving the collection of a peripheral blood sample (see Appendix I). Exposure to substances that may cause false-positive reactions should be noted.

The Procedure

A venipuncture is performed and the sample collected in a red-topped tube or other blood collection tube, depending on laboratory preference. The sample must be handled gently to avoid hemolysis, and sent promptly to the laboratory.

Aftercare and Nursing Observations

Care and assessment following the procedure are the same as for any study involving the collection of a peripheral blood sample.

TABLE 4–3. **Diseases Associated With Human Leukocyte Antigens**

Disease	Associated Antigen
Ankylosing spondylitis	B27
Reiter's syndrome	B27
Diabetes mellitus (juvenile, or insulin-dependent)	Bw15, B8
Multiple sclerosis	A3, B7, B18
Acute anterior uveitis	B27
Grave's disease	B8
Juvenile rheumatoid arthritis	B27
Celiac disease	B8
Psoriasis vulgaris	B13, Bw17
Myasthenia gravis	B8
Dermatitis herpetiformis	B8
Autoimmune chronic active hepatitis	B8

HUMAN LEUKOCYTE ANTIGENS (HLA)

Background Information

All nucleated cells have human leukocyte antigens (HLA) on their surface membranes. Although sometimes described as "white cell antigens," HLA characterize virtually all cell types except red blood cells. HLA consist of a glycoprotein chain and a globulin chain. They are classified into five series designated A, B, C, D, and DR (D-related), each series containing 10 to 20 distinct antigens. A, B, C, and D antigens characterize the membranes of virtually all cells except mature red blood cells; DR antigens seem to reside only on B-lymphocytes and macrophages (see Chapter 3).

The clinical use of this information is mainly in predicting compatibility of donor/recipient tissues and platelets. In donor/recipient HLA tests, a match is sought between the two HLA types. It has been found that HLA matching improves the chances of survival of transplated tissue when the donor and recipient are blood relatives. HLA matching is much less predictive when the donor and recipient are unrelated.[22]

Some antigens have been identified with specific diseases (Table 4–3). Arthritic disorders, for example, have been closely linked to HLA-B27. In addition, HLA typing is valuable in determining parentage. If the HLA phenotypes of a child and one parent are known, it is possible to assess fairly accurately whether or not a given individual is the other parent.[23]

Clinical Applications Data

Reference Values

HLA combinations vary according to certain races and populations. The most common B antigens in American whites, for example, are B7, B8, and B12.

In American blacks, the most common of the B series are Bw17, Bw35, and a specificity characterized as 1AG. This is in contrast to African blacks, whose most common B antigens are B7, Bw17, and 1AG. Similar variations among the A antigens also have been found among various races and populations.

Indications/Purposes for HLA Tests

■ Determination of donor/recipient compatibility for tissue transplantation, especially when they are blood relatives
■ Determination of compatibility of donor platelets in individuals who will receive multiple transfusions over a long period of time
■ Support for diagnosing HLA-associated diseases (Table 4–3), especially when signs and symptoms are inconclusive
■ Determination of biological parentage

Client Preparation

Client preparation is the same as that for any study involving the collection of a peripheral blood sample (see Appendix I).

The Procedure

A venipuncture is performed and the sample collected in a green-topped tube or other blood collection device, depending on laboratory preference. The sample is sent promptly to the laboratory performing the test (not all laboratories are equipped to do so).

Aftercare and Nursing Observations

Care and assessment following the procedure are the same as for any study involving the collection of a peripheral blood sample.

REFERENCES

1. Widmann, FK: Clinical Interpretation of Laboratory Tests, ed 9. FA Davis, Philadelphia, 1983, p 195.
2. Pittiglio, DH, Baldwin, JA, Sohmer, PR: Modern Blood Banking and Transfusion Practices. FA Davis, Philadelphia, 1983, pp 90–93.
3. Widmann, op cit, p 195.
4. Pittiglio et al, op cit, p 91.
5. Widmann, op cit, p 196.
6. Ibid, p 198.
7. Pittiglio et al, op cit, pp 106–113.
8. Ibid, p 107.
9. Widmann, op cit, p 198.
10. Pittiglio, et al, op cit, pp 124–125.
11. Widmann, op cit, pp 198–200.
12. Pittiglio et al, op cit, p 139.
13. Widmann, op cit, p 201.
14. Ibid, p 204.
15. Pittiglio et al, op cit, pp 81–83.
16. Ibid.
17. Ibid, p 82.
18. Widmann, op cit, pp 205–206.

19. *Ibid*, p 207.
20. *Ibid*, pp 206–207.
21. Pittiglio et al, *op cit*, p 82.
22. *Ibid*, p 229.
23. *Ibid*, pp 226–232.

BIBLIOGRAPHY

Barrett, JT: Textbook of Immunology, ed 3. CV Mosby, St Louis, 1978.
Beare, PG, Rahr, VA, and Ronshausen, CA: Nursing Implications of Diagnostic Tests, ed 2. JB Lippincott, Philadelphia, 1985.
Bio-Science Handbook, ed 12. Bio-Science Laboratories, Van Nuys, CA, 1977.
Braunstein, H: Outlines of Pathology. CV Mosby, St Louis, 1982.
Byrne, CJ, Saxton, DF, Pelikan, PK, and Nugent, PM: Laboratory Tests: Implications for Nursing Care, ed 2. Addison-Wesley, Menlo Park, CA, 1986.
Fischbach, FT: A Manual of Laboratory Diagnostic Tests, ed 3. JB Lippincott, Philadelphia, 1988.
Frohlich, ED: Pathophysiology: Altered Regulatory Mechanisms in Disease. JB Lippincott, Philadelphia, 1972.
Groer, ME, and Shekleton, ME: Basic Pathophysiology: A Conceptual Approach, ed 2. CV Mosby, St Louis, 1983.
Kee, JL: Laboratory and Diagnostic Tests with Nursing Implications, ed 2. Appleton & Lange, Norwalk, CT, 1987.
Luckmann, J and Sorensen, KC: Medical-Surgical Nursing: A Psychophysiologic Approach, ed 3. WB Saunders, Philadelphia, 1987.
Malseed, R: Pharmacology: Drug Therapy and Nursing Considerations, ed 2. JB Lippincott, Philadelphia, 1985.
Mathewson, MK: Pharmacotherapeutics: A Nursing Process Approach. FA Davis, Philadelphia, 1986.
Nurse's Reference Library: Diagnostics, ed 2. Springhouse Corporation, Springhouse, PA, 1986.
Pagana, KD and Pagana, TJ: Diagnostic Testing and Nursing Implications: A Case Study Approach, ed 2. CV Mosby, St Louis, 1986.
Selkurt, EE: Basic Physiology for the Health Sciences. Little, Brown, Boston, 1975.
Tilkian, SM, Conover, MB, and Tilkian, AG: Clinical Implications of Laboratory Tests, ed 4. CV Mosby, St. Louis, 1987.
Wallach, J: Interpretation of Diagnostic Tests, ed 4. Little, Brown & Co, Boston, 1986.
Widmann, FK: Pathobiology: How Diseases Happen, Little, Brown & Co, Boston, 1978.

5

BLOOD
CHEMISTRY

TESTS COVERED

First number, background information; second number, clinical applications data

INTRODUCTION

The blood transports innumerable substances that participate in and reflect ongoing metabolic processes. Relatively few of these substances are routinely measured. Some materials are analyzed to provide information about specific organs and processes; other substances reflect the summed effects of numerous metabolic events.[1] "Chemistry" includes measurement of glucose, proteins, lipids, enzymes, electrolytes, hormones, vitamins, toxins, and other substances that may indicate derangement of normal physiological processes. In recent years, the diagnosis of various disorders associated with abnormal blood chemistries has become more rapid and accurate with the use of automated analyzers that can measure multiple chemistry components in a single blood sample.

CARBOHYDRATES

Background Information

The body acquires most of its energy from oxidative metabolism of glucose. Glucose, a simple six-carbon sugar, enters the diet as part of the sugars sucrose, lactose, and maltose, and as the major constituent of the complex polysaccharides called dietary starch. Complete oxidation of glucose yields carbon dioxide (CO_2), water, and energy that is stored as adenosine triphosphate (ATP).

If glucose is not immediately metabolized, it can be stored in the liver or muscle as glycogen. Unused glucose also may be converted by the liver into fatty acids, which are stored as triglycerides, or into amino acids, which can be used for protein synthesis. The liver is pivotal in distributing glucose as needed for immediate fuel or as indicated for storage or for structural purposes. If available glucose or glycogen is insufficient for energy needs, the liver can synthesize glucose from fatty acids or even from protein-derived amino acids.[2]

Glucose fuels most cell and tissue functions. Thus, adequate glucose is a critical requirement for homeostasis. Many cells can derive some energy from burning fatty acids, but this energy pathway is less efficient than burning glucose and generates acid metabolites (e.g., ketones) that are harmful if they accumulate in the body. Many hormones (Table 5–1) participate in maintaining blood glucose levels in steady-state conditions or in response to stress. Measuring blood glucose indicates whether the regulation is successful. Pronounced departure from normal, either too high or too low, indicates abnormal homeo-

TABLE 5–1. Hormones That Influence Blood Glucose Levels

Hormone	Tissue of Origin	Metabolic Effect	Effect on Blood Glucose
Insulin	Pancreatic β cells	1. Enhances entry of glucose into cells 2. Enhances storage of glucose as glycogen, or conversion to fatty acids 3. Enhances synthesis of proteins and fatty acids 4. Suppresses breakdown of protein into amino acids, of adipose tissue into free fatty acids	Lowers
Somatostatin	Pancreatic D cells	1. Suppresses glucagon release from α cells (acts locally) 2. Suppresses release of insulin, pituitary tropic hormones, gastrin, and secretin	Lowers
Glucagon	Pancreatic α cells	1. Enhances release of glucose from glycogen 2. Enhances synthesis of glucose from amino acids or fatty acids	Raises
Epinephrine	Adrenal medulla	1. Enhances release of glucose from glycogen 2. Enhances release of fatty acids from adipose tissue	Raises
Cortisol	Adrenal cortex	1. Enhances synthesis of glucose from amino acids or fatty acids 2. Antagonizes insulin	Raises
ACTH	Anterior pituitary	1. Enhances release of cortisol 2. Enhances release of fatty acids from adipose tissue	Raises
Growth hormone	Anterior pituitary	1. Antagonizes insulin	Raises
Thyroxine	Thyroid	1. Enhances release of glucose from glycogen 2. Enhances absorption of sugars from intestine	Raises

From Widmann, FK: Clinical Interpretation of Laboratory Tests, ed 9. FA Davis, Philadelphia, 1983, p 239, with permission.

stasis and should initiate a search for the etiology.[3] The numerous causes of abnormal blood glucose levels are summarized in Table 5–2.

Two major methods are used to measure blood glucose—chemical and enzymatic. Chemical methods employ the nonspecific reducing properties of the glucose molecule. In enzymatic methods, glucose oxidase reacts with its specific substrate, glucose, liberating hydrogen peroxide whose effects are then measured. Values are 5 to 15 mg/dl higher for the reducing (chemical) methods than for enzymatic techniques because blood contains other reducing substances in addition to glucose. Urea, for example, can contribute up to 10 mg/dl in normal serum and even more when uremia exists. Several different indicator systems are used for automated enzymatic methods, yielding somewhat different normal values.[4]

It should also be noted that in the past, blood glucose values were given in

TABLE 5–2. **Causes of Altered Blood Glucose Levels**

Causes of Hyperglycemia	Causes of Hypoglycemia
Persistent	
Diabetes mellitus	Insulinoma
Hemochromatosis	Addison's disease
Cushing's syndrome	Hypopituitarism
Hyperthyroidism	Galactosemia
Acromegaly, gigantism	Ectopic insulin production from
Obesity	tumors (adrenal carcinoma,
Chronic pancreatitis	retroperitoneal sarcomas,
Pancreatic adenoma	pleural fibrous
	mesotheliomas)
	Starvation
Transient	
Pheochromocytoma	Malabsorption syndrome
Pregnancy (gestational diabetes)	Postgastrectomy "dumping syndrome"
Severe liver disease	Acute alcohol ingestion
Acute stress reaction	Severe liver disease
Shock, trauma	Severe glycogen storage diseases
Convuslions, eclampsia	Stress-related catecholamine excess
	("functional" hypoglycemia)
	Hereditary fructose intolerance
	Myxedema
Drugs	
Glucagon	Salicylates
Adrenal corticosteroids	Antituberculosis agents
Oral contraceptives	Sulfonylureas
Estrogens	Sulfonamides
Thyroid hormones	Insulin
Anabolic steroids	Ethanol
Thiazide diuretics	Clofibrate
Loop diuretics	MAO inhibitors
Propranolol	
Antipsychotic drugs	
Hydantoins	
Clonidine	
Dextrothyroxine	
Niacin	

terms of whole blood. Today, most laboratories measure serum or plasma glucose levels. Because of its higher water content, serum contains more dissolved glucose and the resultant values are 1.15 times higher than those for whole blood. Serum or plasma should be separated promptly because red and white blood cells continue to metabolize glucose. In blood with very high white cell levels, excessive glycolysis may actually lower glucose results. Arterial, capillary, and venous blood samples have comparable glucose levels in a fasting individual. After meals, venous levels are lower than those in arterial or capillary blood.[5]

BLOOD GLUCOSE (CLINICAL APPLICATIONS DATA, p. 136)

Blood glucose (serum glucose, plasma glucose) is measured in a variety of situations. In the fasting state, the serum glucose level gives the best indication of overall glucose homeostasis.[6] Fasting blood glucose (fasting blood sugar, FBS) levels greater than 140 to 150 mg/dl on two or more occasions may be considered diagnostic of diabetes mellitus if other possible causes of hyperglycemia are eliminated as sources of the elevation (see Table 5–2, p. 133). Randomly drawn (i.e., nonfasting) serum glucose levels of greater than 200 mg/dl also may be pathognomonic of diabetes mellitus.[7]

Blood glucose levels also may be measured at regular intervals throughout the day to monitor responses to diet and medications in those persons diagnosed with abnormalities of glucose metabolism. Such monitoring may be done in a hospital setting or in the home with kits specially designed for self-monitoring of blood glucose. Serial blood glucose levels also are used to determine insulin requirements in clients with uncontrolled diabetes mellitus and for individuals receiving total parenteral or enteral nutritional support.

In addition to situations characterized by actual or potential elevations in blood sugar, glucose levels are evaluated in individuals suspected or known to have hypoglycemia. A fasting blood sugar as low as 50 mg/dl in men or 35 mg/dl in women is diagnostic of abnormal hypoglycemia.[8]

TWO-HOUR POSTPRANDIAL BLOOD GLUCOSE (CLINICAL APPLICATIONS DATA, p. 138)

The 2-hour postprandial blood glucose (postprandial blood sugar, PPBS) reflects the metabolic response to a carbohydrate challenge.[9] In normal individuals, the blood sugar returns to the fasting level within 2 hours. Elevated levels, expecially if greater than 200 mg/dl, may indicate diabetes mellitus or other impairment of glucose metabolism that may result in hyperglycemia.

In contrast, postprandial hypoglycemia appears to result from delayed or exaggerated response to the insulin secreted in relation to dietary blood sugar rise. It may occur as an early event in individuals with non–insulin-dependent diabetes mellitus (NIDDM, type II diabetes mellitus) or due to gastrointestinal malfunction. Frequently, no cause is demonstrated and the hypoglycemia is considered "functional." Postprandial hypoglycemia differs from fasting hypoglycemia (i.e., hypoglycemia that occurs after 10 or more hours without food) in that the latter nearly always has pathological significance. It results from either overproduction of insulin or undermobilization of glucose and is most commonly seen in clients with tumors of the pancreatic beta cells (insulinoma), liver disease, and chronic alcohol ingestion.[10]

The 2-hour postprandial blood glucose is usually performed in the morning, 2 hours after the client has eaten a breakfast containing at least 100 g of carbohydrate. Insulin and other medications are administered as usual. Thus, the postprandial blood glucose is more convenient for nonhospitalized clients because meals and medications are not delayed by travel to the laboratory or other setting where the sample will be obtained.

The test is also simpler to perform than the oral glucose tolerance test (see next section), and is largely replacing that test whenever diabetes mellitus is suspected.

GLUCOSE TOLERANCE TESTS

Glucose tolerance tests (GTTs) are used to evaluate the response to a carbohydrate challenge throughout a 3- to 5-hour period. When a glucose load is presented, the normal individual's blood insulin level will rise in response to it, with peak levels occurring 30 to 60 minutes after the carbohydrate challenge. Blood glucose levels, although elevated immediately after the carbohydrate challenge, will return to normal fasting levels 2 to 3 hours later. For individuals in whom abnormal hypoglycemia or gastrointestinal malabsorption are suspected, the test may be extended to a 5-hour period.[11-13]

Several methods may be used to perform a glucose tolerance test. The oral, intravenous and cortisone glucose tolerance tests are discussed in this section. Tolerance tests also may be done for pentose, lactose, galactose, and D-xylose.

Oral Glucose Tolerance Test (Clinical Applications Data, p. 139)

The oral glucose tolerance test (OGTT) is used for individuals who are able to eat and who are not known to have problems with gastrointestinal malabsorption. The client should be in a normal nutritional state and should be capable of normal physical activity (i.e., not immobilized or on bed rest), since carbohydrate depletion and inactivity may impair glucose tolerance. In addition, drugs which affect blood glucose levels (see Table 5–2, p. 133) should not be taken for several days prior to the test. Because oral glucose tolerance testing is affected by so many variables, the results are subject to many different diagnostic interpretations.[14]

The oral glucose tolerance test may be performed using blood samples only or with urine samples as well. The urine is normally negative for sugar throughout the test; that is, since the average renal threshold for glucose is 180 mg/dl, the plasma glucose level must be approximately 180 mg/dl before sugar appears in the urine. Renal threshold levels vary, however, and urine testing during an OGTT may show how much glucose the individual spills, if any, at various blood glucose levels. As long as renal threshold is not surpassed by blood glucose levels, all of the glucose presented to the kidneys is reabsorbed from the glomerular filtrate by the renal tubules, provided that renal function is normal.

It should be noted that persons with fasting blood sugars of greater than 150 mg/dl or postprandial blood glucose levels of greater than 200 mg/dl should not receive the glucose load required for this test.

Intravenous Glucose Tolerance Test (Clinical Applications Data, p. 141)

The intravenous glucose tolerance test (IVGTT) is essentially the same as the OGTT, except that the carbohydrate challenge is administered intravenously instead of orally. Since the results are somewhat difficult to interpret, the IVGTT is used only in certain clinical situations or for research purposes.

Cortisone Glucose Tolerance Test (Clinical Applications Data, p. 142)

The cortisone glucose tolerance test combines administration of a carbohydrate challenge with a cortisone challenge. Cortisone enhances the synthesis of glucose from amino acids and fatty acids (gluconeogenesis) and, when administered with a glucose load, may produce an abnormal GTT that would not otherwise be evident. The cortisone GTT is used only in certain clinical situations and for research purposes.

GLYCOSYLATED HEMOGLOBIN (CLINICAL APPLICATIONS DATA, p. 142)

Throughout the red blood cell's life span, the hemoglobin molecule incorporates glucose onto its beta chain. Glycosylation is irreversible and occurs at a stable rate. The amount of glucose permanently bound to hemoglobin depends on the blood sugar level. Thus, the level of glycosylated hemoglobin, designated Hgb A_{1c}, reflects the average blood sugar over a period of several weeks.

The test is used to evaluate the overall adequacy of diabetic control and provides information that may be missed by individual blood and urine glucose tests. Insulin-dependent diabetics, for example, may have undetected periods of hyperglycemia alternating with postinsulin periods of normoglycemia or even hypoglycemia. High Hbg A_{1c} levels reflect inadequate diabetic control in the preceding 3 to 5 weeks. After normoglycemic levels are stabilized, Hgb A_{1c} levels return to normal in about 3 weeks.[15]

In addition to providing a more accurate assessment of overall blood glucose control, the test is more convenient for diabetic clients because it is performed only every 5 to 6 weeks and because there are no dietary or medication restrictions prior to the test.

TOLBUTAMIDE TOLERANCE TEST (CLINICAL APPLICATIONS DATA, p. 143)

Tolbutamide (Orinase) is a hypoglycemia agent that produces hypoglycemia by stimulating the beta cells of the pancreas to secrete and release insulin. An intravenous infusion of tolbutamide raises the serum insulin and causes a rapid decrease in the blood glucose level. Thus, the test demonstrates the pancreatic beta cell response to drug-induced stimulation. It should be noted that the test may be performed with glucagon or leucine instead of tolbutamide for clients who are sensitive to sulfonylureas or sulfonamides.

Clinical Applications Data

BLOOD GLUCOSE (BACKGROUND INFORMATION, p. 134)
Reference Values

	Children	Adults
Whole Blood	50 to 90 mg/dl	60 to 100 mg/dl
Serum/Plasma	60 to 105 mg/dl	70 to 110 mg/dl

Values may vary depending on the laboratory method used (see pp. 133 to 134).

Interfering Factors

- Elevated urea levels and uremia may lead to falsely elevated levels
- Extremely elevated white blood counts may lead to falsely decreased values
- Failure to follow dietary restrictions prior to a fasting blood glucose may lead to falsely elevated values
- Administration of insulin or oral hypoglycemic agents within 8 hours of a fasting blood glucose may lead to falsely decreased values

Indications/Purposes for Blood Glucose

- Routine screening for diabetes mellitus
  - ☐ Fasting blood glucose levels greater than 140 to 150 mg/dl on two or more occasions may be considered diagnostic of diabetes mellitus if other possible causes of hyperglycemia are eliminated as sources of elevation (see Table 5–2, p. 133)
  - ☐ Random (nonfasting) blood glucose levels of greater than 200 mg/dl may be pathognomonic of diabetes mellitus
- Clinical symptoms of hypoglycemia or hyperglycemia
- Known or suspected disorder associated with abnormal glucose metabolism (see Table 5–2, p. 133)
- Identification of abnormal hypoglycemia as indicated by a fasting blood sugar as low as 50 mg/dl in men or 35 mg/dl in women
- Monitoring response to therapy for abnormal glucose metabolism
- Determination of insulin requirements (i.e., "insulin coverage")
- Monitoring metabolic response to drugs known to alter blood glucose levels (see Table 5–2, p. 133)
- Monitoring metabolic response to parenteral or enteral nutritional support to determine insulin requirements

Client Preparation

Client preparation is essentially the same as that for any study involving the collection of a peripheral blood sample (see Appendix I). If a fasting sample is to be drawn, food, insulin, and/or oral hypoglycemia agents should be withheld for approximately 8 hours prior to the test (i.e., the client usually takes only water from midnight until the sample is drawn in the morning). For home glucose monitoring, the client should be instructed in correct use of the testing equipment and in the method used to obtain the blood sample.

The Procedure

A venipuncture is performed and the sample is obtained in either a gray- or a red-topped tube depending upon the laboratory performing the test. The sample should be handled gently to avoid hemolysis and transported promptly to the laboratory.

A capillary sample may be obtained in infants and children, as well as in adults for whom venipuncture may not be feasible. Capillary samples also are used for self-monitoring of blood glucose.

Aftercare and Nursing Observations

Care and assessment following the procedure are the same as that for any study involving collection of a peripheral blood sample. Food and medications withheld prior to the test should be resumed after the sample is drawn.

Clients who are fasting prior to the test, especially those who are insulin dependent, should be observed for signs of hypoglycemia.

Two-Hour Postprandial Blood Glucose (Background Information, p. 134)

Reference Values

	Children	Adults	Elderly
Blood	120 mg/dl	Up to 120 mg/dl	Up to 140 mg/dl
Serum/Plasma	150 mg/dl	Up to 140 mg/dl	Up to 160 mg/dl

Values may vary depending on the laboratory method used.

With advancing age, the speed of glucose clearance declines. Two-hour levels in persons who do not have diabetes and those with negative family histories may increase an average of 6 mg/dl for each decade over age 30.[16]

Interfering Factors

- Failure to follow dietary instructions may alter test results
- Smoking and drinking coffee during the 2-hour test period may lead to falsely elevated values
- Strenuous exercise during the 2-hour test period may lead to falsely decreased values

Indications/Purposes for Two-Hour Postprandial Blood Glucose

- Abnormal fasting blood sugar
- Routine screening for diabetes mellitus, as indicated by a blood glucose level greater than the fasting level and especially by a 2-hour level greater than 200 mg/ml
- Identification of postprandial hypoglycemia and differentiation of this state from fasting hypoglycemia, with fasting hypoglycemia almost always indicative of a pathological state (see p. 134)
- Known or suspected disorder associated with abnormal glucose metabolism (see Table 5–2, p. 133)
- Monitoring metabolic response to drugs known to alter blood glucose levels (see Table 5–2, p. 133)

Client Preparation

General client preparation is the same as that for any test involving collection of a peripheral blood sample. Specific preparation includes ingesting a meal (usually breakfast) containing at least 100 g of carbohydrate 2 hours prior to the test. The American Diabetes Association recommends a 300-g carbohydrate diet for 2 to 3 days prior to the test, but this is not universally followed.

The time of the last meal prior to the test should be noted. The client should then fast from food and avoid coffee, smoking, and strenuous exercise until the sample is obtained. Although medications are not withheld for this test, those taken should be noted.

The Procedure

Two hours after the carbohydrate challenge is ingested, a venipuncture is performed and the sample is collected in either a gray- or a red-topped tube depending upon the laboratory performing the test. A capillary sample may be obtained in children and in adults for whom venipuncture may not be feasible. Capillary samples also are used when the test is performed for mass screenings. It should be noted that in some instances a fasting blood sugar level may be obtained prior to the carbohydrate challenge.

Aftercare and Nursing Observations

Care and assessment following the procedure are the same as for any study involving collection of a peripheral blood sample. Usual diet and activities may be resumed.

ORAL GLUCOSE TOLERANCE TEST (BACKGROUND INFORMATION, p. 135)
Reference Values

	Time after Carbohydrate Challenge (hr)			
	½	1	2	3
Whole Blood Glucose	<150 mg/dl	<160 mg/dl	<115 mg/dl	Same as fasting
Serum/Plasma Glucose	<160 mg/dl	<170 mg/dl	<125 mg/dl	Same as fasting
Urine Glucose		Negative throughout test		

Values for children over age 6 are the same as those for adults. Values for elderly individuals are 10 to 30 mg/dl higher at each interval due to the age-related decline in glucose clearance.

Interfering Factors

■ Failure to ingest a diet with sufficient carbohydrate content (e.g., 150 g per day) for at least 3 days prior to the test may result in falsely decreased values
■ Impaired physical activity may lead to falsely increased values
■ Excessive physical activity prior to or during the test may lead to falsely decreased values
■ Smoking prior to or during the test may lead to falsely increased values
■ Ingestion of drugs known to alter blood glucose levels may lead to falsely increased or decreased values (see Table 5–2, p. 133)

Indications/Purposes for Oral Glucose Tolerance Test

■ Abnormal fasting or postprandial blood glucose levels which are not clearly indicative of diabetes mellitus
■ Identification of impaired glucose metabolism without overt diabetes mellitus, which is characterized by a modest elevation in blood glucose after 2 hours and a normal level after 3 hours
■ Evaluation of glucose metabolism in women of childbearing age—especially those are are pregnant—with a history of previous fetal loss, birth of babies weighing 9 pounds or more, or positive family history for diabetes mellitus
■ Support for diagnosing hyperthyroidism and alcoholic liver disease, which

are characterized by a sharp rise in blood glucose followed by a decline to subnormal levels
■ Identification of true postprandial hypoglycemia (5-hour GTT) due to excessive insulin response to a glucose load
■ Support for diagnosing gastrointestinal malabsorption, which is characterized by peak glucose levels lower than what is normally expected and hypoglycemia in the latter hours of the test (5-hour GTT)
■ Identification of abnormal renal tubular function, if glycosuria occurs without hyperglycemia

---

Nursing Alert

■ Individuals with fasting blood sugars of greater than 150 mg/dl or postprandial blood glucose levels greater than 200 mg/dl should not receive the glucose load required for this test
■ If the client vomits the oral glucose preparation, notify the laboratory and physician immediately, and implement any treatment ordered
■ If signs and symptoms of hypoglycemia are observed or reported, obtain a blood sugar immediately, and administer orange juice with 1 teaspoon of sugar or other beverage containing sugar; notify the physician that the test has been terminated

---

Client Preparation

Client Teaching. Explain to the client:

■ the purpose of the test
■ the general procedure for the test, including administration of the glucose and the frequency of collection of blood and urine samples
■ the importance of eating a diet containing at least 150 g carbohydrate per day for 3 days prior to the test (provide sample menus or lists of foods which demonstrate how this may be accomplished)
■ which medications, if any, are to be withheld prior to the test
■ that no food may be eaten after midnight before the test, but that water is not restricted
■ the importance of not smoking or performing strenuous exercise after midnight before the test and until the test is completed
■ symptoms of hypoglycemia and the necessity of reporting such symptoms immediately

Encourage questions and verbalization of concerns about the procedure.

Physical Preparation

■ To the extent possible, ensure that the dietary, exercise, medication, and smoking restrictions are followed
■ Provide containers for collection of urine samples

The Procedure

A venipuncture is performed and a sample is obtained for a fasting blood sugar. At the same time, a second-voided (double-voided) urine sample is collected and tested for glucose. To collect a second-voided specimen, have the client void a half-hour before the required specimen is due. Discard this urine, then collect the second-voided specimen at the designated time.

The glucose load is administered orally. This is a calculated dose, either 1.75 g/kg body weight or 50 g/m² body surface. Several commercial preparations are available that are flavored for palatability. Blood and urine samples are obtained at half-hour, 1-hour, 2-hour, and 3-hour intervals. The second-voided urine specimen is necessary only at the beginning of the test. The client should drink one glass of water each time a urine sample is collected to ensure adequate urinary output for remaining specimens. If the test is extended to 5 hours, additional samples are collected at 4- and 5-hour intervals.

It should be noted that the test may be performed with blood samples only, depending on the desired information to be obtained from the test.

Aftercare and Nursing Observations

Care and assessment following the procedure are essentially the same as that for any test involving the collection of peripheral blood samples. Food and medications withheld prior to the test, as well as usual activities, should be resumed upon its completion.

INTRAVENOUS GLUCOSE TOLERANCE TEST (BACKGROUND INFORMATION, p. 135)

Reference Values

The reference values are the same as those for the OGTT, except that the blood glucose level at the half-hour interval may be 300 to 400 mg/dl due to the direct intravenous administration of the glucose load.

Interfering Factors

■ Those factors that may alter results of an oral glucose tolerance test may also alter the results of an intravenous glucose tolerance test (see p. 139)
■ Infusions of total parenteral nutrition (TPN, hyperalimentation) during the test may lead to falsely elevated values; alternative solutions with less glucose should be infused for at least 3 hours prior to and during the test

Indications/Purposes for Intravenous Glucose Tolerance Test

■ Inability to take or tolerate oral glucose preparations used for the OGTT
■ Suspected gastrointestinal malabsorption problems that interfere with accurate performance of the OGTT
■ Evaluation of blood glucose control without the effects of gastrin, secretin, cholecystokinin, and gastric inhibitory peptide, all of which stimulate insulin production following oral ingestion of glucose

Client Preparation

Client preparation is essentially the same as that for the OGTT. If the person is receiving total parenteral nutrition (TPN, hyperalimentation), an alternative solution with less glucose should be prescribed and infused for at least 3 hours prior to and during the test.

The Procedure

The procedure is essentially the same as that for the OGTT except that an intermittent venous access device (e.g., heparin lock) may be inserted to administer the glucose load and to obtain blood samples. Existing intravenous lines

also may be used to administer the carbohydrate challenge, which is usually 50 percent glucose with the amount to be given determined by the client's weight or body surface.

Aftercare and Nursing Observations

Care and assessment following the procedure are the same as that for the OGTT. If an intermittent venous access device was inserted for the procedure, it should be removed following completion of the test and a pressure bandage applied to the site. Food and medications withheld prior to the test, as well as usual activities, should be resumed upon its completion. Infusions of total parenteral nutrition also should be resumed as ordered.

CORTISONE GLUCOSE TOLERANCE TEST (BACKGROUND INFORMATION, p. 136)

Reference Values

The reference values are similar to those for the OGTT except that the blood glucose level at the 2-hour interval may be 20 mg/dl higher than the client's fasting level.

Indications/Purposes for Cortisone Glucose Tolerance Test

■ Inconclusive results of OGTT when prediabetes or "borderline" diabetes is suspected, with a 2-hour level of greater than 165 mg/dl considered indicative of diabetes

Interfering Factors

■ Those factors that may alter results of an oral glucose tolerance test may also alter the results of a cortisone glucose tolerance test (see p. 139)
■ Failure to administer or take the oral cortisone as prescribed for the test will alter results

Client Preparation

Client preparation is essentially the same as that for OGTT. In addition, the client should be instructed on the purpose and administration of the oral cortisone acetate.

The Procedure

The procedure is the same as that for the OGTT except that cortisone acetate is administered orally 8 hours and again 2 hours before the standard GTT is begun.

Aftercare and Nursing Observations

Care and assessment following the procedure are the same as for the OGTT.

GLYCOSYLATED HEMOGLOBIN (BACKGROUND INFORMATION, p. 136)

Reference Values

Hgb A_{1c} is 3 to 6 percent of hemoglobin.

Interfering Factors

■ Individuals with hemolytic anemia and high levels of young red blood cells may have spuriously low levels

■ Individuals with elevated hemoglobin levels or on heparin therapy may have falsely elevated levels

Indications/Purposes for Glycosylated Hemoglobin

■ Monitoring overall blood glucose control in clients with known diabetes, as the test aids in assessing blood glucose levels over a period of several weeks and provides data that may be missed by random blood or urine glucose tests

☐ With prolonged hyperglycemia, levels of Hbg A_{1c} may rise to as high as 18 to 20 percent

☐ After normoglycemic levels are stabilized, Hgb A_{1c} levels return to normal in about 3 weeks

■ Monitoring adequacy of insulin dosage for blood glucose control, especially that administered by automatic insulin pumps

■ Evaluating the diabetic client's degree of compliance with the prescribed therapeutic regimen, as fasting or adjusting medications shortly prior to the test will not significantly alter results

Client Preparation

Client preparation is the same as that for any test involving collection of a peripheral blood sample (see Appendix I). The client should be informed that fasting or adjusting medications for diabetes shortly prior to the test will not significantly alter results.

The Procedure

A venipuncture is performed and the sample obtained in a lavender-topped tube. The sample must be mixed adequately with the anticoagulant contained in the tube and transported promptly to the laboratory.

Aftercare and Nursing Observations

Care and assessment following the procedure are the same as for any study involving collection of a peripheral blood sample.

TOLBUTAMIDE TOLERANCE TEST (Background Information, p. 136)

Reference Values

A decrease in serum glucose levels is evident within 5 to 10 minutes of administration of the drug. The lowest glucose levels occur in about 20 to 30 minutes and are generally about half of the client's usual fasting level. The glucose level returns to pretest values in 1 to 3 hours.

Interfering Factors

■ Those factors that may alter results of an oral glucose tolerance test may also alter the results of a tolbutamide tolerance test (see p. 139)

Indications/Purposes for Tolbutamide Tolerance Test

■ Evaluation of fasting or postprandial hypoglycemia by assessing the degree of pancreatic beta cell response to drug-induced stimulation

■ Suspected insulinoma (insulin-producing tumor of the pancreatic beta cells) as indicated by glucose levels that drop markedly in response to tolbutamide and take 3 or more hours to return to normal levels

■ Suspected prediabetic state which may be characterized by excessive insulin release, as indicated by glucose levels that are lower than expected but that follow the overall pattern of a normal response to the test

---

Nursing Alert

■ Because of the expected drop in blood sugar levels, the test should be performed with extreme caution—if at all—on individuals with fasting blood sugars of 50 mg/dl or less

■ If the client is allergic to sulfonylureas or sulfonamides, the test should be performed using glucagon or leucine instead of tolbutamide

---

Client Preparation

Client preparation is essentially the same as that for an oral glucose tolerance test (see p. 140). The individual should be informed that venous access will be established with either a continuous infusion or intermittent device and that a medication which lowers blood sugar will be administered. The client should be questioned regarding allergies to sulfonylureas or sulfonamides.

Clients with a history of abnormal hypoglycemia will need to be reassured that they will be monitored closely during the test.

The Procedure

Venous access is established and a sample is obtained for a fasting blood sugar (FBS). The intravenous catheter is then connected to an intermittent device (e.g., heparin lock) or to a continuous intravenous infusion of normal saline at a "keep vein open" (KVO) rate. Tolbutamide 1.0 g mixed in 20 ml sterile water is administered intravenously. Blood glucose samples are obtained via the intravenous catheter at quarter-, half-, three-quarter-, 1-, 1½-, 2-, and 3-hour intervals.

Aftercare

The venous access device is left in place until any danger of hypoglycemia is past. It is then removed and a pressure bandage applied to the site. Food and medications withheld prior to the test, as well as usual activities, should be resumed upon its completion.

Nursing Observations

Pretest

■ Assess the client's level of anxiety about the procedure

■ Inquire about possible allergies to sulfonylureas or sulfonamides

During the Test

■ Observe the client closely for signs and symptoms of hypoglycemia. If it occurs, obtain a stat fasting blood sugar, notify the physician, and initiate an intravenous infusion of 5 percent glucose and water, if ordered.

■ Note any signs or symptoms of sensitivity reaction to tolbutamide. If it occurs, notify the physician and administer drugs as ordered. Maintain an open intravenous line until there is no further danger of adverse drug reaction.

Post-Test

■ Continue to observe for signs and symptoms of hypoglycemia for 2 hours or more, depending on results of the 3-hour interval blood sugar
■ Assess the venipuncture site for signs of hematoma or phlebitis
■ Observe for adequate intake when foods are resumed

PROTEINS

Background Information

Proteins, also called polypeptides, consist of amino acids linked together by peptide bonds. Although all human proteins are constructed from a mere 20 amino acids, variations in chain length, amino acid sequence, and incorporated constituents combine to make possible an almost infinite number of different protein molecules. All cells manufacture proteins, with different proteins characterizing different cell types. The amino acids necessary for these processes enter the body from dietary sources. These amino acids are rapidly distributed to tissue cells, which promptly incorporate them into proteins.

Three fourths of the body's solid matter is protein and, except for hemoglobin, relatively little circulates in whole blood. The major plasma proteins are albumin, the globulins, and fibrinogen. Fibrinogen evolves into insoluble fibrin when blood coagulates. The fluid that remains after coagulation is called serum. Serum and plasma have the same protein composition except that serum lacks fibrinogen and several other coagulation factors (prothrombin, factor VIII, factor V, and factor XIII).

The proteins in circulating blood transport amino acids from one site to another, providing raw materials for synthesis, degradation, and metabolic interconversion. Circulating proteins also function as buffers in acid-base balance, contribute to the maintenance of colloidal osmotic pressure, and aid in transporting lipids, enzymes, hormones, vitamins, and certain minerals.

Most plasma proteins originate in the liver. Hepatocytes synthesize fibrinogen, albumin, and 60 to 80 percent of the globulins. The remaining globulins are immunoglobulins (antibodies), which are manufactured by the lymphorecticular system. Immunoglobulins are studied as part of the immune system (see Chapter 3), while fibrinogen is usually studied as part of a coagulation work-up (see Chapter 2). The focus of this section is on the major serum proteins (albumin and nonantibody globulins), binding proteins, and protein metabolites.[17]

SERUM PROTEINS (Clinical Applications Data, p. 152)

General assessment of the serum proteins includes measurement of total protein, albumin, globulin, and the albumin/globulin (A/G) ratio. Although these tests are being replaced by serum protein electrophoresis (see Chapter 3, p. 90), they may still be ordered for screening purposes or as components of multitest chemistry profiles, as they provide an overall picture of protein homeostasis.

TABLE 5-3. **Causes of Altered Total Serum Proteins**

Causes of Increased Levels	Causes of Decreased Levels
Kala azar	Renal disease
Dehydration/	Ulcerative colitis
Macroglobulinemias	Water intoxication
Sarcoidosis	Cirrhosis
Drugs	Severe burns
ACTH, corticosteroids	Scleroderma
BSP	Malnutrition
Clofibrate	Hodgkin's disease
Dextran	Hemorrhage
Growth hormone	Drugs
Heparin	Ammonium ion
Insulin	Dextran
X-ray contrast media	Oral contraceptives
Thyroid preparations	Salicylates
Tolbutamide	Pyrazinamide

A number of disorders can cause alterations in serum proteins. Those affecting total protein levels are listed in Table 5-3. Albumin levels show less variation. Except for dehydration, exercise, and effects of certain drugs (e.g., Flaxedil), elevated albumin levels do not occur. Albumin may be decreased in a number of situations which are caused, in general, by (1) decreased hepatic synthesis, (2) excessive renal excretion, (3) increased metabolic degradation, and (4) complex combined disorders. Specific problems associated with hypoalbuminemia are listed in Table 5-4.

Globulin levels show more variation than albumin levels, probably due to the multiple production sites for this protein. Causes of altered globulin levels are listed in Table 5-5 according to the type of globulin affected.

TABLE 5-4. **Causes of Hypoalbuminemia**

Decreased Synthesis
Malnutrition (starvation,
  malabsorption iron deficiency)
Chronic diseases (tuberculosis)
Acute infections (hepatitis, brucellosis)
Chronic liver disease
Collagen disorders (scleroderma, SLE)

Drugs
Tylenol
Imuran
Cytoxan
Heroin
Niacin
Roniacol
Premarin
Estinyl
Enovid
Dextran

Increased Loss
Ascites
Burns (severe)
Nephrotic syndrome
Chronic renal failure

Increased Catabolism
Malignancies (leukemias, advanced tumors)
Trauma

Multifactorial
Cirrhosis
Congestive heart failure
Pregnancy
Toxemia of pregnancy
Diabetes mellitus
Myxedema
Rheumatic fever
Rheumatoid arthritis
Hypocalcemia

TABLE 5–5. Causes of Altered Serum Globulin Levels

Globulin	Causes of Increased Levels	Causes of Decreased Levels
Alpha-1 (α_1)	Pregnancy Malignancies Acute infections Tissue necrosis	Genetic deficiency of alpha-1 antitrypsin
Alpha-2 (α_2)	Acute infections Trauma, burns Advanced malignancies Rheumatic fever Rheumatoid arthritis Acute myocardial infarction Nephrotic syndrome	Hemolytic anemia Severe liver disease
Beta (β)	Hypothyroidism Biliary cirrhosis Nephrotic syndrome Diabetes mellitus Cushing's disease Malignant hypertension	Hypocholesterolemia

Gamma (γ)	Connective tissue diseases (such as systemic lupus erythematosus and rheumatoid arthritis)
	Hodgkin's disease
	Chronic active liver disease
	Drugs
	  Tolinase
	  Tubocurarine
	  Anticonvulsants
		Nephrotic syndrome
		Lymphocytic leukemia
		Lymphosarcoma
		Drugs
		  BCG vaccine
		  Methotrexate

The A/G ratio indicates the balance between total albumin and total globulin and is usually evaluated in relation to the total protein level. A low protein and a reversed A/G ratio (i.e., decreased albumin and elevated globulins) suggests chronic liver disease. A normal total protein with a reversed A/G ratio suggests myeloproliferative disease (e.g., leukemia, Hodgkin's disease) or certain chronic infectious diseases (e.g., tuberculosis, chronic hepatitis).

ALPHA₁-ANTITRYPSIN (Clinical Applications Data, p. 154)

Alpha$_1$-antitrypsin (α-1-AT) is an alpha$_1$-globulin produced by the liver. Its function is inhibition of the proteolytic enzymes trypsin and plasmin, which are released by alveolar macrophages and by bacteria in the lungs. As with many other proteins, the alpha$_1$-antitrypsin molecule has several structural variants. Some of these variant molecules have different electrophoretic mobility and reduced ability to inhibit proteolytic enzymes.

Inherited deficiencies in normal α-1-AT activity are associated with the development, early in life, of lung and liver disorders in which functional tissue is destroyed and replaced with excessive connective tissue. That is, emphysema and cirrhosis may develop in children and young adults who are deficient in α-1-AT, without the usual predisposing factors associated with onset of these disorders. Such deficiencies are seen on serum protein electrophoresis as a flat area where the normal alpha$_1$-globulin hump should be. More detailed physiochemical analysis can demonstrate which variant form is present. Decreased levels of α-1-AT also are seen in nephrotic syndrome and malnutrition.

Persistently elevated levels are associated with chronic inflammatory disorders. Elevated levels also are seen in pregnancy and acute pulmonary infections, as well as with strenuous exercise and stress. Clients taking oral contraceptives also may have elevated levels.

BINDING PROTEINS

Binding proteins are serum proteins that bind substances for transport in the circulation. Those binding proteins discussed in this section are haptoglobin and ceruloplasmin. Transferrin, a beta globulin that binds iron, is discussed in Chapter 1.

Haptoglobin (Clinical Applications Data, p. 154)

Haptoglobin, an alpha$_2$ (α_2) globulin produced in the liver, binds free hemoglobin released by the hemolysis of red blood cells (RBCs) in the bloodstream. Most RBCs are normally removed in the reticuloendothelial system (e.g., liver, spleen) by a process known as extravascular destruction. Approximately 10 percent of red cells are, however, broken down in the circulation (intravascular destruction). This percentage may increase in situations caused by excessive red cell hemolysis (e.g., transfusion reaction, hemolytic anemia).

The free hemoglobin released from intravascular red cell destruction is unstable in plasma and dissociates into components (alpha-beta dimers), which are quickly bound to haptoglobin. Formation of the haptoglobin-hemoglobin complex prevents the renal excretion of plasma hemoglobin and stabilizes the heme-globin bond. The haptoglobin-hemoglobin complex is removed from the circulation by the liver.

There is a limit to the capacity of the haptoglobin-binding mechanism, and a sudden intravascular release of several grams of hemoglobin can exceed binding capacity. Furthermore, because haptoglobin itself is removed from the circulation as a hemoglobin-haptoglobin complex is catabolized by the liver, a decrease in or absence of haptoglobin may be used to indicate increased intravascular red cell hemolysis.

Since haptoglobin is formed in the liver, chronic liver disease with impaired protein synthesis also may result in decreased haptoglobin levels. Although haptoglobin is absent in most newborns, congenital absence of haptoglobin (congenital ahaptoglobinemia) also may occur in a very small percentage of the population.

If haptoglobin is deficient or its binding capacity overwhelmed, unbound hemoglobin dimers are free to be filtered by the renal glomerulus, after which they are reabsorbed by the renal tubules and converted into hemosiderin (a storage form of iron). If renal tubular uptake capacity is exceeded, either free hemoglobin or methemoglobin (a type of hemoglobin with iron in the ferric, instead of the ferrous, form) is excreted in the urine. It should be noted that reabsorption of free hemoglobin may damage the renal tubules due to excessive deposition of hemosiderin.[18]

Elevated haptoglobin levels are seen in inflammatory diseases (e.g., ulcerative colitis, arthritis, pyelonephritis) and in disorders involving tissue destruction (e.g., malignancies, burns, acute myocardial infarction). Steroid therapy may also elevate haptoglobin levels. Elevated levels are not of major clinical significance except to indicate that additional testing may be necessary to determine the source of the elevation.

TABLE 5-6. Causes of Altered Levels of Ceruloplasmin

Causes of Increased Levels	Causes of Decreased Levels
Acute infections	Wilson's disease
Hepatitis	Malabsorption syndromes
Hodgkin's disease	Long-term total parenteral nutrition
Hyperthyroidism	Menkes' kinky hair syndrome
Pregnancy	Nephrosis
Malignancies of bone, lung, stomach	Severe liver disease
Myocardial infarction	Early infancy
Rheumatoid arthritis	
Drugs	
Oral contraceptives	
Estrogens	
Methadone	
Dilantin	

Ceruloplasmin (Cp) (Clinical Applications Data, p. 155)

Ceruloplasmin (Cp) is an alpha$_2$ (α_2) globulin that binds copper for transport within the circulation after it is absorbed from the gastrointestinal tract. Among the disorders associated with abnormal ceruloplasmin levels is Wilson's disease (hepatolenticular degeneration), an inherited disorder characterized by excessive absorption of copper from the gastrointestinal tract, decreased ceruloplasmin, and deposition of copper in the liver, brain, corneas (Kayser-Fleischer rings), and kidneys. In addition to low ceruloplasmin levels, serum copper levels are decreased owing to excessive excretion of unbound copper in the kidneys and deposition of copper in the body tissues. The disorder manifests during the first three decades of life and is fatal unless treatment is instituted.

Other causes of abnormal ceruloplasmin levels are listed in Table 5-6. It should be noted that low ceruloplasmin levels also are associated with malabsorption syndromes and long-term administration of total parenteral nutrition (hyperalimentation) and are related to the hypocupremia that occurs because of decreased copper absorption from the gastrointestinal tract.

PROTEIN METABOLITES

Most nitrogen in the blood resides in proteins, and the amount of nitrogen contained in proteins is high in relation to amino acid content. When proteins are metabolized, the nitrogen-containing components are removed from the amino acids, a process known as deamination. The resulting protein metabolites include urea, creatinine, ammonia, creatine, and uric acid. Levels of these nonprotein nitrogenous compounds reflect various aspects of protein balance and metabolism.

Blood Urea Nitrogen (BUN) (Clinical Applications Data, p. 156)

Urea is a nonprotein nitrogenous compound that is formed in the liver from ammonia. Although urea diffuses freely into both extracellular and intracellular fluid, it is ultimately excreted by the kidneys. Blood urea levels reflect the bal-

TABLE 5-7. **Causes of Altered Urea Levels**

Causes of Increased Levels		Causes of Decreased Levels
Congestive heart failure	**Drugs**	Inadequate dietary protein
Shock	Aspirin	Severe liver disease
Hypovolemia	Acetominophen	Water overload
Urinary tract obstruction	Cancer chemotherapeutic	Nephrotic syndrome
Renal diseases	agents	Pregnancy
Starvation	Antibiotics (amphotericin	Amyloidosis
Infection	B, cephalosporins,	Malabsorption syndromes
Myocardial infarction	aminoglycosides)	
Diabetes mellitus	Thiazide diuretics	**Drugs**
Burns	Indomethacin (Indocin)	IV dextrose
GI bleeding	Morphine	Phenothiazines
Advanced pregnancy	Codeine	Thymol
Nephrotoxic agents	Sulfonamides	
Excessive protein ingestion	Methyldopa (Aldomet)	
Malignancies	Propranolol (Inderal)	
Addison's disease	Guanethidine (Ismelin)	
Gout	Pargyline (Eutonyl)	
Pancreatitis	Lithium carbonate	
Tissue necrosis	Dextran	
Advanced age	Sulfonylureas	

ance between production and excretion of urea. Changes in protein intake, fluid balance, liver function, and renal excretion will affect blood urea levels. Specific causes of alterations are listed in Table 5-7.

Blood urea analysis involves measurement of nirogen; the result is expressed as blood urea nitrogen (BUN). Nitrogen contributes 46.7 percent of the total weight of urea. The concentration of urea can be calculated by multiplying the BUN result by 2.14.[19]

Serum Creatinine (Clinical Applications Data, p. 157)

Creatinine is the end product of creatine metabolism. Creatine, although synthesized largely in the liver, resides almost exclusively in skeletal muscle, where it reversibly combines with phosphate to form the energy storage compound phosphocreatine. This reaction (creatine + phosphate $\rightleftarrows$ phosphocreatine) repeats as energy is released and regenerated, but in the process small amounts of creatine are irreversibly converted to creatinine, which serves no useful function and circulates only for transportation to the kidneys. The amount of creatinine generated in an individual is proportional to the mass of skeletal muscle present; level of muscular activity is not a critical determinant.

Daily generation of creatinine remains fairly constant unless crushing injury or degenerative diseases cause massive muscle damage. The kidneys excrete creatinine very efficiently. Levels of blood and urine flow affect creatinine excretion much less than they influence urea excretion because temporary alterations in renal blood flow and glomerular function can be compensated by increased tubular secretion of creatinine. Thus, serum creatinine is a more sensitive indicator of renal function than is the blood urea nitrogen (BUN).[20]

TABLE 5–8. Causes of Altered Blood Ammonia Levels

Causes of Increased Levels	Causes of Decreased Levels
Liver failure, late cirrhosis	Renal failure
GI hemorrhage	Hypertension
Late congestive heart failure	
Azotemia	***Drugs***
Hemolytic disease of the newborn	Arginine (R-Gene)
Chronic obstructive pulmonary disease	Benadryl
Leukemias	Sodium salts
Reye's syndrome	Acidulin
Inborn enzyme deficiency	MAO inhibitors
Excessive protein ingestion	Antibiotics
Alkalosis	achromycin
	Kantrex
Drugs	Neomycin
Acetazolamide (Diamox)	Potassium salts
Ammonium salts	
Barbiturates	
Colistin (Coly-Mycin)	
Diuretics	
Heparin	
Methicillin	
Tetracycline	
Ethanol	
Morphine	
Isoniazid	

Ammonia (Clinical Applications Data, p. 158)

Blood ammonia comes from two sources: (1) deamination of amino acids during protein metabolism; and (2) degradation of proteins by colon bacteria. The liver converts ammonia to urea, generating glutamine as an intermediary. The kidneys then use glutamine as a source for synthesizing ammonia for renal regulation of electrolyte and acid-base balance. Serum ammonia levels have little effect on renal excretion of ammonia.

Circulating blood normally contains very little ammonia because the liver converts ammonia in the portal blood to urea. When liver function is severely compromised, especially in situations when decreased hepatocellular function is combined with impaired portal blood flow, ammonia levels rise. Both elevated serum ammonia and abnormal glutamine metabolism have been implicated as etiological factors in hepatic encephalopathy (hepatic coma).[21] Additional causes of altered serum ammonia levels are listed in Table 5–8.

Serum Creatine (Clinical Applications Data, p. 158)

Creatine is a nitrogen-containing compound found largely in skeletal muscle, where it functions as an energy source. Its use by muscles results in loss proportionate to the muscle mass and level of muscular activity. Measurement of serum creatine reflects this loss, which is fairly constant under normal conditions but increases markedly in situations involving muscle damage (e.g., muscle injury, muscular dystrophies, dermatomyositis). Other causes of elevations include hyperthyroidism, rheumatoid arthritis and testosterone therapy.

TABLE 5–9. Causes of Altered Uric Acid Levels

Causes of Increased Levels		Causes of Decreased Levels
Excessive dietary purines	**_Drugs_**	Fanconi's syndrome
Polycythemia	Alcohol	Wilson's disease
Gout	Aspirin (<2 g/day)	Yellow atrophy of the liver
Psoriasis	Thiazide diuretics	
Type III hyperlipidemia	Diazoxide (Hyperstat)	**_Drugs_**
Chemotherapy,	Epinephrine	Probenecid
radiation therapy for	Edecrin	Sulfinpyrazone
malignancies	Furosemide	Aspirin (>4 g/day)
von Gierke's disease	Phenothiazines	ACTH, corticosteroids
Sickle cell anemia	Dextran	Coumarin
Pernicious anemia	Methyldopa	Estrogens
Acute tissue destruction	Ascorbic acid	Allopurinol
(infection, starvation,	Aminophylline	Acetohexamide
exercise)	Antibiotics (gentamicin)	Dymelor
Eclampsia,	Griseofulvin	Imuran
hypertension	Rifampin	Clofibrate
Hyperparathyroidism	Dyrenium	Cinchophen
		Taractan
Decreased Excretion		Mannitol
Lactic acidosis		Marijuana
Ketoacidosis		
Renal failure		
Congestive heart failure		

Uric Acid (Clinical Applications Data, p. 159)

Uric acid (urate) is the end product of purine metabolism. Purines are important constituents of nucleic acids; purine turnover occurs continuously in the body, producing substantial amounts of uric acid even in the absence of dietary purine (e.g., meats, legumes, yeasts) intake. Most uric acid is synthesized in the liver and excreted by the kidneys. Serum urate levels are affected by the amount of uric acid produced as well as by the efficiency of renal excretion.

Both gout and urate renal calculi (kidney stones) are associated with elevated uric acid levels. Other disorders and drugs associated with altered uric acid levels are listed in Table 5–9.

Clinical Applications Data

SERUM PROTEINS (Background Information, p. 145)

Reference Values

The reference values for total protein, albumin, and globulin vary slightly across the life cycle and are listed below accordingly. Values for gamma globulins are provided for comparison purposes. All values are reported in g/dl.

Age	Total Protein	Albumin	Globulins	Gamma Globulins
Newborn	5.0–7.1	2.5–5.0	1.2–4.0	0.7–0.9
3 months	4.7–7.4	3.0–4.2	1.0–3.3	0.1–0.5
1 year	5.0–7.5	2.7–5.0	2.0–3.8	0.4–1.2
15 years	6.5–8.6	3.2–5.0	2.0–4.0	0.6–1.2
Adults	6.6–7.9	3.3–4.5	2.0–4.2	0.5–1.6

Albumin/Globulin (A/G) Ratio 1.5:1–2.5:1

Although discussed in Chapter 3, the normal values for serum protein electrophoresis are repeated below for reference purposes. Values are reported as percent of total proteins.

Albumin	Globulins				
	Total	Alpha-1	Alpha-2	Beta	Gamma
52–68	32–48	2.4–5.3	6.6–13.5	8.5–14.5	10.7–21.0

Interfering Factors

■ High serum lipid levels may interfere with accurate testing
■ Numerous drugs may alter protein levels (see Tables 5–3 and 5–4, p. 146

Indications/Purposes for Total Protein, Albumin, Globulin, A/G Ratio

■ Routine screening as part of a complete physical examination, with normal results indicating satisfactory overall protein homeostasis
■ Clinical signs of diseases associated with altered serum proteins (see Tables 5–3, 5–4, and 5–5, pp. 146 and 147)
■ Monitoring response to therapy with drugs that may alter serum protein levels

Client Preparation

Client preparation is the same as that for any test involving collection of a peripheral blood sample (see Appendix I). Some laboratories require an 8-hour fast prior to the test, as well as a low-fat diet for several days before the test, since high serum lipid levels may interfere with accurate testing.

The Procedure

A venipuncture is performed and the sample collected in a red-topped tube. The sample should be handled gently and sent promptly to the laboratory.

Aftercare and Nursing Observations

Care and assessment following the procedure are the same as for any study involving collection of a peripheral blood sample. Any foods withheld prior to the test should be resumed.

ALPHA₁-ANTITRYPSIN (Background Information, p. 147)

Reference Values

159–400 mg/dl

Interfering Factors

■ Strenuous exercise, stress, and oral contraceptives may falsely elevate values
■ Failure to follow dietary restrictions prior to the test may alter results

Indications/Purposes for Alpha₁-Antitrypsin

■ Family history of alpha₁-antitrypsin deficiency
■ Early onset of emphysema in nonsmokers, which may be due to alpha₁-antitrypsin deficiency
■ Unexplained cirrhosis or jaundice, especially in children and young adults, which may be due to alpha₁-antitrypsin deficiency
■ Suspected chronic inflammatory disorder as indicated by persistently elevated alpha₁-antitrypsin levels

Client Preparation

Client preparation is the same as that for any test involving collection of a peripheral blood sample (see Appendix I). The client should fast from food for at least 8 hours prior to the test. Water is not restricted. It also is recommended that oral contraceptives be withheld for 24 hours prior to the study, although this should be confirmed with the person ordering the test.

The Procedure

A venipuncture is performed and the sample collected in a red-topped tube. The sample should be handled gently to avoid hemolysis and sent promptly to the laboratory.

Aftercare and Nursing Observations

Care and assessment following the procedure are the same as for any study involving the collection of a peripheral blood sample. Foods and any drugs withheld prior to the test should be resumed. For those individuals found to be deficient in alpha₁-antitrypsin, medical follow-up and genetic counseling are indicated.

HAPTOGLOBIN (Background Information, p. 148)

Reference Values

Newborn	0–10 mg/dl
Adult	30–160 mg/dl

Interfering Factors

■ Steroid therapy may result in elevated levels

Indications/Purposes for Haptoglobin

■ Known or suspected disorder characterized by excessive red cell hemolysis, as indicated by decreased levels
■ Known or suspected chronic liver disease, as indicated by decreased levels
■ Suspected congenital ahaptoglobinemia, as indicated by decreased levels
■ Known or suspected disorders involving a diffuse inflammatory process or tissue destruction, as indicated by elevated levels

Client Preparation

Client preparation is the same as that for any test involving collection of a peripheral blood sample (see Appendix I).

The Procedure

A venipuncture is performed and the sample collected in a red-topped tube. Some laboratories require that the sample be placed in ice immediately upon collection. The sample should be handled gently to avoid hemolysis, which may alter test results, and sent promptly to the laboratory.

Aftercare and Nursing Observations

Care and assessment following the procedure are the same as for any study involving the collection of a peripheral blood sample.

CERULOPLASMIN (Background Information, p. 149)

Reference Values

Newborn	2–13 mg/dl
Adult	23–50 mg/dl

Indications/Purposes for Ceruloplasmin (Cp)

■ Family history of Wilson's disease (hepatolenticular degeneration)
■ Signs of liver disease combined with neurological changes, especially in a young person, with Wilson's disease indicated by decreased levels
■ Monitoring Cp levels in disorders associated with abnormal values (see Table 5–6, p. 149)
■ Monitoring response to total parenteral nutrition (hyperalimentation), which may lead to decreased levels

Client Preparation

Client preparation is the same as that for any test involving collection of a peripheral blood sample (see Appendix I).

The Procedure

A venipuncture is performed and the sample collected in a red-topped tube. Some laboratories require that the sample be placed in ice immediately upon collection. The sample should be handled gently to avoid hemolysis and sent promptly to the laboratory.

Aftercare and Nursing Observations

Care and assessment following the procedure are the same as for any study involving the collection of a peripheral blood sample. For those individuals in which Wilson's disease is suspected or confirmed, medical follow-up and genetic counseling are indicated.

BLOOD UREA NITROGEN (Background Information, p. 149)

Reference Values

Newborn	4–18 mg/dl
Child	5–18 mg/dl
Adult	6–20 mg/dl

Interfering Factors

■ Therapy with drugs known to alter BUN levels (see Table 5–7, p. 150)

Indications/Purposes for Blood Urea Nitrogen (BUN)

■ Known or suspected disorder associated with impaired renal function, as indicated by increased levels
  □ Obstructive, inflammatory, or toxic damage to the kidneys, nephron loss due to aging, or extrarenal conditions that reduce the glomerular filtration rate (GFR) will increase retention of urea
■ Monitoring the effects of disorders associated with altered fluid balance
  □ Dehydration or hypovolemia due to vomiting, diarrhea, hemorrhage, or inadequate fluid intake will raise the BUN
  □ Fluid overload will decrease the BUN if renal function is adequate
■ Known or suspected liver disease as indicated by decreased levels due to the liver's inability to convert ammonia to urea (80 percent of liver function may be lost before this is evident)
■ Monitoring effects of drugs known to be nephrotoxic or hepatotoxic
■ Monitoring response to various disorders known to result in altered BUN levels (see Table 5–7, p. 150)

Client Preparation

Client preparation is the same as that for any test involving collection of a peripheral blood sample (see Appendix I). Some laboratories require an 8-hour fast prior to the test.

The Procedure

A venipuncture is performed and the sample is obtained in either a gray- or a red-topped tube depending on the laboratory performing the test. The sample should be handled gently to avoid hemolysis and transported promptly to the laboratory.

Aftercare and Nursing Observations

Care and assessment following the procedure are the same as for any study involving the collection of a peripheral blood sample. If restricted prior to the test, usual diet may be resumed.

SERUM CREATININE (Background Information, p. 150)
Reference Values

Children to age 6	0.3–0.6 mg/dl
Children 6 to 18	0.4–1.2 mg/dl
Adults	
Men	0.6–1.3 mg/dl
Women	0.5–1.0 mg/dl

Indications/Purposes for Serum Creatinine

- Known or suspected impairment of renal function, including therapy with nephrotoxic drugs
  - In the absence of disorders affecting muscle mass, elevated creatinine levels indicate decreased renal function
  - Creatinine levels may be normal in situations in which a slow decline in renal function occurs simultaneously with a slow decline in muscle mass, as may occur in elderly individuals (in such situations, a 24-hour urine collection would yield lower than normal excretion levels)
- Along with a blood urea nitrogen (BUN), to provide additional client information
  - An elevated BUN with a normal creatinine usually indicates a non-renal cause for the excessive urea
  - The BUN rises more steeply than creatinine as renal function declines, and falls more rapidly with dialysis
  - With severe, permanent renal impairment, urea levels continue to climb, but creatinine values tend to plateau (at very high circulating creatinine levels, some is excreted through the gastrointestinal tract)
- Known or suspected disorder involving muscles, including crushing injury to muscles
  - In the absence of renal disease, elevated serum creatinine levels are associated with trauma or disorders causing excessive muscle mass (gigantism, acromegaly)
  - Decreased levels are associated with muscular dystrophy

Client Preparation

Client preparation is the same as that for any test involving collection of a peripheral blood sample (see Appendix I). Some laboratories require an 8-hour fast prior to the test.

The Procedure

A venipuncture is performed and the sample collected in a red-topped tube. The sample should be sent promptly to the laboratory.

Aftercare and Nursing Observations

Care and assessment following the procedure is the same as for any study involving the collection of a peripheral blood sample.

AMMONIA (Background Information, p. 151)

Reference Values

40–120 µg/dl
Values vary depending on the laboratory performing the test.

Indications/Purposes for Serum Ammonia

■ Evaluation of advanced liver disease or other disorders associated with altered serum ammonia levels (see Table 5–8, p. 151)
■ Identification of impending hepatic encephalopathy in clients with known liver diseases (e.g., after bleeding from esophageal varices or other gastrointestinal sources, or after excessive ingestion of protein) as indicated by rising levels
■ Monitoring the effectiveness of treatment for hepatic encephalopathy as indicated by declining levels

Client Preparation

Client preparation is essentially the same as that for any study involving the collection of a peripheral blood sample (see Appendix I). An 8-hour fast from food is required prior to the test.

The Procedure

A venipuncture is performed and the sample collected in a green-topped tube. Some laboratories require that the sample be placed in ice immediately upon collection. The sample should be handled gently to avoid hemolysis and sent promptly to the laboratory.

Aftercare and Nursing Observations

Care and assessment following the procedure are the same as for any study involving the collection of a peripheral blood sample. Foods withheld prior to the test should be resumed.

SERUM CREATINE (Background Information, p. 151)

Reference Values

Male	0.1–0.4 mg/dl
Female	0.2–0.7 mg/dl

Interfering Factors

■ Failure to follow dietary restrictions and vigorous exercise within 8 hours of the test may alter results

Indications/Purposes for Serum Creatine

■ Signs and symptoms of muscular disease (e.g., muscle injury, muscular dystrophies, dermatomyositis), as indicated by elevated levels
■ Monitoring the progression of muscle-wasting diseases with serial measurements indicating the rate of muscle deterioration
■ Evaluating the effects of hyperthyroidism and rheumatoid arthritis on muscle tissue

Client Preparation

Client preparation is essentially the same as that for any study involving the collection of a peripheral blood sample (see Appendix I). Food, fluids, and vigorous exercise are not permitted for at least 8 hours prior to the test.

The Procedure

A venipuncture is performed and the sample collected in a red-topped tube. The sample should be handled gently to avoid hemolysis and sent promptly to the laboratory.

Aftercare and Nursing Observations

Care and assessment following the procedure are the same as for any test involving the collection of a peripheral blood sample. Foods and fluids withheld prior to the test, as well as usual activities, should be resumed.

URIC ACID (BACKGROUND INFORMATION, p. 152)

Reference Values

Male	4.0–8.5 mg/dl
Female	2.7–7.3 mg/dl

Interfering Factors

■ Therapy with drugs known to alter uric acid levels (see Table 5–9, p. 152) unless the test is being done to monitor such drug effects

Indications/Purposes for Serum Uric Acid

■ Family history of gout (autosomal dominant genetic disorder) and/or signs and symptoms of gout, with the disorder indicated by elevated levels
■ Known or suspected renal calculi to determine the cause
■ Signs and symptoms of disorders associated with altered uric acid levels (see Table 5–9, p. 152)
■ Monitoring the effects of drugs known to alter uric acid levels (see Table 5–9, p. 152), either as a side effect or as a therapeutic effect
■ Evaluation of the extent of tissue destruction in infection, starvation, excessive exercise, malignancies, chemotherapy, or radiation therapy
■ Evaluation of possible liver damage in eclampsia, as indicated by elevated levels

Client Preparation

Client preparation is the same as that for any study involving the collection of a peripheral blood sample (see Appendix I). Some laboratories require an 8-hour fast from food prior to the test.

The Procedure

A venipuncture is performed and the sample collected in a red-topped tube. The sample should be handled gently to avoid hemolysis and sent promptly to the laboratory.

Aftercare and Nursing Observations

Care and assessment following the procedure are the same as for any study involving the collection of a peripheral blood sample. Foods withheld prior to the test should be resumed.

LIPIDS

Background Information

Lipids are carbon- and hydrogen-containing compounds that are insoluble in water but soluble in organic solvents. Biologically important categories of lipids are the neutral fats (e.g., triglycerides), the conjugated lipids (e.g., phospholipids), and the sterols (e.g., cholesterol). Lipids function in the body as sources of energy for various metabolic processes. Other functions include contributing to the formation of cell membranes, bile acids, and various hormones.

Lipids are derived from both dietary sources and internal body processes. Almost the entire fat portion of the diet consists of triglycerides, which are combinations of three fatty acids and one glycerol molecule. Triglycerides are found in foods of both animal and plant origin. The usual diet also includes small quantities of phospholipids, cholesterol, and cholesterol esters. Phospholipids and cholesterol esters contain fatty acids. In contrast, cholesterol does not contain fatty acids, but its sterol nucleus is synthesized from their degradation products. Since cholesterol has many of the physical and chemical properties of other lipids, it is included as a dietary fat. It should be noted that cholesterol occurs only in foods of animal origin.

Nearly all dietary fats are absorbed into the lymph. Ingested triglycerides are emulsified by bile and then broken down into fatty acids and glycerol by pancreatic and enteric lipases. The fatty acids and glycerol then pass through the intestinal mucosa and are resynthesized into triglycerides which aggregate and enter the lymph as minute droplets called chylomicrons. Although chylomicrons are composed primarily of triglycerides, cholesterol and phospholipids absorbed from the gastrointestinal tract also contribute to their composition (Table 5–10).

Chylomicrons are transported through lymphatic channels to the thoracic duct and empty into venous blood at the juncture of the jugular and subclavian veins. Immediately after fat ingestion, chylomicron blood levels rise. With normal fat ingestion and metabolism, however, chylomicrons should disappear from circulating blood several hours after eating. It is abnormal to find chylo-

TABLE 5–10. Lipoprotein Composition

	Triglyceride %	Cholesterol %	Phospholipid %	Protein %	Electrophoretic Mobility
Chylomicrons	85–95	3–5	5–10	1–2	Remain at origin
Very low-density lipoproteins	60–70	10–15	10–15	10	α_2-Lipoprotein Pre-β-lipoprotein
Low-density lipoproteins	5–10	45	20–30	15–25	β-Lipoprotein
High-density lipoproteins	Very little	20	30	50	α_1-Lipoprotein

From Widmann, FK: Clinical Interpretation of Laboratory Tests, ed 9. FA Davis, Philadelphia, 1983, p 256, with permission.

microns in fasting serum. Chylomicrons are removed from the blood by the actions of circulating lipoprotein lipases and by the liver.

In addition to dietary sources of lipids, the body itself is able to produce various fats. Unused glucose and amino acids, for example, may be converted into fatty acids by the liver. Similarly, nearly all body cells are capable of forming phospholipids and cholesterol, although most of the endogenous production of these lipids occurs in the liver or intestinal mucosa.

As lipids are insoluble in water, special transport mechanisms are required for circulation in the blood. Free fatty acids travel through blood combined with albumin and in this form are called nonesterified fatty acids. Very little free fatty acid is normally present in the blood; therefore, the major lipid components found in serum are triglycerides, cholesterol, and phospholipids. These lipids exist in blood as macromolecules complexed with specialized proteins (apoproteins) to form lipoproteins.

Lipoproteins are classified according to their density, which results from the amounts of the various lipids they contain (see Table 5–10). The least dense lipoproteins are those with the highest triglyceride levels. Lipoprotein densities also are reflected in the electrophoretic mobility of the various types. As with the formation of other endogenous lipids, most lipoproteins are formed in the liver.[22,23]

FREE FATTY ACIDS (FFA) (CLINICAL APPLICATIONS DATA, p. 167)

Free fatty acids (FFA) travel through the blood combined with albumin and in this form are called nonesterified fatty acids (NEFA). Normally, approximately three fatty acid molecules are combined with each molecule of albumin. If, however, the need for fatty acid transport is great (e.g., in situations when needed carbohydrates are not available or cannot be used for energy), as many as 30 fatty acids can combine with one albumin molecule. Thus, although blood levels of FFA are never very high, they will rise impressively following stimuli to release fat.

The most common causes of elevated levels are untreated diabetes mellitus, prolonged fasting or malnutrition, and stimulation by hormones that promote the release of fatty acids from body tissues. It should be noted that the same stimuli that elevate FFA will, in most cases, also elevate serum triglycerides and may produce alterations in lipoprotein levels. Specific causes of both elevated and decreased FFA, including drugs, are listed in Table 5–11.

TABLE 5–11. **Causes of Altered Free Fatty Acid Levels**

Causes of Increased Levels	Causes of Decreased Levels
Diabetes mellitus	*Drugs*
Starvation	Aspirin
Pheochromocytoma	Clofibrate
Acute alcohol intoxication	Glucose
Chronic hepatitis	Insulin
Acute renal failure	Neomycin
Glycogen storage disease	Streptozocin
Hypoglycemia	
Hypothermia	
Hormones	
ACTH	
Cortisone	
Epinephrine, norepinephrine	
GH	
TSH	
Thyroxine	
Drugs	
Amphetamines	
Chlorpromazine	
Isoproterenol	
Reserpine	
Tolbutamide	
Caffeine	
Nicotine	

TRIGLYCERIDES (CLINICAL APPLICATIONS DATA, p. 168)

Triglycerides, which are combinations of three fatty acids and one glycerol molecule, are used in the body to provide energy for various metabolic processes, with excess amounts stored in adipose tissue. Fatty acids readily enter and leave the triglycerides of adipose tissue, providing raw materials needed for conversion to glucose (gluconeogenesis) or for direct combustion as an energy source. Although fatty acids originate in the diet, many also derive from unused glucose and amino acids that the liver and, to a smaller extent, the adipose tissue convert into storage energy.

Altered triglyceride levels are associated with a variety of disorders and also are affected by hormones and certain drugs, including alcohol (Table 5–12). Diets high in calories, fats, and/or carbohydrates will elevate serum triglyceride levels, which is considered a risk factor for atherosclerotic cardiovascular disease.

TOTAL CHOLESTEROL (CLINICAL APPLICATIONS DATA, p. 169)

Cholesterol is necessary for the formation of cell membranes and is a component of the materials that render the skin waterproof. Cholesterol also contributes to the formation of bile salts, adrenal cortical steroids, estrogens, and androgens.

Cholesterol has two sources: (1) that obtained from the diet (exogenous cholesterol); and (2) that which is synthesized in the body (endogenous choles-

TABLE 5–12. **Disorders and Drugs Associated With Altered Triglyceride Levels**

Elevated Levels	Decreased Levels
Primary hyperlipoproteinemia	Acanthocytosis
Atherosclerosis	Cirrhosis
Hypertension	Inadequate dietary protein
Myocardial infarction	Hyperthyroidism
Diabetes mellitus	Hyperparathyroidism
Obstructive jaundice	
Hypothyroidism (primary)	
Hypoparathyroidism	
Nephrotic syndrome	
Chronic obstructive pulmonary disease	
Down's syndrome	
von Gierke's disease	
Drugs	*Drugs*
Alcohol	Clofibrate
Cholestyramine	Dextrothyroxine
Corticosteroids	Heparin
Colestipol	Pergonal
Oral contraceptives	Sulfonylureas
Thyroid preparations	Norethindrone
Estrogen	Androgens
Furosemide	Niacin
Miconazole	Anabolic steroids
	Ascorbic acid

terol). Although most body cells can form some cholesterol, most is produced by the liver and the intestinal mucosa. Because cholesterol is continuously synthesized, degraded, and recycled, it is probable that very little dietary cholesterol enters directly into metabolic reactions.

Altered cholesterol levels are associated with a variety of disorders and also are affected by hormones and certain drugs (Table 5–13). Excessive dietary intake of cholesterol and saturated fatty acids will elevate total cholesterol levels, whereas consumption of unsaturated fatty acids will decrease them. There also is an inherited tendency toward increased cholesterol levels. Elevated total cholesterol levels are associated with atherosclerotic cardiovascular disease.

PHOSPHOLIPIDS (CLINICAL APPLICATIONS DATA, p. 171)

Phospholipids consist of one or more fatty acid molecules and one phosphoric acid radical, and usually have a nitrogenous base. The three major types of body phospholipids are the lecithins, the cephalins, and the sphingomyelins. In addition to dietary sources of phospholipids, nearly all body cells are capable of forming these lipids. Most endogenous phospholipids are formed, however, in the liver and intestinal mucosa. The phospholipids are transported together in circulating blood in the form of lipoproteins.

Phospholipids are important for the formation of cell membranes and for transporting fatty acids through the intestinal mucosa into lymph. Phospholipids also serve as donors of phosphate groups for intracellular metabolic processes and may act as carriers in active transport systems. Saturated lecithins

TABLE 5–13. **Disorders and Drugs Associated With Altered Cholesterol Levels**

Elevated Levels	Decreased Levels
Familial hyperlipoproteinemia	Malabsorption syndromes
Atherosclerosis	Liver disease
Hypertension	Hyperthyroidism
Myocardial infarction	Cushing's syndrome
Obstructive jaundice	Pernicious anemia
Hypothyroidism (primary)	Carcinomatosis
Nephrosis	
Xanthomatosis	
Pregnancy	
Oophorectomy	
Drugs	*Drugs*
ACTH	Antidiabetic agents
Corticosteroids	Cholestyramine
Androgens	Clofibrate
Bile salts	Colchicine
Catecholamines	Colestipol
Phenothiazines	Estrogen
Oral contraceptives	Dextrothyroxine
Salicylates	Dilantin
Thiouracils	Glucagon
Vitamins A and D (excessive)	Haldol
	Heparin
	Kanamycin
	Neomycin
	Nitrates, nitrites
	PAS

are essential for pulmonary gas exchange, while the cephalins are major constituents of thromboplastin, which is necessary to initiate the clotting process. Sphingomyelin is present in large quantities in the nervous system and acts as an insulator around nerve fibers.[24]

Phospholipids may be measured as part of an overall lipid evaluation, but the significance of altered levels is not completely understood. A direct relationship between elevated phospholipids and atherosclerotic cardiovascular disease has not been demonstrated.

Alterations in phospholipid levels may be seen in situations similar to those in which serum triglycerides and cholesterol also are abnormal. For example, elevated levels are associated with diabetes mellitus, nephrotic syndrome, chronic pancreatitis, obstructive jaundice, and early starvation. Decreased levels are seen in clients with primary hypolipoproteinemia, severe malnutrition and malabsorption syndromes, and cirrhosis. Antilipemic drugs (e.g., clofibrate) may lower phospholipid levels, and epinephrine, estrogens, and chlorpromazine tend to elevate them.

Another clinical application of phospholipid data is the use of the lecithin/sphingomyelin (L/S) ratio in estimating fetal lung maturity, with adequate lung maturity indicated by lecithin levels greater than those for sphingomyelin by a ratio of 2:1 or greater (see Chapter 10).

LIPOPROTEIN AND CHOLESTEROL FRACTIONATION (CLINICAL APPLICATIONS DATA, p. 172)

Lipids are transported in the blood as lipoproteins—complex molecules consisting of triglycerides, cholesterol, phospholipids, and proteins. Lipoproteins exist in several forms that reflect the different concentrations of their constituents. These forms, or fractions, are classified according to either their densities or their electrophoretic mobility.

The lipoprotein fractions in relation to density are (1) chylomicrons, (2) very low-density lipoproteins (VLDL), (3) low-density lipoproteins (LDL), and (4) high-density lipoproteins (HDL). The least dense lipoproteins—chylomicrons and VLDL—contain the highest levels of triglycerides and lower amounts of cholesterol and protein. LDL and HDL contain the lowest amounts of triglycerides and relatively higher amounts of cholesterol and protein (see also Table 5–10, p. 161).

Lipoprotein densities correspond to electrophoretic mobility patterns of the several lipoprotein fractions. The two main fractions of lipoproteins, as identified by electrophoresis, are alpha and beta. Alpha lipoproteins, which approxi-

TABLE 5–14. **Conditions Associated With Altered Levels of Lipoprotein Fractions**

Lipoprotein	Increased Level	Decreased Level

Chylomicrons	Ingested fat
	Ingested alcohol
	Types I and V
	  hyperlipoproteinemia
		Not applicable—normal
		  value is zero

VLDL	Ingested fat Ingested carbohydrate Ingested alcohol All types of hyperlipoproteinemia Exogenous estrogens Diabetes mellitus Hypothyroidism (primary) Nephrotic syndrome Alcoholism Pancreatitis Pregnancy	Abetalipoproteinemia Cirrhosis Hypobetalipoproteinemia

LDL-cholesterol	Ingested cholesterol
	Ingested saturated fatty
	  acids
	Types II and III
	  hyperlipoproteinemia
	Hypothyroidism (primary)
	Biliary obstruction
	Nephrotic syndrome
		Types I and V
		  hyperlipoproteinemia
		Hypobetalipoproteinemia
		Abetalipoproteinemia
		Hyperthryoidism
		Cirrhosis

HDL-cholesterol	Ingested alcohol (moderate
	  amounts)
	Chronic hepatitis
	Hypothyroidism (primary)
	Early biliary cirrhosis
	Biliary obstruction
		All types of
		  hyperlipoproteinemia
		Exogenous estrogens
		Hyperthyroidism
		Cirrhosis
		Tangier disease

mate the high-density lipoproteins (alpha$_1$), migrate with the alpha globulins. The beta lipoproteins, which reflect the very low-density lipoproteins (prebeta) and the low-density lipoproteins (beta), migrate with the beta globulins. Chylomicrons remain at the origin.

The cholesterol content of the HDL and LDL fractions also can be determined by measuring total cholesterol remaining after one fraction has been removed. It should be noted, however, that HDL-cholesterol does not correlate well with the total cholesterol concentration, is higher in women than in men, and tends to be inversely proportional to triglyceride levels. High HDL-cholesterol and low LDL-cholesterol levels are predictive of a lessened risk of cardiovascular disease, whereas high LDL-cholesterol and low HDL-cholesterol levels are considered risk factors for atherosclerotic cardiovascular disease. Further, many health care providers believe that an adequate lipid assessment need

TABLE 5-15. Clinicopathological Significance of Lipoprotein Phenotypes

Phenotype	Familial Syndrome	May Occur Secondary To	Remarks
I	Abdominal pain Eruptive xanthomas Lipemia retinalis Early vascular disease absent	Insulin-dependent diabetes Lupus erythematosus Dysglobulinemias Pancreatitis	Lipoprotein lipase is deficient
II	Early, severe vascular disease Prominent xanthomas	High-cholesterol diet Nephrotic syndrome Porphyria Hypothyroidism Dysglobulinemias Obstructive liver diseases	Familial trait is autosomal-dominant; homozygotes are especially severely affected
III	Accelerated vascular disease, onset in adulthood Xanthomas, palmar yellowing Abnormal glucose tolerance Hyperuricemia	Hypothyroidism Dysglobulinemias Uncontrolled diabetes	Diet, lipid-lowering drugs very effective
IV	Accelerated vascular disease, onset in adulthood Abnormal glucose tolerance Hyperuricemia	Obesity High alcohol intake Oral contraceptives Diabetes Nephrotic syndrome Glycogen storage disease	Weight loss lowers VLDL High-fat diet may convert to type V
V	Abdominal pain Pancreatitis Eruptive xanthomas Abnormal glucose tolerance Vascular disease not associated	High alcohol intake Diabetes Nephrotic syndrome Pancreatitis Hypercalcemia	Weight loss does not lower VLDL

From Widmann, FK: Clinical Interpretation of Laboratory Tests, ed 9. FA Davis, Philadelphia, 1983, p 260, with permission.

include only (1) total cholesterol, (2) HDL-cholesterol, (3) serum triglycerides, and (4) estimate of chylomicron concentration.

Specific conditions associated with altered levels of lipoprotein fractions are listed in Table 5–14.

LIPOPROTEIN PHENOTYPING (CLINICAL APPLICATIONS DATA, p. 173)

Lipoprotein phenotyping is an extension of the information obtained through lipoprotein fractionation (see pp. 165 and 166), and provides another approach to correlating laboratory findings with disease.

Six different lipoprotein distribution patterns (phenotypes) are seen in serums with high levels of cholesterol and/or triglycerides. These phenotypes, which are referred to by their assigned numbers, have been correlated with genetically determined abnormalities (familial or primary hyperlipoproteinemias) and with a variety of acquired conditions (secondary hyperlipoproteinemias).

Phenotype descriptions have proven useful in classifying diagnoses and in evaluating treatment and preventive regimens. Most hyperlipemic serums can be categorized into lipoprotein phenotypes without performing electrophoresis if the following are known: (1) chylomicron status, (2) serum triglyceride level, (3) total cholesterol, and (4) HDL-cholesterol.

Useful information about chylomicron status and VLDL content of serum with excessive triglycerides may be obtained by observing the appearance of serum or plasma after 12 to 16 hours of refrigeration. Uniform turbidity means elevated VLDL without significant chylomicrons. A layer of "cream" atop a turbid specimen indicates elevation of both chylomicrons and VLDL, while a layer of "cream" atop a clear specimen means elevated chylomicrons without excess VLDL.[25]

Table 5–15 shows the clinical significance of each of the lipoprotein phenotypes as primary familial syndromes and as secondary occurrences caused by disorders that alter lipid metabolism.

Clinical Applications Data

FREE FATTY ACIDS (BACKGROUND INFORMATION, p. 161)
Reference Values

Free fatty acids	0.3–1.0 mEq/l

Interfering Factors

- Ingestion of alcohol within 24 hours of the test may result in falsely elevated values
- Failure to follow dietary restrictions prior to the test may alter values
- Ingestion of drugs known to alter FFA levels, unless the test is being done to evaluate such effects (see Table 5–11, p. 162)

Indications/Purposes for Free Fatty Acids

- Support for diagnosing uncontrolled or untreated diabetes mellitus, as indicated by elevated levels

■ Evaluation of response to treatment for diabetes, as indicated by declining levels
■ Suspected malnutrition, as indicated by elevated levels
■ Known or suspected disorder associated with excessive hormone production (see Table 5–11, p. 162), as indicated by elevated levels
■ Evaluation of response to therapy with drugs known to alter FFA levels (see Table 5–11, p. 162)

Client Preparation

Client preparation is essentially the same as that for any study involving the collection of a peripheral blood sample (see Appendix I). The client should abstain from alcohol for 24 hours and from food for at least 8 hours prior to the test; water is not restricted. Drugs known to affect FFA levels (see Table 5–11, p. 162) may be withheld prior to the test, although this may not always be done if the therapeutic effect on FFA levels is being evaluated.

The Procedure

A venipuncture is performed and the sample collected in a red-topped tube. The sample should be sent immediately to the laboratory.

Aftercare and Nursing Observations

Care and assessment following the procedure are the same as for any study involving the collection of a peripheral blood sample. Foods and any drugs withheld prior to the test should be resumed.

TRIGLYCERIDES (BACKGROUND INFORMATION, p. 162)
Reference Values

Age	Value in mg/dl
Infant	5–40
2–20 years	10–140
20–40 years	10–140 (women)
	10–150 (men)
40–60 years	10–180 (women)
	10–190 (men)

Values for serum triglycerides may vary according to the laboratory performing the test. In addition, values have been found to vary in relation to race, income level, level of physical activity, dietary habits and geographic location, as well as in relation to age and sex, as shown here.

Interfering Factors

■ Failure to follow usual diet for 2 weeks prior to the test may yield results that do not accurately reflect client status
■ Ingestion of alcohol 24 hours prior and food 12 hours prior to the test may falsely elevate levels

■ Ingestion of drugs known to alter triglyceride levels within 24 hours of the test, unless the test is being done to evaluate such effects (see Table 5–12, p. 163)

Indications/Purposes for Serum Triglycerides

■ As a component of a complete physical examination, especially for individuals over age 40 and/or who are obese, to estimate the degree of risk for atherosclerotic cardiovascular disease
■ Family history of hyperlipoproteinemia (hyperlipidemia)
■ Known or suspected disorders associated with altered triglyceride levels (see Table 5–12, p. 163)
■ Monitoring response to drugs known to alter triglyceride levels

Client Preparation

General client preparation is the same as that for any procedure involving collection of a peripheral blood sample (see Appendix I). For this test, the client should ingest a normal diet such that no weight gain or loss will occur for 2 weeks before the study, and should abstain from alcohol for 24 hours and from foods for 12 hours prior to the test. Water is not restricted.

It is also recommended that drugs that may alter triglyceride levels be withheld for 24 hours prior to the test, although this should be confirmed with the person ordering the study.

The Procedure

A venipuncture is performed and the sample collected in a red-topped tube. The sample should be sent promptly to the laboratory.

Aftercare and Nursing Observations

Care and assessment following the procedure are the same as for any study involving the collection of a peripheral blood sample. Foods and any drugs withheld prior to the test should be resumed.

TOTAL CHOLESTEROL (BACKGROUND INFORMATION, p. 162)
Reference Values

Age	Values in mg/dl
Under 25 years	125–200
25–40 years	140–250
40–50 years	160–260
50–65 years	170–265
Over 65 years	175–280

Values for total cholesterol may vary according to the laboratory performing the test. In addition, values have been found to vary according to sex, race, income level, level of physical activity, dietary habits, and geographic location, as well as in relation to age as shown here.

Interfering Factors

■ Ingestion of alcohol 24 hours prior and food 12 hours prior to the test may falsely elevate levels
■ Ingestion of drugs known to alter cholesterol levels within 12 hours of the test, unless the test is being done to evaluate such effects (see Table 5–13, p. 164)

Indications/Purposes for Total Cholesterol

■ As a component of a complete physical examination, especially for individuals over age 40 and/or who are obese, to estimate the degree of risk for atherosclerotic cardiovascular disease
  □ In general, the desirable blood cholesterol level is less than 200 mg/dl
  □ Cholesterol levels of 200 to 240 mg/dl are considered borderline, and the person is considered at high risk if other factors such as obesity and smoking are present; for the latter individuals, additional tests such as lipoprotein and cholesterol fractionation (see p. 172) should be done
  □ Cholesterol levels of greater than 250 mg/dl place the person at definite high risk for cardiovascular disease and require treatment; additional tests such as lipoprotein and cholesterol fractionation should be done
■ Family history of hypercholesterolemia and/or cardiovascular disease
■ Known or suspected disorders which are associated with altered cholesterol levels (see Table 5–13, p. 164)
■ Monitoring response to dietary treatment of hypercholesterolemia and support for decisions regarding need for drug therapy (cholesterol levels may fall with diet modification alone over a period of 6 months, only to return gradually to previous levels)
■ Monitoring response to drugs known to alter cholesterol levels (see Table 5–13, p. 164)

Client Preparation

General client preparation is the same as that for any procedure involving collection of a peripheral blood sample (see Appendix I). For this test, the client should abstain from alcohol for 24 hours and from foods for 12 hours prior to the study. Water is not restricted.

It also is recommended that drugs that may alter cholesterol levels be withheld for 12 hours prior to the test, although this should be confirmed with the person ordering the study.

The Procedure

A venipuncture is performed and the sample collected in a red-topped tube. The sample should be sent promptly to the laboratory.

Aftercare and Nursing Observations

Care and assessment following the procedure are the same as for any study involving the collection of a peripheral blood sample. Food and any drugs withheld prior to the test should be resumed.

PHOSPHOLIPIDS (BACKGROUND INFORMATION, p. 163)

Reference Values

150–380 mg/dl
Values may vary depending on the laboratory performing the test.

Interfering Factors

■ Ingestion of alcohol 24 hours prior to and food 12 hours prior to the test may falsely elevate levels
■ Ingestion of drugs known to alter phospholipid levels within 12 hours of the test, unless the test is being done to evaluate such effects
□ Antilipemic drugs (e.g., clofibrate) may lower phospholipid levels
□ Epinephrine, estrogens, and chlorpromazine tend to elevate phospholipid levels

Indications/Purposes for Serum Phospholipids

■ Known or suspected disorders that cause or are associated with altered lipid metabolism
□ Altered phospholipid levels are seen in situations similar to those in which serum triglycerides and cholesterol also are altered (see Tables 5–12 and 5–13, pp. 163 and 164)
□ Elevated levels are associated with diabetes mellitus, nephrotic syndrome, chronic pancreatitis, obstructive jaundice, and early starvation
□ Decreased levels are seen in primary hypolipoproteinemia, severe malnutrition, malabsorption syndromes, and cirrhosis
■ Support for identifying problems related to fat metabolism and transport
□ Phospholipid formation parallels deposition of triglycerides in the liver, and severely decreased levels result in low levels of lipoproteins that are essential for fat transport
■ Abnormal bleeding of unknown origin, with decreased cephalin (a type of phospholipid), a possible contributor to low levels of thromboplastin
■ Suspected neurological disorder, which may be associated with decreased levels of sphingomyelin (a type of phospholipid)

Client Preparation

General client preparation is the same as that for any procedure involving collection of a peripheral blood sample (see Appendix I). For this test, the client should abstain from alcohol for 24 hours and from food for 12 hours prior to the study; water is not restricted.

It also is recommended that drugs that may alter phospholipid levels be withheld for 12 hours prior to the test, although this should be confirmed with the person ordering the study.

The Procedure

A venipuncture is performed and the sample collected in a red-topped tube. The sample should be sent promptly to the laboratory.

Aftercare and Nursing Observations

Care and assessment following the procedure are the same as for any study involving the collection of a peripheral blood sample. Foods and any drugs withheld prior to the test should be resumed.

LIPOPROTEIN AND CHOLESTEROL FRACTIONATION (BACKGROUND INFORMATION, p. 165)

Reference Values

Total Lipoproteins	400–800 mg/dl	
Lipoprotein Fractions		
Chylomicrons	0	
VLDL or Prebeta	3–32	
LDL or Beta	38–40	
HDL or Alpha₁	20–48	
LDL- and HDL-Cholesterol		

Age	LDL-Cholesterol	HDL-Cholesterol
To 25 years	73–138 mg/dl	32–57 mg/dl
25–40 years	90–180 mg/dl	32–60 mg/dl
40–50 years	100–185 mg/dl	33–60 mg/dl
50–65 years	105–190 mg/dl	34–70 mg/dl
Over 65 years	105–200 mg/dl	35–75 mg/dl

HDL-cholesterol values are normally lower in men than in women, with an average range of 22–68 mg/dl.

Interfering Factors

- Failure to follow usual diet for 2 weeks prior to the test may yield results that do not accurately reflect client status
- Ingestion of alcohol 24 hours prior and food 12 hours prior to the test may alter results
- Excessive exercise 12 hours prior to the test may alter results (regular exercise has been found to lower HDL-cholesterol levels)
- Numerous drugs may alter results, including those that are known to alter lipoprotein components (see Tables 5–12 and 5–13, pp. 163 and 164)

Indications/Purposes for Lipoprotein and Cholesterol Fractionation

- Serum cholesterol levels of greater than 250 mg/dl which indicate high risk for cardiovascular disease and the need for further evaluation and possible treatment (see p. 170)
- Estimation of the degree of risk for cardiovascular disease
  - ☐ Individuals with LDL-cholesterol levels greater than 160 mg/dl are considered to be at high risk
  - ☐ Individuals at or above the upper reference range for HDL-cholesterol have half the average risk, while those at or near the bottom have two, three, or more times the average risk
- Known or suspected disorders associated with altered lipoprotein levels (see Table 5–14, p. 165)
- Evaluation of response to treatment for altered levels and support for decisions regarding the need for drug therapy (LDL-cholesterol levels may decrease with dietary modification alone; if not, drug treatment is recommended)

Client Preparation

General client preparation is the same as that for any procedure involving collection of a peripheral blood sample (see Appendix I). For this test, the client should ingest a normal diet such that no weight gain or loss will occur for 2 weeks before the study, and should abstain from alcohol for 24 hours and from food for 12 hours prior to the test; water is not restricted. The client also should avoid excessive exercise for at least 12 hours prior to the test.

It also is recommended that drugs which may alter lipoprotein components be withheld for 24 to 48 hours prior to the test (see Tables 5–12 and 5–13, pp. 163 and 164), although this should be confirmed with the person ordering the study.

The Procedure

A venipuncture is performed and the sample collected in a red-topped tube. The sample should be sent promptly to the laboratory.

Aftercare and Nursing Observations

Care and assessment following the procedure are the same as for any study involving the collection of a peripheral blood sample. Food and any drugs withheld prior to the test, as well as usual activities, should be resumed.

LIPOPROTEIN PHENOTYPING (BACKGROUND INFORMATION, p. 167)
Reference Values

	Phenotype					
	I	IIa	IIb	III	IV	V
Frequency	Very rare	Common	Common	Uncommon	Very common	Rare
Chylomicrons	↑↑↑	Nl	Nl	Nl or ↑	Nl	↑↑
Pre-β-Lipoproteins (approximates VLDL)	↑	↑↑	↑	(these two bands merge)	↑↑↑	↑↑
β-Lipoproteins (approximates LDL)	↓	↑↑	↑↑		Nl or ↑	Nl or ↓
α_1-Lipoproteins (approximates HDL)	↓	Nl	Nl	Nl	Nl or ↓	Nl or ↓
Total cholesterol	Nl or ↑	↑↑	↑↑	↑↑	Nl or ↑	↑↑
Total triglycerides	↑↑↑	Nl	↑	↑↑ or ↑↑↑	↑↑ or ↑↑↑	↑↑↑
Refrigerated serum or plasma	"Cream"/ clear or turbid	Clear	+ or ++ turbid	+++ turbid	++ turbid	"Cream"/ ++ turbid

Nl = normal
From Widmann, FK: Clinical Interpretation of Laboratory Tests, ed 9. FA Davis, Philadelphia, 1983, p. 259, with permission.

Interfering Factors

■ Failure to follow usual diet for 2 weeks prior to the test may yield results that do not accurately reflect client status

■ Ingestion of alcohol 24 hours prior and food 12 hours prior to the test may alter results

■ Excessive exercise 12 hours prior to the test may alter results

■ Numerous drugs, including those that are known to alter lipoprotein components (see Tables 5–12, 5–13, and 5–15; pp. 163, 164, and 166), may alter results

Indications/Purposes for Lipoprotein Phenotyping

■ Further evaluation of elevated serum cholesterol levels and results of lipoprotein and cholesterol fractionation (see p. 172)

■ Family history of primary hyperlipoproteinemia (hyperlipidemia)

■ Identification of the client's specific lipoprotein phenotype

■ Known or suspected disorders associated with the several lipoprotein phenotypes (see Table 5–15, p. 166)

Client Preparation

General client preparation is the same as that for any study involving collection of a peripheral blood sample (see Appendix I). For this test, the client should ingest a normal diet such that no weight gain or loss will occur for 2 weeks before the study, and should abstain from alcohol for 24 hours and from food 12 hours prior to the test; water is not restricted. The client also should avoid excessive exercise for at least 12 hours prior to the test.

It also is recommended that drugs that may alter lipoprotein components be withheld for 24 to 48 hours or longer prior to the test (see Tables 5–12, 5–13, and 5–15, pp. 163, 164, and 166), although this should be confirmed with the person ordering the study.

The Procedure

A venipuncture is performed and the sample collected in either a red- or a lavender-topped tube, depending on the laboratory's procedure for determining lipoprotein phenotypes. The sample should be sent to the laboratory immediately.

Aftercare and Nursing Observations

Care and assessment following the procedure are the same as for any study involving the collection of a peripheral blood sample. Food and any drugs withheld prior to the test, as well as usual activities, should be resumed.

BILIRUBIN

Background Information (Clinical Applications Data, p. 176)

Bilirubin is a degradation product of the pigmented heme portion of hemoglobin. Old, damaged, and abnormal erythrocytes are removed from the circulation by the spleen and to some extent by the liver and bone marrow. The heme component of the red blood cells is oxidized to bilirubin by the reticuloendothelial cells and released into the blood.

In the blood, the fat-soluble bilirubin binds to albumin as unconjugated (prehepatic) bilirubin for transport to the liver. In the liver, hepatocytes detach bilirubin from albumin and conjugate it with glucuronic acid, which renders the bilirubin water soluble. Most of the conjugated (posthepatic) bilirubin is excreted into the hepatic ducts and then into bile. Only small amounts of conjugated bilirubin diffuse from the liver back into the blood. Thus, most circulating bilirubin is normally in the unconjugated form.

Bilirubin is an excretory product that serves no physiological function in bile or blood. Once the conjugated bilirubin in bile enters the intestine, most is converted to a series of urobilinogen compounds and excreted into the stool as stercobilinogen after oxidation. A lesser amount is recycled to the liver and either returned to bile or excreted in the urine as urobilinogen, which is oxidized to urobilin.

Bilirubin and its degradation products are pigments and provide the yellow tinge of normal serum, the yellow-green hue of bile, the brown color of stools, and the yellow color of urine. Abnormally elevated serum bilirubin levels will produce jaundice; obstruction to biliary excretion of bilirubin may produce light-colored stools and dark urine.

The terms "indirect" and "direct," which are used to describe unconjugated (prehepatic) and conjugated (posthepatic) bilirubin, respectively, derive from the methods of testing for their presence in serum. Conjugated bilirubin is described as direct (direct-reacting) because it is water soluble and can be measured without any modification. Unconjugated bilirubin must be rendered soluble with alcohol or other solvents before the test can be done and is thus referred to as indirect (indirect-reacting).

Serum bilirubin concentration is affected by hemoglobin metabolism, liver function, and biliary tract dynamics. If there is increased destruction of red cells, increased amounts of bilirubin will be formed. This may cause unconjugated (prehepatic, indirect) bilirubin levels to rise somewhat, but the normal liver has ample excretory capacity to prevent excessive accumulation in the serum. It should be noted that in such situations, fecal and urinary urobilinogen levels rise owing to the liver's compensatory increase in bilirubin conjugation and excretion.

In contrast, impaired liver function will cause dramatic increases in serum bilirubin levels (hyperbilirubinemia). Bilirubin must be in the conjugated form for normal excretion via bile, stools, and urine. When the liver is unable to conjugate bilirubin adequately, serum levels of unconjugated bilirubin rise. Disorders in which excessive hemolysis of red cells is combined with impaired liver function also produce hyperbilirubinemia. An example is physiological jaundice of the newborn, in which the increased destruction of red cells, common after birth, is combined with the immature liver's inability to conjugate sufficient bilirubin. Kernicterus, a complication of newborn hyperbilirubinemia, occurs when unconjugated bilirubin is deposited in brain tissue.

Impaired excretion of conjugated (posthepatic, direct) bilirubin from the liver into the bile ducts or from the biliary tract itself will cause this form of bilirubin to be reabsorbed from the liver into the blood with resultant elevated serum levels. Since conjugated bilirubin is water soluble and readily crosses the renal glomerulus, excessive amounts may be excreted in the urine. The stools, however, will be lighter in color because of diminished amounts of conjugated bilirubin in the gut.

Whenever impaired liver function is combined with bile duct obstruction (e.g., cirrhosis, hepatitis, hepatic cancer), both unconjugated and conjugated bilirubin levels are elevated.[26]

TABLE 5–16. **Causes of Elevations in Indirect and Direct Bilirubin Levels**

Increased Indirect (Unconjugated) Bilirubin
Hemolysis: Hemoglobinopathies; spherocytosis; G-6-PD deficiency; autoimmunity; transfusion reaction
Red cell degradation: Hemorrhage into soft tissues or body cavities; inefficient erythropoiesis; pernicious anemia
Defective hepatocellular uptake or conjugation: Viral hepatitis; hereditary enzyme deficiencies (Gilbert, Crigler-Najjar syndromes); hepatic immaturity, in newborns

Increased Direct (Conjugated) Bilirubin
Intrahepatic disruption: Viral hepatitis; alcoholic hepatitis; chlorpromazine; cirrhosis
Bile duct disease: Biliary cirrhosis; cholangitis (idiopathic, infectious); biliary atresia
Extrahepatic bile duct obstruction: Gallstones; carcinoma of gallbladder, bile ducts, or head of pancreas; bile duct stricture, from inflammation or surgical misadventure

From Widmann, FK: Clinical Intrepretation of Laboratory Tests, ed. 9. FA Davis, Philadelphia, 1983, p 262, with permission.

Sirum bilirubin levels are measured as total bilirubin, indirect bilirubin, and direct bilirubin. Total bilirubin reflects the combination of unconjugated and conjugated bilirubin in the serum, and may be used to screen clients for possible disorders involving bilirubin production and excretion. If total bilirubin is normal, the levels of indirect (unconjugated) and direct (conjugated) bilirubin also are assumed to be normal in most cases.

When total bilirubin levels are elevated, indirect and direct bilirubin levels are measured to determine the source of the overall elevation. Specific causes of elevations in indirect and direct bilirubin are shown in Table 5–16. Numerous drugs also may alter bilirubin levels.

Clinical Applications Data (Background Information, p. 174)

Reference Values

Total Bilirubin	
Newborn	2.0–6.0 mg/dl
48 hours	6.0–7.0 mg/dl
5 days	4.0–12.0 mg/dl
1 month to adult	0.3–1.2 mg/dl
Indirect Bilirubin (unconjugated, prehepatic)	
1 month to adult	0.3–1.1 mg/dl
Direct Bilirubin (conjugated, posthepatic)	
1 month to adult	0.1–0.4 mg/dl

Interfering Factors

■ Prolonged exposure of the client, as well as the blood sample, to sunlight and to ultraviolet light reduces serum bilirubin levels

■ Failure to follow dietary restrictions prior to the test
  ☐ Fasting normally lowers indirect bilirubin levels
  ☐ In Gilbert's syndrome, a congenital defect in bilirubin degradation, chronically elevated levels of indirect bilirubin increase dramatically in the fasting state
■ Numerous drugs may elevate bilirubin levels (e.g., steroids, sulfonamides, sulfonylureas, barbiturates, antineoplastic agents, propylthiouracil, allopurinol, antibiotics, gallbladder dyes, caffeine, theophylline, indomethacin, and any drugs that are considered hepatotoxic); it is recommended that such drugs be withheld for 24 hours prior to the test, if possible

Indications/Purposes for Bilirubin

■ Known or suspected hemolytic disorders, including transfusion reactions, as indicated by elevated total and indirect bilirubin levels (see also Table 5–16, p. 176)
  ☐ Hemolysis alone rarely causes indirect bilirubin levels higher than 4 or 5 mg/dl
  ☐ If hemolysis is combined with impaired or immature liver function, levels may rise more dramatically
■ Confirmation of observed jaundice
  ☐ Jaundice manifests when serum levels of indirect or direct bilirubin reach 2 to 4 mg/dl
■ Determination of the cause of jaundice (e.g., liver dysfunction, hepatitis, biliary obstruction, carcinoma)
  ☐ Support for diagnosing liver dysfunction as evidenced by elevated direct and total bilirubin levels, or by elevation of all three levels if bile duct drainage also is impaired
  ☐ Support for diagnosing biliary tract obstruction as evidenced by elevated direct and total bilirubin levels, or by elevation of all three levels if liver function is impaired

Client Preparation

General client preparation is the same as that for any study involving collection of a peripheral blood sample (see Appendix I). For these tests, the client should fast from foods for at least 4 hours prior to the test; water is not restricted.

Because many drugs may alter bilirubin levels (see section on Interfering Factors), a medication history should be obtained. It is recommended that those drugs that may alter test results be withheld for 24 hours prior to the test, although this should be confirmed with the person ordering the study.

The Procedure

A venipuncture is performed and the sample obtained in a red-topped tube. The sample should be handled gently to avoid hemolysis and sent immediately to the laboratory. The sample should not be exposed for prolonged periods to sunlight (i.e., more than 1 hour), ultraviolet light, or fluorescent lights. In infants, a capillary sample is obtained by heelstick.

Aftercare and Nursing Observations

Care and assessment following the procedure are the same as for any study involving the collection of a peripheral blood sample. Food and any drugs withheld prior to the test should be resumed.

ENZYMES

Background Information

Enzymes are catalysts that enhance reactions without directly participating in them. Individual enzymes, each of which has its own substrate and product specificity, exist for nearly all the metabolic reactions that maintain body functions.

Enzymes are normally intracellular molecules. Because certain metabolic reactions occur in many tissues, the enzymes involved exist in many cell types. Enzymes with more restricted metabolic functions are found in only one or several specialized cell types. The presence of enzymes in circulating blood indicates cellular changes that have permitted their escape into extracellular fluid. The continuous synthesis and destruction of the cells of the enzymes' origins will, for example, allow small amounts of enzymes to appear in the blood. Cellular disruption due to damage by disease, toxins, or trauma, as well as increased cell wall permeability, also will elevate serum enzyme levels. Additional causes of elevated enzyme levels are an increase in the number or activity of enzyme-containing cells and decreases in normal excretory or degradation mechanisms.

Decreased serum enzyme levels rarely have diagnostic significance because so few enzymes are present in substantial quantity. Enzyme levels may decline if the number of synthesizing cells declines, if there is generalized or specific restriction in protein synthesis (enzymes are proteins), or if excretion or degradation increases.

Very few enzymes are studied routinely. Although highly specialized enzyme analysis is applied to the study of many genetically determined diseases, most diagnostic enzyme studies involve only those enzymes whose changing values in serum provide inferential or confirmatory evidence of various pathological processes. A major goal of enzyme analysis is to localize disease processes to specific organs, preferably to specific functional subdivisions or even to specific cellular activities. Enzymes unique to a single cell type or found only in a few sites are particularly useful in this regard. The source of elevations of those enzymes with widespread distribution also can be determined by partitioning total activity into isoenzyme fractions. Isoenzymes are different forms of a single enzyme with immunological, physical, or chemical characteristics distinctive for their tissue of origin.

Efforts to standardize the study of enzymes (enzymology) have led to new terminology for naming and measuring enzymes. The Commission on Enzymes of the International Union of Biochemistry (IUB) has classified enzymes according to their biochemical functions, assigning to each a numerical designation that embodies class, subclass, and specification number. The IUB has also assigned descriptive names according to the specific reaction catalyzed and, in many cases, a practical name useful for common reference. One result of this is that enzymes that have been studied for years have been renamed according to the new terminology. For example, the liver enzyme that was formerly called glutamic-oxaloacetic transaminase (GOT) is now named aspartate aminotransferase (AST).

Another attempt to standardize enzymology is the introduction of International Units (IU) for reporting enzyme activity. One IU of an enzyme is the amount that will catalyze transformation of one μmol of substrate per minute under defined conditions. The actual amounts vary among enzymes, and the IU is not a single universally applicable value that can be used to compare enzymes of different characteristics.[27]

In this section, enzymes associated with organs and tissues such as the liver, pancreas, bone, heart, and muscle are discussed. Enzymes specific to red and white blood cells are included in Chapter 1.

ALANINE AMINOTRANSFERASE (ALT, SGPT) (CLINICAL APPLICATIONS DATA, p. 189)

Alanine aminotransferase (ALT), formerly known as glutamic-pyruvic transaminase (GPT), catalyzes the reversible transfer of an amino group between the amino acid, alanine, and alpha-ketoglutamic acid. Hepatocytes are virtually the only cells with high ALT concentrations, although the heart, kidneys, and skeletal muscles contain moderate amounts.

Elevated serum ALT levels are considered a sensitive index of liver damage due to a variety of disorders and numerous drugs, including alcohol. Elevations may also be seen in nonhepatic disorders such as muscular dystrophy, extensive muscular trauma, myocardial infarction, congestive heart failure, and renal failure, although the increase in ALT produced by these disorders is not as great as that produced by conditions affecting the liver.

This test was formerly known as serum glutamic-pyruvic transaminase (SGPT).

ASPARTATE AMINOTRANSFERASE (AST, SGOT) (CLINICAL APPLICATIONS DATA, p. 190)

Aspartate aminotransferase (AST), formerly known as glutamic-oxaloacetic transaminase (GOT), catalyzes the reversible transfer of an amino between the amino acid, aspartate, and alpha-ketoglutamic acid. ALT exists in large amounts in both liver and myocardial cells, and in smaller but significant amounts in skeletal muscles, kidneys, pancreas, and brain.

Serum AST rises when there is cellular damage to the tissues in which the enzyme is found. When heart muscle suffers ischemic damage, serum AST rises within 6 to 8 hours; peak values occur at 24 to 48 hours and decline to normal within 72 to 96 hours. Elevation of AST occurs midway in the time sequence between that of creatine phosphokinase (CPK), which rises very early and falls within 48 hours, and lactic dehydrogenase (LDH), which begins rising 12 hours or more after infarction and remains elevated for a week or more. Elevation of AST cannot be used as the single enzyme indicator for myocardial infarction, as it also rises in several other conditions included in the differential diagnosis of heart attack. Other disorders associated with elevated AST, and the magnitude of those elevations, are listed in Table 5–17. It should also be noted that numerous drugs, especially those known to be hepatotoxic or nephrotoxic, may elevate AST levels.[28]

The test for AST was formerly known as serum glutamic-oxaloacetic transaminase (SGOT).

ALKALINE PHOSPHATASE (ALP) (CLINICAL APPLICATIONS DATA, p. 191)

Phosphatases are enzymes that cleave phosphate from compounds with a single phosphate group. Those that are optimally active at pH 9 are grouped under the name alkaline phosphatase (ALP).

Alkaline phosphatase is elaborated by a number of tissues. Liver, bone, and intestine are the major isoenzyme sources. During pregnancy, the placenta also is an abundant source of ALP, while certain cancers elaborate small amounts of a distinctive form of ALP called the Regan enzyme. Additional sources of ALP

TABLE 5–17. **Conditions Affecting Serum Aspartate Aminotransferase Levels**

Pronounced Elevation (5 or more times normal)
Acute hepatocellular damage
Myocardial infarction
Shock
Acute pancreatitis
Infectious mononucleosis

Moderate Elevation (3–5 times normal)
Biliary tract obstruction
Cardiac arrhythmias
Congestive heart failure
Liver tumors
Chronic hepatitis
Muscular dystrophy
Dermatomyositis

Slight Elevation (up to 3 times normal)
Pericarditis
Cirrhosis, fatty liver
Pulmonary infarction
Delirium tremens
Cerebrovascular accident
Hemolytic anemia

Adapted from Widmann, FK: Clinical Interpretation of Laboratory Tests, ed 9. FA Davis, Philadelphia, 1983, p 297.

are the proximal tubules of the kidneys, lactating mammary glands, and the granulocytes of circulating blood (see Chapter 1, section on Leukocyte Alkaline Phosphatase).

Bone ALP predominates in normal serum, along with a modest amount of hepatic isoenzyme, which is believed to derive largely from epithelium of the intrahepatic biliary ducts, rather than from hepatocytes themselves. Levels of intestinal ALP vary; most people have relatively little, but isolated elevations of this enzyme have been observed. Intestinal ALP enters the blood very briefly while fats are being digested and absorbed, but intestinal disease rarely affects serum ALP levels.

Measurements of ALP are helpful in liver disease or bone disease. Serum ALP levels rise with increased bone growth, increased bone destruction, and abnormal proportions of both. Hepatic ALP levels are highest in disorders that cause obstruction or inflammation of the hepatobiliary tract, whereas disorders involving the liver parenchyma itself cause much less elevation. Conditions associated with elevated serum ALP levels, and the magnitude of those elevations, are listed in Table 5–18.[29] Numerous drugs also may elevate serum ALP levels.

Decreased levels are seen in cretinism, secondary growth retardation, scurvy, achondroplasia and, rarely, hypophosphatasia. Drugs known to decrease serum ALP levels include clofibrate, Imuran, and fluorides.

ALKALINE PHOSPHATASE ISOENZYMES

If serum alkaline phosphatase (ALP) levels are elevated, but the clinical picture does not provide enough information to determine the origin of the

TABLE 5–18. Conditions Associated With Elevated Serum ALP Levels

Pronounced Elevation (5 or more times normal)
Advanced pregnancy
Biliary obstruction
Biliary atresia
Cirrhosis
Osteitis deformans
Osteogenic sarcoma
Hyperparathyroidism (primary, or secondary to chronic renal disease)
Paget's disease
Infusion of albumin of placental origin

Moderate Elevation (3 to 5 times normal)
Granulomatous or infiltrative liver diseases
Infectious mononucleosis
Metastatic tumors in bone
Metabolic bone diseases (rickets, osteomalacia)
Extrahepatic duct obstruction

Mild Elevation (up to 3 times normal)
Viral hepatitis
Chronic active hepatitis
Cirrhosis (alcoholic)
Healing fractures
Early pregnancy
Growing children
Large doses of vitamin D
Congestive heart failure

excess, ALP isoenzymes are evaluated. The major ALP isoenzymes derive from liver, bone, intestine, and placenta.

ALP isoenzymes may be partitioned by electrophoresis or by exploiting differences in physical properties on optimal substrates. Electrophoresis has been applied with only modest success. Hepatic and intestinal isoenzymes are easier to differentiate with this method than are hepatic and bone enzymes. Since hepatic ALP is more heat resistant than bone ALP, the most common way to differentiate between these two isoenzymes is by heating the serum to 56°C.

Evaluation of ALP isoenzymes usually focuses on measuring those of hepatic origin which are not affected by bone growth or pregnancy. These are 5' -nucleotidase, leucine aminopeptidase, and gamma glutamyl transpeptidase.

5'-Nucleotidase (5'-N) (Clinical Applications Data, p. 192)

5'-nucleotidase (5'-N), an isoenzyme of alkaline phosphatase, is a specific phosphomonoesterase formed in the hepatobiliary tissues. Elevated serum 5'-N levels are associated with biliary cirrhosis, carcinoma of the liver and biliary structures, and choledocholithiasis or other biliary obstruction.

Leucine Aminopeptidase (LAP) (Clinical Applications Data, p. 192)

Leucine aminopeptidase (LAP), an isoenzyme of alkaline phosphatase, is widely distributed in body tissues, with greatest concentrations found in hepatobiliary tissues, pancreas, and small intestine.

Elevated levels are associated with biliary obstruction due to gallstones, tumors including those of the head of the pancreas, strictures, and atresia. Advanced pregnancy and therapy with drugs containing estrogen and progesterone also may raise LAP levels.

Gamma Glutamyl Transpeptidase (GGT) (Clinical Applications Data, p. 193)

Gamma glutamyl transpeptidase (GGT), an isoenzyme of alkaline phosphatase, catalyzes the transfer of glutamyl groups among peptides and amino acids. Hepatobiliary tissues and renal tubular and pancreatic epithelium contain large amounts of GGT. Other sources include the prostate gland, brain, and heart.

Most GGT in serum derives from hepatobiliary sources, and elevated levels point to hepatobiliary disease. Pronounced elevations are seen with obstructive disorders of the hepatobiliary tract and in hepatocellular carcinoma. Modest elevations occur with hepatocellular degeneration (e.g., cirrhosis), and with pancreatic or renal cell damage or neoplasms. Other disorders associated with elevated GGT levels include congestive heart failure, acute myocardial infarction (after 4 to 10 days), hyperlipoproteinemia (type IV), diabetes mellitus with hypertension, and epilepsy.

Serum GGT levels also rise in response to ingestion of alcohol, barbiturates, and phenytoin. For this reason, serum GGT measurement is gaining clinical significance as an indicator of alcohol use. About 60 to 80 percent of individuals considered to have alcohol-abuse problems will have elevated GGT levels, whether or not other signs of liver damage are present.

Late pregnancy and oral contraceptives may produce lower than normal values.

Isocitrate Dehydrogenase (ICD) (Clinical Applications Data, p. 194)

Isocitrate dehydrogenase (ICD) catalyzes the decarboxylation of isocitrate in the Krebs cycle. This enzyme is important in controlling the rate of the cycle, which must be precisely adjusted to meet the energy needs of cells. ICD is found in the liver, heart, skeletal muscle, placenta, platelets, and erythrocytes.

Elevated levels are seen in early viral hepatitis, cancer of the liver, intrahepatic and extrahepatic obstruction, biliary atresia, cirrhosis, and pre-eclampsia. Hepatotoxic drugs also may cause elevated levels. Although ICD is found in the heart, serum levels usually are not elevated in acute myocardial infarction.

Ornithinecarbamoyl Transferase (OCT) (Clinical Applications Data, p. 195)

Ornithinecarbamoyl transferase (OCT), formerly known as ornithine transcarbamoylase, catalyzes ornithine to citrulline in the urea cycle prior to its link with the citric acid cycle. Its importance stems from its role in the conversion of ammonia to urea by the liver.

Elevated levels are seen in clients with viral hepatitis, cholecystitis, cirrhosis, cancer of the liver, obstructive jaundice, and mushroom poisoning. Hepatotoxic drugs and chemicals also may cause elevated levels. Decreased levels may be seen in inherited disorders associated with a partial block in the urea cycle.

Serum Amylase (Clinical Applications Data, p. 196)

Amylase is a digestive enzyme that splits starch into disaccharides such as maltose. Although many cells have amylase activity (e.g., liver, small intestine,

TABLE 5-19. Causes of Elevated Serum Amylase

Pronounced Elevation (5 or more times normal)
Acute pancreatitis
Pancreatic pseudocyst
Macrocmylasemia
Morphine administration

Moderate Elevation (3 to 5 times normal)
Advanced carcinoma of the head of the pancreas
Mumps
Parotitis
Perforated peptic ulcer (sometimes)
Duodenal obstruction

Mild Elevation (up to 3 times normal)
Chronic pancreatitis (nonadvanced)
Renal failure
Common bile duct obstruction
Gastric resection

Adapted from Widmann, FK: Clinical Interpretation of Laboratory Tests, ed 9. FA Davis, Philadelphia, 1983, p 298.

skeletal muscle, fallopian tubes), amylase circulating in normal serum derives from the parotid glands and the pancreas. Unlike many other enzymes, amylase activity is primarily extracellular; it is secreted into saliva and the duodenum where it splits large carbohydrate molecules into smaller units for further digestive action by intestinal enzymes.

Elevations in serum amylase are generally seen in pancreatic inflammations, which cause disruption of pancreatic cells and absorption of the extracellular enzyme from the intestine and peritoneal lymphatics. Serum amylase levels will also rise sharply following administration of drugs that constrict pancreatic duct sphincters. The most common offender is morphine, and this drug is never indicated for individuals with abdominal pain that could be of pancreatic or biliary tract origin. Other drugs that may produce elevated serum amylase levels are codeine, chlorthiazides, aspirin, pentazocine, corticosteroids, oral contraceptives, pancreozymin, and secretin. Specific causes of elevated serum amylase, and the magnitude of the elevations produced, are listed in Table 5-19.

Serum amylase levels are decreased in the presence of high blood glucose levels, which may be due to diabetes mellitus or to intravenous glucose infusions. Decreased levels also are seen in clients having disorders involving loss of functional pancreatic tissue such as advanced chronic pancreatitis and advanced cystic fibrosis. Liver disease, liver abscess, toxemia of pregnancy, severe burns, and cholecystitis also are associated with decreased serum amylase levels.

SERUM LIPASE (CLINICAL APPLICATIONS DATA, p. 197)

Lipases split triglycerides into fatty acids and glycerol. Different lipolytic enzymes have different specific substrates, but overall activity is collectively described as lipase. Serum lipase derives primarily from pancreatic lipase, which is secreted into the duodenum and participates in fat digestion. Pancreatic lipase is quite distinct from lipoprotein lipases, which clear the blood of chylomicrons after fats are absorbed.

Elevated serum lipase levels point more specifically to pancreatic inflammation and remain elevated longer than do serum amylase levels. Lipase is not excreted in the urine. Acute pancreatitis, early carcinoma of the pancreas, and obstruction of the pancreatic duct are associated with elevated serum lipase levels. Other possible sources of elevations include perforated peptic ulcer, acute cholecystitis, and early renal failure. Drugs that lead to elevated levels include morphine, cholinergic drugs, and heparin.

Serum lipase levels are decreased in disorders involving loss of functional pancreatic tissue such as advanced chronic pancreatitis, cystic fibrosis, and advanced carcinoma of the pancreas. Viral hepatitis and disorders in which bile salts are decreased also may produce low serum lipase levels, as will protamine and intravenous infusions of saline.

ACID PHOSPHATASE (ACP) (CLINICAL APPLICATIONS DATA, p. 198)

Phosphatases are enzymes that cleave phosphate from compounds with a single phosphate group. Those that are optimally active at pH 5 are grouped under the name "acid phosphatase" (ACP).

Many tissues (kidneys, spleen, liver, bone) contain acid phosphatase, but the prostate gland, red blood cells (RBCs), and platelets are especially rich in this activity. Two isoenzymes, prostatic fraction and RBC/platelet fraction, are diagnostically significant. These isoenzymes differ from one another in preferred substrate and in the degree to which they are inhibited by various additives during laboratory testing. Normal serum contains more RBC/platelet than prostatic ACP, and small changes in prostatic fraction may be difficult to detect. Tartaric acid inhibits prostatic ACP. Thus, many laboratories report tartrate-inhibitable ACP as well as total ACP, in an effort to focus more specifically on the prostatic fraction.

Prostatic ACP is elevated in 50 to 75 percent of individuals with prostatic carcinoma that has extended beyond the gland. Prostatic cancer usually metastasizes to bone, but intrapelvic extension may also elevate ACP values. Cancers that remain within the gland cause ACP elevation only in 10 to 25 percent of those affected. Other causes of elevated prostatic ACP include metastatic bone cancer, Paget's disease, osteogenesis imperfecta, hyperparathyroidism, and multiple myeloma. It should be noted that benign hyperplasia, inflammation, or ischemic damage to the prostate rarely cause elevated ACP levels. Decreased levels of prostatic ACP are seen after estrogen therapy for prostatic carcinoma and in clients with Down's syndrome.

RBC/platelet ACP may be elevated in those having Gaucher's disease, Niemann-Pick disease, hemolytic anemia, sickle cell crisis, thrombocytosis, acute myelogenous leukemia, renal insufficiency, and liver disease. Administration of androgens in females and of clofibrate in both sexes also will produce elevated levels. Decreased levels are associated with ingestion of alcohol, fluorides, oxalates, and phosphates.

ALDOLASE (CLINICAL APPLICATIONS DATA, p. 199)

Aldolase is a glycolytic enzyme that catalyzes the breakdown of 1,6-diphosphate into triose phosphate. It is found in many body tissues, but is most diagnostically significant in disorders of skeletal and cardiac muscle, liver, and pancreas. Three isoenzymes have been identified: A, originating in skeletal and cardiac muscle; B, originating in liver, kidneys, and white blood cells; and C, originating in brain tissue. Isoenzyme C probably lacks diagnostic capability because it does not cross the blood-brain barrier.

Pronounced elevations in aldolase levels are seen in disorders involving muscles such as Duchenne's muscular dystrophy, polymyositis, dermatomyositis, and trichinosis, and in severe crush injuries. Moderate increases are associated with acute hepatitis, neoplasms, and leukemias; a mild increase may be demonstrated in clients with acute myocardial infarction. Hepatotoxic drugs, insecticides, and antihelmintics also may cause elevations. It should be noted that aldolase is not elevated in those with multiple sclerosis or myasthenia gravis, both of which are of neural origin.

Decreased aldolase levels are seen in disorders in which muscle cells are lost such as late muscular dystrophy. Phenothiazines also may cause decreases.

CREATINE PHOSPHOKINASE (CPK) AND ISOENZYMES (CLINICAL APPLICATIONS DATA, p. 201)

Creatine phosphokinase (CPK), also called creatine kinase (CK), catalyzes the reversible exchange of phosphate between creatine and adenotriphosphate (ATP). Important in intracellular storage and release of energy, CPK exists almost exclusively in skeletal muscle, heart muscle, and, to a lesser extent, brain. No CPK is found in the liver. Anything that damages skeletal or cardiac muscle will elevate serum CPK levels. Brain injury affects serum CPK levels much less, probably because relatively little enzyme crosses the blood-brain barrier.

Spectacular CPK elevations occur in the early phases of muscular dystrophy, but CPK elevation diminishes as the disease progresses and muscle mass decreases. Levels of CPK may be normal to low in late, severe cases. Women heterozygous for the gene causing Duchenne's muscular dystrophy have, on the average, higher CPK levels than unaffected women, but this distinction is not sufficiently clear-cut to identify the carrier state reliably. Values two to four times normal also may follow such stimuli as prolonged vigorous exercise, deep intramuscular injections, delirium tremens, and surgical procedures in which muscle is transected or compressed.

Acute myocardial infarction releases CPK into the serum within the first 48 hours, and values return to normal in about 3 days. Recurrent elevation suggests reinfarction or extension of the ischemic damage, provided there is no other muscle source contributing to circulating CPK. An elevated serum CPK level helps to differentiate myocardial infarction from congestive heart failure and conditions associated with liver damage. Hypothyroidism also may cause high serum CPK levels. Additional causes of elevated CPK, and the magnitude of those elevations, are listed in Table 5–20.

The CPK molecule consists of two parts, which may be identical or dissimilar. These two constituent chains are called M (muscle) and B (brain). Three diagnostically significant isoenzymes have been identified in relation to the two main components of CPK. Brain CPK (CPK-BB, CPK_1) is almost entirely BB; cardiac CPK (CPK-MB, CPK_2) contains 60 percent MM and 40 percent MB; skeletal muscle CPK (CPK-MM, CPK_3) contains about 90 percent MM and 10 percent MB. The isoenzyme normally present in serum is almost entirely MM, and only CPK-MM (CPK_3) rises when skeletal muscle is damaged. In contrast, serum CPK-MB (CPK_2) rises only when heart muscle is damaged.

In the differential diagnosis of myocardial infarction, the presence of CPK-MB is a potent indicator of myocardial damage but not necessarily of myocardial infarction. Both total CPK and the MB fraction may rise in severe angina or extensive reversible ischemic damage. Absence of CPK-MB does not rule out infarction. There could have been damage to only a few cells, or blood supply near the damaged area might be so poor that the enzyme cannot enter the circulation. Elevated CPK-MB levels also may be missed if the study is done too late. The MB isoenzyme remains only briefly in the serum; it appears in the first 6 to 24 hours, and is usually gone in 72 hours.[30]

TABLE 5-20. Causes of Elevated Creatine Phosphokinase

Pronounced Elevation (5 or more times normal)
Early muscular dystrophy (CPK-MM, CPK_3)
Acute myocardial infarction (CPK-MB, CPK_2)
Severe angina (CPK-MB, CPK_2)
Polymyositis (CPK-MM, CPK_3)
Cardiac surgery

Moderate Elevation (2 to 4 times normal)
Vigorous exercise
Deep intramuscular injections
Surgical procedures affecting skeletal muscles
Delerium tremens
Convulsive seizures
Dermatomyositis
Alcoholic myopathy
Hypothyroidism
Pulmonary infarction
Acute agitated psychosis

Mild Elevations (up to 2 times normal)
Late pregnancy
Women heterozygous for the gene causing Duchenne's muscular dystrophy (CPK-MM, CPK_3)
Brain injury (CPK-BB, CPK_1)

Adapted from Widmann, FK: Clinical Interpretation of Laboratory Tests, ed 9. FA Davis, Philadelphia, 1983, p 300.

Drugs that may produce elevated CPK levels include anticoagulants, morphine, alcohol, salicylates in high doses, amphotericin-B, clofibrate, and certain anesthetics. Any medication administered intramuscularly also will elevate CPK. In addition to late muscular dystrophy, decreased levels are seen in early pregnancy.

LACTIC DEHYDROGENASE AND ISOENZYMES (LDH) (CLINICAL APPLICATIONS DATA, p. 202)

Lactic dehydrogenase (LDH) catalyzes the reversible conversion of lactic acid to pyruvic acid within cells. Because many tissues contain LDH, elevated total LDH is considered a nonspecific indication of cellular damage unless other clinical data make the tissue origin obvious. Pronounced elevations in total LDH are seen in clients with megaloblastic anemia, metastatic cancer (especially if the liver is involved), shock, hypoxia, hepatitis, and renal infarction. Moderate elevations occur in those with myocardial and pulmonary infarctions, hemolytic conditions, leukemias, infectious mononucleosis, delirium tremens, and muscular dystrophy. Mild elevations are associated with most liver diseases, nephrotic syndrome, hypothyroidism, and cholangitis.

The most useful diagnostic information is obtained by analyzing the five isoenzymes of LDH through electrophoresis. These isoenzymes are specific to certain tissues. The heart and erythroctes are rich sources of LDH_1 and LDH_2; however, the brain is a source of LDH_1, LDH_2, and LDH_3. The kidneys contain LDH_3 and LDH_4; the liver and skeletal muscle contain LDH_4 and LDH_5. Certain glands (thyroid, adrenal, and thymus), the pancreas, spleen, lungs, lymph nodes, and white blood cells contain LDH_3, whereas the ileum is an additional source of LDH_5.

Damage to the tissues rich in the several LDH isoenzymes will produce serum elevations accordingly. Myocardial infarction, for example, elevates LDH_1 and LDH_2. It should also be noted that pulmonary infarctions are associated with elevated LDH_3, LDH_4, and LDH_5.

Situations in which isoenzyme analysis is most useful include distinguishing myocardial infarction from lung or liver problems, diagnosing myocardial infarction in ambiguous settings such as the postoperative period or during severe shock, and in hemolysis at a time of bone marrow hypoplasia.

Normally, serum contains more LDH_2 than LDH_1. Damage to tissues rich in LDH_1, however, will cause this ratio to reverse. The reversed ratio (i.e., LDH_1 greater than LDH_2) is an important diagnostic finding that occurs whether or not total LDH is elevated. The reversal is short-lived. In myocardial infarction, for example, the LDH_1 to LDH_2 ratio returns to normal within a week of the

TABLE 5–21. LDH Isoenzymes: Tissue Sources and Common Causes of Elevations

Isoenzyme	Tissue Sources	Common Causes of Elevations
LDH_1	Heart Erythrocytes Brain	Acute myocardial infarction Red cell hemolysis Cerebrovascular accident Renal infarction Muscular dystrophy
LDH_2	Heart Erythrocytes Brain	Acute myocardial infarction Lymphoproliferative disorders Cerebrovascular accident Shock Muscular dystrophy
LDH_3	Brain Kidneys Glands (thyroid, adrenal, thymus) Pancreas Spleen Lungs Lymph nodes Leukocytes	Lymphoproliferative disorders Shock Infectious mononucleosis Acute pancreatitis Renal necrosis Pneumonia Pulmonary infarction
LDH_4	Liver Kidneys Skeletal muscles	Pulmonary infarction Pneumonia Shock Hepatitis Cirrhosis Pancreatitis Infectious mononucleosis Muscular dystrophy Acute glomerulonephritis Renal necrosis
LDH_5	Liver Ileum Skeletal muscles	Pulmonary infarction Hepatitis Cirrhosis Liver trauma Shock Infectious mononucleosis Dermatomyositis Muscular dystrophy

infarction even though total LDH may remain elevated.[31] The tissue sources of LDH isoenzymes and common causes of elevations are summarized in Table 5–21.

It should also be noted that numerous drugs may elevate LDH levels: anabolic steroids, anesthetics, aspirin, alcohol, fluorides, narcotics, clofibrate, mithramicin, and procainamide.

ALPHA-HYDROXYBUTYRIC DEHYDROGENASE (α-HBD, HBD) (CLINICAL APPLICATIONS DATA, p. 203)

Alpha-hydroxybutyric dehydrogenase (α-HBD, HBD) is an enzyme similar to two isoenzymes of lactic dehydrogenase (LDH): LDH_1 and LDH_2. The α-HBD test, however, is cheaper and easier to perform than LDH isoenzyme electrophoresis. Moreover, HBD levels remain elevated for 18 days following acute myocardial infarction, providing a diagnosis when the client has delayed seeking treatment or has not had classic signs and symptoms.

In addition to HBD elevations associated with acute myocardial infarction, increased levels are seen in clients with megaloblastic and hemolytic anemias, leukemias, lymphomas, melanomas, muscular dystrophy, nephrotic syndrome, and acute hepatocellular disease.

CHOLINESTERASES (CLINICAL APPLICATIONS DATA, p. 204)

Cholinesterases hydrolyze concentrated acetylcholine and also cleave other choline esters. Two types of cholinesterase are measured: (1) acetylcholinesterase ("true" cholinesterase) and (2) pseudocholinesterase. Acetylcholinesterase (AcCHS) is found at nerve endings and in erythrocytes; very little is found in the serum. Its substrate specificity is limited to acetylcholine and it is optimally active against very low concentrations of it. Pseudocholinesterase (CHS) derives from the liver and is normally found in the serum in substantial amounts. It is active against acetylcholine and other choline esters. CHS is unusual in that diagnostically significant change is depression, not elevation.

Both cholinesterases are inhibited by organophosphorus compounds. Declining CHS levels offer a sensitive index of exposure to organic phosphate insecticides. Red cell AcCHS levels decline with severe exposure; serum CHS changes occur early. When exposure ceases, serum CHS rises before red cell AcCHS returns to normal. Serum CHS is less useful than red cell AcCHS in indicating prior exposure.

CHS levels also decline in clients hepatocellular diseases, especially acutely destructive processes, but CHS measurement contributes little to the overall evaluation of such problems and is not used to diagnose them.

An important application of information about CHS is in evaluating individuals for genetic variations of the enzyme prior to surgery in which succinylcholine, an inhibitor of acetycholine, is to be used to induce anesthesia. Persons homozygous for the abnormal form of CHS have depressed total serum activity and their enzyme does not inactivate succinylcholine; persons who receive the drug during surgery may experience prolonged respiratory depression. Presence of the abnormal form is determined by exposing the enzyme to dibucaine. Normal CHS is inhibited by dibucaine, while the abnormal CHS is found to be "dibucaine-resistant."[32]

RENIN (CLINICAL APPLICATIONS DATA, p. 205)

Renin is an enzyme released by the juxtoglomerular apparatus of the kidney in response to decreased extracellular fluid volume, serum sodium, and renal perfusion pressure. It catalyzes the conversion of angiotensinogen, produced by the liver, to angiotensin I. Angiotensin I is then converted to angiotensin II in the lungs. Angiotensin II elevates systemic blood pressure by causing vasoconstriction and by stimulating the release of aldosterone.

Elevated renin levels are seen in renovascular and malignant hypertension, hypovolemia, adrenal hypofunction (Addison's disease), salt-wasting disorders, end-stage renal disease, renin-producing renal tumors, and secondary hyperaldosteronism. Decreased levels are associated with primary hyperaldosteronism, hypervolemia, excessive salt ingestion or retention, excessive adrenocortical steroid levels due to either disease or drug therapy, and excessive licorice ingestion. Renin levels may be high, low, or normal in those having essential hypertension.

Renin released by the kidneys is found initially in the renal veins. Thus, the output of renin by each kidney may be determined by obtaining samples directly from the right and left renal veins and comparing the results with that obtained from an inferior vena cava sample. This test is indicated when renal artery stenosis is suspected, as the kidney affected by decreased perfusion will release higher amounts of renin. Renal vein assay for renin is performed using fluoroscopy and involves cannulation of the femoral vein and injection of dye to aid in visualizing the renal veins. Because this is an invasive procedure, a signed consent is required.

Clinical Application Data

ALANINE AMINOTRANSFERASE **(ALT, SGPT)** (BACKGROUND INFORMATION, p. 179)

Reference Values

10–30 IU/ml
1–36 U/ml
5–35 Sigma Frankel U/ml
5–25 mU/ml–Wroblewski
8–50 mU/ml at 30°C–Karmen
4–36 U/l at 37°C (SI units)

Reference values vary among laboratories and according to the method used for reporting results.

Interfering Factors

■ Numerous drugs, including alcohol, may falsely elevate levels

Indications/Purposes for Alanine Aminotransferase

■ Known liver disease or liver damage due to hepatotoxic drugs
  □ Markedly elevated levels (sometimes as high as 20 times normal) are considered confirmatory of liver disease
  □ A sudden drop in serum ALT levels in the presence of acute illness after extreme elevation of blood levels (e.g., as seen in severe viral or toxic hepatitis) is an ominous sign and indicates that so many cells have been damaged that no additional source of enzyme remains

■ Monitoring response to treatment for liver disease, with tissue repair indicated by gradually declining levels

Client Preparation

General client preparation is the same as that for any study involving collection of a peripheral blood sample (see Appendix I). For this test, the client should abstain from alcohol for at least 24 hours prior to the study.

Because many drugs may alter ALT levels, a medication history should be obtained. It is recommended that drugs that may alter test results be withheld for 12 hours prior to the test, although this should be confirmed with the person ordering the study.

The Procedure

A venipuncture is performed and the sample is collected in a red-topped tube. The sample should be handled gently to avoid hemolysis and transported promptly to the laboratory.

Aftercare and Nursing Observations

Care and assessment following the procedure are the same as for any study involving the collection of a peripheral blood sample. Any drugs withheld prior to the test should be resumed.

ASPARTATE AMINOTRANSFERASE (AST, SGOT) (BACKGROUND INFORMATION, p. 179)

Reference Values

Newborn	16–72 U/l
6 months	20–43 U/l
1 year	16–35 U/l
5 years	19–28 U/l
Adult men	8–46 U/l
Adult women	7–34 U/l

Interfering Factors

■ Numerous drugs may falsely elevate levels

Indications/Purposes for Aspartate Aminotransferase

■ Suspected disorders or injuries involving the liver, myocardium, kidneys, pancreas or brain, with elevated levels indicating cellular damage to tissues in which AST is normally found (see Table 5–17, p. 180)
  □ In myocardial infarction, AST rises within 6 to 8 hours, peaks at 24 to 48 hours, and declines to normal within 72 to 96 hours
■ Monitoring response to therapy with potentially hepatotoxic or nephrotoxic drugs
■ Monitoring response to treatment for various disorders in which AST may be elevated, with tissue repair indicated by declining levels

Client Preparation

General client preparation is the same as that for any study involving collection of a peripheral blood sample (see Appendix I).

Because many drugs alter AST levels, a medication history should be obtained. It is recommended that any drugs that may alter test results be withheld for 12 hours prior to the test, although this should be confirmed with the person ordering the study.

The Procedure

A venipuncture is performed and the sample is collected in a red-topped tube. The sample should be handled gently to avoid hemolysis and transported promptly to the laboratory.

Aftercare and Nursing Observations

Care and assessment following the procedure are the same as that for any study involving the collection of a peripheral blood sample. Any drugs withheld prior to the test should be resumed, pending test results.

ALKALINE PHOSPHATE (ALP) (BACKGROUND INFORMATION, p. 179)
Reference Values

General Reference Levels	
Newborn	50–65 U/l
Child	20–150 U/l
Adult	20–90 U/l

	Bessey-Lowry Method	Bodansky Method	King-Armstrong Method
Child	3.4–9.0 U/ml	5–14 U/dl	15–30 U/dl
Adult	0.8–2.3 U/ml	1.5–4.5 U/dl	4–13 U/dl

Interfering Factors

■ Numerous drugs, including intravenous albumin, may falsely elevate levels
■ Clofibrate, Imuran, and fluorides may falsely decrease levels

Indications/Purposes for Serum Alkaline Phosphatase

■ Signs and symptoms of various disorders associated with elevated ALP levels (e.g., biliary obstruction, hepatobiliary disease, bone disease including malignant processes) (see also Table 5–18, p. 181)
■ Differentiation of obstructive biliary disorders from hepatocellular disease, with greater elevations of ALP seen in the former
■ Known renal disease to determine effects on bone metabolism
■ Signs of growth retardation in children

Client Preparation

Client preparation is the same as that for any test involving collection of a peripheral blood sample (see Appendix I). As many drugs may alter ALP levels, a medication history should be obtained.

The Procedure

A venipuncture is performed and the sample collected in a red-topped tube. The sample should be handled gently to avoid hemolysis and transported promptly to the laboratory.

Aftercare and Nursing Observations

Care and assessment following the procedure are the same as for any study involving the collection of a peripheral blood sample.

5'-NUCLEOTIDASE (5'-N) (BACKGROUND INFORMATION, p. 181)

Reference Values

0–1.6 U
0.3–3.2 Bodansky U

Indications/Purposes for 5'-Nucleotidase

■ Elevated alkaline phosphatase of uncertain etiology
  □ Elevated 5'-N levels support the diagnosis of hepatobiliary disorders as the source of the elevated alkaline phosphatase
  □ Normal levels support the diagnosis of bone disease as the source of the elevated alkaline phosphatase

Client Preparation

Client preparation is the same as that for any test involving collection of a peripheral blood sample (see Appendix I).

The Procedure

A venipuncture is performed and the sample collected in a red-topped tube. The sample should be handled gently to avoid hemolysis and transported promptly to the laboratory.

Aftercare and Nursing Observations

Care and assessment following the procedure are the same as for any study involving the collection of a peripheral blood sample.

LEUCINE AMINOPEPTIDASE (LAP) (BACKGROUND INFORMATION, p. 181)

Reference Values

Male	80–200 U/ml
Female	75–185 U/ml

Values may vary depending on the units of measure used by the laboratory performing the test.

Interfering Factors

■ Advanced pregnancy and therapy with drugs containing estrogen and progesterone may falsely elevate levels

Indications/Purposes for Leucine Aminopeptidase

■ Elevated alkaline phosphatase of uncertain etiology
  □ Elevated levels support the diagnoses of hepatobiliary and/or pancreatic disease as the source of the elevated alkaline phosphatase
  □ Normal levels support the diagnosis of bone disease as the source of the elevated alkaline phosphatase

Client Preparation

Client preparation is the same as that for any test involving collection of a peripheral blood sample (see Appendix I). Some laboratories require the client to fast from food for 8 hours prior to the test.

The Procedure

A venipuncture is performed and the sample collected in a red-topped tube. The sample should be handled gently to avoid hemolysis and transported promptly to the laboratory.

Aftercare and Nursing Observations

Care and assessment following the procedure are the same as for any study involving the collection of a peripheral blood sample. Any food withheld prior to the test should be resumed.

GAMMA GLUTAMYL TRANSPEPTIDASE (GGT) (BACKGROUND INFORMATION, p. 182)

Reference Values

Men	6–37 U/l
Women over age 45	6–37 U/l
Women under age 45	5–27 U/l

Interfering Factors

■ Alcohol, barbiturates, and phenytoin may elevate GGT levels
■ Late pregnancy and oral contraceptives may produce lower than normal values

Indications/Purposes for Gamma Glutamyl Transpeptidase

■ Elevated alkaline phosphatase of uncertain etiology
  □ Pronounced elevations are seen in clients with obstructive disorders of the hepatobiliary tract and hepatocellular carcinoma

☐ Modest elevations occur with hepatocellular degeneration (e.g., cirrhosis) and with pancreatic or renal cell damage or neoplasms

☐ Other disorders associated with elevated GGT levels include congestive heart failure, acute myocardial infarction (after 4 to 10 days), hyperlipoproteinemia (type IV), diabetes mellitus with hypertension, and epilepsy

☐ Normal levels in the presence of elevated alkaline phosphatase support the diagnosis of bone disease

■ Known or suspected alcohol abuse, including monitoring individuals participating in alcohol-abstinence programs

☐ About 60 to 80 percent of individuals considered to have alcohol-abuse problems will have elevated GGT levels, whether or not other signs of liver damage are present

☐ Moderate increases in GGT levels occur with low alcohol intake

☐ A significant sustained rise occurs with ingestion of six or more drinks per day

☐ Normal levels return within 2 to 6 weeks of abstinence from alcohol

Client Preparation

Client preparation is essentially the same as that for any test involving collection of a peripheral blood sample (see Appendix I). Some laboratories require the client to fast from food for 8 hours prior to the test.

When the test is done to determine if the liver is the source of elevated alkaline phosphatase, the client should abstain from alcohol for 2 to 3 weeks prior to the test. This restriction may not apply when the test is used to monitor compliance with alcohol-abstinence programs. The client's reported intake (or nonintake) of alcohol should, however, be noted.

The Procedure

A venipuncture is performed and the sample collected in a red-topped tube. The sample should be handled gently to avoid hemolysis and transported promptly to the laboratory.

Aftercare and Nursing Observations

Care and assessment following the procedure are the same as that for any study involving the collection of a peripheral blood sample. Any food withheld prior to the test should be resumed.

ISOCITRATE DEHYDROGENASE (ICD) (BACKGROUND INFORMATION, p. 182)

Reference Values

Neonate	4–28 U/l
Adult	1.2–7 U/l

Interfering Factors

■ Numerous drugs, including those that are hepatotoxic, may cause elevated levels

Indications/Purposes for Isocitrate Dehydrogenase

■ Elevated serum aspartate aminotransferase (ALT, SGOT) and/or alkaline phosphatase of uncertain etiology
  □ Elevated ICD levels are seen in early viral hepatitis, cancer of the liver, intrahepatic and extrahepatic obstruction, biliary atresia, cirrhosis, and pre-eclampsia
■ Therapy with potentially hepatotoxic drugs which may lead to elevated ICD levels early in the course of treatment

Client Preparation

General client preparation is the same as that for any study involving collection of a peripheral blood sample (see Appendix I).

Because many drugs may alter ICD levels, a medication history should be obtained. It is recommended that any drugs that may alter test results be withheld for 24 hours prior to the test, although this should be confirmed with the person ordering the study.

The Procedure

A venipuncture is performed and the sample collected in a red-topped tube. The sample should be handled gently to avoid hemolysis and transported promptly to the laboratory.

Aftercare and Nursing Observations

Care and assessment following the procedure are the same as for any study involving the collection of a peripheral blood sample. Any drugs withheld prior to the test should be resumed, pending test results.

ORNITHINECARBAMOYL TRANSFERASE (OCT) (BACKGROUND INFORMATION, p. 182)

Reference Values

0–500 Sigma Units
8–20 mIU/ml
8–20 U/l

Interfering Factors

■ Hepatotoxic drugs and chemicals may produce elevated levels

Indications/Purposes for Ornithinecarbamoyl Transferase

■ Elevated serum alkaline phosphatase (ALP) of uncertain etiology
  □ Elevated OCT levels are seen in viral hepatitis, cholecystitis, cirrhosis, cancer of the liver, and obstructive jaundice
■ Therapy with hepatotoxic drugs or exposure to hepatotoxic chemicals, with early effects indicated by elevated OCT levels
■ Suspected mushroom poisoning as indicated by elevated levels

Client Preparation

General client preparation is the same as that for any study involving collection of a peripheral blood sample (see Appendix I).

Because many drugs may alter OCT levels, a medication history should be obtained. It is recommended that any drugs that may alter test results be withheld for 24 hours prior to the test, although this should be confirmed with the person ordering the study.

The Procedure

A venipuncture is performed and the sample collected in a red-topped tube. The sample should be handled gently to avoid hemolysis and transported promptly to the laboratory.

Aftercare and Nursing Observations

Care and assessment following the procedure are the same as for any study involving the collection of a peripheral blood sample. Any drugs withheld prior to the test should be resumed, pending test results.

SERUM AMYLASE (BACKGROUND INFORMATION, p. 182)
Reference Values

Children	60–160 Somogyi U/dl
	111–296 SIU/l
Adults	80–180 Somogyi U/dl
	45–200 dye U/dl

Values may vary according to the laboratory performing the test.

Interfering Factors

■ A number of drugs may produce elevated levels (e.g., morphine, codeine, chlorthiazides, aspirin, pentazocine, corticosteroids, oral contraceptives, pancreozymin, and secretin)
■ High blood glucose levels, which may be due to diabetes mellitus or intravenous glucose solutions, may lead to decreased levels

Indications/Purposes for Serum Amylase

■ Diagnosis of early acute pancreatitis
  □ Serum amylase begins rising within 6 to 24 hours after onset and returns to normal in 2 to 7 days
  □ Urine amylase levels may remain elevated for several days after serum amylase levels return to normal
■ Detection of blunt trauma or inadvertent surgical trauma to the pancreas as indicated by elevated levels
■ Diagnosis of macroamylasemia, a disorder seen in alcoholism, malabsorption syndrome, and other digestive problems in which there are circulating complexes of amylase and high molecular weight dextran (findings include high serum amylase and negative urine amylase)

■ Support for diagnosing other disorders associated with elevated serum amylase levels (see Table 5–19, p. 183)
■ Support for diagnosing disorders associated with decreased amylase levels such as advanced chronic pancreatitis, advanced cystic fibrosis, liver disease, liver abscess, toxemia of pregnancy, severe burns, and cholecystitis

Client Preparation

General client preparation is the same as that for any study involving collection of a peripheral blood sample (see Appendix I).

As many drugs may alter serum amylase levels, a medication history should be obtained. It is recommended that any drugs that may alter test results be withheld for 12 to 24 hours prior to the test, although this should be confirmed with the person ordering the study.

The Procedure

A venipuncture is performed and the sample collected in a red-topped tube. The sample should be handled gently to avoid hemolysis and transported promptly to the laboratory.

Aftercare and Nursing Observations

Care and assessment following the procedure are the same as for any study involving the collection of a peripheral blood sample. Any drugs withheld prior to the test should be resumed, pending test results.

SERUM LIPASE (BACKGROUND INFORMATION, p. 183)

Reference Values

Infants	9–105 IU/l at 37°C
Children	20–136 IU/l at 37°C
Adults	0–1.5 U/ml (Cherry-Crandall)
	14–280 mIU/ml
	14–280 SIU/l

Values may vary according to the laboratory performing the test.

Interfering Factors

■ Morphine, cholinergic drugs, and heparin may lead to elevated levels
■ Protamine and intravenous infusions of saline may lead to decreased levels

Indications/Purposes for Serum Lipase

■ Diagnosis of acute pancreatitis, especially if the client has been ill for more than 3 days
  □ Serum amylase levels may return to normal after 3 days, but serum lipase remains elevated for approximately 10 days after onset
■ Support for diagnosing pancreatic carcinoma, especially if there is a sustained moderate elevation in serum lipase levels

■ Support for diagnosing other disorders associated with elevated serum lipase levels (e.g., peptic ulcer, acute cholecystitis, and early renal failure)
■ Support for diagnosing disorders associated with decreased serum lipase levels (e.g., advanced chronic pancreatitis, cystic fibrosis, advanced carcinoma of the pancreas, and viral hepatitis)

Client Preparation

Client preparation is the same as that for any test involving collection of a peripheral blood sample (see Appendix I). The client should fast from food for at least 8 hours prior to the test.

It is recommended that drugs that may alter test results be withheld for 12 to 24 hours prior to the test, although this should be confirmed with the person ordering the study.

The Procedure

A venipuncture is performed and the sample collected in a red-topped tube. The sample should be handled gently to avoid hemolysis and transported promptly to the laboratory.

Aftercare and Nursing Observations

Care and assessment following the procedure are the same as for any study involving the collection of a peripheral blood sample. Food and any drugs withheld prior to the test should be resumed.

ACID PHOSPHATASE (ACP) (BACKGROUND INFORMATION, p. 184)

Reference Values

Newborn	10.4–16.4 U/ml (King-Armstrong)
1 month–13 years	0.5–11.0 U/ml (King-Armstrong)
	6.4–15.2 U/l
Adults	0–6 U/ml (Shinowara-Jones-Reinhart)
	0–0.8 IU/l (SI Units)
	0.1–2.0 U/dl (Gutman)
	0.5–2.0 U/dl (Bodansky)
	0.1–5.0 U/dl (King-Armstrong)
	0.1–0.8 U/dl (Bessey-Lowry)
	0–0.56 U/ml (Roy)

Interfering Factors

■ Prostatic massage or rectal examination within 48 hours of the test may cause elevated levels
■ Administration of androgens in females and of clofibrate in either sex may produce elevated levels
■ Ingestion of alcohol, fluorides, oxalates, and phosphates may result in decreased levels

Indications/Purposes for Serum Acid Phosphatase

■ Enlarged prostate gland, especially if prostatic carcinoma is suspected
  ☐ Prostatic ACP is elevated in 50 to 75 percent of individuals with prostatic carcinoma that has extended beyond the gland
  ☐ Cancers that remain within the gland cause ACP elevation in only 10 to 25 percent of those affected
  ☐ Benign hyperplasia, inflammation, or ischemic damage to the prostate rarely causes elevated ACP levels
■ Evaluation of the effectiveness of treatment of prostatic carcinoma
  ☐ ACP levels fall to normal within 3 to 4 days of successful estrogen therapy
  ☐ Recurrent elevation strongly suggests that bone metastases are active
■ Support for diagnosing other disorders associated with elevated prostatic ACP levels (e.g., metastatic bone cancer, Paget's disease, osteogenesis imperfecta, hyperparathyroidism, and multiple myeloma)
■ Known or suspected hematologic disorder
  ☐ Elevated RBC/platelet ACP is seen in hemolytic anemia, sickle cell crisis, thrombocytosis, and acute leukemia
  ☐ Support for diagnosing other disorders associated with increased RBC/platelet ACP (e.g., renal insufficiency, liver disease, Gaucher's disease, and Niemann-Pick disease)

Client Preparation

Client preparation is the same as that for any test involving collection of a peripheral blood sample (see Appendix I).

It is recommended that any drugs that may alter test results be withheld for 12 to 24 hours prior to the test, although this should be confirmed with the person ordering the study.

The Procedure

A venipuncture is performed and the sample collected in a red-topped tube. The sample should be handled gently to avoid hemolysis and transported promptly to the laboratory. If the test cannot be performed within a few hours, the serum should be frozen.

Aftercare and Nursing Observations

Care and assessment following the procedure are the same as for any study involving the collection of a peripheral blood sample. Any drugs withheld prior to the test should be resumed.

ALDOLASE (BACKGROUND INFORMATION, p. 184)

Reference Values

Newborns	5.2–32.8 U/dl (Sibley-Lehninger)
Children	2.6–16.4 U/dl (Sibley-Lehninger)
Adult	1.3–8.2 U/dl (Sibley-Lehninger)
Men	3.1–7.5 IU at 37°C
Women	2.7–5.3 IU at 37°C

Interfering Factors

- Hepatotoxic drugs, insecticides, and antihelminthics may cause elevated levels
- Phenothiazines may cause decreased levels

Indications/Purposes for Aldolase

- Family history of Duchenne's muscular dystrophy
  - ☐ Aldolase levels rise before clinical signs appear, thus permitting early diagnosis
- Signs and symptoms of neuromuscular disorders, to differentiate muscular disorders from neurological disorders
  - ☐ Pronounced elevations are seen in clients having Duchenne's muscular dystrophy, polymyositis, dermatomyositis, trichinosis, and severe crush injuries
  - ☐ Decreased aldolase levels are seen in those with late muscular dystrophy, owing to loss of muscle cells
  - ☐ Aldolase is not elevated in those with multiple sclerosis or myasthenia gravis, both of which are of neural origin
- Support for diagnosing other disorders associated with elevated aldolase levels
  - ☐ Moderate increases are associated with acute hepatitis, neoplasms, and leukemia
  - ☐ Mild elevations are seen in acute myocardial infarction (peak elevation occurs in 24 hours, with gradual return to normal within 1 week)
- Evaluating response to exposure to hepatotoxic drugs or chemicals, with liver damage indicated by elevated levels

Client Preparation

Client preparation is the same as that for any test involving collection of a peripheral blood sample (see Appendix I).

It is recommended that drugs that may alter test results be withheld for 12 to 24 hours prior to the test, although this should be confirmed with the person ordering the study.

The Procedure

A venipuncture is performed and the sample collected in a red-topped tube. The sample should be handled gently to avoid hemolysis and transported promptly to the laboratory.

Aftercare and Nursing Observations

Care and assessment following the procedure are the same as for any study involving the collection of a peripheral blood sample. Any drugs withheld prior to the test should be resumed.

CREATININE PHOSPHOKINASE (CPK) AND ISOENZYMES (BACKGROUND INFORMATION, p. 185)

Reference Values

Total CPK	
Newborns	10–300 IU/l
	30–100 U/l
Children	15–50 U/l
Adult Men	5–55 U/ml
	20–50 IU/l
	55–170 U/l (SI Units)
	5–35 µg/ml
Adult Women	5–25 U/ml
	10–37 IU/l
	30–135 U/l (SI Units)
	5–25 µg/ml
Isoenzymes	
CPK-BB (CPK$_1$)	0
CPK-MB (CPK$_2$)	0–7 IU/l
CPK-MM (CPK$_3$)	5–70 IU/l

Interfering Factors

- Vigorous exercise, deep intramuscular injections, delirium tremens, and surgical procedures in which muscle is transected or compressed may produce elevated levels
- Drugs that may produce elevated CPK levels include anticoagulants, morphine, alcohol, salicylates in high doses, amphotericin-B, clofibrate, and certain anesthetics
- Early pregnancy may produce decreased levels

Indications/Purposes for Creatine Phosphokinase and Isoenzymes

- Signs and symptoms of acute myocardial infarction
  - ☐ Acute myocardial infarction releases CPK into the serum within the first 48 hours and values return to normal in about 3 days
  - ☐ CPK levels rise before aspartate aminotransferase (AST, SGOT) and lactic dehydrogenase (LDH) levels rise
  - ☐ The isoenzyme CPK-MB (CPK$_2$) rises only when the heart muscle is damaged; it appears in the first 6 to 24 hours and is usually gone in 72 hours
  - ☐ Both total CPK and the MB fraction may rise in severe angina or extensive reversible ischemic damage
  - ☐ Recurrent elevation of CPK suggests reinfarction or extension of ischemic damage
  - ☐ An elevated CPK level helps to differentiate myocardial infarction from congestive heart failure and conditions associated with liver damage
- Family history of Duchenne's muscular dystrophy
  - ☐ Spectacular CPK elevations occur in the early phases of muscular dystrophy, even before clinical signs or symptoms appear
  - ☐ CPK elevation diminishes as the disease progresses and muscle mass decreases

■ Signs and symptoms of other disorders associated with elevated CPK levels (see Table 5–20, p. 186)

Client Preparation

Client preparation is the same as that for any test involving collection of a peripheral blood sample (see Appendix I).

It is recommended that any drugs that may alter test results be withheld for 12 to 24 hours prior to the test, although this should be confirmed with the person ordering the study. Vigorous exercise and intramuscular injections also should be avoided for 24 hours before the test.

The Procedure

A venipuncture is performed and the sample collected in a red-topped tube. The sample should be handled gently to avoid hemolysis and transported promptly to the laboratory.

Aftercare and Nursing Observations

Care and assessment following the procedure are the same as that for any study involving the collection of a peripheral blood sample. Any drugs withheld prior to the test, as well as usual activities, may be resumed unless otherwise ordered by the physician.

LACTIC DEHYDROGENASE (LDH) AND ISOENZYMES (BACKGROUND INFORMATION, p. 186)

Reference Values

Total LDH	80–120 U (Wacker)
	71–207 IU/l
	150–450 U (Wroblewski)
LDH Isoenzymes	
LDH_1	29–37%
LDH_2	42–48%
LDH_3	16–20%
LDH_4	2–4%
LDH_5	0.5–1.5%

Values may vary according to the laboratory performing the test.

Interfering Factors

■ Numerous drugs may produce elevated LDH levels (e.g., anabolic steroids, anesthetics, aspirin, alcohol, fluorides, narcotics, clofibrate, mithramicin, and procainamide)

Indications/Purposes for Lactic Dehydrogenase (LDH) and Isoenzymes

■ Confirmation of acute myocardial infarction or extension thereof, as indicated by elevation (usually) of total LDH, elevation of LDH_1 and LDH_2, and reversal of the LDH_1:LDH_2 ratio within 48 hours of the infarction

■ Differentiation of acute myocardial infarction from pulmonary infarction and liver problems, which elevate LDH_4 and LDH_5
■ Confirmation of red cell hemolysis or renal infarction, especially as indicated by reversal of the $LDH_1:LDH_2$ ratio
■ Confirmation of chronicity in liver, lung, and kidney disorders, as evidenced by LDH levels that remain persistently high
■ Evaluation of the effectiveness of cancer chemotherapy (LDH levels should fall with successful treatment)
■ Evaluation of the degree of muscle wasting in muscular dystrophy (LDH levels rise early in this disorder and approach normal as muscle mass is reduced by atrophy)
■ Signs and symptoms of other disorders associated with elevation of the several LDH isoenzymes (see Table 5–21, p. 187)

Client Preparation

Client preparation is the same as that for any test involving collection of a peripheral blood sample (see Appendix I).

It is recommended that drugs that may alter test results be withheld for 12 to 24 hours prior to the test, although this should be confirmed with the person ordering the study.

The Procedure

A venipuncture is performed and the sample collected in a red-topped tube. The sample should be handled gently to avoid hemolysis and transported promptly to the laboratory.

Aftercare and Nursing Observations

Care and assessment following the procedure are the same as for any study involving the collection of a peripheral blood sample. Any drugs withheld prior to the test should be resumed.

ALPHA-HYDROXYBUTYRIC DEHYDROGENASE (α-HBD, HBD) (BACKGROUND INFORMATION, p. 188)

Reference Values

70–300 IU/l
140–350 U/ml
Values may vary according to the laboratory performing the test.

Indications/Purposes for Alpha-Hydroxybutyric Dehydrogenase

■ Suspected "silent" myocardial infarction or otherwise atypical myocardial infarction in which the client delayed seeking care
  □ HBD levels remain elevated for 18 days following acute myocardial infarction (i.e., when other cardiac enzymes have returned to normal levels)
■ Support for diagnosing other disorders associated with elevated HBD levels (e.g., megaloblastic and hemolytic anemias, leukemias, lymphomas, melanomas, muscular dystrophy, nephrotic syndrome, and acute hepatocellular disease)

Client Preparation

Client preparation is the same as that for any test involving collection of a peripheral blood sample (see Appendix I).

The Procedure

A venipuncture is performed and the sample collected in a red-topped tube. The sample should be handled gently to avoid hemolysis and transported promptly to the laboratory.

Aftercare and Nursing Observations

Care and assessment following the procedure are the same as for any study involving the collection of a peripheral blood sample.

CHOLINESTERASES (BACKGROUND INFORMATION, p. 188)

Reference Values

Acetylcholinesterase (AcCHS)	0.5–1.0 pH units
Pseudocholinesterase (CHS)	0.5–1.3 pH units
Men	274–532 IU/dl
Women	204–500 IU/dl

Interfering Factors

■ Numerous drugs may falsely decrease cholinesterase levels (e.g., caffeine, theophylline, quinidine, quinine, barbiturates, morphine, codeine, atropine, epinephrine, phenothiazines, folic acid, and vitamin K)

Indications/Purposes for Cholinesterase Determinations

■ Suspected exposure to organic phosphate insecticides
  □ Red cell AcCHS levels decline with severe exposure; serum CHS decreases occur earlier
  □ When exposure ceases, serum CHS rises before red cell AcCHS returns to normal
  □ Red cell AcCHS levels are more useful than serum CHS levels in determining prior exposure
■ Impending use of succinylcholine during anesthesia
  □ Persons homozygous for the abnormal form of CHS have depressed total serum activity and their enzyme does not inactivate succinylcholine, with the abnormal CHS indicated as "dibucaine-resistant"

Client Preparation

Client preparation is the same as that for any study involving collection of a peripheral blood sample (see Appendix I).

As many drugs may alter cholinesterase levels and activity, a medication history should be obtained. It is recommended that those drugs that may alter test results be withheld for 12 to 24 hours prior to the test, although this should be confirmed with the person ordering the study.

The Procedure

A venipuncture is performed and the sample collected in a red-topped tube. The sample should be handled gently to avoid hemolysis and transported promptly to the laboratory.

Aftercare and Nursing Observations

Care and assessment following the procedure are the same as for any study involving the collection of a peripheral blood sample. Any medications withheld prior to the test should be resumed.

RENIN (BACKGROUND INFORMATION, p. 188)

Reference Values

Peripheral vein	0.4–4.5 ng/ml/hr (normal salt intake, upright position)
	1.5–1.6 ng/ml/hr or more (normal salt intake, recumbent position)
Renal vein assay	Difference between each renal sample and the vena cava sample should be <1.4–1.

Values for peripheral vein samples should be substantially higher (e.g., 2.9–24 ng/ml/hr) in clients who are sodium depleted and in the upright position. These values also may vary according to the laboratory performing the test.

Interfering Factors

■ Failure to follow dietary restrictions, if ordered, prior to the test
■ Failure to take prescribed diuretics, if ordered, prior to the test
■ Failure to maintain required positioning (e.g., upright versus recumbent) for at least 2 hours prior to the test
■ High-dose adrenocortical steroid therapy, excessive salt intake, and excessive licorice ingestion may produce decreased levels

Indications/Purposes for Renin

■ Assessment of renin production by the kidneys when client has hypertension of unknown etiology or when other disorders associated with altered renin levels are suspected
  □ Elevated renin levels are seen in renovascular and malignant hypertension, adrenal hypofunction (Addison's disease), salt-wasting disorders, end-stage renal disease, renin-producing renal tumors, and secondary hyperaldosteronism
  □ Decreased levels are associated with primary hyperaldosteronism, hypervolemia, excessive salt ingestion or retention, excessive adrenocortical steroid levels due to either disease or drug therapy, and excessive licorice ingestion
  □ Renin levels may be high, low, or normal in essential hypertension
  □ In primary hyperaldosteronism, plasma renin levels are decreased, even with salt depletion prior to the test (results should be evaluated in relation to the serum aldosterone level, which is elevated in primary hyperaldosteronism)
■ Suspected renal artery stenosis as the cause of hypertension, as indicated by renal vein output of renin by the affected kidney more than 1.4 times that of the vena cava sample

---

Nursing Alert

■ The renal vein assay for renin should be performed with extreme caution, if at all, in clients with allergies or previous exposure to radiographical dyes

---

Client Preparation

Client preparation varies according to the method for obtaining the sample and factors to be controlled (e.g., salt-depletion).

1. *Peripheral Vein, Normal Salt Intake.* Client preparation is essentially the same as that for any test involving collection of a peripheral blood sample. The client should follow a normal diet with adequate salt and potassium intake. Licorice intake and certain medications may be restricted for 2 weeks or more prior to the test, although this should be confirmed with the person ordering the study. The position relevant to the type of sample (e.g., upright versus recumbent) should be maintained for 2 hours prior to the test.
2. *Peripheral Vein, Sodium-Depleted.* Client preparation is the same as just described, except that a diuretic is administered for 3 days prior to the study and dietary sodium is limited to "no added salt" (approximately 3 g per day). Sample menus should be provided. The purpose of the diuretic therapy and sodium restriction should be explained, and client understanding and ability to follow pretest preparation ascertained.
3. *Renal Vein Assay*

   Client Teaching. Explain to the client:

■ the purpose of the study
■ that a "no added salt" diet must be followed for 3 days prior to the study
■ that prescribed diuretics must be taken for 3 days prior to the study
■ other restrictions in diet (e.g., licorice) or drugs necessary prior to the study
■ that the test will be performed in the radiology department by a physician and takes about 30 minutes
■ the general procedure including the sensations to be expected (momentary discomfort as the local anesthetic is injected, sensation of warmth as dye is injected)
■ whether or not premedications will be given
■ posttest assessment routines (e.g., frequent vital signs) and activity restrictions

Encourage questions and verbalization of concerns appropriate to the client's age and mental status.
The client should be questioned regarding possible allergies to radiographical dyes.
Ensure that signed consent has been obtained.

   Physical Preparation

■ To the extent possible, ensure that the dietary and medication regimens and restrictions are followed
■ Assist the client to maintain the upright position (standing or sitting) for 2 hours prior to the test, if ordered, to stimulate renin secretion
■ Take and record vital signs and have the client void; provide a hospital gown
■ Administer premedication, if ordered
■ Obtain a stretcher for client transport

The Procedure

The procedure varies with the method for obtaining the sample.

1. *Peripheral Vein.* A venipuncture is performed and the sample collected in a chilled lavender-topped tube. The tube should be inverted gently several times to promote adequate mixing with the anticoagulant, placed in ice, and sent to the laboratory immediately.
2. *Renal Vein.* The client is assisted to the supine position on the fluoroscopy table, and a site is selected for femoral vein catheterization. The skin may be shaved (if necessary), cleansed with an antiseptic, draped with sterile covers, and injected with a local anesthetic.

   A catheter is inserted into the femoral vein and advanced to the renal veins under fluoroscopical observation. Radiographical dye may be injected into the inferior vena cava at this point to aid in identification of the renal veins. A renal vein is entered and a blood sample obtained. The other renal vein is then entered and a second blood sample obtained. The catheter is then retracted into the inferior vena cava and a third sample obtained.

   The samples are placed in chilled lavender-topped tubes that are labeled to identify collection sites. The tubes should be inverted gently several times to promote adequate mixing with the anticoagulant, placed in ice, and sent to the laboratory immediately.

   The femoral catheter is removed after the third sample is obtained, and pressure is applied to the site for 10 minutes. A pressure dressing is then applied.

Aftercare and Nursing Observations

1. *Peripheral Vein.* Care and assessment following the procedure are the same as for any study involving the collection of a peripheral blood sample. Pretest diet and medications, which may have been modified or restricted prior to the study, should be resumed.
2. *Renal Vein.* The client should remain on bed rest for 8 hours following the procedure. Vital signs are taken and recorded according to the following schedule: every 15 minutes for 1 hour; every 30 minutes for 1 hour; and every hour for 4 hours. The catheterization site is observed for bleeding or hematoma each time vital signs are checked. Previous diet and medications are resumed.

HORMONES

Background Information

Hormones are chemicals that control the activities of responsive tissues. Some hormones exert their effects in the vicinity of their release; others are released into the extracellular fluids of the body and affect distant tissues. Similarly, some hormones affect only specific tissues (target tissues), while others affect nearly all cells of the body. Chemically, hormones are classified as polypeptides, amines, and steroids.

Hormones act on responsive tissues by (1) altering the rate of synthesis and secretion of enzymes or other hormones; (2) affecting the rate of enzymatic catalysis; and (3) altering the permeability of cell membranes. Once the hormone has accomplished its function, its rate of secretion normally decreases. This is known as negative feedback. After sufficient reduction in hormonal effects, negative feedback decreases and the hormone is again secreted.

Hypophyseal Hormones

The hypophysis, also known as the pituitary gland, lies at the base of the brain in the sella turcica and is connected to the hypothalamus by the hypophyseal stalk. The hypophysis has two distinct portions: (1) the adenohypophysis (anterior pituitary); and (2) the neurohypophysis (posterior pituitary). The adenohypophysis arises from upward growth of pharyngeal epithelium in the embryo, whereas the neurohypophysis arises from the downward growth of the hypothalamus in the embryo.

Almost all hormonal secretion from the hypophysis is controlled by the hypothalamus. Neurohypophyseal hormones are formed in the hypothalamus and travel down nerve fibers to the neurohypophysis, where they are stored and then released into the circulation in response to feedback mechanisms. Adenohypophyseal hormone secretion is controlled by releasing and inhibiting factors which are secreted by the hypothalamus and carried to the adenohypophysis by the hypothalamic-hypophyseal portal vessels. Those hypothalamic releasing/inhibiting factors identified thus far include (1) thyrotropin-releasing hormone (TRH); (2) corticotropin-releasing hormone (CRH); (3) gonadotropin-releasing hormone (GnRH), also known as luteinizing hormone releasing hormone (LHRH) and follicle-stimulating hormone releasing factor; (4) growth hormone releasing hormone (GHRH); (5) growth hormone inhibiting hormone (GHIH); and (6) prolactin inhibitory hormone (PIH). A releasing factor for melanocyte-stimulating hormone also is believed to exist. The releasing factors will either stimulate or inhibit the adenohypophysis in releasing its hormones.

The adenohypophysis consists of three major cell types: (1) acidophils, (2) basophils, and (3) chromophobes. The acidophils secrete growth hormone (GH), also called somatotropic hormone (STH, SH) or somatotropin; and prolactin (HPLR), also known as luteotropic hormone (LTH), lactogenic hormone, or lactogen. The basophils secrete adrenocorticotropic hormone (ACTH), also known as adrenocorticotropin and corticotropin; thyroid-stimulating hormone (TSH), also known as thyrotropin; follicle-stimulating hormone (FSH); luteinizing hormone (LH), also known as interstitial cell–stimulating hormone (ICSH); and melanocyte-stimulating hormone (MSH). The chromophobes, which constitute about half of the adenohypophyseal cells, are resting cells capable of transformation to either acidophils or basophils.

The hormones stored and released by the neurohypophysis include antidiuretic hormone (ADH), also known as vasopressin, and oxytocin. Radioimmunoassays are used to determine blood levels of the hypophyseal hormones.

GROWTH HORMONE (GH, STH, SH) (CLINICAL APPLICATIONS DATA, p. 227)

Growth hormone (GH), also known as somatotropic hormone (STH, SH) or somatotropin, is secreted in episodic bursts, usually during early sleep. The effects of GH occur throughout the body. GH promotes skeletal growth by stimulating hepatic production of proteins. It also affects lipid and glucose metabolism. Under the influence of growth hormone, free fatty acids enter the circulation for use by muscle; hepatic glucose production (gluconeogenesis) also rises. Growth hormone also increases blood flow to the renal cortex and the glomerular filtration rate; the kidney excretes more calcium and less phosphate than usual. GH is believed to antagonize insulin.

Deficiencies in GH are apparent only in childhood. Children with GH deficiency have very small statures but normal body proportions. The child also may be deficient in other hypophyseal hormones, and this disorder is known as "pituitary dwarfism." Other causes of decreased GH levels include pituitary tumors, craniopharyngiomas, and pituitary damage or trauma. Decreased levels of GH also are associated with hyperglycemia and tuberculosis meningitis. Adrenal corticosteroids and chlorpromazine also may produce decreased levels.

Excessive levels of growth hormone are apparent in all ages. Excess GH in children causes the long bones of the skeleton to enlarge and produces gigantism. In adults, the bones of the skull, hands, and feet thicken to produce the physical appearance of acromegaly. In this disorder, the internal organs, skeletal muscle, and heart muscle hypertrophy. Nerves and cartilage also enlarge and may produce nerve compression and joint disorders. The usual cause of excessive levels of GH is acidophil or chromophobe tumors of the adenohypophysis.

Hypoglycemia and a variety of drugs (e.g., amphetamines, arginine, dopamine, levodopa, methyldopa, beta blockers, histamine, nicotinic acid, estrogens), as well as physical activity and stress also may elevate GH levels.[33]

GROWTH HORMONE STIMULATION TESTS (CLINICAL APPLICATIONS DATA, p. 228)

Baseline levels of growth hormone (GH) are affected by many factors and may be misleading at times. Stimulation tests are done to determine responsiveness to substances that normally stimulate GH secretion such as arginine and L-dopa. Insulin also may be given to induce hypoglycemia, which in turn stimulates GH secretion. It has been found that blood sugar levels less than 50 mg/dl will cause GH levels to rise 10 times or more in normal individuals. It should be noted that idiosyncratic responses to the different stimulants may occur. Thus, it may be necessary to perform two or three different stimulation tests before arriving at diagnostic conclusions.[34]

GROWTH HORMONE SUPPRESSION TEST (CLINICAL APPLICATIONS DATA, p. 229)

Hyperglycemia suppresses growth hormone (GH) secretion in normal individuals. This principle is used in evaluating individuals with abnormally elevated levels and those who are believed to be hypersecreting GH but who show normal levels on routine serum GH determinations. Administration of a glucose load that produces hyperglycemia should decrease serum GH levels within 1 to 2 hours. In individuals who are hypersecreting GH, a decrease in serum GH will not occur in response to hyperglycemia. It should be noted that the test may need to be repeated to confirm results.

PROLACTIN (HPRL, LTH) (CLINICAL APPLICATIONS DATA, p. 230)

Prolactin (HPRL), also known as luteotropic hormone (LTH), lactogenic hormone, or lactogen, is secreted by the acidophil cells of the adenohypophysis. It is unique among hormones in that it responds to inhibition via the hypothalamus rather than to stimulation; that is, prolactin is secreted except when influenced by the hypothalamic inhibiting factor, which is believed to be the neurotransmitter, dopamine.

The only known function of prolactin is to induce milk production in a female breast already stimulated by high estrogen levels. Once milk production is established, lactation can continue without elevated prolactin levels. Prolactin levels rise late in pregnancy, peak with the initiation of lactation, and surge each time a woman breastfeeds. The function of prolactin in males is not known.

Elevated prolactin levels are seen in clients with reduced dopamine levels and with damage to the hypothalamus or pituitary stalk. Episodic elevations also may occur in response to sleep, stress, exercise, and hypoglycemia. Thyroid-stimulating hormone (TSH) enhances prolactin release; primary hypothyroidism often causes hyperprolactinemia by provoking TSH hypersecretion. Elevated prolactin levels also are seen in pituitary adenomas, lung or kidney tumors with ectopic prolactin production, liver disease, and chronic alcoholism. A number of drugs may produce elevated levels; these include estrogens, oral contraceptives, reserpine, alpha-methyldopa, phenothiazines, haloperidol, tricyclic antidepressants, and procainamide derivatives.

Excessive circulating prolactin disturbs sexual function in both men and women. Women experience amenorrhea and anovulation, and may have inappropriate milk secretion (galactorrhea). Men experience impotence, which occurs even when testosterone levels are normal, and, sometimes, gynecomastia.[35]

Decreased levels, which are not as frequently seen, occur with postpartum hypophyseal infarction (Sheehan's syndrome) and may be seen in clients receiving dopamine, apomorphine, and ergot alkaloids.

ADRENOCORTICOTROPIC HORMONE (ACTH) (CLINICAL APPLICATIONS DATA, p. 231)

Adrenocorticotropic hormone (ACTH), also known as adrenocorticotropin and corticotropin, is secreted by the basophils of the adenohypophysis. ACTH stimulates the adrenal cortex to secrete (1) glucocorticoids, of which cortisol predominates; (2) adrenal androgens, which are converted by the liver to testosterone; and (3) to a lesser degree, mineralocorticoids, of which aldosterone predominates. ACTH secretion is closely linked to melanocyte-stimulating hormone; it also is thought to stimulate pancreatic beta cells and the release of growth hormone.

ACTH release, which is stimulated by its corresponding hypothalamic releasing factor, occurs episodically in relation to decreased circulating levels of glucocorticoid, increased stress, and hypoglycemia. ACTH levels also vary diurnally; highest levels occur upon awakening, decrease throughout the day, and then begin to rise again a few hours before awakening. Circulating aldosterone levels may influence ACTH secretion to some extent; however, androgens are believed to have no effect on ACTH levels.

Elevated plama ACTH levels are seen in pituitary adenomas, in which ACTH secretion continues despite elevated circulating levels of glucocorticoids and mineralocorticoids. Increased levels also may be due to nonendocrine malignant tumors (e.g., certain lung cancers), which produce ACTH autonomously. Cushing's syndrome includes all disorders characterized by excessive adrenal corticosteroid production. About 70 percent of these cases involve pituitary oversecretion of ACTH; 25 percent are usually due to benign or malignant adrenal tumors, in response to which ACTH levels are usually low due to normal feedback mechanisms. In contrast, adrenal cortical hypofunction (Addison's disease) will lead to elevated plasma ACTH levels.

Decreased ACTH levels are associated with adrenal cortical hyperplasia or tumors, panhypopituitarism and hypothalamic dysfunction. Therapy with adrenal corticosteroids also results in decreased ACTH levels. Other drugs that may lead to decreased ACTH levels include estrogens, calcium gluconate, amphetamines, spironolactone, and ethanol. These drugs elevate circulating cortisol levels and, thus, ACTH levels are lowered owing to normal feedback mechanisms.

It should be noted that ACTH assays are expensive to perform and are not universally available.

Thyroid-Stimulating Hormone (TSH) (Clinical Applications Data, p. 232)

Thyroid-stimulating hormone (TSH), also called thyrotropin, is produced by the basophil cells of the adenohypophysis in response to stimulation by its hypothalamic releasing factor, thyrotropin-releasing hormone (TRH). TRH responds to decreased circulating levels of thyroid hormones, as well as to intense cold, psychological tension, and increased metabolic need, and stimulates the adenohypophysis to secrete TSH. TSH accelerates all aspects of hormone production by the thyroid gland and enhances prolactin release. Measuring TSH provides useful information about both hypophyseal and thyroid gland function.

Hypersecretion of TSH by the adenohypophysis (e.g., due to TSH-secreting pituitary tumors) causes hyperthyroidism due to excessive stimulation of the thyroid gland. Elevated TSH levels also are seen with prolonged emotional stress and are more common in colder climates. Primary hypothyroidism (i.e., hypothyroidism due to disorders involving the thyroid gland itself) will lead to elevated TSH levels due to normal feedback mechanisms. TSH levels are normally elevated at birth. Drugs that may lead to elevated TSH levels include lithium carbonate and potassium iodide.

It should be noted that increased TSH secretion is associated with excess secretion of exophthalmos-producing substance, which also originates in the adenohypophysis. This substance promotes water storage in the retro-orbital fat pads and causes the eyes to protrude, a common sign of hyperthyroidism. Exophthalmos sometimes persists after the hyperthyroidism is corrected and also may occur in persons with normal thyroid function.

Hyposecretion of TSH due to pituitary or hypothalamic dysfunction will produce secondary hypothyroidism. Primary hyperthyroidism due to disorders involving the thyroid gland will lead to decreased TSH levels due to normal feedback mechanisms. Drugs that may lead to low TSH levels include aspirin, adrenal corticosteroids, and heparin.

TSH levels are normal in situations in which the functional ability of the thyroid gland is normal but the thyroid hormone levels are low, a phenomenon that is seen in clients with severe illnesses with protein deficiency (thyroid hormones are proteins) such as neoplastic disease, severe burns, trauma, liver disease, renal failure, and cardiovascular problems. The deficiency of thyroid hormone produces a hypometabolic state. Excess TSH production is not stimulated, however, because circulating thyroid levels are appropriate to the client's metabolic needs (i.e., the person is metabolically euthyroid). Treatment involves correcting the underlying causes. The apparent hypothyroidism is not treated, however, as such treatment could be devastating to a severely debilitated person.

TSH is measured by radioimmunoassay. Immunological cross-reactivity occurs with glycoprotein hormones such as human chorionic gonadotropin (hCG), follicle-stimulating hormone (FSH), and luteinizing hormone (LH). Thus, TSH levels may be artificially high in the presence of hydatidiform mole, choriocarcinoma, embryonal carcinoma of the testes, pregnancy, and postmenopausal states characterized by high FSH and LH levels.[36]

TSH Stimulation Test (Clinical Applications Data, p. 233)

The TSH stimulation test is used to evaluate the thyroid-pituitary-hypothalamic feedback loop. In this test, a purified form of hypothalamic thyrotropin-releasing hormone (TRH) is administered intravenously. Normally, TRH will stimulate the adenohypophysis to release TSH (thyroid-stimulating hormone), which, in turn, causes hormonal release from the thyroid gland. A normal response (e.g., elevated TSH levels) indicates that the adenohypophysis is capable of responding to TRH stimulation. If thyroid hormones also are measured as part of the test, elevated levels indicate that the thyroid gland is capable of responding to TSH stimulation.

Failure of TSH levels to rise is seen in clients with primary hypopituitarism, in which the adenohypophysis is unable to respond to TRH. In those with primary hyperthyroidism, TSH levels are low but can be elevated by TRH administration. When TRH elicits no response in such clients, it indicates that thyroid hormone production is occurring independently, without normal control by the hypothalamic-hypophyseal axis. In primary hypothyroidism, TSH levels are elevated; administration of TRH will produce even greater increases but thyroid gland hormonal response will remain depressed.

FOLLICLE-STIMULATING HORMONE (FSH) (CLINICAL APPLICATIONS DATA, p. 234)

Follicle-stimulating hormone (FSH) is secreted by the basophil cells of the adenohypophysis in response to stimulation by hypothalamic gonadotropin releasing hormone (GnRH), which also is called luteinizing hormone releasing hormone (LHRH) and follicle-stimulating hormone releasing factor. FSH affects gonadal function in both men and women. In women, FSH promotes maturation of the graafian (germinal) follicle, causing estrogen secretion and allowing the ovum to mature. In men, FSH partially controls spermatogenesis, but the presence of testosterone also is necessary. GnRH secretion, which in turn stimulates FSH secretion, is stimulated by decreased estrogen and testosterone levels. Isolated FSH elevation also may occur when there is failure to produce spermatozoa, even though testosterone production is normal. FSH production is inhibited by rising estrogen and testosterone levels.

During childhood, FSH levels are normally low but begin to rise as puberty approaches. Surges of FSH occur initially during sleep, but as puberty advances, daytime levels also rise. During childbearing years, FSH levels in women vary according to the menstrual cycle. Decreased FSH levels after puberty are associated with male and female infertility. After the reproductive years, estrogen and testosterone levels decline, causing FSH levels to rise in response to normal feedback mechanisms.

Excessive FSH secretion is associated with precocious puberty in children, pituitary tumors, ovarian or testicular failure, polycystic ovary disease, postviral orchitis, adrenogenital syndrome in females, Turner's syndrome in females, Klinefelter's syndrome in males, and early acromegaly. Administration of clomiphene results in elevated FSH levels by preventing the hypothalamus from recognizing normally inhibitory levels of estrogen and testosterone.

Decreased levels are associated with hypothalamic lesions, panhypopituitarism, neoplasms of the testes, ovaries and adrenal glands with excessive sex hormone production (sex hormones are steroids), anorexia nervosa, cirrhosis, and renal disease. Therapy with estrogens and progesterone will decrease FSH levels, as will the phenothiazines.[37]

LUTEINIZING HORMONE (LH, ICSH) (CLINICAL APPLICATIONS DATA, p. 235)

Luteinizing hormone (LH), also known as interstitial cell–stimulating hormone (ICSH), is secreted by the basophil cells of the adenohypophysis in response to stimulation by gonadotropin releasing hormone (GnRH), the same hypothalamic releasing factor that stimulates follicle-stimulating hormone (FSH) release. LH affects gonadal function in both men and women. In women, a surge of LH occurs at the midpoint of the menstrual cycle and is believed to be induced by high estrogen levels. LH causes the ovum to be expelled from the ovary and stimulates development of the corpus luteum and progesterone production. As progesterone levels rise, LH production decreases. In men, LH stimulates the interstitial cells of Leydig, located in the testes, to produce testosterone.

During childhood, LH levels are decreased and are lower than those of FSH. Similarly, LH levels rise after those of FSH as puberty approaches. During childbearing years, LH levels in women vary according to the menstrual cycle but remain fairly constant in men. Decreased LH levels after puberty are associated with male and female infertility. After the reproductive years, as gonadal hormones decline, LH levels rise in response to normal feedback mechanisms. The rise in LH levels, however, is not as marked as that for FSH levels.

Elevated and decreased serum LH levels are associated with essentially the same disorders as altered FSH levels (see p. 212). In contrast to FSH, however, LH levels are stimulated by estrogen. Thus, drugs and disorders that elevate blood estrogen levels (e.g., ovarian tumors and drugs containing estrogen) will tend to cause elevated LH levels. Progesterone and testosterone, on the other hand, may lead to decreased LH levels.

FSH/LH CHALLENGE TESTS

The hypothalamic-hypophyseal-gonadal axis can be evaluated by administering drugs and hormones known to affect specfic hormonal interactions. These include clomiphene, gonadotropin releasing hormone (GnRH), human chorionic gonadotropin, and progesterone.

Clomiphene, a drug used to treat infertility, prevents the hypothalamus from recognizing normally inhibitory levels of estrogen and testosterone. Consequently, the hypothalamus will continue to secrete GnRH, which will, in turn, continue to stimulate the adenohypophysis to secrete follicle-stimulating hormone (FSH) and luteinizing hormone (LH). After 5 days of clomiphene, both FSH and LH levels will rise, usually 50 to 100 percent above baseline levels. In anovulatory women whose ovaries are normal, clomiphene often enhances FSH and LH levels such that ovulation is induced. If FSH and LH levels do not rise with clomiphene administration, either hypothalamic or hypophyseal dysfunction is indicated. The source of the dysfunction may be identified by administering purified GnRH. If FSH and LH levels rise, the pituitary gland is normal but hypothalamic function is impaired. FSH and LH levels that do not rise indicate hypophyseal dysfunction.

Human chorionic gonadotropin (hCG), a placental hormone with effects similar to those of LH, is used to evaluate testicular activity in men with low testostrone levels. Elevated testosterone levels after hCG administration indicate that testicular function is normal, but hypothalamic-pituitary activity is impaired. Failure of testosterone levels to rise suggests primary testicular dysfunction.

Progesterone, a hormone secreted by the ovary, is used to evaluate amenorrhea. In the normal menstrual cycle, the progesterone surge that follows ovulation inhibits GnRH secretion, and hormonal levels decline. Menstrual bleeding, also called withdrawal bleeding, occurs when the estrogen-stimulated endometrium experiences a drop in hormonal stimulation. This normal situation can be simulated by administering oral or intramuscular progesterone to amenorrheic women already exposed to adequate estrogen levels. If menstrual bleeding occurs, the underlying cause of the amenorrhea is failure to ovulate. Lack of bleeding in response to progesterone administration indicates (1) inadequate estrogen production, due to either primary ovarian failure or inadequate pituitary secretion of FSH; (2) hypothalamic dysfunction with defective GnRH secretion; (3) impaired hypophyseal response to GnRH; or (4) abnormal uterine response to hormonal stimulation. These possibilities can be distinguished by administering estrogen to stimulate the endometrium and then repeating the progesterone challenge. If bleeding occurs, then either ovarian failure or inadequately responsive hypothalamic-hypophyseal activity is the underlying cause of the amenorrhea. Measuring FSH, LH, and estrogen levels helps further to diagnose the problem.[38]

ANTIDIURETIC HORMONE (ADH) (CLINICAL APPLICATIONS DATA, p. 236)

Antidiuretic hormone (ADH), also known as vasopressin, is formed by the hypothalamus but stored in the neurohypophysis (posterior pituitary gland). ADH is released in response to increased serum osmolality or decreased blood volume. Although as little as a 1 percent change in serum osmolality will stimulate ADH secretion, blood volume must decrease by approximately 10 percent for ADH secretion to be induced. Psychogenic stimuli (e.g., stress, pain, anxiety) also may stimulate ADH release, but the mechanism by which this occurs is unclear.

ADH acts on the epithelial cells of the distal convoluted tubules and collecting ducts of the kidneys, making them permeable to water. Thus, with ADH more water is absorbed from the glomerular filtrate into the bloodstream. Without ADH, water remains in the filtrate and is excreted, producing very dilute urine. In contrast, maximal ADH secretion produces very concentrated urine. ADH also is believed to stimulate mild contractions in the pregnant uterus and to aid in promoting milk ejection in lactation, functions similar to those of oxytocin, which also is secreted by the hypothalamus and released by the neurohypophysis.

Diabetes insipidus (DI) occurs when ADH secretion or response is inadequate, and may be of neurogenic or nephrogenic origin. Neurogenic (central) DI is caused by impaired hypothalamic-hypophyseal regulation of ADH. This most commonly occurs because of cerebral trauma, neoplasms, inflammations, or surgical ablation of the pituitary. Individuals with DI excrete large amounts of hypotonic urine. Thirst is the body's response to this fluid loss. If the person is unable to ingest sufficient fluid, or if the thirst center is impaired, severe dehydration may result.

Nephrogenic DI occurs when there is decreased renal responsiveness to ADH stimulation. One cause of nephrogenic DI is psychogenic polydipsia. In this disorder, the person consumes large amounts of fluid and excretes massive volumes of hypotonic urine, which ultimately causes the tubular epithelium to lose its responsiveness to ADH. Nephrogenic DI also may be caused by various disorders affecting the renal tubules. It should be noted that serum ADH levels may be elevated in nephrogenic DI due to normal feedback mechanisms. Overhydration, decreased serum osmolality, and hypervolemia also decrease ADH secretion, as do alcohol, phenytoin drugs, beta-adrenergic drugs, and morphine antagonists.

Excessive ADH levels are associated with the syndrome of inappropriate ADH secretion (SIADH). In SIADH, water is reabsorbed into the body despite decreased serum osmolality and increased blood volume. SIADH may be due to impaired hypothalamic-hypophyseal regulation of ADH with failure of the negative feedback system or secretion of ADH-active material of non-pituitary origin. The latter is seen in various types of cancer in which there is ectopic hormone production (e.g., oat cell lung cancer, thymoma, lymphoma, leukemia, and carcinomas of the pancreas, prostate gland, and intestine). SIADH also is common in pulmonary disorders such as tuberculosis and pneumonia, and may occur in individuals on positive pressure ventilation. Disorders involving the central nervous system (e.g., brain tumors and infections), thyroid gland, and adrenal gland also may lead to excessive ADH secretion, as will pain, stress, and anxiety. Drugs that elevate ADH levels include acetaminophen, barbiturates, cholinergic agents, clofibrate, estrogens, nicotine, oral hypoglycemia agents, cytotoxic agents (e.g., vincristine), tricyclic antidepressants, oxytocin, Tegretol, and thiazide diuretics.[39]

Thyroid and Parathyroid Hormones

The thyroid gland synthesizes and releases thyroxine (T_4) and triiodothyronine (T_3) in response to stimulation by thyroid-stimulating hormone, which is secreted by the adenohypophysis. The thyroid gland synthesizes its hormones from iodine and the essential amino acid tyrosine. Most of the body's iodine is ingested as iodide through dietary intake and is absorbed into the bloodstream from the gastrointestinal tract. One third of the absorbed iodide enters the thyroid gland; the remaining two thirds are excreted in the urine. In the thyroid gland, enzymes oxidize iodide to iodine.

The thyroid gland secretes a protein, thyroglobulin, into its follicles. Thyroglobulin has special properties that allow the tyrosine contained in its molecule to react with iodine to form thyroid hormones. The thyroid hormones thus formed are stored in the follicles of the gland as the thyroglobulin-thyroid hormone complex called colloid.

When thyroid hormones are released into the bloodstream, they are split from thyroglobulin as a result of the action of proteases, which are secreted by thyroid cells in response to stimulation by thyroid-stimulating hormone. Much more T_4 than T_3 is secreted into the bloodstream. Upon entering the bloodstream, both immediately combine with plasma proteins, mainly thyroxine-binding globulin (TBG), but also albumin and prealbumin. Although more than 99 percent of both T_4 and T_3 are bound to TBG, physiological activity of both hormones results from only the unbound ("free") molecules. It should also be noted that TBG has greater affinity for T_4 than for T_3, which allows for more rapid release of T_3 from TBG for entry into body cells. T_3 is thought to exert at least 65 to 75 percent of thyroidal hormone effects, and it is believed by some that T_4 has no endocrine activity at all until it is converted to T_3, which occurs when one iodine molecule is removed from T_4.[40]

The main function of thyroid hormones is to increase the metabolic activities of most tissues by increasing the oxidative enzymes in the cells. This, in turn, causes increased oxygen consumption and increased utilization of carbohydrates, proteins, fats, and vitamins. Thyroid hormones also mobilize electrolytes and are necessary for the conversion of carotene to vitamin A. Although the mechanism is not known, thyroid hormones are essential for the development of the central nervous system. Thyroid-deficient infants may suffer irreversible brain damage (cretinism). Thyroid deficiency in adults (myxedema) produces diffuse psychomotor retardation, which is reversible with hormone replacement. Thyroid hormones also are thought to increase the rate of parathyroid hormone secretion.

Alterations in thyroid hormone production may be caused by disorders affecting the hypothalamus, which secretes thyrotropin-releasing hormone (TRH) in response to circulating T_4 and T_3 levels, the pituitary gland, or the thyroid gland itself. Such alterations may affect all body systems. "Hypothyroidism" is the general term for the hypometabolic state induced by deficient thyroid hormone secretion, whereas "hyperthyroidism" indicates excessive production of thyroid hormones.

An additional hormone produced by the thyroid gland is calcitonin, which is secreted in response to high serum calcium levels. Calcitonin causes an increase in calcium resorption by bone, thus lowering serum calcium.[41]

A number of tests pertaining to thyroid hormones may be performed, some of which may be grouped as a "thyroid screen" (e.g., T_4, T_3, and THS). It should also be noted that a "T_7" is sometimes ordered. This is interpreted as a T_4 plus a T_3, since there is no substance such as T_7. Before it was possible to measure thyroid hormones directly, serum iodine measurements (e.g., protein-bound iodine) were used as indicators of thyroid function. These tests were severely affected by organic and inorganic iodine contaminants, and are no longer used to any great extent. Similarly, measurement of thyroidal uptake of radioactive iodine (^{131}I) has been replaced by direct measurements of T_4 and TSH.[42]

Thyroxine (T_4) (Clinical Applications Data, p. 238)

Thyroxine (T_4) is measured by competitive protein binding or by radioimmunoassay. In competitive protein binding, the affinity between T_4 and thyroxine-binding globulin (TBG) is exploited. Reagent TBG fully saturated with radiolabeled T_4 is incubated with T_4 extracted from the client's serum. The T_4 from the test serum displaces the radiolabeled T_4 in the amount present. This procedure is known as T_4 by displacement (T_4 D), T_4 by competitive binding (T_4 CPB), and T_4 Murphy-Pattee (T_4 MP). T_4 measured by radioimmunoassay (T_4 RIA) is the preferred method to measure T_4 because it is not affected by circulating iodinated substances.

Most T_4 (99.97 percent) in the serum is bound to TBG. The remainder circulates as unbound ("free") T_4 (FT_4) and is responsible for all of the physiological activity of thyroxine. Because FT_4 is not dependent on normal levels of TBG, as is the case with total serum thyroxine, FT_4 levels are considered the most accurate indicator of thyroxine and its thyrometabolic activity. It is difficult, however, to measure FT_4 directly because quantitites are so small and the interference from bound T_4 is great. Free hormone levels are, therefore, usually calculated by multiplying the values for total T_4 and by the T_3 uptake ratio (see p. 217). The result is expressed as the free thyroxine index (FT_4 I). The free hormone index varies directly with the amount of circulating hormone and inversely with the amount of unsaturated TBG present in the serum.[43]

T_4 and FT_4 are elevated in most types of hyperthyroidism. An exception is T_3 thyrotoxicosis, in which levels of bound and free thyroxine are usually normal. Ingesting thyroxine also will elevate T_4 levels. The circulating T_4 level is directly affected by the quantity of thyroid-binding proteins present in the blood. Estrogens increase the amount of TBG in the serum, and thus, elevated T_4 levels are seen in pregnancy and in women receiving estrogen therapy or with estrogen-secreting tumors. Heroin and methadone may also produce increased T_4 levels. It should be noted that T_4 levels are higher in newborn infants and children and do not approach adult levels until adolescence.

T_4 and FT_4 are decreased in most types of hypothyroidism and in early thyroiditis. Thyroxine levels also may be decreased in pituitary and hypothalamic dysfunction. Any disorder that depresses serum proteins will decrease T_4 levels. Thus, decreased T_4 is frequently seen in severe illnesses due to metastatic cancer, liver disease, renal disease, diabetes mellitus, cardiovascular problems, burns, and trauma. Androgens and glucocorticoids depress TBG synthesis and will result in lower T_4 levels. Other drugs that result in low T_4 levels include heparin, salicylates, phenytoin anticonvulsants, sulfonamides, and antithyroid drugs such as propylthiouracil.

TRIIODOTHYRONINE (T_3) (CLINICAL APPLICATIONS DATA, p. 239)

Although produced in smaller quantities than thyroxine (T_4), triiodothyronine (T_3) is physiologically more significant. The competitive protein-binding techniques that are useful in measuring T_4 are not used to measure T_3, as it is present in smaller amounts and has less affinity for thyroxine-binding globulin (TBG) than T_4. Thus, T_3 is measured only by radioimmunoassay (T_3 RIA).

As with T_4, most T_3 (99.7 percent) in the serum is bound to TBG. The remainder circulates as unbound ("free") T_3 (FT_3) and is responsible for all of the physiological activity of triiodothyronine. Since FT_3 is not dependent on normal levels of TBG, as is the case with total T_3, FT_3 levels are the most accurate indicators of thyrometabolic activity. FT_3 levels may be calculated by multiplying total T_3 levels by the T_3 uptake ratio (see below).

T_3 and FT_3 levels are elevated in most types of hyperthyroidism, which also elevates T_4 and FT_4. In fact, there is no point in measuring T_3 in clients with elevated T_4 levels, because T_3 will always be high as well. Measurement of T_3 levels is most useful in diagnosing a subclass of hyperthyroidism, T_3 thyrotoxicosis, which occurs in about 5 percent of thyrotoxic persons. In this disorder, excessive amounts of T_4 are converted to T_3 resulting in normal T_4 levels and elevated T_3 levels. T_3 determinations may also be useful in the early diagnosis of hyperthyroidism characterized by elevated T_4 and T_3 levels because T_3 and FT_4 levels rise before T_4 levels do.

Reverse T_3 (rT_3), a variant form of T_3, is derived from T_4 when an iodine molecule is removed by a different reaction than usual. Reverse T_3 has its three iodines at the 3, 3′, and 5′ positions, instead of at the 3, 5, and 3′ positions of active T_3. Reverse T_3 serves no known physiological function but has been found to be elevated in severe illness with protein deficiency. In such disorders, T_4 and T_3 levels are decreased and the client shows signs of hypothyroidism. The rise in rT_3 levels is thought to be due to an increase in the metabolic pathways leading to its production. Differentiation of true hypothyroidism from this "euthyroid sick" syndrome is critical, since unnecessary treatment for hypothyroidism could be devasting to these individuals.[44]

T_3 UPTAKE (RT_3 U) (CLINICAL APPLICATIONS DATA, p. 240)

The T_3 uptake (RT_3 U) test evaluates the quantity of thyroxine-binding globulin (TBG) present in the serum and the quantity of thyroxine (T_4) bound to it. In the T_3 uptake procedure, a known amount of resin containing radiolabeled T_3 is added to a sample of the client's serum. Normally, TBG in the serum is not fully saturated with thyroid hormones; the saturation level varies in relation to the amounts of TBG and thyroid hormones present. In the T_3 uptake test, the radiolabeled T_3 will bind with available TBG sites. Results of the test are determined by measuring the percentage of labeled T_3 which remains bound to the resin after all available sites on TBG have been filled. It should be noted that the percentage of T_3 bound to the resin is inversely proportional to the percentage TBG saturation in the serum.

Results of the T_3 uptake test are evaluated in relation to serum levels of total T_4 and T_3, and also are used in calculating free T_3 and T_4 indices. For these calculations, the T_3 uptake ratio (RT_3 UR) is used, a ratio obtained by dividing the client's RT_3 U level by the RT_3 U level determined from a pool of normal serum.

THYROXINE-BINDING GLOBULIN (TBG) (CLINICAL APPLICATIONS DATA, p. 241)

Thyroxine-binding globulin (TBG) may be measured directly by radioimmunoassay. Estrogens elevate serum TBG levels; thus, women who are pregnant, who are receiving estrogen therapy or oral contraceptives, or who have estrogen-secreting tumors will have higher TBG levels. Androgens and cortico-steroids decrease TBG levels. TBG also is decreased in clients with low overall serum protein levels and hereditary abnormalities of globulin synthesis.

THYROID-STIMULATING IMMUNOGLOBULINS (TSI, TSIg) (CLINICAL APPLICATIONS DATA, p. 242)

The globulin formerly known as long-acting thyroid stimulator (LATS) is one of the biologically unique autoantibodies whose effect is to stimulate the target cell. Now called thyroid-stimulating immunoglobulins (TSI, TSIg), these antibodies react with the cell surface receptor that usually combines with TSH. The TSI reacts with the receptors, activates intracellular enzymes, and promotes epithelial cell activity that operates outside the feedback regulation for TSH. It has been found that 50 to 80 percent of individuals with thyrotoxicosis have elevated TSI levels. It is also believed that elevated TSI levels may be involved in the etiology of exophthalmos.

CALCITONIN (CLINICAL APPLICATIONS DATA, p. 242)

Calcitonin, also called thyrocalcitonin, is secreted by the parafollicular or C cells of the thyroid gland in response to elevated serum calcium levels. Its role is not completely understood, but the following functions are known: (1) it antagonizes the effects of parathormone and vitamin D; (2) it inhibits osteo-clasts that reabsorb bone so that calcium continues to be laid down and not reab-sorbed into the blood; and (3) it increases renal clearance of magnesium and inhibits tubular reabsorption of phosphates. The net result is that calcitonin decreases serum calcium levels.

Persons with medullary carcinoma of the thyroid have elevated calcitonin levels, while their serum calcium levels remain normal. Elevated calcitonin levels also are seen in cancers involving the breast, lung, and pancreas owing to ectopic calcitonin production by tumor cells. Calcitonin levels also may be elevated in response to primary and secondary hyperparathyroidism. The latter is associated with chronic renal failure.

PARATHYROID HORMONE (PTH) (CLINICAL APPLICATIONS DATA, p. 243)

Parathyroid hormone (parathormone, PTH) is secreted by the parathyroid glands in response to decreased levels of circulating calcium. Actions of PTH include (1) mobilizing calcium from bone into the bloodstream, along with phosphates and protein matrix; (2) promoting renal tubular reabsorption of cal-cium and depression of phosphate reabsorption, thereby reducing calcium excretion and increasing phosphate excretion by the kidneys; (3) decreasing renal secretion of hydrogen ions which leads to increased renal excretion of bicarbonate and chloride; and (4) enhancing renal production of active vitamin D metabolites, causing increased calcium absorption in the small intestine. The net result of PTH action is maintenance of adequate serum calcium levels.

Elevated PTH levels may occur in primary hyperparathyroidism due to hyperplasia or tumor of the parathyroid glands. High PTH levels are also seen in secondary hyperparathyroidism, which is most commonly due to renal dis-ease with its accompanying hypocalcemia, hyperphosphatemia, and impaired vitamin D metabolism. Other causes of elevated PTH include malignant tumors, which produce ectopic PTH, and malabsorption syndromes.

Decreased PTH levels are associated with hypoparathyroidism, most com-monly due to removal of the parathyroid glands during thyroid gland or other neck surgery. Elevated serum calcium levels, especially those due to malignant processes, also will lead to decreased PTH production. Hypomagnesemia has been found to depress PTH production as well as tissue responsiveness to PTH. Autoimmune destruction of the parathyroids, a rare disorder also will produce decreased PTH levels.[45]

Adrenal Hormones

Adrenal hormones are secreted by two functionally and embryologically distinct portions of the adrenal gland. The adrenal cortex, which is of mesodermal origin, secretes three types of steroids: (1) glucocorticoids, which affect carbohydrate metabolism; (2) mineralocorticoids, which promote potassium excretion and sodium retention by the kidneys; and (3) adrenal androgens, which the liver converts to testosterone. Cortisol is the predominant glucocorticoid, while aldosterone is the predominant mineralocorticoid. Production and secretion of cortisol and the adrenal androgens is stimulated by adrenocorticotropin (ACTH). Although ACTH also may enhance aldosterone production, the usual stimulants are either increased serum potassium or decreased serum sodium.

The adrenal medulla, which constitutes only about one-tenth of the volume of the adrenal glands, derives from the ectoderm and physiologically belongs to the sympathetic nervous system. The hormones secreted by the adrenal medulla are epinephrine and norepinephrine, which are collectively known as the catecholamines. Epinephrine is secreted in response to sympathetic stimulation, hypoglycemia, or hypotension. Most norepinephrine is manufactured by and secreted from sympathetic nerve endings; only a small amount is normally secreted by the adrenal medulla.[46]

CORTISOL (CLINICAL APPLICATIONS DATA, p. 244)

Cortisol (hydrocortisone), the predominant glucocorticoid, is secreted in response to stimulation by ACTH. Ninety percent of cortisol is bound to cortisol-binding globulin (CBG) and albumin; the free portion is responsible for its physiological effects. Cortisol stimulates gluconeogenesis, mobilizes fats and proteins, antagonizes insulin, and suppresses inflammation. Cortisol secretion varies diurnally, with highest levels seen upon awakening and lowest levels occurring late in the day. Bursts of cortisol excretion also may occur at night.

Elevated cortisol levels occur in Cushing's syndrome, in which there is excessive production of adrenal corticosteroids. Cushing's syndrome may be due to pituitary adenoma, adrenal hyperplasia, benign or malignant adrenal tumors, and nonendocrine malignant tumors which secrete ectopic ACTH. Therapy with adrenal corticosteroids also may produce cushingoid signs and symptoms. Elevated cortisol levels are additionally associated with stress, hyperthyroidism, obesity, and diabetic ketoacidosis.

Circulating plasma cortisol levels are affected by the level of protein binding. Excess estrogens, for example, may increase CBG, thereby promoting high absolute levels of cortisol. Thus, elevated cortisol levels are seen in pregnancy and in individuals on estrogen therapy or oral contraceptives. Lithium carbonate, methadone, and ethyl alcohol also may produce elevated cortisol levels.

Decreased cortisol levels occur with Addison's disease, in which there is deficient production of adrenal corticosteroids. Addison's disease is usually due to idiopathic adrenal hypofunction, although it may also be seen in pituitary hypofunction, hypothyroidism, tuberculosis, metastatic cancer involving the adrenal glands, amyloidosis, and hemochromatosis. Addison's disease may occur after withdrawal of corticosteroid therapy due to drug-induced atrophy of the adrenal glands. Drugs that may lead to decreased cortisol levels include levodopa, barbiturates, phenytoin (Dilantin), and androgens.

CORTISOL/ACTH CHALLENGE TESTS

A variety of tests that stimulate or suppress cortisol/ACTH levels may be used further to evaluate individuals with signs and symptoms of adrenal hypofunction or hyperfunction or abnormal cortisol levels.

Dexamethasone is a potent glucocorticoid that suppresses ACTH and cortisol production. In the rapid dexamethasone test, 1 mg of oral dexamethasone is given at midnight; cortisol levels are then measured at 8 A.M. Normally, plasma cortisol should be no more than 5 to 10 μg/dl after dexamethasone administration. A 5-hour urine collection test for 17-hydroxycorticoids (17-OHCS), metabolites of glucocorticoids, also may be collected as part of the test. Elevated plasma cortisol levels in response to dexamethasone administration are associated with Cushing's syndrome.

Metyrapone is a drug that inhibits certain enzymes required to convert precursor substances into cortisol. When the drug is administered, plasma cortisol levels decrease and ACTH levels subsequently increase in response. The test mainly involves measurement of urinary excretion of 17-OHCS, which should rise if the adenohypophysis is normally responsive to decreased cortisol levels. Plasma cortisol levels are measured to ensure that sufficient suppression has been induced by the metyrapone such that test results will be valid.

Insulin-induced hypoglycemia (serum glucose of 50 mg/dl or less) also will stimulate ACTH production. Adenohypophyseal response to hypoglycemia is usually measured indrectly by plasma cortisol levels because the test is more universally available. A normal response is an increase of 6 μg/dl or more over baseline cortisol levels. Lack of response to hypoglycemic stimulation indicates either pituitary or adrenal hypofunction. These two can be differentiated by either directly measuring plasma ACTH levels or by administering ACTH preparations and observing cortisol response.

Purified exogenous ACTH or synthetic ACTH preparations (e.g., cosyntropin) may be used diagnostically to stimulate cortisol secretion. The usual response is an increase in plasma cortisol levels of 7 to 18 μg/dl over baseline levels within 1 hour of ACTH administration. Lack of response indicates adrenal insufficiency.[47]

ALDOSTERONE (CLINICAL APPLICATIONS DATA, p. 245)

Aldosterone, the predominant mineralocorticoid, is secreted by the zona glomerulosa of the adrenal cortex in response to decreased serum sodium, decreased blood volume, and increased serum potassium. It is thought that altered serum sodium and potasium levels directly stimulate the adrenal cortex to release aldosterone. In addition, decreased blood volume and altered sodium and potassium levels stimulate the juxtaglomerular apparatus of the kidney to secrete renin. Renin is subsequently converted to angiotensin II, which then stimulates the adrenal cortex to secrete aldosterone. In normal states, adrenocorticotropic hormone (ACTH) does not play a major role in aldosterone secretion. In disease or stress states, however, ACTH also may enhance aldosterone secretion.

Aldosterone increases sodium reabsorption in the renal tubules, the gastrointestinal tract, salivary glands, and sweat glands. This subsequently results in increased water retention, blood volume, and blood pressure. Aldosterone also increases potassium excretion by the kidneys in exchange for the sodium ions that are retained.

Excessive aldosterone levels are categorized as primary and secondary hyperaldosteronism. Primary hyperaldosteronism represents inappropriate aldosterone secretion, which is usually due to benign adenomas or bilateral hyperplasia of the aldosterone-secreting zona glomerulosa cells. Excessive aldosterone is secreted independently of control by the renin-angiotensin system. A hallmark of primary hyperaldosteronism is low plasma renin levels (see p. 205).

Secondary hyperaldosteronism indicates an appropriate response to pathological changes in blood volume and electrolytes (i.e., decreased serum sodium or increased serum potassium). Common causes of secondary hyperaldosteronism include congestive heart failure, cirrhosis, nephrotic syndrome, chronic obstructive pulmonary disease, and renal artery stenosis. In secondary hyperaldosteronism, plasma renin levels are elevated. Presenting features of both primary and secondary hyperaldosteronism include low serum potassium, high-normal or slightly elevated serum sodium, metabolic alkalosis, and hypertension. Elevated aldosterone levels also are associated with upright body position, stress, and late pregnancy. Drugs that may lead to elevated aldosterone levels include diuretics, Apresoline, Hyperstat, and nitroprusside.

Hypernatremia and hypokalemia will decrease aldosterone secretion as will excessive licorice ingestion. Decreased aldosterone levels may be seen in diabetes mellitus and toxemia of pregnancy. Drugs that may produce decreased aldosterone levels include propranolol and fludrocortisone (Florinef).

ALDOSTERONE CHALLENGE TESTS

In normal individuals, increased serum sodium levels and blood volume suppress aldosterone secretion. In primary aldosteronism, however, this response is not seen. Serum sodium levels may be elevated through ingestion of a high-sodium diet for approximately 4 days or by infusing 2 liters of normal saline intravenously. If there is appropriate control of aldosterone levels through negative feedback systems and the renin-angiotensin system, plasma aldosterone levels will be low normal or decreased in response to the increased sodium load. Fludrocortisone acetate (Florinef), a synthetic mineralocorticoid, will produce the same effect after 3 days of administration. Aldosterone challenges are used to differentiate between primary and secondary hyperaldosteronism.[48]

CATECHOLAMINES (CLINICAL APPLICATIONS DATA, p. 246)

The adrenal medulla, a component of the sympathetic nervous system, secretes epinephrine and norepinephrine, which are collectively known as the catecholamines. A third catecholamine, dopamine, is secreted in the brain where it functions as a neurotransmitter.

Epinephrine (adrenalin) is secreted in response to generalized sympathetic stimulation, hypoglycemia, or arterial hypotension. It increases the metabolic rate of all cells, heart rate, arterial blood pressure, and blood glucose and free fatty acid levels; peripheral resistance and blood flow to the skin and kidneys are decreased.

Norepinephrine is secreted by sympathetic nerve endings, as well as by the adrenal medulla, in response to sympathetic stimulation and the presence of tyramine. It decreases the heart rate, while increasing peripheral vascular resistance and arterial blood pressure. Normally, norepinephrine is the predominant catecholamine.

The only clinically significant disorder involving the adrenal medulla is the catecholamine-secreting tumor, pheochromocytoma. Catecholamine-producing tumors also may originate along sympathetic paraganglia; these are known as functional paragangliomas. Pheochromocytomas may release catecholamines, primarily epinephrine, continuously or intermittently. Since the most common sign of pheochromocytoma is arterial hypertension, measurement of plasma catecholamines (or the urinary metabolites thereof) is indicated in evaluating new-onset hypertension.[49]

Shock, stress, hyperthyroidism, strenuous exercise, and smoking may produce elevated plasma catecholamines. Levels also vary diurnally and with postural changes. Because the adrenal glands secrete catecholamines in episodic bursts, several plasma determinations may be necessary for accurate diagnostic interpretation.

Drugs that elevate plasma catecholamine levels include dopamine, levophed, sympathomimetics, tricyclic antidepressants, alpha-methyldopa, hydralazine, quinidine, and Isuprel. Drugs which may lead to decreased levels include ganglionic and adrenergic blocking agents (e.g., hexamethonium, guanethidine, and reserpine). A diet high in amines (e.g., bananas, nuts, cereal grains, tea, coffee, cocoa, aged cheese, beer, ale, certain wines, avocados, fava beans) may falsely elevate plasma catecholamines, but the effect is more likely to be seen in relation to certain urinary metabolites.

Gonadal Hormones

The gonadal hormones, secreted primarily by the ovaries and testes, include estrogens, progesterone, and testosterone. These hormones are essential for normal sexual development and reproductive function in men and women. All gonadal hormones are steroids, and their molecular structures and those of the adrenal corticosteroids are quite similar. Moreover, small amounts of the gonadal hormones or precursors thereof are secreted by the adrenal glands in both males and females.

Secretion of gonadal hormones is regulated via the hypothalamic-hypophyseal system. When blood levels of gonadal hormones decline, the hypothalamus is stimulated to release gonadotropin-releasing hormone (GnRH), which then stimulates the adenohypophysis to release its gonadotropic hormones. These tropic hormones are called, in both men and women, follicle-stimulating hormone (FSH) and luteinizing hormone (LH), even though the ovarian follicle and corpus luteum are unique to females.

ESTROGENS (CLINICAL APPLICATIONS DATA, p. 248)

Estrogens are secreted in large amounts by the ovaries and, during pregnancy, by the placenta. Minute amounts are secreted by the adrenal glands and, possibly, by the testes. Estrogens induce and maintain the female secondary sex characteristics, promote growth and maturation of the female reproductive organs, influence the pattern of fat deposition that characterizes the female form, and cause early epiphyseal closure. They also promote retention of sodium and water by the kidneys and sensitize the myometrium to oxytocin.

Elevated estrogen levels are associated with ovarian and adrenal tumors as well as estrogen-producing tumors of the testes. Elevations also are seen in precocious puberty and cirrhosis. Decreased levels are associated with primary and secondary ovarian failure, Turner's syndrome, hypopituitarism, adrenogenital syndrome, Stein-Leventhal syndrome, anorexia nervosa, and menopause. Estrogen levels vary in relation to the menstrual cycle. Therapy with estrogen-containing drugs and adrenal corticosteroids will elevate levels, while clomiphene will decrease them.

Many different types of estrogens have been identified, but only three are present in the blood in measurable amounts: estrone, estradiol, and estriol. Estrone (E_1) is the immediate precursor of estradiol (E_2), which is the most biologically potent. In addition to ovarian sources, estriole (E_3) is secreted in large amounts by the placenta during pregnancy from precursors produced by the fetal liver. Through radioimmunoassay, plasma levels of E_2 and E_3 may be determined. Total plasma estrogen levels are difficult to measure and are not routinely done.

PROGESTERONE (CLINICAL APPLICATIONS DATA, p. 249)

Progesterone is secreted in nonpregnant females during the latter half of the menstrual cycle by the corpus luteum and in large amounts by the placenta during pregnancy. It also is secreted in minute amounts by the adrenal cortex in both males and females. Progesterone prepares the endometrium for implantation of the fertilized ovum, decreases myometrial excitability, stimulates proliferation of the vaginal epithelium, and stimulates growth of the breasts during pregnancy. Although progesterone may promote sodium and water retention, its effect is weaker than that of aldosterone, which it directly antagonizes. The net effect is loss of sodium and water from the body.

Abnormally elevated progesterone levels are associated with precocious puberty, ovarian tumor or cysts, and adrenocortical hyperplasia and tumors. Elevated levels also may be seen with estrogen, progesterone, or adrenocortical therapy. Decreased levels are associated with panhypopituitarism, ovarian failure, Turner's syndrome, adrenogenital syndrome, Stein-Leventhal syndrome, placental insufficiency, fetal abnormality or demise, threatened abortion, and toxemia of pregnancy.

TESTOSTERONE (CLINICAL APPLICATIONS DATA, p. 250)

Testosterone is produced in the mature male by the Leydig cells of the testes. Minute amounts also are secreted by the adrenal glands in males and females, and by the ovaries in females. In the male fetus, testosterone is secreted by the genital ridges and fetal testes.

Testosterone is produced in response to stimulation by luteinizing hormone (LH), which is secreted by the adenohypophysis in response to stimulation by gonadotropin-releasing hormone (GnRH). Testosterone promotes development of the male sex organs and testicular descent in the fetus, induces and maintains secondary sexual characteristics in males, promotes protein anabolism and bone growth, and enhances sodium and water retention to some degree.

Elevated testosterone levels in males are associated with precocious puberty, testicular tumors, and benign prostatic hypertrophy. In females, elevated levels are associated with adrenogenital syndrome, adrenal tumors or hyperplasia, Stein-Leventhal syndrome, ovarian tumors or hyperplasia, and luteomas of pregnancy. Levels may be elevated in both men and women with nonendocrine tumors that produce adrenocorticotropic hormone (ACTH) ectopically. Administration of testosterone, thyroid and growth hormones, clomiphene, and barbiturates also may lead to elevated levels. Decreased levels are associated with testicular failure, hypopituitarism, Kleinfelter's syndrome, cryptorchidism (failure of testicular descent), and cirrhosis. Therapy with estrogens and aldactone also may produce decreased levels. Testosterone levels vary diurnally, with highest levels occurring in the early morning.

Placental Hormones

During pregnancy, the placenta secretes estrogens, progesterone, human chorionic gonadotropin (hCG), and human placental lactogen (hPL). Estrogens and progesterone, which are not specific to pregnancy, are discussed in the preceding sections. In contrast, hCG and hPL are fairly specific to pregnancy but levels also may be altered in individuals with trophoblastic tumors (e.g., hydatidiform mole, choriocarcinoma) and tumors that ectopically secrete placental hormones.

HUMAN CHORIONIC GONADOTROPIN (hCG) (CLINICAL APPLICATIONS DATA, p. 251)

Human chorionic gonadotropin (hCG) is a glycoprotein that is unique to the developing placenta. Its presence in blood and urine has been used for decades to detect pregnancy. Tests using rabbits, frogs, and rats, however, have now been replaced by immunological tests that employ antibodies to hCG. Earlier immunological tests were not always reliable since the antibody used could cross-react with other glycoprotein hormones such as luteinizing hormine (LH). Furthermore, it was sometimes not possible to obtain reliable results until 4 to 8 weeks after the first missed period. Currently, more sensitive and specific tests use antibody that reacts only with the beta subunit of hCG, not with other hormones. The most sensitive of the radioimmunoassays for hCG can detect elevated levels within 8 to 10 days after conception, even before the first missed period.

Since hCG is associated with the developing placenta it is secreted at increasingly higher levels during the first 2 months of pregnancy, declines during the third and fourth months, and then remains relatively stable until term. Levels return to normal within 1 to 2 weeks of termination of pregnancy. Human chorionic gonadotropin prevents the normal involution of the corpus luteum at the end of the menstrual cycle and stimulates it to double in size and produce large quantities of estrogen and progesterone. hCG also is thought to stimulate the testes of the male fetus to produce testosterone and to induce descent of the testicles into the scrotum.

In addition to pregnancy, elevated hCG levels are associated with hydatidiform mole, choriocarcinoma, and testicular epithelioma. Elevated levels also may be seen in nonendocrine tumors which produce hCG ectopically (e.g., carcinomas of the stomach, liver, pancreas, and breast; multiple myeloma; and malignant melanoma). Decreased levels are seen in intrauterine fetal demise, threatened abortion, and incomplete abortion.[50]

HUMAN PLACENTAL LACTOGEN (hPL) (CLINICAL APPLICATIONS DATA, p. 252)

Human placental lactogen (hPL), also known as human chorionic somatotropin (hCS), is produced by the placenta but exerts its known effect on the mother. Human placental lactogen causes decreased maternal sensitivity to insulin and utilization of glucose, thus increasing the glucose available to the fetus. It also promotes release of maternal free fatty acids for utilization by the fetus. hPL also is thought to stimulate the action of growth hormone in protein deposition, promote breast growth and preparation for lactation, and maintain the pregnancy by altering the endometrium.

Human placental lactogen rises steadily through pregnancy, maintaining a high plateau during the last trimester. Blood levels of hPL correlate with placental weight and tend to be high in diabetic mothers. Levels also may be elevated in multiple pregnancy and Rh isoimmunization, as well as in nonendocrine tumors that secrete ectopic hPL. Decreased hPL levels are associated with intrauterine fetal growth retardation, toxemia of pregnancy, impending abortion, hydatidiform mole, and choricocarcinoma.

During pregnancy, hPL levels vary greatly with the individual as well as on a day-to-day basis. Thus, serial determinations may be necessary with the client serving as her own control.[51]

Pancreatic Hormones

The islets of Langerhans, the endocrine cells of the pancreas, produce at least three glucose-related hormones: (1) insulin, which is produced by the beta cells; (2) glucagon, which is produced by the alpha cells; and (3) somatostatin, which is produced by the delta cells.

The overall effect of insulin is to promote glucose utilization and energy storage. It does this by enhancing glucose and potassium entry into most body cells, stimulating glycogen synthesis in liver and muscle, promoting the conversion of glucose to fatty acids and triglycerides, and enhancing protein synthesis. It exerts its effects by interacting with cell surface receptors.

In contrast to insulin, glucagon increases blood glucose levels by stimulating the breakdown of glycogen and the release of glucose stored in the liver. Somatostatin inhibits secretion of both insulin and glucagon. It also inhibits release of growth hormone, thyroid-stimulating hormone and adrenocorticotropic hormone by the adenohypophysis, and may decrease production of parathormone, calcitonin, and renin. In addition, it is thought to inhibit secretion of gastric acid and gastrin. The exact physiological roles of glucagon and somatostatin are unknown.

Blood levels of insulin are measured by radioimmunoassay and may be determined in most laboratories. Samples for blood glucagon levels require special handling and tests for its presence may not be routinely available in all laboratories. Somatostatin may be measured but this test is not routinely done. C-peptide, a metabolically inactive peptide chain formed during the conversion of proinsulin to insulin, may be measured to provide an index of beta cell activity not affected by exogenous insulin.[52]

INSULIN (CLINICAL APPLICATIONS DATA, p. 253)

Insulin is secreted by the beta cells in response to elevated blood glucose, certain amino acids, ketones, fatty acids, cortisol, growth hormone, glucagon, gastrin, secretin, cholecystokinin, gastric inhibitory peptide, estrogen, and progesterone. Because of normal feedback mechanisms, high insulin levels will inhibit secretion of insulin. Elevated blood levels of somatostatin, epinephrine, and norepinephrine also will inhibit insulin secretion.

Abnormally elevated serum insulin levels are seen with insulin- and proinsulin-secreting tumors (insulinomas), with reactive hypoglycemia in developing diabetes mellitus, and with excessive administration of exogenous insulin. Decreased levels are associated with beta cell failure and may be seen with pheochromocytoma with excessive production of catecholamines.

A blood glucose level is usually obtained with the serum insulin determination. Serum insulin levels also may be measured when glucose tolerance tests are performed (see p. 135).

C-PEPTIDE (CLINICAL APPLICATIONS DATA, p. 254)

Measurement of C-peptide, which is done using radioimmunoassay techniques, provides an index of beta cell activity that is unaffected by the administration of exogenous insulin. As the beta cells release insulin, they also release equimolar amounts of metabolically inactive C-peptide. Injectable insulin preparations are purified to remove C-peptide. Furthermore, injected insulin elevates immunoreactive serum insulin levels and suppresses pancreatic secretion of endogenous insulin and C-peptide. That is, while exogenous insulin will elevate serum insulin levels, C-peptide levels will be either unaffected or decreased. C-peptide determinations may be done to augment or confirm results of serum insulin measurements.[53]

GLUCAGON (CLINICAL APPLICATIONS DATA, p. 255)

Glucagon is secreted by the alpha cells of the islets of Langerhans in response to decreased blood glucose levels. Its actions are opposed by insulin. Elevated glucagon levels are associated with conditions that produce actual hypoglycemia or a physiological need for greater blood glucose (e.g., trauma, infection, starvation, excessive exercise), and with insulin lack. Thus, elevated glucagon levels may be found in severe or uncontrolled diabetes mellitus, despite hyperglycemia.

Glucagon is thought to be metabolized in the kidneys. Thus, renal failure or rejection of a transplanted kidney may result in increased serum glucagon levels. Other causes of elevated glucagon levels include glucagonoma, acute pancreatitis, and pheochromocytoma. Infusion of arginine also elevates blood glucagon levels and may be used to confirm deficiency states.

Decreased glucagon levels are seen with elevated blood glucose levels not associated with insulin lack (e.g., after ingesting food), and with loss of pancreatic tissue due to chronic pancreatitis, carcinoma of the pancreas, or surgical resection of the pancreas.

Gastric and Intestinal Hormones

The stomach and intestine secrete various enzymes and hormones that aid in the digestive process. The hormones secreted include gastrin, cholecystokinin, secretin, and gastric inhibitory peptide (GIP). Of these, only gastrin is currently of diagnostic significance.

Gastrin is secreted by the gastrin cells (G cells) of the gastric antrum, the pylorus, and the proximal duodenum in response to vagal stimulation and the presence of food (especially protein) in the stomach. Gastrin stimulates the secretion of acidic gastric juice and pepsin, and the release of pancreatic enzymes. It also stimulates motor activities of the stomach and intestine, increases pyloric relaxation, constricts the gastroesophageal sphincter, and promotes the release of insulin.

Cholecystokinin is secreted by the duodenal mucosa in response to the presence of fats. It opposes the actions of gastrin, stimulates contraction of the gallbladder, relaxes the sphincter of Oddi, and with secretin, controls pancreatic secretions. Secretin is secreted by the duodenal mucosa in response to the presence of peptides and acids in the duodenum. It also opposes the actions of gastrin, and with cholecystokinin, controls pancreatic secretions. GIP inhibits gastric motility and secretion, and stimulates secretion of insulin.

GASTRIN (CLINICAL APPLICATIONS DATA, p. 256)

Measurement of serum gastrin levels, which is done using radioimmunoassay techniques, is indicated when disorders producing elevated levels are suspected. The disorder most commonly associated with excessive gastrin secretion is Zollinger-Ellison syndrome, in which a gastrin-producing tumor (gastrinoma) leads to a condition characterized by peptic ulceration. Most gastrinomas are found in the nonendocrine portions of the pancreas, although a small percentage are found in the duodenal area. G-cell hyperplasia also may cause elevated serum gastrin levels. Excessive gastrin secretion will occur due to normal feedback mechanisms in disorders associated with decreased gastric acid production due to cellular destruction or atrophy (e.g., gastric carcinoma and age-related changes in gastric acid secretion). Elevated levels also may be seen in gastric and duodenal ulcers in which gastric acid secretion is actually normal or low, pernicious anemia, uremia, and chronic gastritis. Decreased gastrin levels are associated with true gastric hyperacidity as may occur with stress ulcers.

It should be noted that both protein ingestion and calcium infusions will elevate serum gastrin levels in certain situations. Thus, these substances may be used to provoke gastrin secretion when a single serum determination is inconclusive. In the secretagogue provocation test, a fasting serum gastrin sample is drawn and the client is then given a high-protein test meal. A postprandial blood sample is then obtained. In individuals with duodenal or gastric ulcers, gastrin levels will be markedly higher than in normal persons after protein-stimulated gastrin secretion. Likewise, an infusion of calcium gluconate will produce elevated serum gastrin levels in a person with gastrinoma due to gastrin production by tumor cells. This effect is not seen in individuals with peptic ulcer disease.

Clinical Applications Data

GROWTH HORMONE (GH, STH, SH) (BACKGROUND INFORMATION, p. 208)
Reference Values

Newborns	15–40 ng/ml
Children	0–10 ng/ml
Adults	0–10 ng/ml

Values may vary according to the laboratory performing the test.

Interfering Factors

- Hyperglycemia and therapy with drugs such as adrenal corticosteroids and chlorpromazine may cause falsely decreased levels
- Hypoglycemia, physical activity, stress, and a variety of drugs (e.g., amphetamines, arginine, dopamine, levodopa, methyldopa, beta blockers, histamine, nicotinic acid, estrogens) may cause falsely elevated levels

Indications/Purposes for Growth Hormone

- Growth retardation in children with decreased levels indicative of pituitary etiology

■ Monitoring response to treatment of growth retardation due to growth hormone deficiency
■ Suspected disorder associated with decreased growth hormone (e.g., pituitary tumors, craniopharyngiomas, tuberculosis meningitis, and pituitary damage or trauma
■ Gigantism in children with increased levels indicative of pituitary etiology
■ Support for diagnosing acromegaly in adults as indicated by elevated levels, and which is frequently due to acidophil or chromophobe tumors of the adenophyophysis

Client Preparation

Client preparation is essentially the same as that for any study involving collection of a peripheral blood sample (see Appendix I). The client should be informed that the test will be performed on two consecutive days, between the hours of 6 and 8 A.M. The client should fast from food and avoid strenuous exercise for 12 hours before each sample is drawn. Additionally, it is recommended by some that the client be maintained on bed rest for 1 hour before each sample is obtained.

Because many drugs may affect serum GH levels, a medication history should be obtained. It is recommended that those drugs that alter test results be withheld for 12 hours prior to the study, although this should be confirmed with the person ordering the test.

The Procedure

The test is performed on two consecutive days, between the hours of 6 and 8 A.M. A venipuncture is performed and the sample collected in a red-topped tube. The sample should be handled gently to avoid hemolysis and sent immediately to the laboratory.

Aftercare and Nursing Observations

Care and assessment following the procedure are the same as for any study involving the collection of a peripheral blood sample. Food and any medications withheld prior to the test, as well as usual activities, should be resumed.

GROWTH HORMONE STIMULATION TESTS (BACKGROUND INFORMATION, p. 209)
Reference Values

Arginine	
Men	>10 ng/ml
Women	>15 ng/ml
L-dopa or insulin	>7 ng/ml above baseline level

Interfering Factors

■ Factors that may affect serum growth hormone determinations (see p. 227) may also alter results of growth hormone stimulation tests

Indications/Purposes for Growth Hormone Stimulation Tests

■ Low or undetectable serum GH levels, with GH deficiency or adult pan-hypopituitarism confirmed by no increase after administration of the stimulant
■ Confirmation of the diagnosis of acromegaly as evidenced by reduced GH output after L-dopa is administered as a stimulant (i.e., an idiosyncratic response is seen in acromegaly)

Nursing Alert

■ If insulin is used as the stimulant, the client should be observed carefully during and after the test for signs and symptoms of extreme hypoglycemia

---

Client Preparation

Initial client preparation is the same as that for serum GH determinations. The client should be weighed on the day of the test, as dosage of the stimulant is weight-determined. Because several blood samples will be obtained and because certain of the stimulants (i.e., insulin and arginine) are administered intravenously, the client should be informed that an intermittent venous access device (e.g., heparin lock) will be inserted.

The Procedure

An intermittent venous access device is inserted, usually at about 8 A.M., and a venous sample is obtained and placed in a red-topped tube. The sample is handled gently to avoid hemolysis and sent to the laboratory immediately.

The stimulant is then administered. L-dopa is administered orally; arginine and insulin are administered intravenously in a saline infusion. If insulin is used to lower blood sugar, an ampule of 50 percent glucose should be on hand in the event that severe hypoglycemia occurs.

After the stimulant is administered, three blood samples are obtained via the venous access device at 30-minute intervals. The samples are placed in red-topped tubes and sent to the laboratory immediately upon collection.

Aftercare and Nursing Observations

Care and assessment following the procedure are essentially the same as for serum GH determinations. If an intermittent venous access device was inserted for the procedure, it should be removed following completion of the test and a pressure bandage applied to the site. If insulin was used as the stimulant, dietary intake should be resumed as soon as possible after the test is completed, and the client observed for signs of hypoglycemia.

GROWTH HORMONE SUPPRESSION TEST (BACKGROUND INFORMATION, p. 209)

Reference Values

< 3 ng/dl

Interfering Factors

- Factors that may affect serum growth hormone determinations (see p. 227) may also alter results of growth hormone suppression tests

Indications/Purposes for Growth Hormone Suppression Test

- Elevated serum GH levels
- Signs of GH hypersecretion with serum GH levels within normal limits
- Confirmation of GH hypersecretion as indicated by decreased response to GH suppression

Client Preparation

Initial client preparation is the same as that for serum GH determinations. The client should be informed that it will be necessary to drink an oral glucose solution and that two blood samples will be obtained.

The Procedure

A venipuncture is performed and a sample collected in a red-topped tube. The sample is handled gently to avoid hemolysis and sent to the laboratory immediately.

The glucose solution (usually 100 g) is administered orally. If the client is unable to drink or retain the glucose solution, the physician is notified. Intravenous glucose may be administered, if necessary, to perform the test.

After 1 to 2 hours, depending on laboratory procedures, a second blood sample is collected in a red-topped tube and sent to the laboratory immediately.

Aftercare and Nursing Observations

Care and assessment following the procedure are the same as that for serum GH determinations.

PROLACTIN (HPRL, LTH) (BACKGROUND INFORMATION, p. 209)
Reference Values

Children	1–20 ng/ml
Men	1–20 ng/ml
Women	
Nonlactating	1–25 ng/ml
Menopausal	1–20 ng/ml

Interfering Factors

- Therapy with drugs such as estrogens, oral contraceptives, reserpine, alpha-methyldopa, phenothiazines, haloperidol, tricyclic antidepressants, and procainamide derivatives may produce elevated levels
- Episodic elevations may occur in response to sleep, stress, exercise, and hypoglycemia
- Therapy with dopamine, apomorphine, and ergot alkaloids may produce decreased levels

Indications/Purposes for Serum Prolactin

■ Sexual dysfunction in men and women of unknown etiology, since excessive circulating prolactin may indicate the source of the problem (e.g., damage to the hypothalamus, pituitary adenoma)

■ Failure of lactation in the postpartum period and/or suspected postpartum hypophyseal infarction (Sheehan's syndrome), as indicated by decreased levels

■ Suspected tumor involving the lungs or kidneys with elevated levels indicating ectopic prolactin production

■ Support for diagnosing primary hypothyroidism as indicated by elevated levels

Client Preparation

Client preparation is the same as for any study involving collection of a peripheral blood sample (see Appendix I).

Since many drugs may alter serum prolactin levels, a medication history should be obtained. It is recommended that drugs that may alter test results be withheld for 12 to 24 hours prior to the test, although this should be confirmed with the person ordering the study.

The Procedure

A venipuncture is performed and the sample collected in a red-topped tube. The sample should be handled gently to avoid hemolysis and transported promptly to the laboratory.

Aftercare and Nursing Observations

Care and assessment following the procedure are the same as that for any study involving the collection of a peripheral blood sample. Any medications withheld prior to the test should be resumed.

ADRENOCORTICOTROPIC HORMONE (ACTH) (BACKGROUND INFORMATION, p. 210)

Reference Values

BioScience Labs	<80 pg/ml at 8 A.M.
Mayo Clinic	<120 pg/ml at 6 to 8 A.M.

Normal values vary according to the laboratory performing the test. Results are usually evaluated in relation to other tests of adrenal-hypophyseal function (e.g., plasma cortisol).

Interfering Factors

■ ACTH levels vary diurnally; highest levels occur upon awakening, decrease throughout the day, and then begin to rise again a few hours before awakening

■ Numerous drugs may lead to decreased ACTH levels (e.g., adrenal corticoste-

roids, estrogens, calcium gluconate, amphetamines, spironolactone, and ethanol)
■ Stress, exercise, and blood glucose levels may affect results

Indications/Purposes for Plasma ACTH

■ Signs and symptoms of adrenal cortical dysfunction
 ☐ Elevated ACTH levels with low cortisol levels indicate adrenal cortical hypoactivity (Addison's disease)
 ☐ Low ACTH levels with high cortisol levels indicate adrenal cortical hyperactivity (Cushing's syndrome) due to benign or malignant adrenal tumors
 ☐ High ACTH levels, without diurnal variation, combined with high cortisol levels indicate adrenal cortical hyperfunction due to excessive ACTH production (e.g., due to pituitary adenoma and nonendocrine malignant tumors in which there is ectopic ACTH production)
 ☐ Decreased ACTH levels are associated with panhypopituitarism, hypothalamic dysfunction, and long-term adrenal corticosteroid therapy

Client Preparation

General client preparation is the same as that for any study involving collection of a peripheral blood sample (see Appendix I). For this test, the client should follow a low-carbohydrate diet for 48 hours and fast from food for 12 hours prior to the test. In addition, strenuous exercise should be avoided for 12 hours prior to the test, and 1 hour of bed rest is necessary immediately before the test. Medications that may alter test results should be withheld for at least 24 to 48 hours, or longer, prior to the study, although this should be confirmed with the person ordering the test.

The client should be informed that it may be necessary to obtain more than one sample, and that samples must be obtained at specific times to detect peak and trough levels of ACTH.

The Procedure

Between 6 and 8 A.M. (peak ACTH secretion time), a venipuncture is performed and the sample collected in a green-topped tube. The sample must be placed in a container of ice and sent to the laboratory immediately. When ACTH hypersecretion is suspected, a second sample may be obtained between 8 and 10 P.M. to determine if diurnal variation in ACTH levels is occurring.

Aftercare and Nursing Observations

Care and assessment following the procedure are the same as for any study involving the collection of a peripheral blood sample. Foods and any medications withheld prior to the test, as well as usual activities, should be resumed.

THYROID-STIMULATING HORMONE (TSH) (BACKGROUND INFORMATION, p. 211)
Reference Values

Newborns	<25 µIU/ml by day 3
Children and adults	<10 µIU/ml
	$<10^{-3}$ IU/l (SI Units)

Interfering Factors

■ Aspirin, adrenal corticosteroids, and heparin may produce decreased TSH levels
■ Lithium carbonate and potassium iodide may produce elevated TSH levels
■ Falsely increased levels may occur in hydatidiform mole, choriocarcinoma, embryonal carcinoma of the testes, pregnancy, and postmenopausal states characterized by high FSH and LH levels

Indications/Purposes for Thyroid-Stimulating Hormone

■ Signs and symptoms of hypothyroidism or hyperthyroidism and/or suspected pituitary or hypothalamic dysfunction
   ☐ Elevated levels are seen with primary hypothyroidism
   ☐ Decreased or undetectable levels are associated with secondary hypothyroidism due to pituitary or hypothalamic hypofunction
   ☐ Decreased levels are seen with primary hyperthyroidism
   ☐ Elevated levels may indicate secondary hyperthyroidism due to pituitary hyperactivity (e.g., due to tumor)
■ Differentiation of functional euthyroidism from true hypothyroidism in debilitated individuals, with the former indicated by normal levels.

Client Preparation

Client preparation is the same as that for any study involving collection of a peripheral blood sample (see Appendix I). It is recommended that those drugs which are known to alter TSH levels be withheld for 12 to 24 hours prior to the test, although this should be confirmed with the person ordering the study.

The Procedure

A venipuncture is performed and the sample is collected in a red-topped tube. The sample should be handled gently to avoid hemolysis and transported promptly to the laboratory.

Aftercare and Nursing Observations

Care and assessment following the procedure are the same as for any study involving the collection of a peripheral blood sample. Any medications withheld prior to the test should be resumed.

TSH Stimulation Test (Background Information, p. 211)

Reference Values

TSH levels rise within 15 to 30 minutes of thyrotropin-releasing hormome (TRH) administration, peak at 2.5 to 4 times normal, and return to baseline levels within 2 to 4 hours. Thyroid hormone secretion (e.g., T_3 and T_4), which should be increased by 50 to 75 percent, will occur in 1 to 4 hours.

Indications/Purposes for TSH Stimulation Test

■ Low or undetectable serum TSH levels and/or hypothyroidism or hyperthyroidism of unknown etiology or type
   ☐ A normal or delayed TSH response in persons with low baseline TSH levels and signs of hypothyroidism indicates hypothalamic dysfunction or

disruption of the hypothalamic-hypophyseal portal circulation and confirms the diagnosis of tertiary hypothyroidism

☐ A decreased or absent TSH response in persons with low baseline TSH levels and signs of hypothyroidism indicates hypopituitarism and confirms the diagnosis of secondary hypothyroidism

☐ A normal or increased TSH response in clients with elevated baseline TSH levels and signs of hypothyroidism, with persistently decreased thyroid gland hormone levels, confirms the diagnosis of primary hypothyroidism

☐ A decreased or absent TSH response in persons with low baseline TSH levels and signs of hyperthyroidism, with persistently elevated thyroid gland hormone levels, indicates that thyroid hormone production is occurring autonomously and confirms the diagnosis of primary hyperthyroidism

Client Preparation

Initial client preparation is the same as that for serum determinations of thyroid-stimulating hormone. Because several blood samples will be obtained and because the TRH will be administered intravenously, the client should be informed that an intermittent venous access device (e.g., heparin lock) may be inserted.

The Procedure

The procedure varies somewhat according to the laboratory performing the test. One example of the procedure is described subsequently.

An intermittent venous access device is inserted and a venous sample is obtained and placed in a red-topped tube. The sample is handled gently to avoid hemolysis and sent promptly to the laboratory. The sample should be labeled either with the time drawn or as the baseline sample.

A bolus of TRH is then administered intravenously through the access device. Additional blood samples are obtained via the access device one half, 1, 2, 3, and 4 hours after administration of the TRH. Each sample is placed in a red-topped tube, labeled, and sent to the laboratory.

Aftercare and Nursing Observations

Care and assessment following the procedure are essentially the same as for serum TSH determinations. If an intermittent venous access device was inserted for the procedure, it should be removed following completion of the test and a pressure bandage applied to the site.

FOLLICLE-STIMULATING HORMONE (FSH) (BACKGROUND INFORMATION, p. 212)

Reference Values

Children	5–10 mIU/ml
Men	10–15 mIU/ml
Women (menstruating)	
Early in cycle	5–25 mIU/ml
Midcycle	20–30 mIU/ml
Luteal phase	5–25 mIU/ml
Women (menopausal)	40–250 mIU/ml

Results should be evaluated in relation to other tests of gonadal function.

Interfering Factors

- In menstruating women, values vary in relation to the phase of the menstrual cycle
- Values are higher in postmenopausal women
- Administration of the drug clomiphene may result in elevated FSH levels
- Therapy with estrogens, progesterone, and phenothiazines may result in decreased FSH levels

Indications/Purposes for Follicle-Stimulating Hormone

- Evaluation of ambiguous sexual differentiation in infants
- Evaluation of early sexual development in girls under age 9 or boys under age 10, with precocious puberty associated with elevated levels
- Evaluation of failure of sexual maturation in adolescence
- Evaluation of sexual dysfunction or changes in secondary sexual characteristics in men and women
  - ☐ Elevated levels are associated with ovarian or testicular failure, with polycystic ovary disease, following viral orchitis, and with Turner's syndrome in females and Klinefelter's syndrome in males
  - ☐ Decreased levels may be seen with neoplasms of the testes, ovaries, and adrenal glands, which result in excessive production of sex hormones
- Suspected pituitary or hypothalamic dysfunction
  - ☐ Elevated levels may be seen in pituitary tumors
  - ☐ Decreased levels are associated with hypothalamic lesions and panhypopituitarism
- Suspected early acromegaly as indicated by elevated levels
- Suspected disorders associated with decreased FSH levels such as anorexia nervosa and renal disease

Client Preparation

Client preparation is the same as that for any study involving collection of a peripheral blood sample (see Appendix I). It is recommended that those drugs that are known to alter FSH levels be withheld for 12 to 24 hours prior to the test, although this should be confirmed with the person ordering the study. In women, the phase of the menstrual cycle should be ascertained if possible.

The Procedure

A venipuncture is performed and the sample collected in a red-topped tube. The sample should be handled gently to avoid hemolysis and transported to the laboratory immediately.

Aftercare and Nursing Observations

Care and assessment following the procedure are the same as for any study involving the collection of a peripheral blood sample. Any medications withheld prior to the test should be resumed.

LUTEINIZING HORMONE (LH, ICSH) (BACKGROUND INFORMATION, p. 212)

Reference Values

Children	5–10 mIU/ml
Men	5–20 mIU/ml

Women (menstruating)	
Early in cycle	5–25 mIU/ml
Midcycle	40–80 mIU/ml
Luteal phase	5–25 mIU/ml
Women (menopausal)	>75 mIU/ml

Results should be evaluated in relation to other tests of gonadal function.

Interfering Factors

■ In menstruating women, values vary in relation to the phase of the menstrual cycle
■ Values are higher in postmenopausal women
■ Drugs containing estrogen tend to cause elevated LH levels
■ Drugs containing progesterone and testosterone may lead to decreased levels

Indications/Purposes for Serum Luteinizing Hormone

■ Evaluation of male and female infertility, as indicated by decreased levels
■ Support for diagnosing infertility due to anovulation as evidenced by lack of the midcycle LH surge
■ Evaluating response to therapy to induce ovulation
■ Suspected pituitary or hypothalamic dysfunction
  □ Elevated levels may be seen in pituitary tumors
  □ Decreased levels are associated with hypothalamic lesions and pan-hypopituitarism

Client Preparation

Client preparation is the same as that for any study involving collection of a peripheral blood sample (see Appendix I). It is recommended that any drugs that are known to alter LH levels be withheld for 12 to 24 hours prior to the test, although this should be confirmed with the person ordering the study. In women, the phase of the menstrual cycle should be ascertained if possible.

If the test is being performed to detect ovulation, the client should be informed that it may be necessary to obtain a series of samples over a period of several days to detect peak LH levels.

The Procedure

A venipuncture is performed and the sample collected in a red-topped tube. The sample should be handled gently to avoid hemolysis and transported promptly to the laboratory.

Aftercare and Nursing Observations

Care and assessment following the procedure are the same as for any study involving the collection of a peripheral blood sample. Any medications withheld prior to the test should be resumed.

ANTIDIURETIC HORMONE (ADH) (BACKGROUND INFORMATION, p. 214)

Reference Values

2.3–3.1 pg/ml

Interfering Factors

■ Alcohol, phenytoin drugs, beta-adrenergic drugs, and morphine antagonists may lead to decreased ADH secretion
■ Acetaminophen, barbiturates, cholinergic agents, clofibrate, estrogens, nicotine, oral hypoglycemic agents, cytotoxic agents (e.g., vincristine), tricyclic antidepressants, oxytocin, Tegretol, and thiazide diuretics may lead to increased ADH secretion
■ Pain, stress, and anxiety may lead to increased ADH secretion
■ Failure to follow dietary and exercise restrictions prior to the test may alter results

Indications/Purposes for Serum Antidiuretic Hormone

■ Polyuria and/or altered serum osmolality of unknown etiology to identify possible alterations in ADH secretion as the cause
■ Central nervous system trauma, surgery, or disease that may lead to impaired secretion of ADH
■ Differentiation of neurogenic (central) diabetes insipidus from nephrogenic diabetes insipidus
  □ Neurogenic diabetes insipidus is characterized by decreased ADH levels
  □ ADH levels may be elevated in nephrogenic diabetes insipidus if normal feedback mechanisms are intact
■ Known or suspected malignancy associated with syndrome of inappropriate ADH secretion (e.g., oat cell lung cancer, thymoma, lymphoma, leukemia, and carcinoma of the pancreas, prostate gland, and intestine) with the disorder indicated by elevated ADH levels
■ Known or suspected pulmonary conditions associated with syndrome of inappropriate ADH secretion (e.g., tuberculosis, pneumonia, and positive pressure mechanical ventilation) with the disorder indicated by elevated ADH levels

Client Preparation

Client preparation is essentially the same as that for any study involving collection of a peripheral blood sample (see Appendix I). The client should fast from food and avoid strenuous exercise for 12 hours before the sample is obtained. It is recommended that drugs that may alter ADH levels be withheld for 12 to 24 hours prior to the study, although this should be confirmed with the person ordering the test.

The Procedure

A venipuncture is performed and the sample collected in a plastic red-topped tube. Plastic is used because contact with glass causes degradation of ADH. The sample should be handled gently to avoid hemolysis and sent to the laboratory immediately.

Aftercare and Nursing Observations

Care and assessment following the procedure are the same as for any study involving collection of a peripheral blood sample. Food and any medications withheld prior to the test, as well as usual activities, should be resumed.

THYROXINE (T₄) (BACKGROUND INFORMATION, p. 216)

Reference Values

T₄D	
Newborns	11.0–23.0 µg/dl
1 to 4 months old	7.5–16.5 µg/dl
4 to 12 months old	5.5–14.5 µg/dl
Children	5.0–13.5 µg/dl
Adults	4.5–13.0 µg/dl
T₄ RIA	4.0–12.0 µg/dl
FT₄	0.9–2.3 ng/dl
FT₄ I	3.8–14.9

Values may vary according to the laboratory performing the test. Results should be evaluated in relation to other tests of thyroid function.

Interfering Factors

- Results of T_4 D may be altered by circulating iodinated substances; T_4 RIA is not similarly affected
- Pregnancy, estrogen therapy, or estrogen-secreting tumors may produce elevated T_4 levels
- Ingestion of thyroxine will elevate T_4 levels
- Heroin and methadone may produce elevated T_4 levels
- Androgens, glucocorticoids, heparin, salicylates, phenytoin anticonvulsants, sulfonamides, and antithyroid drugs such as propylthiouracil may lead to decreased T_4 levels

Indications/Purposes for Thyroxine

- Signs of hypothyroidism or hyperthyroidism and/or neonatal screening for congenital hypothyroidism (required in many states)
  - ☐ Decreased T_4 and FT_4 levels indicate hypothyroid states and also may be seen in early thyroiditis
  - ☐ Elevated T_4 and FT_4 levels indicate hyperthyroid states
  - ☐ Normal T_4 and FT_4 levels in clients with signs of hyperthyroidism may indicate T_3 thyrotoxicosis
  - ☐ Normal FT_4 levels are seen in pregnancy, while T_4 and thyroxine-binding globulin (TBG) usually are elevated
- Monitoring response to therapy for hypothyroidism or hyperthyroidism
  - ☐ Elevated T_4 and FT_4 levels indicate response to treatment for hypothyroidism
  - ☐ Decreased T_4 and FT_4 levels indicate response to treatment for hyperthyroidism
- Evaluating thyroid response to protein deficiency associated with severe illnesses (e.g., metastatic cancer, liver disease, renal disease, diabetes mellitus, cardiovascular disorders, burns, and trauma)
  - ☐ T_4 is decreased in such disorders owing to a deficiency of thyroxine-binding globulin (TBG), a protein
  - ☐ FT_4 I is normal, if thyroid function is normal, since FT_4 I is not dependent on TBG levels

Client Preparation

Client preparation is essentially the same as that for any study involving collection of a peripheral blood sample (see Appendix I). It is usually recommended that thyroid medications should be withheld for 1 month before the test, and that other drugs that may alter thyroxine levels be withheld for at least 24 hours prior to the study. This should be confirmed, however, with the person ordering the test.

For infants, explain to the parent(s) the purpose of the test and that it may need to be repeated in 3 to 6 weeks due to normal changes in infant thyroid hormone levels.

The Procedure

A venipuncture is performed and the sample collected in a red-topped tube. The sample should be handled gently to avoid hemolysis and transported promptly to the laboratory.

For neonatal screening, the sample is obtained by heel stick. A multiple neonatal screening kit is usually employed; the directions provided with the kit must be followed carefully.

Aftercare and Nursing Observations

Care and assessment following the procedure are the same as for any study involving collection of a peripheral blood sample. Any medications withheld prior to the test should be resumed.

TRIIODOTHYRONINE (T_3) (BACKGROUND INFORMATION, p. 217)
Reference Values

T_3 RIA	
Newborns	90–170 ng/dl
Adults	80–200 ng/dl
FT_3	0.2–0.6 ng/dl
rT_3	38–44 ng/dl

Indications/Purposes for Triiodothyronine

■ Support for diagnosing hyperthyroidism in clients with normal T_4 levels, with early hyperthyroidism and T_3 thyrotoxicosis indicated by elevated T_3 levels in the presence of normal T_4 levels

■ Support for diagnosing "euthyroid sick" syndrome in severely ill clients with protein deficiency, as indicated by low T_3 levels, normal FT_3 levels, and elevated rT_3 levels

Client Preparation

Client preparation is essentially the same as that for any study involving collection of a peripheral blood sample (see Appendix I).

The Procedure

A venipuncture is performed and the sample collected in a red-topped tube. The sample should be handled gently to avoid hemolysis and transported promptly to the laboratory

Aftercare and Nursing Observations

Care and assessment following the procedure are the same as for any study involving collection of a peripheral blood sample.

T₃ Uptake RT₃ U (Background Information, p. 217)

Reference Values

T₃ resin uptake	25–35%
T₃ uptake ratio	0.1–1.35

Interfering Factors

■ Drugs that alter thyroxine-binding globulin (TBG) levels or that compete for TBG binding sites may affect test results
  ☐ Estrogens may lead to increased TBG levels
  ☐ Androgens and glucocorticoids may lead to decreased TBG levels
  ☐ Salicylates and phenytoin anticonvulsants compete with T_4 for TBG binding sites
■ Results may vary during pregnancy when TBG levels are usually elevated

Indications/Purposes for T₃ Uptake

■ Signs of hypothyroidism or hyperthyroidism
  ☐ Decreased levels (indicating a low percentage of radiolabeled T_3 remaining) indicate low serum T_4 levels and hypothyroidism
  ☐ Elevated levels (indicating a high percentage of radiolabeled T_3 remaining) indicate high serum T_4 levels and hyperthyroidism
■ Known or suspected problems associated with altered TBG levels (e.g., hereditary abnormality of TBG synthesis, drug therapy, pregnancy, and disorders associated with decreased serum proteins)
  ☐ Elevated levels may indicate low TBG levels
  ☐ Decreased levels may indicate elevated TBG levels
■ Monitoring response to therapy with drugs that compete with T_4 for TBG binding sites
  ☐ Elevated levels may indicate that TBG binding sites are saturated with competing drugs
■ Calculation of free T_3 and T_4 indices (see pp. 216 and 217)

Client Preparation

Client preparation is essentially the same as that for any study invovling collection of a peripheral blood sample (see Appendix I). It is recommended that drugs that alter TBG levels or compete for TGB binding sites be withheld for 12 to 24 hours prior to the test, although this should be confirmed with the person ordering the study.

The Procedure

A venipuncture is performed and the sample collected in a red-topped tube. The sample should be handled gently to avoid hemolysis and transported promptly to the laboratory.

Aftercare and Nursing Observations

Care and assessment following the procedure are the same as for any study involving collection of a peripheral blood sample. Any medications withheld prior to the test should be resumed.

THYROXINE-BINDING GLOBULIN (TBG) (BACKGROUND INFORMATION, p. 217)
Reference Values

12–18 μg/dl

Interfering Factors

■ Estrogens elevate serum TBG levels and, thus, women who are pregnant, who are receiving estrogen therapy or oral contraceptives, or who have estrogen-secreting tumors will have higher TBG levels
■ Androgens and corticosteriods decrease serum TBG levels

Indications/Purposes for Thyroxine-Binding Globulin

■ Signs and symptoms of hypothyroidism or hyperthyroidism in conditions associated with altered TBG levels (e.g., pregnancy) to differentiate true thyriod disorders from problems related to altered TBG levels
■ Diagnosis of hereditary abnormality of globulin systhesis is indicated by decreased levels

Client preparation

Client preparation is essentially the same as that for any study involving collection of a peripheral blood sample (see Appendix I). It is recommended that drugs that may alter TBG levels be withheld for 12 to 24 hours prior to the test, although this should be confirmed with the person ordering the study.

The Procedure

A venipuncture is performed and the sample is collected in a red-topped tube. The sample should be handled gently to avoid hemolysis and transported promply to the laboratory.

Aftercare and Nursing Observations

Care and assessment following the procedure are the same as for any study involving collection of a peripheral blood sample. Any medications withheld prior to the test should be resumed.

THYROID-STIMULATING IMMUNOGLOBULINS (TSI, TSIg) (BACKGROUND INFORMATION, p. 218)

Reference Values

TSI is not normally detected in the serum, although it may be found in the serum of about 5 percent of people without apparent hyperthyroidism or exophthalmos.

Interfering Factors

■ Administration of radioactive iodine preparations within 24 hours of the test may alter results

Indications/Purposes for Thyroid-Stimulating Immunoglobulins

■ Known or suspected thyrotoxicosis with elevated levels found in 50 to 80 percent of affected individuals
■ Determination of possible etiology of exophthalmos as indicated by elevated levels
■ Monitoring response to treatment for thyrotoxicosis with possible relapse indicated by elevated levels

Client Preparation

Client preparation is essentially the same as that for any study involving collection of a peripheral blood sample (see Appendix I). The client should not have received any radioactive iodine preparations within 24 hours of the test.

The Procedure

A venipuncture is performed and the sample collected in a red-topped tube. The sample should be handled gently to avoid hemolysis and transported promptly to the laboratory.

Aftercare and Nursing Observations

Care and assessment following the procedure are the same as that for any study involving collection of a peripheral blood sample.

CALCITONIN (BACKGROUND INFORMATION, p. 242)

Reference Values

Males	<0.155 ng/ml
Females	<0.105 ng/ml

Interfering Factors

■ Failure to fast from food for 8 hours prior to the test may alter results

Indications/Purposes for Calcitonin

■ Support for diagnosing medullary carcinoma of the thyroid gland as indicated by elevated calcitonin levels, when serum calcium levels are normal (further verification may require raising the serum calcium level by intravenous infusion of calcium or pentagastrin and measuring the level to which plasma calcitonin rises in response; a rise of 0.105 to 0.11 ng/ml is to be expected)
■ Altered serum calcium levels of unknown etiology that may be due to a disorder associated with altered calcitonin levels
  □ Elevated calcitonin levels are seen in cancers involving the breast, lung, and pancreas due to ectopic calcitonin production by tumor cells
  □ Elevated calcitonin levels also are seen in primary hyperparathyroidism and in secondary hyperparathyroidism due to chronic renal failure

Client Preparation

Client preparation is essentially the same as that for any study involving collection of a peripheral blood sample (see Appendix I). For this test, the client should fast from food for at least 8 hours prior to collection of the sample.

The Procedure

A venipuncture is performed and the sample collected in a green-topped tube. The sample should be handled gently to avoid hemolysis and transported promptly to the laboratory.

Aftercare and Nursing Observations

Care and assessment following the procedure are the same as for any study involving collection of a peripheral blood sample. Foods withheld prior to the test should be resumed.

PARATHYROID HORMONE (PTH) (BACKGROUND INFORMATION, p. 218)

Reference Values

2.3–2.8 mmol/l
PTH is measured by radioimmunoassay. As the antibody used for the assay directly affects the results, values will vary according to the laboratory performing the test.

Interfering Factors

■ Failure to fast from food for 8 hours prior to the test may alter results

Indications/Purposes for Parathyroid Hormone

■ Suspected hyperparathyroidism
  □ Elevated levels occur in primary hyperparathyroidism due to hyperplasia or tumor of the parathyroid glands
  □ Elevated levels also may occur in secondary hyperparathyroidism (usually due to chronic renal failure, malignant tumors that produce ectopic PTH, and malabsorption syndromes)
■ Suspected surgical removal of the parathyroid glands or incidental damage to them during thyroid or neck surgery, as indicated by decreased levels

■ Evaluation of parathyroid response to altered serum calcium levels, with elevated serum calcium levels, especially those due to malignant processes, leading to decreased PTH production

■ Evaluation of parathyroid response to other disorders that may lead to decreased PTH production (e.g., hypomagnesemia, autoimmune destruction of the parathyroid glands)

Client Preparation

Client preparation is essentially the same as that for any study involving collection of a peripheral blood sample (see Appendix I). For this test, the client should fast from food for at least 8 hours prior to collection of the sample.

The Procedure

A venipuncture is performed and the sample collected in a red-topped tube. A sample for serum calcium also may be obtained. The sample(s) should be handled gently to avoid hemolysis and transported promptly to the laboratory.

Aftercare and Nursing Observations

Care and assessment following the procedure are the same as for any study involving collection of a peripheral blood sample. Foods withheld prior to the test should be resumed.

CORTISOL (BACKGROUND INFORMATION, p. 219)

Reference Values

	8 A.M.	4 P.M.
Children	15–25 µg/dl	5–10 µg/dl
Adults	9–24 µg/dl	3–12 µg/dl

Interfering Factors

■ The time of day the test is performed may alter results because cortisol levels vary diurnally, with highest levels seen upon awakening and lowest levels occurring late in the day

■ Stress and excessive physical activity may produce elevated levels

■ Pregnancy, therapy with estrogen-containing drugs, lithium carbonate, methadone, and ethyl alcohol may lead to elevated cortisol levels

■ Therapy with levodopa, barbiturates, phenytoin (Dilantin), and androgens may produce decreased levels

■ Failure to follow dietary restrictions, if ordered, may alter test results

Indications/Purposes for Cortisol Assay

■ Suspected adrenal hyperfunction (Cushing's syndrome) due to a variety of causes (see p. 219), as indicated by elevated levels that do not vary diurnally

■ Evaluation of effects of disorders associated with elevated cortisol levels (e.g., hyperthyroidism, obesity, and diabetic ketoacidosis)

- Suspected adrenal hypofunction (Addison's disease) due to a variety of causes (see p. 219), as indicated by decreased levels
- Monitoring response to therapy with adrenal corticosteroids
  - ☐ Elevated levels are seen in clients receiving adrenal corticosteroid therapy
  - ☐ Decreased levels may occur for months after therapy is discontinued, resulting from drug-induced atrophy of the adrenal glands

Client Preparation

General client preparation is the same as that for any study involving collection of a peripheral blood sample (see Appendix I). Some laboratories require an 8-hour fast and activity restriction prior to the test. Medications that may alter cortisol levels should be withheld for 12 to 24 hours prior to the study, although this should be confirmed with the person ordering the test.

The client should be informed that it may be necessary to obtain more than one sample, and that samples must be obtained at specific times to detect peak and trough levels of cortisol.

The Procedure

At approximately 8 A.M., a venipuncture is performed and the sample is collected in a green-topped tube. The sample should be handled gently to avoid hemolysis and sent promptly to the laboratory. If cortisol hypersecretion is suspected, then a second sample may be obtained at approximately 4 P.M. to determine if diurnal variation in cortisol levels is occurring.

Aftercare and Nursing Observations

Care and assessment following the procedure are the same as for any study involving the collection of a peripheral blood sample. Food and any medications withheld prior to the test, as well as usual activities, should be resumed.

ALDOSTERONE (BACKGROUND INFORMATION, p. 245)
Reference Values

Supine	3–9 ng/dl
Standing	5–30 ng/dl

Interfering Factors

- Upright body posture (see under Client Preparation), stress, and late pregnancy may lead to increased levels
- Therapy with diuretics, Apresoline, Hyperstat, and nitroprusside may lead to elevated levels
- Excessive licorice injection may produce decreased levels, as may therapy with propranolol and fludrocortisone (Florinef)
- Altered serum electrolyte levels affect aldosterone secretion
  - ☐ Decreased serum sodium and elevated serum potassium increase aldosterone secretion
  - ☐ Elevated serum sodium and decreased serum potassium suppress aldosterone secretion

Indications/Purposes for Plasma Aldosterone

■ Suspected hyperaldosteronism as indicated by elevated levels
  □ Primary aldosteronism (e.g., due to benign adenomas or bilateral hyper-plasia of the aldosterone-secreting zona glomerulosa cells) is indicated by elevated aldosterone and low plasma renin levels (see pp. 189 and 205)
  □ Secondary hyperaldosteronism (e.g., due to changes in blood volume and serum electrolytes, congestive heart failure, cirrhosis, nephrotic syndrome, chronic obstructive pulmonary disease, and renal artery stenosis) is indicated by elevated aldosterone and plasma renin levels
■ Suspected hypoaldosteronism (e.g., as seen in diabetes mellitus and toxemia of pregnancy) as indicated by decreased levels
■ Evaluation of hypertension of unknown etiology

Client Preparation

General client preparation is the same as that for any study involving collection of a peripheral blood sample (see Appendix I). The client should not have ingested licorice for 2 weeks prior to the test. Medications that alter plasma aldosterone levels also may be withheld for up to 2 weeks prior to the test, although this should be confirmed with the person ordering the study.

If hospitalized, the client should be told not to get out of bed in the morning until the sample has been obtained, and that it may be necessary to obtain a second sample after he or she has been up for about 2 to 4 hours.

Nonhospitalized individuals should be instructed when to report to the laboratory in relation to the length of time to be upright prior to the test.

The Procedure

A venipuncture is performed and the sample is collected in a red-, green-, or lavender-topped tube, depending on laboratory procedures. The client's position and length of time the position was held should be noted on the laboratory request form. The sample(s) should be handled gently to avoid hemolysis and sent to the laboratory immediately. A sample for plasma renin also may be obtained in conjunction with the test.

Aftercare and Nursing Observations

Care and assessment following the procedure are the same as for any study involving the collection of a peripheral blood sample. Any medications withheld prior to the test should be resumed.

CATECHOLAMINES (BACKGROUND INFORMATION, p. 221)

Reference Values

Epinephrine and norepinephrine	100–500 ng/l
Epinephrine	
Supine	0–110 pg/ml
Standing	0–140 pg/ml
Norepinephrine	
Supine	70–750 pg/ml
Standing	200–1700 pg/ml

Results are usually evaluated in relation to urinary measurements of catecholamine metabolites. Several measurements of plasma levels also may be indicated.

Interfering Factors

- Catecholamine levels vary diurnally and with postural changes
- Shock, stress, hyperthyroidism, strenuous exercise, and smoking may produce elevated plasma catecholamines
- Dopamine, Levophed, sympathomimetic drugs, tricyclic antidepressants, alpha-methyldopa, hydralazine, quinidine, and Isuprel may produce elevated levels
- A diet high in amines (e.g., bananas, nuts, cereal grains, tea, coffee, cocoa, aged cheese, beer, ale, certain wines, avocados, and fava beans) may produce elevated plasma catecholamine levels, although this effect is more likely to be seen in relation to certain urinary metabolites

Indications/Purposes for Plasma Catecholamines

- Hypertension of unknown etiology and/or suspected pheochromocytoma or paragangliomas
  - ☐ Identification of pheochromocytoma as the cause of hypertension as indicated by elevated combined catecholamine and epinephrine levels
  - ☐ Support for diagnosing paragangliomas as indicated by elevated combined catecholamine and norepinephrine levels

Client Preparation

General client preparation is the same as that for any study involving collection of a peripheral blood sample (see Appendix I). For this test, the client should fast for 12 hours and abstain from smoking for 24 hours prior to the test. Vigorous exercise should be avoided, with provision made for rest in a recumbent position for at least 1 hour prior to the study.

Medications that may alter test results, especially over-the-counter cold preparations containing sympathomimetics, may be withheld for up to 2 weeks prior to the test, although this should be confirmed with the person ordering the study. The need for dietary restriction of amine-rich foods for 48 hours prior to the test should be confirmed with the laboratory performing the test or the person ordering it.

If samples are to be obtained via an intermittent venous access device (e.g., heparin lock), the client should be informed of its purpose and that it may be inserted as long as 24 hours prior to the test.

The Procedure

If more than one sample is to be obtained, a heparin lock should be inserted 12 to 24 hours prior to the test; the stress of repeated venipunctures could falsely elevate levels.

For hospitalized individuals, a sample of venous blood should be collected in a chilled lavender-topped tube between 6 and 8 A.M. For nonhospitalized clients, the first sample should be obtained after approximately 1 hour of rest in a recumbent position. The sample is handled gently to avoid hemolysis, packed on ice, and sent to the laboratory immediately.

The client should then be assisted to stand for 10 minutes, after which a second sample is obtained. The time(s) of collection and position of the client should be noted on the laboratory request form.

Aftercare and Nursing Observations

If an intermittent venous access device was inserted, it should be removed after completion of the test and a pressure bandage applied to the site. Foods and any medications withheld prior to the test, as well as usual activities, should be resumed.

ESTROGENS (BACKGROUND INFORMATION, p. 222)
Reference Values

Estradiol (E_2)	
Children under 6 years	3–10 pg/ml
Adults	
Men	12–34 pg/ml
Women (menstruating)	
Early cycle	24–68 pg/ml
Midcycle	50–186 pg/ml
Late cycle	73–149 pg/ml
Estriol (E_3)	
Weeks of pregnancy	
30–32	2–12 ng/ml
33–35	3–19 ng/ml
36–38	5–27 ng/ml
39–40	10–30 ng/ml

Interfering Factors

■ In menstruating women, estrogen levels vary in relation to the menstrual cycle
■ Therapy with estrogen-containing drugs and adrenal corticosteroids will elevate levels, whereas clomiphene will decrease them

Indications/Purposes for Estrogen

■ Infertility or amenorrhea of unknown etiology, with primary or secondary ovarian failure indicated by low estradiol (E_2) levels
■ Establishment of the time of ovulation
■ Evaluation of response to therapy for infertility
■ Suspected precocious puberty with the disorder indicated by elevated estradiol (E_2) levels
■ Suspected estrogen-producing tumors, as indicated by consistently high estradiol (E_2) levels without normal cyclic variations
■ High-risk pregnancy with suspicion of fetal growth retardation, placental dysfunction or impending fetal jeopardy, as indicated by decreased estriol (E_3) levels relative to the stage of pregnancy

Client Preparation

Client preparation is the same as that for any study involving collection of a peripheral blood sample (see Appendix I). It is recommended that those drugs that are known to alter estrogen levels be withheld for 12 to 24 hours prior to the test, although this should be confirmed with the person ordering the study.

In menstruating women, the phase of the menstrual cycle should be ascertained if possible. If the test is being done to detect ovulation, the client should be informed that it may be necessary to obtain a series of samples over a period of several days to detect the normal variation in estrogen levels.

The Procedure

A venipuncture is performed and the sample is collected in a red-topped tube. The sample should be handled gently to avoid hemolysis and transported promptly to the laboratory.

Aftercare and Nursing Observations

Care and assessment following the procedure are the same as for any study involving the collection of a peripheral blood sample. Any medications withheld prior to the test should be resumed.

PROGESTERONE (BACKGROUND INFORMATION, p. 223)

Reference Values

Adults	
Males	<100 ng/dl
Females (menstruating)	
Follicular phase	<150 ng/dl
Luteal phase	300–1,200 ng/dl
Females (pregnant)	
First trimester	1,500–5,000 ng/dl
Second and third trimesters	8,000–20,000 ng/dl
Females (menopausal)	10–22 ng/dl

Interfering Factors

- In menstruating women, progesterone levels vary in relation to the menstrual cycle
- Therapy with estrogen, progesterone, or adrenal corticosteroids may produce elevated levels

Indications/Purposes for Plasma Progesterone

- Infertility of unknown etiology with failure to ovulate, indicated by low levels throughout the menstrual cycle
- Evaluation of response to therapy for infertility
- Support for diagnosing disorders associated with elevated progesterone levels (e.g., prococious puberty, ovarian tumors or cysts, and adrenocortical hyperplasia and tumors)
- High-risk pregnancy with suspicion of placental dysfunction, fetal abnormality, impending fetal jeopardy, threatened abortion, or toxemia of pregnancy, as indicated by lower than expected levels for the stage of pregnancy
- Support for diagnosing disorders associated with decreased progesterone levels (e.g., panhypopituitarism, Turner's syndrome, adrenogenital syndrome, and Stein-Leventhal syndrome)

Client Preparation

Client preparation is the same as that for any study involving collection of a peripheral blood sample (see Appendix I). It is recommended that any drugs that may alter progesterone levels be withheld for 12 to 24 hours prior to the test, although this should be confirmed with the person ordering the study.

In menstruating women, the phase of the menstrual cycle should be ascertained if possible. If the test is being done to detect ovulation, the client should be informed that it may be necessary to obtain a series of samples over a period of several days to detect the normal variation in progesterone levels.

The Procedure

A venipuncture is performed and the sample collected in a green-topped tube. The sample should be handled gently to avoid hemolysis and transported promptly to the laboratory.

Aftercare and Nursing Observations

Care and assessment following the procedure are the same as for any study involving the collection of a peripheral blood sample. Any medications withheld prior to the test should be resumed.

TESTOSTERONE (BACKGROUND INFORMATION, p. 223)

Reference Values

Children	0.12–0.16 ng/ml
Adults	
Males	
Under age 60	3.9– 7.9 ng/ml
Over age 60	1.5– 3.1 ng/dl
Females	
Menstruating	0.25–0.67 ng/ml
Menopausal	0.21–0.37 ng/ml

Interfering Factors

- Testosterone levels vary diurnally, with highest levels occurring in the early morning
- Administration of testosterone, thyroid and growth hormones, clomiphene, and barbiturates may lead to elevated levels
- Therapy with estrogens and Aldactone may produce decreased levels

Indications/Purposes for Testosterone

- In males, support for diagnosing precocious puberty, testicular tumors, and benign prostatic hypertrophy, as indicated by elevated levels
- In females, support for diagnosing adrenogenital syndrome, adrenal tumors or hyperplasia, Stein-Leventhal syndrome, ovarian tumors or hyperplasia, and luteomas of pregnancy, as indicated by elevated levels
- In males and females, support for diagnosing nonendocrine tumors that pro-

duce adrenocorticotropic hormone (ACTH) ectopically, as indicated by elevated levels without diurnal variation

■ In males, support for diagnosing infertility, with testicular failure indicated by decreased levels

■ Support for diagnosing other disorders associated with decreased testosterone levels (e.g., hypopituitarism, Kleinfelter's syndrome, cryptorchidism [failure of testicular descent], and cirrhosis)

Client Preparation

Client preparation is the same as that for any study involving collection of a peripheral blood sample (see Appendix I). It is recommended that drugs that may alter testosterone levels be withheld for 12 to 24 hours prior to the test, although this should be confirmed with the person ordering the study.

The Procedure

A venipuncture is performed and the sample collected in either a red- or a green-topped tube, depending on the laboratory performing the test. The sample should be handled gently to avoid hemolysis and transported promptly to the laboratory.

Aftercare and Nursing Observations

Care and assessment following the procedure are the same as for any study involving the collection of a peripheral blood sample. Any medications withheld prior to the test should be resumed.

HUMAN CHORIONIC GONADOTROPIN (hCG) (BACKGROUND INFORMATION, p. 224)

Reference Values

Nonpregnant	<3 mIU/ml
Pregnant	
8–10 days	5–40 mIU/ml
1 month	100 mIU/ml
2 months	100,000 mIU/ml
4 months–term	50,000 mIU/ml

Indications/Purposes for Human Chorionic Gonadotropin

■ Early detection of pregnancy (i.e., within 8 to 10 days of conception) especially in women with a history of infertility or habitual abortion

■ Prediction of outcome in threatened abortion (levels below 10,000 mIU/ml are highly predictive that abortion will occur)

■ Suspected intrauterine fetal demise or incomplete abortion as indicated by decreased levels

■ Suspected hydatidiform mole or choriocarcinoma as indicated by elevated levels

■ Suspected testicular tumor as indicated by elevated levels

■ Support for diagnosing nonendocrine tumors that produce hCG ectopically (e.g., carcinoma of the stomach, liver, pancreas, and breast; multiple myeloma; and malignant melanoma), as indicated by elevated levels
■ Monitoring the effectiveness of treatment for malignancies associated with ectopic hCG production, as indicated by decreasing levels

Client Preparation

Client preparation is the same as that for any study involving collection of a peripheral blood sample (see Appendix I).

The Procedure

A venipuncture is performed and the sample collected in a red-topped tube. The sample should be handled gently to avoid hemolysis and sent promptly to the laboratory.

Aftercare and Nursing Observations

Care and assessment following the procedure are the same as for any study involving the collection of a peripheral blood sample.

HUMAN PLACENTAL LACTOGEN (hPL) (BACKGROUND INFORMATION, p. 224)
Reference Values

Males	<0.5 μg/ml
Females	
Nonpregnant	<0.5 μg/ml
Pregnant	
5–27 weeks	<4.6 μg/ml
28–31 weeks	2.4–6.1 μg/ml
32–35 weeks	3.7–7.7 μg/ml
36 weeks–term	5.0–8.6 μg/ml
Diabetic at term	10–12 μg/ml

Interfering Factors

■ During pregnancy, hPL levels vary greatly with the individual, as well as on a day-to-day basis
■ Levels tend to be higher in diabetic mothers, multiple gestation, and Rh isoimmunization

Indications/Purposes for Human Placental Lactogen

■ Detection of placental insufficiency as evidenced by low hPL levels in relation to gestational age
■ Support for diagnosing intrauterine growth retardation due to placental insufficiency, as indicated by hPL levels less than 4 μg/ml, especially when blood estrogen levels are low
■ Prediction of outcome in threatened abortion as indicated by lower than expected levels for the stage of pregnancy

■ Support for diagnosing hydatidiform mole and choriocarcinoma as indicated by decreased levels

■ Support for diagnosing malignancies associated with elevated levels (e.g., nonendocrine tumors that secrete ectopic hPL)

■ Monitoring the effectiveness of treatment for malignancies associated with ectopic hPL production, as indicated by decreasing levels

Client Preparation

Client preparation is the same as that for any study involving collection of a peripheral blood sample (see Appendix I). The pregnant client should be informed that several determinations may be necessary throughout the pregnancy.

The Procedure

A venipuncture is performed and the sample is collected in a red-topped tube. The sample should be handled gently to avoid hemolysis and sent promptly to the laboratory.

Aftercare and Nursing Observations

Care and assessment following the procedure are the same as for any study involving the collection of a peripheral blood sample.

INSULIN (BACKGROUND INFORMATION, p. 225)

Reference Values

Fasting	8.0–15.0 μU/ml or 0.3–0.6 ng/ml
After 100 g glucose	
½ hour	25–231 μU/ml
1 hour	18–276 μU/ml
2 hours	16–166 μU/ml
3 hours	4–38 μU/ml
Insulin-to-glucose ratio	<0.3:1

Interfering Factors

■ Administration of insulin or oral hypoglycemic agents within 8 hours of the test may lead to falsely elevated levels

■ Failure to follow dietary restrictions prior to the test may lead to falsely elevated levels

■ Therapy with drugs containing estrogen and progesterone may produce elevated levels

Indications/Purposes for Serum Insulin

■ Evaluation of postprandial ("reactive") hypoglycemia of unknown etiology
  □ Support for diagnosing early or developing non–insulin-dependent diabetes mellitus as indicated by excessive production of insulin in relation to blood glucose levels (best demonstrated with glucose tolerance tests or 2-hour postprandial tests)

☐ Confirmation of functional hypoglycemia (i.e., no known physiological cause for the hypoglycemia) as indicated by circulating insulin levels appropriate to changing blood glucose levels
■ Evaluation of fasting hypoglycemia of unknown etiology
☐ Support for diagnosing insulinoma as indicated by sustained high levels of insulin and absence of blood glucose related variations
■ Evaluation of uncontrolled insulin-dependent diabetes mellitus
☐ Differentiation between insulin-resistant diabetes, in which insulin levels are high, and non–insulin-resistant diabetes, in which insulin levels are low
■ Support for diagnosing pheochromocytoma as indicated by decreased levels

Client Preparation

Client preparation is the same as that for the related blood glucose test (e.g., fasting blood glucose, glucose tolerance test) with which the serum insulin determination is performed (see pp. 137 to 142).

The Procedure

The general procedure is the same as that for the related blood glucose test. Blood samples for serum insulin determinations are obtained in red-topped tubes and then packed in ice. The samples should be handled gently to avoid hemolysis and sent immediately to the laboratory.

Aftercare and Nursing Observations

Care and assessment following the procedure are the same as for the related blood glucose test. The client should be observed for signs of hypoglycemia, which may occur in response to fasting or excessive blood glucose load. Foods and any medications withheld prior to the test should be resumed.

C-PEPTIDE (BACKGROUND INFORMATION, p. 226)
Reference Values

0.9–4.2 ng/ml

Indications/Purposes for C-Peptide

■ Suspected excessive insulin administration in either diabetic or nondiabetic individuals, as indicated by low C-peptide and elevated serum insulin levels
■ Determination of beta cell function when insulin antibodies preclude accurate measurement of serum insulin production (insulin antibodies are most common in diabetic clients receiving exogenous insulin prepared from animal extracts)
■ Support for diagnosing insulinoma, especially when the tumor secretes more proinsulin than active hormone, because the normal correlation between insulin and C-peptide will be altered

Client Preparation

Client preparation is the same as that for any test involving collection of a peripheral blood sample (see Appendix I). Some laboratories may require that the client fast from food for 8 hours prior to the test.

The Procedure

A venipuncture is performed and the sample collected in a red-topped tube. The sample is handled gently to avoid hemolysis and sent promptly to the laboratory.

Aftercare and Nursing Observations

Care and assessment following the procedure are the same as for any study involving collection of a peripheral blood sample. The client's usual diet may be resumed.

GLUCAGON (BACKGROUND INFORMATION, p. 226)

Reference Values

50–200 pg/ml

Interfering Factors

■ Trauma, infection, starvation, and excessive exercise may lead to elevated levels, as will acute pancreatitis, pheochromocytoma, uncontrolled diabetes mellitus, and uremia

■ Failure to follow dietary restrictions prior to the test may lead to falsely decreased levels

Indications/Purposes for Glucagon Determination

■ Suspected glucagonoma as indicated by elevated levels (as high as 1000 pg/ ml) in the absence of diabetic ketoacidosis, uremia, pheochromocytoma, or acute pancreatitis

■ Confirmation of glucagon deficiency related to loss of pancreatic tissue due to chronic pancreatitis, pancreatic neoplasm, or surgical resection (arginine infusion, which would normally lead to elevated glucagon levels, may be used for further confirmation of the deficiency state)

■ Suspected renal transplant rejection, as indicated by rising plasma glucagon levels (glucagon levels may rise markedly several days before serum creatinine begins to rise)

Client Preparation

General client preparation is the same as that for any test involving collection of a peripheral blood sample (see Appendix I). For this test, the client should fast from foods for 8 hours prior to the study. Water is permitted.

The Procedure

A venipuncture is performed and the sample is collected in either a green- or a lavender-topped tube, depending on the laboratory performing the test. The sample should be handled gently to avoid hemolysis and sent to the laboratory immediately.

Aftercare and Nursing Observations

Care and assessment following the procedure are the same as for any test involving collection of a peripheral blood sample. The client's usual diet should be resumed as soon as possible after the sample has been obtained.

GASTRIN (BACKGROUND INFORMATION, p. 227)

Reference Values

Fasting	50–150 pg/ml
Postprandial	80–170 pg/ml

Postprandial values may vary according to the test method used.

Interfering Factors

■ Protein ingestion and calcium infusions will elevate serum gastrin levels in some situations; these substances may be used for "challenge tests" of gastrin secretion

Indications/Purposes for Serum Gastrin

■ Suspected gastrinoma (Zollinger-Ellison syndrome) as indicated by markedly elevated levels (e.g., greater than 1000 pg/ml) and by marked response to calcium challenge
■ Support for diagnosing gastric carcinoma, pernicious anemia, or G-cell hyperplasia as indicated by elevated levels
■ Differential diagnosis of peptic ulcer disease from other disorders, since gastrin levels may be normal but will rise in response to protein challenge

Client Preparation

General client preparation is the same as that for any test involving collection of a peripheral blood sample (see Appendix I). For this test, the client should fast from food for 12 hours prior to the study. Water is not restricted. It also is recommended that medications be withheld for 12 to 24 hours prior to the test, although this should be confirmed with the person ordering the study.

The Procedure

A venipuncture is performed and the sample collected in a red-topped tube. The sample should be packed in ice, handled gently to avoid hemolysis, and transported immediately to the laboratory.

Aftercare and Nursing Observations

Care and assessment following the procedure is the same as for any test involving collection of a peripheral blood sample. The client's usual diet and medications should be resumed.

ELECTROLYTES

Background Information

Electrolytes are substances that dissociate into electrically charged ions when dissolved. Cations carry positive charges, while anions carry negative charges. Both affect the electrical and osmolal (i.e., the number of particles dissolved in a fluid) functioning of the body. Body fluids always contain equal numbers of positive and negative charges, but the nature of the ions, the number of charges present on a single molecule, and the nature and mobility of the charged molecules differ enormously among body fluid compartments (e.g., intracellular versus extracellular).

Not all charged particles are ions. Proteins, for example, carry a net negative charge. Whenever fluid contains protein, there must be accompanying cations. Similarly, not all solutes found in plasma are ions. Urea and glucose, for example, do not dissociate; they do not contribute to electrical activity of fluids and membranes, and contribute only moderately to plasma osmolality.

Electrolyte quantities and the balance among them in the body fluid compartments are controlled by (1) oxygen and carbon dioxide exchange in the lungs; (2) absorption, secretion, and excretion of many substances by the kidneys; and (3) secretion of regulatory hormones by the endocrine glands.

Quantitatively, the most important body fluid ions are sodium, potassium, chloride, and bicarbonate. These ions are measured in routine serum electrolyte determinations. Other serum ions that may be measured include calcium, magnesium, and phosphorus.[54]

SERUM SODIUM (Na) (CLINICAL APPLICATIONS DATA, p. 265)

Sodium (Na, Na^+) is the most abundant cation in extracellular fluid and, along with its accompanying chloride and bicarbonate anions, accounts for 92 percent of serum osmolality. Sodium plays a major role in maintaining homeostasis through a variety of functions, which include (1) maintenance of osmotic pressure of extracellular fluid; (2) regulation of renal retention and excretion of water; (3) maintenance of acid-base balance; (4) regulation of potassium and chloride levels; (5) stimulation of neuromusuclar reactions; and (6) maintenance of systemic blood pressure. Serum sodium levels may be affected by a variety of disorders and drugs (Table 5–22) and are evaluated in relation to other serum electrolyte and blood chemistry results. Tests of urinary sodium and osmolality also may be necessary for complete interpretation. It should be noted that falsely decreased serum sodium levels may occur with elevated serum triglyceride levels and myeloma proteins.

SERUM POTASSIUM (K) (CLINICAL APPLICATIONS DATA, p. 266)

Potassium (K, K^+) is the most abundant intracellular cation; much smaller amounts are found in the blood. Potassium is essential for the transmission of electrical impulses in cardiac and skeletal muscle. In addition, it helps to maintain the osmolality and electroneutrality of cells, functions in enzyme reactions that transform glucose into energy and amino acids into proteins, and participates in the maintenance of acid-base balance.

Numerous disorders and drugs may affect serum potassium levels. As shown in Table 5–23, the clinical problems associated with altered serum potassium levels may be categorized as (1) inappropriate cellular metabolism, (2) altered renal excretion, and (3) altered intake. False elevations in serum potassium may occur with vigorous pumping of the hand after tourniquet application for venipuncture, in hemolyzed samples, or with high platelet counts during clotting. Falsely decreased levels are seen in anticoagulated samples left at room temperature.

Altered serum potassium levels are of particular concern due to their effects on cardiac impulse conduction, especially when the client also is taking medications that affect cardiac conduction. The combination of low serum potassium

TABLE 5-22. Disorders and Drugs Associated with Altered Serum Sodium and Extracellular Fluid (ECF) Levels

Increased Serum Sodium (Hypernatremia)	Decreased Serum Sodium (Hyponatremia)
Total Body Sodium Normal, ECF Volume Low	*Total Body Sodium and ECF Volume Low, but Total Body Sodium Proportionately Lower*
Hypovolemia	Addison's disease
Dehydration	Salt-losing renal disorders
Fever	Gastrointestinal fluid loss (nasogastric
Thyrotoxicosis	suction, vomiting, diarrhea, fistula,
Hyperglycemic hyperosmolar	paralytic ileus)
nonketotic syndrome	Diaphoresis
Diabetes insipidus	Diuresis
Hyperventilation	Burns
Mechanical ventilation without	Ascites
humidification	Massive pleural effusion
	Diabetic ketoacidosis
Total Body Sodium Increased Proportionately More Than ECF Volume	*Total Body Sodium Normal and ECF Volume Normal too High*
Excessive salt ingestion	Acute water intoxication
Inappropriate or incorrect	Syndrome of inappropriate ADH secretion
intravenous therapy with	Glucocorticoid deficiency
fluids containing sodium	Severe total body potassium depletion
Cushing's syndrome	
Hyperaldosteronism	
Total Body Sodium Low With ECF Volume Proportionately Lower	*Total Body Sodium and ECF Volume Increased, but ECF Proportionately Greater*
Gastroenteritis	Acute renal failure with water overload
Osmotic diuresis	Congestive heart failure
Diaphoresis	Cirrhosis
	Nephrotic syndrome
Drugs	*Drugs*
Adrenal corticosteroids	Lithium carbonate
Methyldopa (Aldomet)	Vasopressin
Hydralazine (Apresoline)	Diuretics (thiazides, Mannitol, ethacrynic
Reserpine (Serpasil)	acid, furosemide)
Cough medicines	

Adapted from Widmann, FK: Clinical Interpretation of Laboratory Tests, ed 9. FA Davis, Philadelphia, 1983, p 289.

(hypokalemia) and therapy with digitalis preparations, for example, can produce serious consequences due to increased ventricular irritability.

It should also be noted that potassium is a very changeable ion, moving easily between intracellular and extracellular fluids. An example of this is seen in states of acidosis and alkalosis. In acidosis (decreased serum pH), potassium moves from the cells into the blood; in alkalosis (increased serum pH), the reverse occurs.

TABLE 5–23. **Disorders and Drugs Associated With Altered Serum Potassium Levels**

Increased Serum Potassium (Hyperkalemia)	Decreased Serum Potassium (Hypokalemia)
Inappropriate Cellular Metabolism Acidosis Insulin deficiency Hypoaldosteronism Cell necrosis (trauma, burns, hemolysis, antineoplastic therapy) Addison's disease	*Inappropriate Cellular Metabolism* Alkalosis Insulin excess Familial periodic paralysis Rapid cell generation (leukemia, treated megaloblastic anemia) Chronic excessive licorice ingestion
Decreased Renal Excretion Acute renal failure Chronic interstitial nephritis Tubular unresponsiveness to aldosterone Hypoaldosteronism	*Increased Excretion* Gastrointestinal loss (vomiting, diarrhea, nasogastric suction, fistula) Excessive diuresis Hyperaldosteronism Laxative abuse Hypomagnesemia Renal tubular acidosis Diaphoresis Thyrotoxicosis Cushing's syndrome
Increased Potassium Intake Salt substitutes Potassium supplements (oral or intravenous) Potassium salts of antibiotics Transfusion of old banked blood	*Decreased Potassium Intake* Anorexia nervosa Diet deficient in meat and vegetables Clay eating (binds potassium and prevents absorption) Intravenous therapy with inadequate potassium supplementation
Drugs Potassium chloride Potassium-sparing diuretics Aldosterone antagonists Potassium preparations of antibiotics Amphotericin-B Tetracycline Heparin Epinephrine Marijuana Isoniazid	*Drugs* Furosemide Ethacrynic acid Thiazide diuretics Insulin Aspirin Prednisone Cortisone Gentamicin Polymyxin B Lithium carbonate Kayexalate Ammonium chloride Aldosterone Laxatives

Adapted from Widmann, FK: Clinical Interpretation of Laboratory Tests, ed 9. FA Davis, Philadelphia, 1983, p 290.

SERUM CHLORIDE (Cl) (CLINICAL APPLICATIONS DATA, p. 267)

Chloride (Cl, Cl^-) is the most abundant anion in extracellular fluid. It participates with sodium in the maintenance of water balance and aids in the regulation of osmotic pressure. It also contributes to gastric acid (HCl) for digestion and for activation of enzymes. Its most important function is in the maintenance of acid-base balance. In certain forms of metabolic acidosis, for example, serum chloride levels may rise in response to decreased serum bicarbonate levels; this is known as hyperchloremic acidosis. If bicarbonate levels fall and serum chloride concentration remains relatively normal, however, a gap between measured cations (i.e., sodium and potassium) and measured anions (i.e., chloride and bicarbonate) will occur. This condition often is called anion gap acidosis (see also p. 262).

Chloride also helps to maintain acid-base balance through the chloride-bicarbonate shift mechanism, in which chloride ions enter red blood cells in exchange for bicarbonate. Bicarbonate leaves the red blood cells in response to carbon dioxide, which is released from the tissues into venous blood and absorbed into the red blood cells. The carbon dioxide is subsequently converted into carbonic acid, which dissociates into bicarbonate and hydrogen ions. When the bicarbonate concentration in the red blood cells exceeds that of the plasma, bicarbonate diffuses into the blood, and chloride enters the red blood cells to

---

TABLE 5–24. Disorders and Drugs Associated With Altered Serum Chloride Levels

Increased Serum Chloride (Hyperchloremia)	Decreased Serum Chloride (Hypochloremia)
Acidosis	Alkalosis
Hyperkalemia	Hypokalemia
Hypernatremia	Hyponatremia
Dehydration	Gastrointestinal loss (vomiting, diarrhea,
Eclampsia	nasogastric suction, fistula)
Renal failure (severe)	Diuresis
Congestive heart failure	Hypoventilation (especially due to
Hyperventilation (especially due to	chronic obstructive pulmonary
neurogenic hyperventilation	disease)
related to head injury)	Acute infections
Cushing's syndrome	Burns
Hyperaldosteronism	Heat stroke
Anemia	Fever
Hypoproteinemia	Diabetic ketoacidosis
Serum sickness	Pyelonephritis
Hyperparathyroidism	Addisonian crisis
Excessive dietary salt	Starvation
Jejunoileal bypass	Inadequate chloride intake
Gastric carcinoma	
Drugs	**Drugs**
Potassium chloride	Ethacrynic acid (Edecrin)
Ammonium chloride	Furosemide (Lasix)
Acetazolamide (Diamox)	Thiazide diuretics
Methyldopa (Aldomet)	Bicarbonate
Diazoxide (Hyperstat)	
Guanethidine (Ismelin)	

supply the anions necessary for electroneutrality. For this reason, the chloride content of red blood cells in venous blood is slightly higher than that of arterial red blood cells.

Numerous disorders and drugs may alter serum chloride levels (Table 5–24).

SERUM BICARBONATE (HCO_3) (CLINICAL APPLICATIONS DATA, p. 268)

Bicarbonate (HCO_3, HCO_3^-) is the major extracellular buffer in the blood; it functions with carbonic acid (H_2CO_3) in maintaining acid-base balance. Normally, the ratio of bicarbonate to dissolved carbon dioxide (CO_2), which derives from H_2CO_3, is 20 to 1. If this ratio is altered, acid-base imbalance occurs. Additional CO_2, for example, will cause increased acidity (falling pH), while loss of CO_2 will produce alkalinity (rising pH). Similarly, additional bicarbonate will lead to alkalosis, while loss of bicarbonate will produce acidosis.

The lungs control regulation of CO_2 levels. Bicarbonate levels are under renal control; the kidneys regulate both the generation of bicarbonate ions and their rate of urinary excretion. Bicarbonate also participates with chloride in the bicarbonate-chloride shift mechanism involving red blood cells (see also p. 260).

Measurement of serum bicarbonate ion concentration may be done directly or indirectly by means of total CO_2 content, since over 90 percent of blood CO_2

TABLE 5–25. Disorders and Drugs Associated With Altered Serum Bicarbonate Levels

Increased Serum Bicarbonate	Decreased Serum Bicarbonate
Metabolic alkalosis	Metabolic acidosis
Compensated metabolic alkalosis	Compensated metabolic acidosis
Respiratory acidosis (slightly elevated or normal)	Respiratory alkalosis (slightly low or normal)
Compensated respiratory acidosis	Compensated respiratory alkalosis
Hypoventilation	Hyperventilation
Chronic obstructive pulmonary disease	Diarrhea
Vomiting	Dehydration
Nasogastric suction	Severe malnutrition
Diuresis	Burns
Aldosteronism	Myocardial infarction
Congestive heart failure	Acute ethanol intoxication
Hypokalemia	Shock
Cushing's syndrome	Renal disease
Pulmonary edema	Hyperthyroidism
Drugs:	*Drugs:*
Aldosterone	Triamterene (Dyrenium)
ACTH	Acetazolamide (Diamox)
Sodium bicarbonate abuse	Calcium chloride
Milk-alkali syndrome	Ammonium chloride
Adrenal corticosteroids	Salicylate toxicity
Viomycin	Paraldehyde
Thiazide diuretics	Sodium citrate

exists in the ionized bicarbonate form. Bicarbonate also is measured as part of blood gas determinations (see p. 273). Numerous disorders, especially those involving acid-base imbalance, and drugs are associated with altered serum bicarbonate levels (Table 5–25).

ANION GAP

The results of serum levels of sodium, potassium, chloride, and bicarbonate may be used to calculate the "anion gap." The anion gap refers to the normal discrepancy between unmeasured (i.e., those not routinely measured) cations and anions in the blood. Unmeasured anions include the negative charges contributed by serum proteins and those of phosphates, sulfates, and other metabolites. Unmeasured anions normally total about 24 mEq/l. Cations not routinely measured include calcium and magnesium, and together they account for about 7 mEq/l. Because there are normally more unmeasured anions than cations, the difference between the two is called the anion gap. This is normally 12 to 18 mEq/l.

The anion gap may be determined by subtracting the sum of routinely measured anions, chloride and bicarbonate, from the sum of routinely measured cations, sodium and potassium (i.e., [Na + K] − [Cl + HCO₃]). The concept of anion gap allows consideration of metabolic derangements without measuring specific metabolites. An increase in the anion gap is seen in acidotic states in

TABLE 5–26. Disorders and Drugs Associated With Altered Serum Calcium Levels

Increased Levels (Hypercalcemia)	Decreased Levels (Hypocalcemia)
Acidosis	Alkalosis
Hyperparathyroidism	Hypoparathyroidism
Cancers involving bone	Pseudohypoparathyroidism
Paget's disease of bone	Inadequate dietary intake of calcium
Prolonged immobility	and/or vitamin D
Leukemia	Vitamin D–resistant rickets
Multiple myeloma	Malabsorption syndromes
Lymphomas	Hypoproteinemia
Hyperproteinemia	Laxative abuse
Polycythemia vera	Acute pancreatitis
Bone growth or active bone formation	Burns
Vitamin D intoxication	Osteomalacia
Hyperthyroidism (severe)	Peritonitis
	Pregnancy
	Overwhelming infections
	Hypomagnesemia
	Renal failure
	Phosphate excess
Drugs	*Drugs*
Thiazide diuretics	Barbiturates
Hormones (androgens, progestins, estrogens)	Anticonvulsants
Vitamin D	Acetazolamide (Diamox)
Calcium supplements	Adrenal corticosteroids
Milk-alkali syndrome	Cytotoxic drugs

which there is no compensatory rise in chloride levels. Examples of anion gap acidosis include diabetic ketoacidosis, lactic adicosis due to either tissue hypoxia (type A) or renal or hepatic metabolic defect (type B), and excessive alcohol ingestion.[55]

SERUM CALCIUM (Ca) (CLINICAL APPLICATIONS DATA, p. 269)

Calcium (Ca, Ca^{++}) is the most abundant cation in the body and participates in virtually all vital processes. About half the total amount of calcium circulates as free ions which participate in blood coagulation, neuromuscular conduction, intracellular regulation, glandular secretion, and control of skeletal and cardiac muscle contractility. The remaining calcium is bound to circulating proteins and plays no physiological role. Serum calcium measurement includes both ionized and protein-bound calcium.

Calcium ions undergo continuous turnover, with bone serving as the major reservoir. Serum contains only a small amount at any one time, but the serum level reflects overall calcium metabolism. Calcium levels are largely regulated by the parathyroid glands and vitamin D. Other substances affecting calcium levels include estrogens and androgens, calcitonin, and ingested carbohydrates. Increased or decreased serum proteins also may affect levels of protein-bound calcium.[56]

Table 5–26 shows the various disorders and drugs associated with altered calcium levels. It should be noted that abnormal serum calcium may produce cardiac dysrhythmias. Furthermore, serum calcium levels have a reciprocal relationship with serum phosphate levels; if one rises, the other tends to fall.

TABLE 5–27. **Disorders and Drugs Associated With Altered Serum Phosphorus/Phosphate Levels**

Increased Levels (Hyperphosphatemia)	Decreased Levels (Hypophosphatemia)
Diabetic ketoacidosis	Recovery phase of diabetic ketoacidosis
Renal failure	Renal tubular acidosis
Vitamin D intoxication	Hypocalcemia
Hypercalcemia	Vitamin D deficiency
Prolonged immobilization	Hyperparathyroidism
Hypoparathyroidism	Carbohydrate ingestion
Pseudohypoparathyroidism	Malnutrition
Bone growth or active bone formation	Malabsorption syndromes
Hyperthyroidism	Hypothyroidism
Acromegaly	Hypopituitarism
Sarcoidosis	Alcholism
Pyloric obstruction	Prolonged vomiting and diarrhea
	Rickets, osteomalacia
Drugs	*Drugs*
Sodium phosphate	Acetazolamide (Diamox)
Milk-alkali syndrome	Aluminum hydroxide
Heparin	Insulin
Diphenylhydantoin (Dilantin)	Epinephrine
Pituitrin	
Androgens	

SERUM PHOSPHORUS/PHOSPHATE (P) (CLINICAL APPLICATIONS DATA, p. 271)

Phosphorus (P), the dominant intracellular anion, is measured in serum as phosphate (HPO_4^{--}, $H_2PO_4^-$). Results are reported as inorganic phosphorus (Pi). Phosphates are vital constituents of nucleic acids, intracellular energy storage compounds, intermediary compounds in carbohydrate metabolism and various regulatory compounds, including that which modulates dissociation of oxygen from hemoglobin. Phosphorus also aids in regulation of calcium levels and functions as a buffer in the maintenance of acid-base balance. It contributes to the mineralization of bones and teeth, promotes renal tubular reabsorption of glucose, and, as a component of phospholipids, aids in fat transport.

As with calcium, phosphorus ions undergo continuous turnover, with bone serving as the major reservoir. Serum contains a relatively small amount of phosphorus at any given time. Phosphorus levels are largely regulated by the parathyroid glands and vitamin D, and are normally reciprocal to those of serum calcium. The equilibrium between serum phosphate levels and intracellular stores is affected by carbohydrate metabolism and blood pH. When persons with diabetic ketoacidosis are treated with insulin, for example, phosphate enters the cells along with glucose and potassium. Phosphate excretion is controlled by the kidneys. Disorders and drugs associated with altered phosphorus levels are listed in Table 5–27. Note that several disorders associated with decreased phosphorus levels are the same as those causing elevated serum calcium levels (e.g., hyperparathyroidism).

TABLE 5–28. Disorders and Drugs Associated With Altered Serum Magnesium Levels

Increased Levels (Hypermagnesemia)	Decreased Levels (Hypomagnesemia)
Addison's disease	Hyperaldosteronism
Adrenalectomy	Hypokalemia
Renal failure	Hypocalcemia
Diabetic ketoacidosis	Diabetic ketoacidosis (resolving)
Dehydration	Alcholism, cirrhosis
Hypothyroidism	Hyperthyroidism
Hyperparathyroidism	Hypoparathyroidism
	Acute pancreatitis
	Gastrointestinal loss (vomiting, diarrhea, nasogastric suction, fistula)
	Malabsorption syndromes
	Malnutrition
	Nephrotic syndrome
	Toxemia of pregnancy
	High-phosphate diet
Drugs	*Drugs*
Antacids and laxatives containing magnesium	Thiazide diuretics
Salicylates	Ethacrynic acid (Edecrin)
Lithium carbamate	Calcium gluconate
	Amphotericin B
	Neomycin
	Insulin
	Aldosterone
	Ethanol

Serum Magnesium (Mg) (Clinical Applications Data, p. 272)

Magnesium (Mg, Mg^{++}) is an essential nutrient found in bone and muscle. In the blood, magnesium is most abundant in the red blood cells, with relatively little found in the serum. Magnesium functions in (1) control of sodium, potassium, calcium, and phosphorus; (2) carbohydrate, lipid, and protein utilization; and (3) activation of enzyme systems that enable B vitamins to function. Magnesium also increases intestinal absorption of calcium and is required for bone and cartilage formation. It is essential for oxidative phosphorylation, nucleic acid synthesis, and blood clotting.

Magnesium is so abundant in foods that dietary deficiency is rare. Decreased serum magnesium levels are seen, however, in chronic alcoholism. Elevated levels most commonly occur in renal failure. A variety of other disorders and drugs also are associated with altered magnesium levels (Table 5–28). It should be noted that altered magnesium levels are associated with cardiac dysrhythmias, especially decreased levels, which may lead to excessive ventricular irritability.

Clinical Applications Data

Serum Sodium (Na) (Background Information, p. 257)
Reference Values

Infants	134–150 mEq/l
Children	135–145 mEq/l
Adults	135–145 mEq/l
	135–142 mmol/l (SI Units)

Interfering Factors

■ Elevated serum triglyceride levels and myeloma proteins may lead to falsely decreased levels
■ Adrenal corticosteroids, methyldopa, hydralazine, reserpine, and cough medicines may lead to increased levels
■ Lithium, vasopressin, and diuretics may lead to decreased levels

Indications/Purposes for Serum Sodium

■ Routine electrolyte screening in acute and critical illness
■ Determination of whole body stores of sodium, since the ion is predominantly extracellular
■ Known or suspected disorder associated with altered fluid and electrolyte balance (see Table 5-22, p. 258)
■ Estimation of serum osmolality which is normally 285 to 310 mOsm/kg, by using the formula shown below:

$$\text{Serum osmolality} = 2(Na^+) + \frac{\text{glucose}}{20} + \frac{\text{BUN}}{3}$$

Note: If the value for serum osmolality is greater than 2.0 to 2.3 times the value for serum sodium, then hyperglycemia, uremia, or metabolic acidosis should be suspected

■ Evaluating the effects of drug therapy on serum sodium levels (e.g., diuretic therapy)

Client Preparation

Client preparation is the same as that for any study involving collection of a peripheral blood sample (see Appendix I).

Because many drugs may alter serum sodium levels, a medication history should be obtained. It is recommended that any drugs that may alter test results be withheld for 12 to 24 hours prior to the test, although this should be confirmed with the person ordering the study.

The Procedure

A venipuncture is performed and the sample collected in a red-topped tube. The sample should be handled gently to avoid hemolysis and transported promptly to the laboratory.

Aftercare and Nursing Observations

Care and assessment following the procedure are the same as for any study involving the collection of a peripheral blood sample. Any medications withheld prior to the test should be resumed.

SERUM POTASSIUM (K) (BACKGROUND INFORMATION, p. 257)

Reference Values

3.5–5.0 mEq/l

Interfering Factors

■ False elevations may occur with vigorous pumping of the hand after tourniquet application for venipuncture, in hemolyzed samples, or with high platelet counts during clotting
■ Falsely decreased levels are seen in anticoagulated samples left at room temperature
■ Numerous drugs may produce elevated and decreased levels (see Table 5–23, p. 259)

Indications/Purposes for Serum Potassium

■ Routine electrolyte screening in acute and critical illness
■ Known or suspected disorder associated with altered fluid and electrolyte balance, especially renal disease, disorders of glucose metabolism, trauma, and burns (see Table 5–23, p. 259)
■ Known or suspected acidosis of any etiology, as potassium moves from the cells into the blood in acidotic states
■ Evaluation of cardiac dysrhythmias to determine if altered serum potassium level is contributing to the problem (e.g., the combination of low serum potassium and therapy with digitalis preparations may lead to ventricular irritability)
■ Evaluation of the effects of drug therapy (e.g., diuretics) on serum potassium levels
■ Evaluation of response to treatment for abnormal serum potassium levels

---

Nursing Alert

■ Because of the effects of serum potassium levels on cardiac impulse conduction, abnormal values should be reported to the physician immediately so that treatment may be instituted

---

Client Preparation

Client preparation is the same as that for any study involving collection of a peripheral blood sample (see Appendix I).

As many drugs may alter serum potassium levels, a medication history should be obtained. It is recommended that those drugs that may alter test results be withheld for 12 to 24 hours prior to the test, although this should be confirmed with the person ordering the study.

The Procedure

A venipuncture is performed and the sample collected in a red-topped tube. Vigorous pumping of the hand after tourniquet application should be avoided, as this may lead to falsely elevated results. The sample should be handled gently to avoid hemolysis, which may also falsely elevate results, and transported immediately to the laboratory.

Aftercare and Nursing Observations

Care and assessment following the procedure are the same as for any study involving the collection of a peripheral blood sample. Any medications withheld prior to the test should be resumed.

SERUM CHLORIDE (Cl) (BACKGROUND INFORMATION, p. 260)
Reference Values

Newborns	94–112 mEq/l
Infants	95–110 mEq/l
Children	98–105 mEq/l
Adults	95–105 mEq/l
	340–370 mg/dl
	98–106 mmol/l (SI units)

Interfering Factors

■ Drugs such as potassium chloride, ammonium chloride, acetazolamide (Diamox), methyldopa (Aldomet), diazoxide (Hyperstat), and guanethidine (Ismelin) may lead to elevated levels
■ Drugs such as ethacrynic acid (Edecrin), furosemide (Lasix), thiazide diuretics, and bicarbonate may lead to decreased levels

Indications/Purposes for Serum Chloride

■ Routine electrolyte screening in acute and critical illness
■ Known or suspected disorder associated with altered acid-base and/or fluid and electrolyte balance
■ Support for diagnosing disorders associated with altered serum chloride levels (see Table 5–24, p. 260)
■ Differentiation of the type of acidosis (hyperchloremic versus anion gap acidosis), with serum chloride levels remaining relatively normal in anion gap acidosis
■ Evaluation of the effects of drug therapy on serum chloride levels (see Table 5–24, p. 260)

Client Preparation

Client preparation is the same as that for any study involving collection of a peripheral blood sample (see Appendix I).

Because many drugs may alter serum chloride levels, a medication history should be obtained. It is recommended that those drugs that may alter test results be withheld for 12 to 24 hours prior to the test, although this should be confirmed with the person ordering the study.

The Procedure

A venipuncture is performed and the sample collected in a red-topped tube. The sample should be handled gently to avoid hemolysis and transported promptly to the laboratory.

Aftercare and Nursing Observations

Care and assessment following the procedure are the same as for any study involving the collection of a peripheral blood sample. Any medications withheld prior to the test should be resumed.

SERUM BICARBONATE (HCO_3) (BACKGROUND INFORMATION, p. 261)
Reference Values

Peripheral vein	19–25 mEq/l
Arterial sample	22–26 mEq/l

Interfering Factors

■ Numerous drugs may alter serum bicarbonate levels (see Table 5–25, p. 261)

Indications/Purposes for Serum Bicarbonate

■ Routine electrolyte screening in acute and critical illness
■ Known or suspected disorder associated with altered acid-base and/or fluid and electrolyte balance
■ Support for diagnosing disorders associated with altered serum bicarbonate levels (see Table 5–25, p. 261)

TABLE 5–29. Blood Gases in Acid-Base Imbalances

	pH	pCO$_2$	HCO$_3^-$	BE
Respiratory acidosis	↓	↑	Normal	Normal
with compensation	Sl. ↓ or normal	↑	↑	↑
Respiratory alkalosis	↑	↓	Normal	Normal
with compensation	Sl. ↑ or normal	↓	↓	↓
Metabolic acidosis	↓	Normal	↓	↓
with compensation	Sl. ↓ or normal	↓	↓	↓
Metabolic alkalosis	↑	Normal	↑	↑
with compensation	Sl. ↑ or normal	↑	↑	↑
Mixed respiratory and metabolic acidosis	↓	↑	↓	↓

Sl. = slightly

■ Determination of the degree of compensation in acidotic and alkalotic states (Table 5–29)
■ Evaluation of the effects of drug therapy on serum bicarbonate levels

Client Preparation

Client preparation is the same as that for any study involving collection of a peripheral blood sample (see Appendix I).

As many drugs may alter serum bicarbonate levels, a medication history should be obtained. It is recommended that drugs that may alter test results be withheld for 12 to 24 hours prior to the test, although this should be confirmed with the person ordering the study.

The Procedure

A venipuncture is performed and the sample collected in a red-topped tube. The sample should be handled gently to avoid hemolysis and transported promptly to the laboratory.

Aftercare and Nursing Observations

Care and assessment following the procedure are the same as for any study involving the collection of a peripheral blood sample. Any medications withheld prior to the test should be resumed.

SERUM CALCIUM (Ca) (BACKGROUND INFORMATION, p. 263)
Reference Values

Children	<12.0 mg/dl
	<6.0 mEq/l
Adults	9–11 mg/dl
	4.5–5.5 mEq/l

Interfering Factors

■ Values are higher in children because of growth and active bone formation
■ Numerous drugs may alter serum calcium levels (see Table 5–26, p. 262)
■ Increased or decreased serum protein levels may alter results

Indications/Purposes for Serum Calcium

■ Evaluating the effects of various disorders on overall calcium metabolism, especially diseases involving bone (see Table 5–26, p. 262)
■ Detection of parathyroid gland loss after thyroid or other neck surgery, as indicated by decreased levels
■ Monitoring the effects of renal failure on calcium levels, which are usually decreased in the disorder
■ Evaluation of cardiac dysrhythmias to determine if altered serum calcium level is contributing to the problem
■ Evaluation of coagulation disorders to determine if altered serum calcium level is contributing to the problem
■ Monitoring the effects of various drugs on serum calcium levels (see Table 5–26, p. 262)
■ Evaluating the effectiveness of treatment for abnormal calcium levels, especially in deficiency states

---

Nursing Alert

■ Because altered serum calcium levels may produce cardiac dysrhythmias, abnormal values should be reported to the physician immediately so that treatment may be instituted

---

Client Preparation

Client preparation is the same as that for any study involving collection of a peripheral blood sample (see Appendix I).

Because many drugs may alter serum calcium levels, a medication history should be obtained. It is recommended that drugs that may alter test results be withheld for 12 to 24 hours prior to the test, although this should be confirmed with the person ordering the study.

The Procedure

A venipuncture is performed and the sample collected in a red-topped tube. The sample should be handled gently to avoid hemolysis and transported promptly to the laboratory.

Aftercare and Nursing Observations

Care and assessment following the procedure are the same as for any study involving the collection of a peripheral blood sample. Any medications withheld prior to the test should be resumed.

SERUM PHOSPHORUS/PHOSPHATE (P) (BACKGROUND INFORMATION, p. 264)
Reference Values

Children	<7 mg/dl
Adults	2.4–4.7 mg/dl

Phosphorus is measured in terms of phosphate; the results cannot be expressed in milliequivalents, because different phosphate groups have different valences.

Interfering Factors

■ Phosphate levels are higher in children owing to bone growth and active bone formation
■ Values vary diurnally, being higher at night than in the morning
■ A number of drugs may alter serum phosphate levels (see Table 5–27, p. 263)
■ Hemolysis of the sample may cause falsely elevated values resulting from release of phosphate from red blood cells

Indications/Purposes for Serum Phosphorus/Phosphate

■ Support for diagnosing disorders associated with altered phosphorus/phosphate levels, especially bone disorders, parathyroid disorders, renal disease, and alcoholism (see Table 5–27, p. 263)
■ Monitoring the effects of renal failure on phosphorus levels, which are usually increased in the disorder
■ Support for identification of the cause of growth abnormalities in children
■ Monitoring the effects of various drugs on serum phosphate levels (see Table 5–27, p. 263)

Client Preparation

Client preparation is the same as that for any study involving collection of a peripheral blood sample (see Appendix I).

Because many drugs may alter serum phosphorus/phosphate levels, a medication history should be obtained. It is recommended that any drugs that may alter test results be withheld for 12 to 24 hours prior to the test, although this should be confirmed with the person ordering the study.

The Procedure

A venipuncture is performed and the sample collected in a red-topped tube. The sample should be handled gently to avoid hemolysis, which may falsely elevate levels, and transported promptly to the laboratory.

Aftercare and Nursing Observations

Care and assessment following the procedure are the same as for any study involving the collection of a peripheral blood sample. Any medications withheld prior to the test should be resumed.

Serum Magnesium (Mg) (Background Information, p. 265)

Reference Values

Newborns	1.4–2.9 mEq/l
Children	1.6–2.6 mEq/l
Adults	1.5–2.5 mEq/l
	1.8–3.0 mg/dl

Interfering Factors

■ A number of drugs may alter serum magnesium levels (see Table 5–28, p. 264)
■ Because magnesium is found in red blood cells, hemolysis of the sample may lead to falsely elevated values

Indications/Purposes for Serum Magnesium

■ Determination of magnesium balance in renal failure and chronic alcoholism
■ Evaluation of known or suspected disorders associated with altered magnesium levels (see Table 5–28, p. 264)
■ Evaluation of cardiac dysrhythmias to determine if altered serum magnesium level is contributing to the problem (i.e., decreased magnesium levels may lead to excessive ventricular irritability)
■ Monitoring the effects of various drugs on serum magnesium levels (see Table 5–28, p. 264)

Client Preparation

Client preparation is the same as that for any study involving collection of a peripheral blood sample (see Appendix I).

As many drugs may alter serum magnesium levels, a medication history should be obtained. It is recommended that those drugs that may alter test results be withheld for 12 to 24 hours prior to the test, although this should be confirmed with the person ordering the study.

The Procedure

A venipuncture is performed and the sample collected in a red-topped tube. The sample should be handled gently to avoid hemolysis, which may falsely elevate levels, and transported promptly to the laboratory.

Aftercare and Nursing Observations

Care and assessment following the procedure are the same as for any study involving the collection of a peripheral blood sample. Any medications withheld prior to the test should be resumed.

ARTERIAL BLOOD GASES (ABGs)

Background Information (Clinical Applications Data, below)

Arterial blood gas (ABG) determinations are done not only to determine levels of actual blood gases (i.e., oxygen and carbon dioxide), but also to assess the client's overall acid-base balance. Thus, ABG levels may indicate hypoxia, hypercapnia or hypocapnia, acidosis, alkalosis, and physiological compensation for acid-base imbalance. The components of an ABG determination are discussed as follows:

1. *pH.* pH reflects the number of hydrogen ions in the body and is influenced primarily by the ratio of bicarbonate ions (HCO_3^-) to carbonic acid (H_2CO_3), which is essentially carbon dioxide (CO_2), in the blood. The normal HCO_3^- to CO_2 ratio is 20:1. When the hydrogen ion concentration increases (acidosis), the pH falls; when the hydrogen ion concentration decreases (alkalosis), the pH rises. Bicarbonate levels are regulated by the kidneys, while carbon dioxide levels are controlled by the lungs. Both the lungs and the kidneys will respond to alterations in pH levels by either retaining or excreting carbon dioxide and bicarbonate, respectively.
2. *pO_2.* pO_2 indicates the partial pressure of oxygen in the blood. When oxygen levels are lower than normal, the client is hypoxic. Hypoxemia may be due to either a low cardiac output or impaired lung function.
3. *pCO_2.* pCO_2 indicates the partial pressure of carbon dioxide in the blood, which is regulated by the lungs. Except in cases of compensation for metabolic acid-base imbalances, elevated levels (hypercapnia, hypercarbia) indicate impaired gas exchange in the lungs such that excess CO_2 is not eliminated. Decreased levels (hypocapnia, hypocarbia) indicate increased loss of CO_2 through the lungs (hyperventilation).
4. *HCO_3^-.* HCO_3^- indicates the bicarbonate ion concentration in the blood, which is regulated by the kidneys. Altered levels are associated with metabolic acid-base imbalances or reflect response to respiratory alterations in CO_2 levels.
5. *O_2 Saturation.* O_2 saturation (O_2 Sat, SaO_2) indicates the oxygen content of the blood expressed as percent of oxygen capacity (the amount of oxygen the blood could carry if all of the hemoglobin were fully saturated with oxygen). If the blood is 50 percent saturated, for example, the oxygen content is one half of the oxygen capacity.
6. *Base Excess.* Base excess (BE) usually indicates the difference between the normal serum bicarbonate (HCO_3^-) level and the client's bicarbonate level. Positive values indicate excess bicarbonate relative to normal values, while negative values indicate decreased HCO_3^- levels.

Clinical Applications Data (Background Information, above)

Reference Values

pH	7.35–7.45
pO_2	85–100 mmHg

pCO_2	35–45 mmHs
HCO_3	22–26 mEq/l
O_2 Saturation	95–97%
Base Excess	$+2--2$

Interfering Factors

■ Fever may falsely elevate pO_2 and pCO_2; hypothermia may lower them
■ Suctioning of respiratory passages within 20 to 30 minutes of the test may alter results
■ Excessive heparin in the sample will lower the pH and pCO_2
■ Exposure of the sample to atmospheric air (e.g., air bubbles in the sample) may alter results
■ Exposure of the sample to room temperature for more than 2 minutes may alter test results

Indications/Purposes for Arterial Blood Gases

■ Evaluation of the effectiveness of pulmonary ventilation in maintaining adequate oxygenation and in removing carbon dioxide, especially in disorders such as chronic pulmonary disease, neurological insults, and drug intoxication
■ Evaluation of the effectiveness of cardiac output in maintaining adequate oxygenation, especially in shock and acute myocardial infarction
■ Determination of the need for oxygen therapy (oxygen is generally indicated if the pO_2 is 70 mm Hg or less, except in pulmonary disorders characterized by chronic hypoxemia in which lower oxygen levels may be tolerated by the client without supplemental oxygen)
■ Determination of respiratory failure, which is defined as a pO_2 of 50 mm Hg or less with a pCO_2 of 50 mm Hg or more
■ Determination of acid-base balance, type of imbalance, and degree of compensation (see Table 5–29, p. 269)
■ Determination of need for mechanical ventilation (e.g., elevated or rising pCO_2 levels may indicate the need for mechanical ventilation, especially when pO_2 is decreased)
■ Evaluation of effectiveness of mechanical ventilation and indication for modification of ventilator settings
■ Evaluation of response to weaning from mechanical ventilation

Client Preparation

Client Teaching. Explain to the client:

■ the purpose of the test
■ that repeat determinations may be necessary until cardiopulmonary function and/or acid-base balance are stabilized
■ the method and site for obtaining the sample (e.g., arterial puncture or arterial line sample)
■ any anticipated discomforts (arterial punctures will cause a brief, sharp pain unless a local anesthetic is used)
■ that if an arterial puncture is done, it will be necessary to maintain digital pressure on the puncture site for 5 minutes or more, after which a pressure dressing will be applied

Encourage questions and verbalization of concerns appropriate to the client's age and mental status.

Physical Preparation

- Take the client's temperature. Fever may falsely elevate pO_2 and pCO_2; hypothermia may lower them
- The client should not have had a respiratory therapy treatment, been suctioned, or had ventilator settings changed less than 20 to 30 minutes before the sample is obtained
- If the test is being done to determine the need for oxygen therapy or response to weaning from mechanical ventilation, the client should be off oxygen, off mechanical ventilation, or on a weaning mode for a preset time, which is specified by the person ordering the test
- If the sample is to be obtained by radial artery puncture, the Allen test should be performed to assess patency of the ulnar artery; in the event that thrombosis involving the radial artery occurs after the puncture:
  - [ ] extend the client's wrist over a rolled towel or similar support
  - [ ] ask the client to clench the fist; if the client cannot clench the fist, elevate the hand above heart level
  - [ ] apply digital pressure over both the radial and ulnar arteries
  - [ ] have the client unclench the fist while pressure is maintained on the arteries
  - [ ] observe the palm for blanching, which is the expected response
  - [ ] release pressure on the ulnar artery while continuing to maintain pressure on the radial artery
  - [ ] observe the palm for returning pinkness, which is a positive result
  - [ ] if the palm remains blanched or if return of pinkness takes longer than approximately 5 seconds (a negative result), do not use the wrist for arterial punctures
  - [ ] inform the client's physician of a negative response to the Allen test

The Procedure

The procedure varies slightly with the method for obtaining the sample.

Arterial Puncture. A blood gas collection kit is obtained. If prepackaged kits are not available, obtain a 3 ml syringe, heparin (usually in the concentration of 100 U/ml), 20-G or 21-G needles, povidone-iodine and/or alcohol swabs or sponges, gauze pads, and tape. Fill a plastic or paper cup or a small plastic bag about halfway with ice.

If the syringe is not preheparinized, draw approximately 1 ml of heparin into the syringe, pull the plunger back to about the 3 ml line, and rotate the barrel. Then expel all except approximately 0.1 ml of heparin and change the needle. Excessive heparin in the syringe will lower the pH and pCO_2 of the sample.

Palpate the artery to be used. The radial artery is usually the most accessible, but the brachial and femoral arteries also may be used. If the radial artery is to be used, extend the client's wrist over a rolled towel or similar support.

Cleanse the site to be used with povidone-iodine and allow to dry. It is recommended by some that the iodine solution be removed with an alcohol swab prior to arterial puncture. If the client is allergic to iodine, use only alcohol to prepare the site. Some authorities also advocate anesthetizing the puncture site with a small amount of 1 percent Xylocaine (lidocaine).

Using the heparinized syringe with needle attached, puncture the artery. A 45-degree angle is used for radial artery punctures, while a 60- to a 90-degree angle is used for brachial arteries. A 90-degree angle is generally employed for femoral artery punctures. Advance the needle until blood begins to enter the syringe; it should not be necessary to pull back on the plunger. After 2 to 3 ml of blood have been obtained, withdraw the needle and immediately apply firm pressure to the puncture site with a sterile gauze pad.

Meanwhile, expel any air or air bubbles from the syringe, as mixing with atmospheric air may alter test results. The needle may be plugged by inserting into a rubber cap, or it may be removed and the rubber cap supplied in the blood gas collection kit placed on the hub of the syringe. The sample is then placed in ice to inhibit metabolic blood activity; failure to do this within 2 minutes of collecting the sample will alter test results.

The sample is sent for analysis immediately. On the ABG request form or sample label, note the time the sample was collected, the client's temperature, and whether the client was breathing room air, receiving oxygen, or on mechanical ventilation.

Arterial Line Sample. Obtain a 5 ml and a 3 ml syringe, heparin, gauze pads, and a container of ice. If the 3 ml syringe is not preheparinized, heparinize it as described earlier. Using the stopcock attached to the arterial line and a 5 ml nonheparinized syringe, obtain 5 ml of blood from the line and discard it. Then, using the heparinized syringe, obtain a 2 to 3 ml sample of arterial blood. Expel any excess air, cap the syringe, and place it in ice.

Flush the stopcock syringe port of blood, using the gauze pads to absorb expelled blood and flush solution. Cap the port, and then flush the blood remaining in the arterial line back to the client.

As indicated with arterial punctures, use the ABG request form or sample label to note the time the sample was collected, the client's temperature, and whether the client was breathing room air, receiving oxygen, or on mechanical ventilation. Send the sample for analysis immediately.

Aftercare

For arterial punctures, maintain digital pressure on the site for 5 minutes and then apply a sterile pressure dressing. If the client is receiving anticoagulants or has bleeding tendencies, it may be necessary to apply digital pressure for 10 to 15 minutes.

Nursing Observations

Pretest

■ Assess the client's response to explanations provided
■ Assess the client's degree of anxiety about the procedure
■ Assess the client's response to removal of oxygen or assisted mechanical ventilation
■ Assess the client's response to the Allen test

During the Test

■ Observe the client's response to any discomfort experienced

Post-Test

■ Observe the arterial puncture site for bleeding or hematoma formation every 5 to 10 minutes for one-half hour after the pressure dressing is applied
■ Check for presence of pulses distal to the site when performing site observations, if the brachial or femoral artery was used
■ Check for signs of nerve impairment distal to the site

VITAMINS AND TRACE MINERALS

Background Information

Vitamins are essential organic substances that perform various metabolic functions. Vitamins cannot be synthesized in adequate amounts by the body, and therefore, inadequate dietary intake will cause deficiency diseases. Vitamins are classified as fat soluble and water soluble. The fat-soluble vitamins are vitamins A, D, E, and K. Because these are stored in the body, excessive ingestion of exogenous fat-soluble vitamins may cause abnormally elevated levels. Vitamin C and the B-complex vitamins are water soluble and are not stored in the body.

For diagnostic purposes, blood levels of vitamins A and C and a metabolite of vitamin D are measured. Vitamin B_{12} and folic acid also are measured in studies pertaining to hematologic function (see Chapter 1).

Seven trace minerals are known to be essential to human function even though they are present in minute quantities in the body. These essential minerals are cobalt, copper, iodine, iron, manganese, molybdenum, and zinc. Other trace minerals are found in the body, but their functions remain unclear. These include chromium, fluorine, lithium, arsenic, cadmium, nickle, silicon, tin, and vanadium.

VITAMIN A (CLINICAL APPLICATIONS DATA, p. 278)

Vitamin A is obtained from foods of animal origin such as eggs, milk, butter, and liver. Its precursor, carotene, a yellowish pigment, is obtained from yellow or orange vegetables and fruits and from leafy green vegetables.

Vitamin A promotes normal vision by permitting visual adaptation to light and dark, and prevents nightblindness (xerophthalmia). It also contributes to the growth of bone, teeth, and soft tissues; supports the formation of thyroxine; maintains epithelial cellular membranes; aids in spermatogenesis; and maintains the integrity of skin and mucous membranes as barriers to infection.

Elevated levels are generally seen with excessive intake of vitamin A, and also may be associated with pregnancy, oral contraceptive use, myxedema, nephritis, hyperlipidemia, and hypercholesterolemia of diabetes. Decreased levels are associated with various skin disorders (e.g., acne) and may be due to decreased nutritional intake. Since fats and bile salts are necessary for vitamin A absorption, decreased blood levels may be seen with lipid malabsorption, biliary obstruction, and low-fat diets. Decreased levels also are associated with liver disease and excessive ingestion of mineral oil.

VITAMIN C (CLINICAL APPLICATIONS DATA, p. 279)

Vitamin C (ascorbic acid) functions in many metabolic processes, especially in those related to collagen formation and the stress response. In addition, vitamin C helps to maintain capillary strength, facilitates the release of iron from ferritin for hemoglobin formation and red cell maturation, and may maintain the integrity of the amniotic sac.

Elevated vitamin C levels are associated with excessive intake of the vitamin within 24 hours of the test. Decreased intake produces scurvy with low vitamin C levels. Decreased levels also may be seen in malabsorption syndromes, pregnancy, infections, cancer, and burns.

VITAMIN D (CLINICAL APPLICATIONS DATA, p. 280)

The form of vitamin D most easily and accurately measured is 25-hydroxy-cholecalciferol (vitamin D_3, 25-(OH)D_3, cholecalciferol), a monohydroxylated form that leaves the liver for subsequent dihydroxylation by the kidney. Indirect measurement of vitamin D by serum alkaline phosphatase, calcium and phosphorus determinations preceded 25-(OH)D_3 assays, and may still be used in the diagnosis of disorders of calcium metabolism.

Vitamin D aids in the maintenance of calcium-phosphorus balance and in the deposition of calcium and phosphorus in the bone. It also facilitates absorption of calcium and phosphorus from the small intestine and aids in the renal excretion of phosphorus. Elevated vitamin D levels are associated with excessive ingestion. Decreased levels are seen in malabsorption syndromes, chronic renal failure, hepatobiliary diseases, hypothyroidism, and vitamin D–resistant rickets. Therapy with anticonvulsants and glucocorticoids also may produce decreased levels.

TRACE MINERALS (CLINICAL APPLICATIONS DATA, p. 281)

Seven trace minerals are known to be essential to human function even though they are present in minute quantities in the body. These essential minerals are cobalt, copper, iodine, iron, manganese, molybdenum, and zinc.

Cobalt is a constituent of vitamin B_{12} and is essential to the formation of red blood cells. Copper participates in cytochrome oxidation of tissue cells for energy production, promotes absorption of iron from the intestines and transfer from tissues to plasma, and is essential to hemoglobin formation. It also promotes bone and brain tissue formation and supports the maintenance of myelin. Iodine is an essential component for the synthesis of thyroid hormones. Iron, which is discussed in Chapter 1, is an essential component of hemoglobin.

Manganese functions as a coenzyme in urea formation and in the metabolism of proteins, fats, and carbohydrates. Molybdenum facilitates the enzymatic action of xanthine oxidase and liver aldehyde oxidase in purine catabolism, and functions in the formation of carboxylic acid. Zinc is an essential component of cellular enzymes such as alkaline phosphatase, carbonic anhydrase, lactic dehydrogenase, and carboxypeptidase, which function in protein and carbohydrate metabolism. It also aids in the storage of insulin, functions in deoxyribonucleic acid (DNA) replication, assists in carbon dioxide exchange, promotes body growth and sexual maturation, and may affect lymphocyte formation and cellular immunity.

Other trace minerals are found in the body, but their functions remain unclear. These include chromium, fluorine, lithium, arsenic, cadmium, nickel, silicon, tin, and vanadium.

Deficiencies of trace minerals are likely only in individuals dependent on parenteral nutrition because the normal diet provides adequate intake. Elevated blood levels are usually due to environmental contamination, either in industrial settings or through water pollution.

Clinical Applications Data

VITAMIN A (BACKGROUND INFORMATION, p. 277)

Reference Values

Vitamin A	65–275 IU/dl
	0.15–0.60 mg/ml

Carotene	
Infants	0–40 µg/dl
Children	40–130 µg/dl
Adults	50–300 µg/dl

Interfering Factors

■ Pregnancy and oral contraceptive use may lead to falsely elevated levels, as may hyperlipidemia, hypercholesterolemia of diabetes, myxedema, and nephritis
■ Excessive ingestion of mineral oil, low-fat diets, and liver disease may lead to decreased levels
■ Failure to follow dietary and drug restrictions prior to the test may alter results
■ Excessive exposure of the sample to light may alter results

Indications/Purposes for Vitamin A and Carotene

■ Evaluation of skin disorders, with vitamin A deficiency a possible cause
■ Support for diagnosing xerophthalmia (night blindness) as indicated by decreased levels
■ Suspected vitamin A deficiency due to fat malabsorption or biliary tract disease
■ Support for diagnosing excessive vitamin A and/or carotene ingestion, as indicated by elevated blood levels

Client Preparation

General client preparation is the same as that for any study involving collection of a peripheral blood sample (see Appendix I). For this test, the client should fast from food for 8 hours prior to the study. Water is not restricted. Vitamin supplements containing vitamin A should be withheld for at least 24 hours prior to the test.

The Procedure

A venipuncture is performed and the sample collected in a red-topped tube. The sample should be covered to protect it from light, which may alter test results, handled gently to avoid hemolysis, and sent promptly to the laboratory.

Aftercare and Nursing Observations

Care and assessment following the procedure are the same as for any test involving collection of a peripheral blood sample. The client's usual diet should be resumed. Vitamin supplements may be resumed pending test results.

VITAMIN C (BACKGROUND INFORMATION, p. 277)

Reference Values

Children	0.6–1.6 mg/dl
Adults	0.2–2.0 mg/dl

Interfering Factors

- Excessive intake of vitamin C within 24 hours of the test will produce elevated levels
- Failure to follow dietary restrictions prior to the test may alter results

Indications/Purposes for Vitamin C

- Evaluation of the effects of major stressors (e.g., pregnancy, major surgery, burns, infections, malignancies) on vitamin C levels
- Evaluation of the effects of malabsorption syndromes on vitamin C levels
- Evaluation of the effectiveness of therapy with vitamin C in treating deficiency states

Client Preparation

General client preparation is the same as that for any study involving collection of a peripheral blood sample (see Appendix I). For this test, the client should fast from food for 8 hours prior to the test. Vitamin C preparations also should be withheld for 24 hours prior to the study.

The Procedure

A venipuncture is performed and the sample collected in a black-topped tube. The sample is handled gently to avoid hemolysis and transported promptly to the laboratory.

Aftercare and Nursing Observations

Care and assessment following the procedure are the same as for any test involving collection of a peripheral blood sample. The client's usual diet should be resumed. Vitamin C preparations may be resumed pending test results.

VITAMIN D (BACKGROUND INFORMATION, p. 278)

Reference Values

25-(OH)D$_3$	0.7–3.3 IU/ml
	10–55 ng/ml

Interfering Factors

- Excessive ingestion of vitamin D will lead to elevated levels
- Therapy with anticonvulsants and glucocorticoids may produce decreased levels

Indications/Purposes for Vitamin D

- Differential diagnosis of hypercalcemia due to parathyroid adenoma or vitamin D toxicity
- Confirmation of vitamin D deficiency as the cause of bone disease
- Confirmation of vitamin D deficiency due to malabsorption syndromes, hepatobiliary disease, and chronic renal failure

■ Evidence of interference with vitamin D levels due to anticonvulsant or steroid therapy

Client Preparation

Client preparation is the same as that for any study involving collection of a peripheral blood sample. It is recommended that anticonvulsant and steroid medications be withheld for 24 hours prior to the test, although this should be confirmed by the person ordering the study.

The Procedure

A venipuncture is performed and the sample collected in a red-topped tube. The sample should be handled gently to avoid hemolysis and transported promptly to the laboratory.

Aftercare and Nursing Observations

Care and assessment following the procedure are the same as for any study involving collection of a peripheral blood sample. Medications withheld prior to the test should be resumed.

TRACE MINERALS (BACKGROUND INFORMATION, p. 278)
Reference Values

Cobalt	1 mg/dl
Copper	130–230 mg/dl
Iodine (protein-bound)	4–8 mg/dl
Manganese	4–20 mg/dl
Zinc	50–150 mg/dl
Chromium	0.3–0.85 mg/dl

Indications/Purposes for Trace Minerals

■ Monitoring response to parenteral nutrition, which may lead to deficiencies of trace minerals
■ Suspected exposure to environmental toxins, which may be indicated by elevated levels of trace minerals

Client Preparation

Client preparation is the same as that for any test involving collection of a peripheral blood sample (see Appendix I).

The Procedure

A venipuncture is performed and the sample collected in a metal-free tube. The sample is handled gently to avoid hemolysis and transported immediately to the laboratory.

Aftercare and Nursing Observations

Care and assessment following the procedure are the same as for any test involving collection of a peripheral blood sample.

DRUGS AND TOXIC SUBSTANCES

Background Information

Blood levels of drugs are used to monitor attainment of therapeutic drug levels, compliance with therapeutic regimens, and potential excess dosing. They are also employed in situations when accidental or deliberate drug overdose is suspected. In therapeutic situations, serial samples may be drawn to determine peak (highest) and trough (lowest) blood levels of drugs. Samples for peak drug levels are generally drawn within 30 to 60 minutes of drug administration. Trough levels are drawn immediately before the next dose of the drug is to be given. It is necessary to know as exactly as possible the time the drug was administered or ingested for accurate interpretation of test results.

Many potential toxins are present in the household and in industrial settings. Data regarding circulating levels of toxic substances may be used to diagnose either acute or chronic poisoning with metals or common commercial substances.

Clinical Applications Data
Reference Values

Therapeutic and toxic levels of various drugs are shown in Table 5–30. Toxic doses and effects of industrial and household toxins are listed in Table 5–31.

Indications/Purposes for Blood Levels of Drugs and Toxic Substances

- Determination of therapeutic levels of prescribed drugs, especially those with narrow therapeutic ranges and/or serious toxic effects
- Evaluation of the degree of compliance with the therapeutic regimen
- Known or suspected drug overdose
- Known or suspected exposure to environmental toxins
- Evaluation of chronic exposure to industrial products known to be toxic

Client Preparation

Client preparation is the same as that for any study involving collection of a peripheral blood sample.

The Procedure

A venipuncture is performed and the sample collected in a red-topped tube. The sample should be handled gently to avoid hemolysis and transported to the laboratory immediately. For drug levels, the name of the drug, dosage, and time administered or ingested should be noted on the laboratory request form.

Aftercare and Nursing Observations

Care and assessment following the procedure are the same as for any test involving collection of a peripheral blood sample. It may be necessary to withhold subsequent doses of drugs administered for therapeutic reasons until test results are available, but this should be confirmed with the person prescribing the medication.

Table 5–30. Blood Levels of Drugs

Drug	Peak Time	Duration of Action	Therapeutic Level	Toxic Level
Antibiotics				
Amikacin	IM: ½ hr IV: 15 min	2 days	20–25 µg/ml	35 µg/ml
Gentamicin	IM: ½ hr IV: 15 min	2 days	4–8 µg/ml	12 µg/ml
Kanamycin	½ hr	2 days	20–25 µg/ml	35 µg/ml
Streptomycin	½–1½ hr	5 days	25–30 µg/ml	>30 µg/ml
Tobramycin	IV: 15 min	2 days	2–8 µg/ml	12 µg/ml
Anticonvulsants				
Barbiturates and barbiturate-related				
Amobarbital	IV: 30 sec	10–20 hr	7 µg/ml	30 µg/ml
Pentobarbital	IV: 30 sec	15 hr	4 µg/ml	15 µg/ml
Phenobarbital	15 min	80 hr	10 µg/ml	>55 µg/ml
Primidone	PO: 3 hr	7–14 hr	1 µg/ml	>10 µg/ml
Benzodiazepines				
Clonazepam (Clonopin)	1–4 hr	60 hr	5–70 ng/ml	>70 ng/ml
Diazepam (Valium)	1–4 hr	1–2 days	5–70 ng/ml	>70 ng/ml
Hydantoins				
Phenytoin (Dilantin)	3–12 hr	7–42 hr	10–20 µg/ml	>20 µg/ml
Succinimides				
Ethosuximide (Zarontin)	1 hr	8 days	40–80 µg/ml	100 µg/ml
Miscellaneous				
Carbamazepine (Tegretol)	4 hr	2 days	2–10 µg/ml	12 µg/ml
Bronchodilators				
Aminophylline/theophylline	PO: 2 hr IV: 15 min	8–9 hr	10–18 µg/ml	>20 µg/ml
Cardiac drugs				
Disopyramide (Norpace)	PO: 2 hr	25–30 hr	2–4.5 µg/ml	>9 µg/ml
Quinidine	PO: 1 hr IV: immediate	20–30 hr	2.4–5 µg/ml	>6 µg/ml
Procainamide (Pronestyl)	PO: 1 hr IV: ½ hr	10–20 hr	4–8 µg/ml	>12 µg/ml

TABLE 5–30 — Continued

Drug	Peak Time	Duration of Action	Therapeutic Level	Toxic Level
NAPA (N-acetyl-procainamide, a procainamide metabolite)	—	—	2–8 μg/ml	>30 μg/ml
Lidocaine	IV: immediate	5–10 hr	2–6 μg/ml	>9 μg/ml
Bretylium	15–30 min	6–8 hr	5–10 mg/kg	30 mg/kg
Verapamil	PO: 5 hrs / IV: 3–5 min	8–10 hr / IV: ½–1 hr	5–10 mg/kg	>15 mg/kg
Diltiazem	PO: 2–3 hr	3–4 hr	50–200 ng/ml	>200 ng/ml
Nifedipine	1–3 hr	3–4 hr	5–10 mg	90 mg
Digitoxin	4 hr	30 days	5–30 ng/ml	30 ng/ml
Digoxin	2 hr	7 days	0.5–2 ng/ml	>2.5 ng/ml
Phenytoin (Dilantin)	PO: 2 hr / IV: 1 hr	96 hr	10–18 μg/ml	>20 μg/ml
Salicylates				
Aspirin	15 min	12–30 hr	20 μg/ml / 2–30 mg/dl	40 mg/dl
Narcotics				
Codeine	—	—	—	>0.005 mg/dl
Hydromorphone (Dilaudid)	—	—	—	>0.1 mg/dl
Methadone	—	—	—	>0.2 mg/dl
Meperidine (Demerol)	—	—	—	>0.5 mg/dl
Morphine	—	—	—	>0.005 mg/dl
Barbiturates				
Phenobarbital	—	—	10 μg/ml	55 μg/ml
Amobarbital	—	—	7 μg/ml	30 μg/ml
Pentobarbital	—	—	4 μg/ml	15 μg/ml
Secobarbital	—	—	3 μg/ml	10 μg/ml
Alcohols				
Ethanol	—	—	—	100 mg/dl
Methanol	—	—	—	20 mg/dl
Miscellaneous				
Acetaminophen	—	—	—	>150 μg/ml / 4 hr after ingestion
Phenothiazines	—	—	0.5 μg/ml	1.0 μg/ml

TABLE 5-31. Toxic Doses and Effects of Industrial and Household Toxins

Substance	Toxic Doses	Toxic Effects
Aniline	50 mg/kg	Methemoglobinemia, hepatotoxicity, nephrotoxicity
Arsenic/antimony	5 mg/kg	Gastric hemorrhage, shock
Barium salts	—	Bloody diarrhea, cardiac depression, muscle spasms, respiratory failure, renal failure
Benzene products	50 mg/kg	CNS depression, respiratory failure, cardiac arrest, bone marrow depression, liver damage
Cadmium	>41 ng/ml	Severe gastroenteritis, liver damage, acute renal failure; if inhaled as dust or fumes, pulmonary edema
Carbon tetrachloride	5–10 ml (total)	CNS depression, liver and kidney failure
Chlorate or bromate salts	50 mg/kg	Methemoglobinemia, intravascular hemolysis, acute renal failure
Copper salts	50 mg/kg	Generalized capillary damage, kidney and liver damage
Cyanide	>5 mg total (>0.5 mg/100 ml of blood)	Confusion, dyspnea, convulsions, death from respiratory failure
DDT	50 mg/kg	Fatigue, confusion, ataxia, convulsions, death from respiratory failure
2,4-D	—	Lethargy, diarrhea, cardiac arrest, hyperpyrexia, convulsions, coma
Ergot	5 mg/kg	Gastrointestinal inflammation, renal damage, gangrene of fingers and toes due to persistent peripheral vasoconstriction
Ethylene glycol	>5 mg/kg	CNS depression, death from renal failure or respiratory paralysis
Iron salts	500 mg/kg	Bloody diarrhea, shock, liver damage
Fluoride	50 mg/kg (0.2–0.3 mg/dl of blood)	Hemorrhagic gastroenteritis, tremors, hypocalcemia, shock
Formaldehyde	500 mg/kg	Hemorrhagic gastroenteritis, renal failure, circulatory collapse
Hydrogen sulfide	0.1–0.2% in air	Death from respiratory paralysis
Sodium hypochloride	Several ounces of household bleach	Edema of pharynx, glottis, larynx; perforation of esophagus or stomach, pulmonary edema from fumes
Iodine	5 mg/kg	Bloody diarrhea, renal damage; death from asphyxia or circulatory collapse
Ipecac, syrup or fluid-extract	1–2 oz fluid-extract (14 times more concentrated than the syrup)	Shock due to intractable vomiting and diarrhea, death due to cardiac depression
Isopropyl alcohol	500 mg/kg	Severe CNS depression, death due to respiratory failure or circulatory collapse
Kerosene	500 mg/kg if swallowed; few ml lethal if aspirated	Severe chemical pneumonitis, coma

TABLE 5-31—*Continued*

Substance	Toxic Doses	Toxic Effects
Lead	30 g/kg (>120 μg/ l blood level)	Gastrointestinal inflammation, liver and kidney damage, encephalopathy in children, paralysis of extremities, death due to encephalopathy or peripheral vascular collapse
Lye, sodium and potassium hydroxide	10 g total dose may be fatal	Laryngeal or glottic edema, perforation of esophagus or stomach, severe diarrhea, shock, death
Mercury salts	5 mg/kg	*Acute* Death due to acute renal failure or peripheral vascular collapse *Chronic* Progressive peripheral neuritis, death due to renal failure
Naphthalene (moth balls)	5 gm/kg	CNS excitement or depression, acute hemolytic anemia, convulsions
Nicotine	>5 mg/kg	CNS stimulation followed by depression; vomiting, diarrhea, dyspnea, death from respiratory paralysis
Oxalic acid	50 mg/kg	Shock due to severe gastroenteritis, hypocalcemia, convulsions, renal damage, coma, death
Parathion/ organophosphorus insecticides	>5 mg/kg	Vomiting, diarrhea, generalized muscle weakness, convulsions, coma, death, all due to inhibition of acetylcholinesterase and accumulation of cholinesterase at myoneural junctions
Phosphorus	>5 mg/kg	Penetrating burns; liver, kidney, and cardiac damage
Quartenary ammonium germicides	5 mg/kg	CNS depression, dyspnea, death due to asphyxia
Rotenone	50 mg/kg	Severe hypoglycemia, tremors, convulsions, respiratory stimulation followed by depression, death from respiratory arrest
Silver salts	3.5 to 35 g total dose	Bloody diarrhea, severe corrosion of the gastrointestinal tract, coma, convulsions, death
Strychnine	>5 mg/kg	Stimulation of spinal cord, tetanic convulsions, death in 1–3 hr (with the face fixed in a grin and the body arched in hyperextension) from anoxia
Thallium salts	5 mg/kg (>50 μg/ l blood level)	Hemorrhagic gastroenteritis, encephalopathy (delirium, convulsions, coma), death
Turpentine	500 mg/kg	Aspiration pneumonitis, vomiting, diarrhea, CNS excitement (delirium), stupor, convulsions, coma, death from respiratory failure

REFERENCES

1. Widmann, FK: Clinical Interpretation of Laboratory Tests, ed 9. FA Davis, Philadelphia, 1983, p 237.
2. *Ibid*, pp 237–238.
3. *Ibid*, p 238.
4. *Ibid*.
5. *Ibid*, pp 238–239.
6. *Ibid*, p 240.
7. *Ibid*, p 452.
8. *Ibid*, p 459.
9. *Ibid*, p 240.
10. *Ibid*, pp 454–459.
11. *Ibid*, pp 451–454.
12. Diagnostics, ed 2. Springhouse Corp, Springhouse, PA, 1986, p 242.
13. Fischbach, F: A Manual of Laboratory Diagnostic Tests, ed 3. JB Lippincott, Philadelphia, 1988, p 276.
14. Widmann, *op cit*, p 453.
15. *Ibid*, pp 454–455.
16. *Ibid*, p 454
17. *Ibid*, pp 241–243.
18. Hillman, RS and Finch, CA: Red Cell Manual, ed 5. FA Davis, Philadelphia, 1985, pp 17–21.
19. Widmann, *op cit*, pp 246–247.
20. *Ibid*, p 249.
21. *Ibid*, pp 251–252.
22. *Ibid*, pp 253–258.
23. Guyton, AC: Textbook of Medical Physiology, ed 6. WB Saunders, Philadelphia, 1981, pp 849–850.
24. *Ibid*, pp 856–857.
25. Widmann, *op cit*, pp 257–258.
26. *Ibid*, pp 258–262, 312–314.
27. *Ibid*, pp 293–295.
28. *Ibid*, pp 295–296.
29. *Ibid*, pp 305–306, 316–317.
30. *Ibid*, pp 299–300.
31. *Ibid*, pp 301–303.
32. *Ibid*, pp 298–299
33. *Ibid*, pp 398–400.
34. *Ibid*, p 400.
35. *Ibid*, pp 400–401, 471–473.
36. *Ibid*, pp 428, 433, 435–438.
37. *Ibid*, pp 460–469.
38. *Ibid*, pp 463–464.
39. *Ibid*, pp 402–406.
40. *Ibid*, pp 426–442.
41. Guyton, *op cit*, pp 931–937, 984.
42. Widmann, *op cit*, pp 429–430, 434.
43. *Ibid*, pp 430–433.
44. *Ibid*, pp 427–428, 438–439.
45. *Ibid*, pp 445–448.
46. *Ibid*, p 422.
47. *Ibid*, pp 409–411, 415–416.
48. *Ibid*, pp 417–418.
49. *Ibid*, pp 422–425.
50. *Ibid*, pp 479–481.
51. *Ibid*, pp 481–482.
52. *Ibid*, pp 449, 451
53. *Ibid*, pp 451, 459.
54. *Ibid*, pp 269–270.

55. *Ibid*, pp 277–278, 281–284.
56. *Ibid*, pp 262–264, 445–448.

BIBLIOGRAPHY

Beare, PG, Rahr, VA and Ronshausen, GA: Nursing Implications of Diagnostic Tests, ed 2. JB Lippincott, Philadelphia, 1985.

Bio-Science Handbook, ed 12. Bio-Science Laboratories, Van Nuys, CA, 1977.

Braunstein, H: Outlines of Pathology. CV Mosby, St Louis, 1982.

Byrne, CJ, Saxton, DF, Pelikan, PK and Nugent, PM: Laboratory Tests: Implications for Nursing Care. Addison-Wesley, Menlo Park, CA, 1986.

Carlson, C and Blackwell, B: Behavioral Concepts and Nursing Interventions, ed 2. JB Lippincott, Philadelphia, 1970.

Garza, D and Becan-McBride, K: Phlebotomy Handbook. Appleton-Century-Crofts, Norwalk, CT, 1984.

Goodman, L and Gilman, AG: Pharmacological Basis of Therapeutics, ed. Macmillan, New York, 1985.

Harvey, AM, Johns, RJ, Owens, AH and Ross, RS: The Principles and Practices of Medicine, ed 19. Appleton-Century-Crofts, New York, 1976.

Kee, JL: Laboratory and Diagnostic Tests with Nursing Implications, ed 2. Appleton & Lange, Norwalk, CT, 1987.

Lamb, JO: Laboratory Tests for Clinical Nursing. Robert J Brady, Bowie, MD, 1984.

Levine, DZ: Care of the Renal Patient. WB Saunders, Philadelphia, 1983.

Luckmann, J and Sorensen, KC: Medical-Surgical Nursing: A Psychophysiologic Approach, ed 3. WB Saunders, Philadelphia, 1987.

Mathewson, M: Pharmacotherapeutics: A Nursing Process Approach. FA Davis, Philadelphia, 1986.

Metheny, NM and Snively WD: Nurse's Handbook of Fluid Balance, ed 4. JB Lippincott, Philadelphia, 1983.

Michaels, D: Diagnostic Procedures: The Patient and the Health Care Team. John Wiley & Sons, New York, 1983.

Pagana, KD and Pagana, TJ: Diagnostic Testing and Nursing Implications: A Case Study Approach, ed 2. CV Mosby, St Louis, 1986.

Pagliaro, A and Pagliaro L: Pharmacologic Aspects of Nursing. CV Mosby, St Louis, 1986.

Pilar, FL: Chemistry: The Universal Science. Addison-Wesley, Reading, MA, 1979.

Stryer, L: Biochemistry. WH Freeman & Company, San Francisco, 1971.

Tilkian, SM, Conover, MB and Tilkian, AS: Clinical Implications of Laboratory Tests, ed 4. CV Mosby, St Louis, 1987.

Wallach, J: Interpretation of Diagnostic Tests: A Handbook Synopsis of Laboratory Medicine, ed 4. Little, Brown & Co, Boston, 1986.

Widmann, FK: Pathobiology: How Disease Happens. Little, Brown & Co, Boston, 1978.

Williams, SR: Nutrition and Diet Therapy, ed 4. CV Mosby, St Louis, 1981.

STUDIES OF URINE

OVERVIEW OF URINE FORMATION AND ANALYSIS

Because urine results from filtration of blood, many of the substances carried in the blood also will be found in the urine. The nature and amount of the substances present in urine reflect on-going physiological processes in health and disease states.

The study of urine was one of the earliest approaches to laboratory diagnosis. Ancient physicians carried out very basic tests of urine by observing characteristics of urine that are still studied today: color, odor, turbidity, volume, and sweetness. Indeed, the sweetness of urine was once determined by the tendency of the sample to attract ants! The advent of the microscope and chemical tests for certain constituents of urine expanded the amount of data that could be obtained from studies of urine. The comparative ease of obtaining urine samples also aided in the continuing use of urine analyses as an aid to diagnosis.[1]

Urine is an ultrafiltrate of plasma from which substances essential to the body are reabsorbed and through which those substances not needed are excreted. Normally, 25 percent of the cardiac output perfuses the kidneys each minute. This results in the production of 180 liters of glomerular filtrate per day, 90 percent of which is reabsorbed. In addition to water, substances reabsorbed

289

include glucose, amino acids, and electrolytes. Substances excreted from the body include urea, uric acid, creatinine, and ammonia. The major electrolytes lost are chloride, sodium, and potassium. Other substances found in urine include pigments, enzymes, hormones and their metabolites, vitamins, minerals, and drugs. Red blood cells, white blood cells, epithelial cells, crystals, mucus, and bacteria also may be found in urine.[2,3]

In general, the concentration of most substances normally found in the urine reflects the plasma levels of the substances. If the plasma concentration of a substance is high, more of it will be lost in the urine, in the presence of normal renal function. Conversely, if the plasma concentration is abnormally low, the substance will be reabsorbed. The concentration of substances found in the urine is affected also by factors such as dietary intake, body metabolism, endocrine function, physical activity, body position, and time of day.[4] For these reasons, results of urine tests must be evaluated in relation to the client's history and current health status. For some studies, urine specimens are collected at certain times of day or over 24-hour periods. Dietary intake also may be modified for certain studies.

Urine samples may be obtained through a variety of methods. These are described in Appendix II. Urine studies include routine urinalysis, clearance tests, tubular function tests, concentration tests, and analyses for specific substances such as electrolytes, pigments, enzymes, hormones and their metabolites, protein, and vitamins and minerals. Microbiological and cytological examination of urine also may be performed.

ROUTINE URINALYSIS (UA)

Background Information (Clinical Applications Data, p. 309)

The routine urinalysis has two major components: (1) macroscopic analysis and (2) microscopic analysis. Macroscopic analysis includes examining the urine for overall physical and chemical characteristics. Physical characteristics for which urine is routinely examined include color, appearance (clarity), odor, specific gravity, and pH. Chemical analyses include tests for protein, glucose, ketones, blood, myoglobin, bilirubin, urobilinogen, nitrate, and leukocyte esterases. The microscopic component of a routine urinalysis involves examining the sample for formed elements such as red and white blood cells, epithelial cells, casts, bacteria, mucus, and crystals. These are also termed "urinary sediment."

Urine samples for routine analysis are best collected first thing in the morning. Urine that has accumulated in the bladder overnight is more concentrated, thus allowing for detection of substances that may not be present in more dilute random samples.[5] The sample should be examined within 1 hour of collection. If this is not possible, the sample may be refrigerated until it can be examined. Failure to observe these precautions may lead to invalid results. If, for example, the sample is allowed to stand for long periods of time without refrigeration, the glucose level may drop and ketones dissipate. The color of the urine also may deepen. Similarly, urinary sediment begins deteriorating within 2 hours of collecting the sample. If bacteria are present, they may multiply if the sample is neither examined promptly nor refrigerated. This also may alter the pH of the sample, rendering it more alkaline. If the sample is exposed to light for long periods of time, bilirubin and urobilinogen may be oxidized.[6]

MACROSCOPIC ANALYSIS

Color

The color of urine is due mainly to the presence of the pigment urochrome, which is produced through endogenous metabolic processes. Because urochrome is normally produced at a fairly constant rate, the intensity of the yellow color may indirectly indicate urine concentration and the client's state of hydration.[7,8] Pale urine with a low specific gravity may occur, for example, in a normal person after high fluid intake. It should be noted, however, that an individual with uncontrolled or untreated diabetes also may produce pale urine. The pale urine, in this case, is caused by osmotic diuresis resulting from the excessive glucose load. The client actually may be dehydrated. Further, the specific gravity of the urine from such an individual could be high owing to the presence of excessive glucose.[9] Similarly, deeper-colored urine may not always indicate concentrated urine. The presence of bilirubin may produce darker urine in normally hydrated individuals.

Urine color may be described as pale yellow, straw, light yellow, yellow, dark yellow, and amber. For the most accurate appraisal of urine color, the sample should be examined in good light against a white background. If the sample is allowed to stand at room temperature for any length of time, the urochrome will increase and the color of the sample may deepen.[10]

Numerous factors affect the color of urine (Table 6–1). Certain abnormal colors occur more frequently than others or are of greater significance. As noted, dark yellow urine may be due to the abnormal presence of bilirubin. If excessive bilirubin is present, a yellow foam will appear when the sample is shaken. Blood is a frequent cause of abnormal urine color, although the actual color produced may range anywhere from pink to brownish-black, depending on the amount of blood, length of the time it has been in the urine, and the pH of the urine. If an acidic urine sample containing blood is allowed to stand at room temperature for several hours, the resulting urine color will be brownish-black because of breakdown of hemoglobin. In contrast, a fresh sample of brownish-black urine with red blood cells may indicate glomerular bleeding. Hemoglobin and myoglobin also may produce red urine; however, the specimen is usually clear rather than cloudy, as usually occurs when red cells are present. Numerous drugs and certain foods (e.g., beets and carrots) may cause abnormally colored urine. For this reason, a thorough medication and diet history is essential in evaluating urine coloration.[11]

Appearance (Clarity)

The term "appearance" generally refers to the clarity of the urine sample. Urine is normally clear or slightly cloudy. In alkaline urine, cloudiness may be due to precipitation of phosphates and carbonates. In acidic urine, cloudiness may be due to precipitation of urates, uric acid, or calcium oxalate. The accumulation of uroerythrin, a pink pigment normally present in urine, may produce a pinkish or reddish haze in acidic urine.

The most common substances that may cause cloudy urine are white blood cells, red blood cells, bacteria, and epithelial cells. Presence of these substances may indicate inflammation or infection of the urinary and genital tracts and must be confirmed through microscopic examination (see p. 302). Other substances that may produce cloudy urine are mucus, yeasts, sperm, prostatic fluid, menstrual and vaginal discharges, fecal material, and external substances such as talcum powder and antiseptics.[12] Proper client instruction and specimen collection may aid in reducing the presence of such substances in the urine.

TABLE 6-1. Factors Affecting the Color of Urine

Urine Color	Cause
Very pale yellow	Excessive fluid intake
	Diabetes mellitus
	Diabetes insipidus
	Nephrotic syndrome
	Alcohol
	Diuretics
	Anxiety
Dark yellow, amber	Underhydration
	Bilirubin
	Urobilin
	Carrots
	Phenacetin
	Cascara
	Nitrofurantoin
	Chlorpromazine
	Quinacrine
	Riboflavin
	Sulfasalazine
Orange	Bilirubin
	Pyridium
	Azo- drugs
	Phenothiazine
	Oral anticoagulants
Red	Red blood cells
	Hemoglobin
	Myoglobin
	Porphyrins
	Porphobilinogen
	Many drugs and dyes
	Rifampin
	Phenolsulfonphthalein
	Fuscin
	Beets
	Rhubarb
	Senna
Green	Biliverdin
	Pseudomonas
	Vitamins
	Psychoactive drugs
	Proprietary diuretics
Blue	Nitrofurans
	Proprietary diuretics
	Methylene blue
Brown	Acid hematin
	Myoglobin
	Bile pigments
	Levodopa
	Nitrofurans
	Some sulfa drugs
	Rhubarb
Black, Brownish-black	Melanin
	Homogentisic acid
	Indicans
	Urobilin
	Red blood cells oxidized to methemoglobin
	Levodopa
	Cascara
	Iron complexes
	Phenols

Lymph and fat globules in urine also may yield cloudy specimens. The presence of lymph in the urine is most often associated with obstruction to abdominal lymph flow and rupture of lymphatic vessels into portions of the urinary tract. Fat globules in the urine are most commonly associated with nephrotic syndrome but also may be seen in clients with fractures of the long bones or pelvis.[13]

Odor

Normally, a fresh urine specimen has a faintly aromatic odor. As the specimen stands, the odor of ammonia will predominate owing to the breakdown of urea. Ingestion of certain foods and drugs will impart characterisic odors to urine; this is especially true of asparagus.

Some unusual odors are indicative of certain disease states. Urine with a fruity odor, for example, may indicate ketonuria due to uncontrolled diabetes mellitus or starvation. Other abnormal odors are associated with amino acid disorders. Urine with a "mousey" smell is associated with phenylketonuria (PKU), whereas urine that smells like maple syrup is associated with maple syrup urine disease. Urine with a "fishy" or fetid odor is generally associated with bacterial infection. This odor is especially noticeable when urine is allowed to stand for a period of time. Occasionally, urine may lack an odor. This is seen in acute renal failure due to acute tubular necrosis (ATN) and failure of normal mechanisms of ammonium secretion.[14,15]

Specific Gravity

The specific gravity of urine is an indication of the kidney's ability to reabsorb water and chemicals from the glomerular filtrate. It also aids in evaluating hydration status and in detecting problems related to secretion of antidiuretic hormone. By definition, specific gravity is the density of a liquid compared with that of a similar volume of distilled water when both solutions are at the same or similar temperatures. The normal specific gravity of distilled water is 1.000. The specific gravity of urine is greater than 1.000, and reflects the density of the substances dissolved in the urine. Both the number of particles present and their size influence the specific gravity of urine. Large urea molecules, for example, will influence the specific gravity more than will small sodium and chloride molecules. Similarly, if large amounts of glucose or protein are present in the sample, the specific gravity will be higher.[16]

The specific gravity of the glomerular filtrate is normally 1.010 as it enters Bowman's capsule. A consistent urinary specific gravity of 1.010 usually indicates damage to the renal tubules such that concentrating ability is lost. Urine with a low specific gravity may be seen in clients with overhydration and diabetes insipidus. Urine with a high specific gravity is associated with dehydration, uncontrolled diabetes mellitus, and nephrosis. High specific gravities also may be seen in clients who are receiving intravenous solutions of dextran or other high molecular weight fluids and in those who have received radiological contrast media.

The specific gravity of urine provides preliminary information. For a more thorough evaluation of renal concentrating ability, urine osmolarity may be determined and concentration tests may be performed (see p. 314).[17]

pH

The pH of urine reflects the kidney's ability to regulate the acid-base balance of the body. In general, when too much acid is present in the body (i.e., respiratory or metabolic acidosis), acidic urine (low pH) will be excreted. Conversely, alkaline urine (high pH) will be excreted in states of respiratory or metabolic alkalosis. Various foods and drugs also will affect urinary pH.

The kidney controls the acid-base balance of the body through regulation of hydrogen ion excretion. Various acids are excreted via the glomerulus along with sodium ions. In the renal tubules, bicarbonate ions are reabsorbed and hydrogen ions secreted in exchange for sodium ions. Additional hydrogen ions are excreted as ammonium.

Disorders involving the renal tubules will affect regulation of pH. In renal tubular acidosis, for example, the ability of the distal tubules to secrete hydrogen ions and form ammonia is impaired. Metabolic acidosis results. Similarly, in proximal tubular acidosis, bicarbonate is wasted.

As noted previously, the acidity or alkalinity of the urine generally reflects that of the body. A paradoxical situation may occur, however, in clients with hypokalemic alkalosis, which may occur with prolonged vomiting or excessive use of diuretics. In this situation, an acidic urine may be produced when hydrogen ions are secreted instead of potassium ions (which are deficient) in order to maintain electrochemical neutrality in the renal tubules.[18]

The pH or urine samples must be evaluated in relation to the client's dietary and drug intake. A diet high in meat and certain fruits such as cranberries will produce acidic urine. A diet high in vegetables and citrus fruits will produce an alkaline urine. Drugs such as ammonium chloride and methamine mandelate will produce an acid urine, while sodium bicarbonate, potassium citrate, and acetazolamide will result in alkaline urine.

The changes in urinary pH that occur in relation to ingestion of certain foods and drugs are applied to the treatment of certain urinary tract disorders. Maintenance of an acidic urine may be used in the treatment of urinary tract infections because urea-splitting organisms do not multiply as rapidly in an acidic environment. These same organisms will cause the pH of a urine specimen to rise if it is allowed to stand for a period of time.[19] Acidic urine also helps to prevent the formation of ammonium magnesium kidney stones, which are more likely to form in alkaline urine. Other types of kidney stones are more likely to be prevented if the urine is alkaline. The induction of alkaline urine also may be used in the treatment of urinary tract infections with drugs such as kanamycin, in sulfonamide therapy, and in the treatment of salicylate poisoning.[20]

Urine is generally less acidic following a meal (the "alkaline tide") because of secretion of acids into the stomach. Urine tends to be more acidic in the morning as a result of the mild respiratory acidosis that normally occurs during sleep.[21] Thus, time of day the sample is collected may influence evaluation of urinary pH.

Protein

Urine normally contains only a scant amount of protein, which derives both from the blood and the urinary tract itself. The proteins normally filtered through the glomerulus include small amounts of low molecular weight serum proteins such as albumin. Most of these filtered proteins are reabsorbed by the proximal renal tubules. The distal renal tubules secrete a protein (Tamm-Horsfall glycoprotein) into the urine. Other normal proteins in urine include microglobulin, immunoglobulin light chains, enzymes and proteins from tubular epithelial cells, leukocytes, and other cells shed by the urinary tract. It is noted that more than 200 urinary proteins have been identified.[22]

Normal protein excretion must be differentiated from that due to disease states. Persons who do not have renal disease may have proteinuria after strenuous exercise or when dehydrated. Functional (nonrenal) proteinuria also may be seen in congestive heart failure, cold exposure, and fever.[23]

Postural (orthostatic) proteinuria also may occur in a small percentage of normal individuals. In this situation, the client spills protein while in an upright posture but not when recumbent. Postural proteinuria is evaluated by having the client collect a urine sample upon first arising and then approximately 2 hours later after having been up and about. The second sample should be positive for protein, the first should be negative. Orthostatic proteinuria is generally a benign condition, although the client should be re-evaluated periodically for persistent, nonpostural proteinuria.

Persistent proteinuria is generally indicative of renal disease or of systemic disorders leading to increased serum levels of low molecular weight proteins. Renal disease resulting in proteinuria may be due to damage to the glomerulus or damage to the renal tubules. When the glomerular membrane is damaged, greater amounts of albumin pass into the glomerular filtrate. If damage is more extensive, large globulin molecules also will be excreted. Nephrotic syndrome is an example of renal disease primarily associated with a glomerular damage. In this disorder there is heavy proteinuria accompanied by decreased serum albumin. In contrast, renal disease due to tubular damage is characterized by loss of proteins that are normally reabsorbed by the tubules (i.e., low molecular weight proteins). An example of renal disease primarily associated with tubular damage is pyelonephritis. The proteinuria that occurs in disorders involving the renal tubules is generally not as profound as that associated with glomerular damage.[24,25]

Systemic disorders that result in excessive production or release of hemoglobin, myoglobin, or immunoglobulins may lead to proteinuria and may, in addition, lead to actual renal disease. Myoglobinemia, for example, which may occur with extensive destruction of muscle fibers, will lead to excretion of myoglobin in the urine and may lead to acute renal tubular necrosis.[26] Multiple myeloma, a neoplastic disorder of plasma cells, is another example of a systemic disorder that may cause proteinuria. In this disorder, the blood contains excessive levels of monoclonal immunoglobulin light chains (Bence Jones protein).[27] This protein overflows through the glomerulus in quantities greater than what the renal tubules can absorb. Thus, large amounts of Bence Jones protein appear in the urine. As with myoglobinuria, the excessive amounts of protein may ultimately damage the kidney itself.

Because proteinuria may indicate serious renal or systemic disease, its detection on routine urinalysis must always be further evaluated for possible cause. Proteinuria occurring in the latter months of pregnancy also must be carefully evaluated, as it may indicate serious complications of pregnancy.

Glucose

Normally, glucose is virtually absent from the urine. Although nearly all glucose passes into the glomerular filtrate, most of it is reabsorbed by the proximal renal tubules through active transport mechanisms. In active transport, carrier molecules attach to molecules of other substances (e.g., glucose) and transport them across cell membranes. Usually there are enough carrier molecules to transport all of the glucose from the renal tubules back to the blood. If plasma glucose levels are very high, however, such that carrier mechanisms are overwhelmed, glucose will appear in the urine. The point at which a substance appears in the urine is called its renal threshold.[28] The renal threshold for glucose ranges from 160 to 200 mg/dl, depending on the individual. That is, the blood sugar must rise to its renal threshold level before glucose will appear in the urine.

The most common cause of glycosuria is uncontrolled diabetes mellitus. Because even a normal person may have elevated blood glucose levels immediately after a meal, urine samples for glucose are best collected immediately prior to meals, when the blood sugar should be at its lowest point. Similarly, urine that has been accumulating in the bladder overnight may contain excessive amounts of glucose resulting from increased concentration of urine and perhaps also from something eaten the previous evening. Because a negative test result for urinary sugar may not necessarily indicate a normal blood sugar level, and because there is a great deal of variation in individual renal thresholds for glucose, recent trends for diabetic control have moved away from urinary glucose monitoring to blood glucose monitoring. Evaluation of glucose in routine urine specimens, however, remains a useful screening technique.

In addition to diabetes mellitus, many other disorders may result in glycosuria. In general, these disorders fall into two general categories: (1) those in which the blood sugar is elevated, and (2) those in which the blood sugar is not elevated, but in which renal tubular absorption of glucose is impaired. Disorders that may lead to elevated blood glucose levels, and thus to glycosuria, are listed in Table 6–2, A. In addition, several drugs are known to elevate the blood sugar enough to produce glycosuria. These also are listed in Table 6–2, A.

When renal tubular reabsorption of glucose is impaired, glucose may appear in the urine without actual hyperglycemia. In disorders involving the renal tubules, glycosuria is one of many abnormal findings. Reabsorption of amino

---

TABLE 6–2, A. Disorders and Drugs That May Result in Glycosuria

Glucosuria With High Blood Sugar	Glycosuria Without High Blood Sugar
Diabetes mellitus	Renal tubular dysfunction
Gestational diabetes	Fanconi's syndrome
Acromegaly	Galactosemia
Cushing's syndrome	Cystinosis
Hyperthyroidism	Lead poisoning
Pheochromocytoma	Multiple myeloma
Advanced cystic fibrosis	Pregnancy (must be distinguished from
Hemachromatosis	gestational diabetes)
Severe chronic pancreatitis	
Carcinoma of the pancreas	
Hypothalamic dysfunction	
Brain tumor or hemorrhage	
Massive metabolic derangement	
Severe burns	
Uremia	
Advanced liver disease	
Sepsis	
Cardiogenic shock	
Glycogen storage disease	
Obesity	
Medication-induced hyperglycemia	
Adrenal corticosteroids	
ACTH	
Thiazides	
Oral contraceptives	
Excessive intravenous glucose	
Dextrothyroxine	

TABLE 6–2, B. Drugs That May Produce False-Positive Glucosuria Results

Ascorbic acid	Paraldehyde
Cephalosporins	Penicillins
Chloral hydrate	Salicylates
Skelaxin	Streptomycin
NegGram	Morphine
Terramycin	Levodopa
PABA	Radiographical contrast media

acids, bicarbonate, phosphate, sodium, and water also may be impaired. Disorders associated with altered renal tubular function and glycosuria are listed in Table 6–2, A. Pregnancy represents a special case in which there may be glycosuria without hyperglycemia. During pregnancy, the glomerular filtration rate is increased such that it may not be possible for the renal tubules to reabsorb all of the glucose presented. Glucose may appear in the urine even though blood glucose levels are within normal limits. This situation must be distinguished from actual diabetes, with elevated blood sugar levels, a serious complication of pregnancy.[29]

Certain drugs are known to produce false-positive results when testing for glucose in urine. This is especially true when copper sulfate reduction testing methods (e.g., Clinitest tablets, Benedict solution) are used. These drugs are listed in Table 6-2, B. Allowing urine specimens to remain at room temperature for long periods of time also may produce false-positive results.

The presence of nonglucose sugars in the urine also may produce false-positive results in tests for glycosuria. These sugars include lactose, fructose, galactose, pentose, and sucrose. Lactose may appear in the urine during normal pregnancy and lactation, in lactase deficiency states, and in certain disorders affecting the intestines (e.g., celiac disease, tropical sprue, and kwashiorkor). Fructose may appear in the urine after parenteral feedings with fructose and in clients with inherited enzyme deficiencies, which are generally benign in nature. Galactose in the urine also is associated with certain inherited enzyme deficiencies. Pentose may appear in the urine after ingestion of excessive amounts of fruits. Similarly, sucrose may be found if large amounts of sucrose are ingested, but also may occur in clients with intestinal disorders associated with sucrase deficiency (e.g., sprue).[30]

Glycosuria may, therefore, indicate a number of pathological states or may result from drug and food ingestion. A thorough history and further evaluation through additional laboratory tests are indicated whenever glycosuria occurs.

Ketones

The term "ketones" refers to three intermediate products of fat metabolism: acetone, acetoacetic acid, and beta-hydroxybutyric acid. Measurable amounts of ketones are not normally present in urine. If there is excessive fat metabolism, however, ketones may be found. Excessive fat metabolism may occur in several situations: (1) impaired ability to metabolize carbohydrates, (2) inadequate carbohydrate intake, (3) excessive carbohydrate loss, and (4) increased metabolic demand.[31] The disorder most commonly associated with impaired ability to metabolize carbohydrates is diabetes mellitus. As carbohydrates cannot be used to meet the body's energy needs, fats are burned, thus leading to the presence of ketones in the urine. A similar situation occurs when carbohydrate intake is inadequate to the body's needs. This is seen in weight-reduction diets and starvation. Excessive loss of carbohydrate (e.g., due to vomiting and diarrhea) and increased metabolic demand (e.g., acute febrile conditions and toxic states, especially in infants and children) also may produce ketonuria. Other disorders in which ketones may be found in the urine include lactic acidosis and salicylate toxicity. Ketonuria also has been found after anesthesia and is believed to be due to both decreased food intake prior to surgery and increased metabolic demand in relation to physiological stressors.

As with glucose, ketones in the urine are associated with elevated blood ketone levels. Because ketone bodies are acids, ketonuria may indicate systemic acidosis. Ketones in urine are measured most frequently in clients with diabetes mellitus and in those on weight-reduction diets. The finding of ketones on routine urinalysis requires further follow-up through history and laboratory tests to determine the source. Individuals receiving levodopa, paraldehyde, pyridium, and phthalein compounds may produce false-positive results when tested for ketonuria.

Blood

Blood may be present in the urine as either red blood cells or hemoglobin. If enough blood is present, the color of the sample may range from pink-tinged to red to brownish-black (see p. 291). Very small amounts of blood, although clinically significant, may not be detected unless the sample is tested with reagent strips ("dipsticks") or microscopic examination (see p. 302). The dipstick approach for macroscopic routine urinalysis provides a useful screening approach. Positive results require further evaluation to determine the nature and source of the blood.[32,33]

The presence of red blood cells in urine (hematuria) is relatively common, whereas the presence of hemoglobin in urine (hemoglobinuria) is seen much less frequently. Hematuria is usually associated with disease of or damage to the genitourinary tract. When hematuria is accompanied by significant proteinuria, kidney disease is generally indicated (e.g., acute glomerulonephritis). In contrast, hematuria with only small amounts of protein is associated with inflammation and bleeding of the lower urinary tract (e.g., cystitis).[34] Other disorders commonly associated with hematuria include pyelonephritis, tumors of the genitourinary tract, kidney stones, lupus nephritis, and trauma to the genitourinary tract. Nonrenal causes of hematuria include bleeding disorders and anticoagulant therapy. Hematuria also may occur in healthy individuals after excessive strenuous exercise, owing to damage to the mucosa of the urinary bladder.[35]

Free hemoglobin is not normally found in the urine. Instead, any hemoglobin that could be presented to the glomerulus combines with haptoglobin. The resultant hemoglobin-haptoglobin complex is too large to pass through the glomerular membrane. If the amount of free hemoglobin exceeds the amount of haptoglobin, however, the hemoglobin will pass through the glomerulus and ultimately be excreted into the urine.[36] Any disorder associated with hemolysis of red blood cells and resultant release of hemoglobin may lead to the appearance of hemoglobin in the urine. Common causes of hemoglobinuria include hemolytic anemias, transfusion reactions, trauma to red blood cells by prosthetic cardiac valves, extensive burns, trauma to muscles and blood vessels, and severe infections. Hemoglobinuria also may occur in healthy individuals and is thought to be due to trauma to small blood vessels.[37]

It should be noted that hemoglobin is broken down in the renal tubular cells into ferritin and hemosiderin. Hemosiderin may, therefore, be found in urine a few days after an episode of acute red cell hemolysis. Hemosiderin also is found in the urine of individuals with hemachromatosis, a disorder of iron metabolism.[38]

Bilirubin and Urobilinogen

If the urine sample for routine urinalysis appears dark, or if the client is experiencing jaundice, the specimen may be tested for the presence of bilirubin and excessive urobilinogen. Both of these substances are bile pigments that result from the breakdown of hemoglobin (Fig. 6–1).

The average life span of red blood cells is 120 days. Old and damaged cells are broken down primarily in the spleen and to some extent in the liver. The breakdown products are iron, protein, and protoporphyrin. The body reuses the iron and protein; the protoporphyrin is converted into bilirubin and released into the circulation, where it combines with albumin. This form of bilirubin is called unconjugated or prehepatic bilirubin. It does not pass into the urine, because the complex is insoluble in water and is too large to pass through the glomerular membrane. When circulating unconjugated bilirubin reaches the liver, it is conjugated with glucuronic acid. The conjugated (posthepatic) bilirubin is normally absorbed into the bile ducts, stored in the gallbladder, and ultimately excreted via the intestine.[39] In the intestine, bilirubin is converted into urobilinogen by bacteria. Approximately half of the urobilinogen is excreted in the stools, where it is converted into urobilin; the remaining half is reabsorbed from the intestine back into the bloodstream. From the bloodstream, urobilinogen is either recirculated to the liver and excreted with bile or excreted via the kidneys. Normally, only a small amount of urobilinogen (i.e., less than 4 mg per 24 hours) is found in the urine.[40]

Bilirubin may be found in the urine in liver disease and is usually found in clients who have biliary tract obstructions. Excessive urobilinogen also may be found in the urine of those with liver disease or hemolytic disorders. Urobilinogen is absent from the urine in disorders that cause complete obstruction of the bile ducts (Table 6–3).

Bilirubinuria may occur in clients with liver disease when the integrity of liver cells is disrupted and conjugated bilirubin leaks into the circulation; this may be seen in hepatitis and cirrhosis. In fact, in these disorders, bilirubin may appear in the urine before the client actually becomes jaundiced. It should be noted that if liver function is impaired such that the liver cannot conjugate bilirubin, excessive bilirubin will not be found in the urine. Similarly, excessive bilirubin is not seen in the urine of clients with hemolytic disorders. In these disorders there is marked destruction of red blood cells with resultant high levels of unconjugated bilirubin. The normally functioning liver is unable to conjugate the excessive load, and while serum levels of unconjugated bilirubin rise, urinary bilirubin excretion remains relatively unchanged. This, again, is due to the kidney's inability to excrete unconjugated bilirubin.

If there is bile duct obstruction, the conjugated bilirubin cannot pass from the biliary tract into the intestine. Instead, excess amounts are absorbed into the bloodstream and excreted via the kidneys. Also, because little or no bilirubin passes into the intestine, where urobilinogen is formed, the urine will be negative for urobilinogen. Absence of urobilinogen in urine is associated with complete obstruction of the common bile duct. When absence of urobilinogen is combined with the presence of blood in the stool, carcinoma involving the head of the pancreas may be indicated.[41]

As noted previously, approximately half the urobilinogen formed in the intestines is reabsorbed into the bloodstream. Normally, most of this urobilinogen is circulated to the liver where it is processed and excreted via bile. A smaller amount is excreted in the urine. When liver cells are damaged, excretion

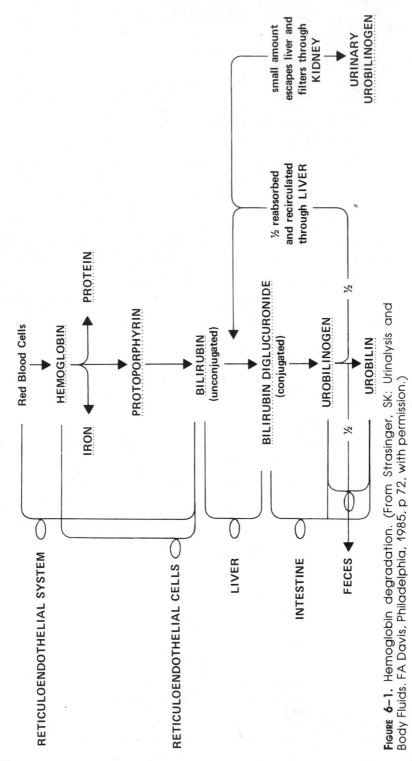

Figure 6-1. Hemoglobin degradation. (From Strasinger, SK: Urinalysis and Body Fluids. FA Davis, Philadelphia, 1985, p 72, with permission.)

TABLE 6-3. Urine Bilirubin and Urobilinogen in Jaundice

	Urine Bilirubin	Urine Urobilinogen
Bile duct obstruction	+++	Negative
Liver damage	+ or −	++
Hemolytic disease	Negative	+++

From Strasinger, SK: Urinalysis and Body Fluids. FA Davis, Philadelphia, 1985, p 73, with permission.

of urobilinogen in bile is decreased, whereas its urinary excretion is increased. This may be seen in clients with cirrhosis, hepatitis, and congestive heart failure with congestion of the liver.

Excessive urobilinogen also appears in the urine in those with hemolytic disorders. As noted, in such disorders the amount of unconjugated bilirubin produced is more than the liver can handle, but the liver attempts to compensate, and increased amounts of urobilinogen are ultimately formed. When this urobilinogen is recirculated back to the liver, however, the liver is unable to process it further and additional amounts are excreted in the urine.

A number of factors may cause spurious results when urine is tested for bilirubin and urobilinogen. Because excessive exposure of a urine sample to light and room air may lead to false-negative results for bilirubin, only fresh urine specimens should be used for this. Large amounts of ascorbic acid and nitrates in the urine also will cause false-negative results. It should also be noted that bilirubin excretion is enhanced in alkalotic states. This also is true of urobilinogen and is due to decreased tubular reabsorption from alkaline urine. Similarly, acidic urine will result in decreased urinary levels of urobilinogen. As noted, urobilinogen is formed by bacterial action in the intestine. Broad-spectrum antibiotics impair this process and result in decreased urobilinogen production. As with bilirubin, high levels of nitrates in the urine also may cause false-negative results in tests for urobilinogen.[42,43]

Nitrite

Testing urine samples for nitrite is a rapid screening method for determining the presence of bacteria in the specimen. This test is based on the fact that nitrate, which is normally present in urine, is converted to nitrite in the presence of bacteria. The test is performed by the dipstick method and, if positive, indicates that clinically significant bacteriuria is present. Positive test results should always be followed by a regular urine culture.

Several factors may interfere with the accuracy of tests for nitrite. First, not all bacteria reduce nitrate to nitrite. Those that do so include the gram-negative bacteria, the organisms most frequently involved in urinary tract infections. Because yeasts and gram-positive bacteria may not convert nitrate to nitrite, the presence of these organisms can cause a false-negative test result.

In order for bacteria to convert nitrate to nitrite, the organisms must be in contact with urinary nitrate for some period of time. Thus, freshly voided random samples or urine that is withdrawn from a Foley catheter may produce false-negative results. The best urine samples for nitrite testing are first morning samples from urine that has been in the bladder overnight. Other causes of false-negative results include inadequate amounts of nitrate in the urine for conver-

n (may occur in individuals who do not eat enough green vegetables), large
amounts of ascorbic acid in the urine, antibiotic therapy, and excessive bacteria
in the urine such that nitrite is further reduced to nitrogen, which is not detected
by the test. False-positive reactions will occur if the container in which the sample is collected is contaminated with gram-negative bacteria.[44,45]

Leukocyte Esterase

Testing urine samples for the presence of leukocyte esterase is a rapid
screening method for determining the presence of certain white blood cells (i.e.,
neutrophils) in the sample and, thus, the possibility of a urinary tract infection.
This test is performed by the dipstick method and is based on the fact that the
esterases present in neutrophils will convert the indoxyl carboxylic acid ester
on the dipstick to indoxyl, which is converted to indigo blue by room air.
Approximately 15 minutes are needed for this reaction to occur if neutrophils
are present. If positive, the test should be followed by a regular urine culture.[46]

Some factors may interfere with the accuracy of tests for leukocyte esterases.
False-positive results may occur if the sample is contaminated with vaginal
secretions.[47] False-negative results may occur if there are high levels of protein
and ascorbic acid in the urine. If the urine contains excessive amounts of yellow
pigment, a positive reaction will be indicated by a change to green instead of
blue.[48]

Microscopic Analysis

The microscopic component of a routine urinalysis involves examining the
sample for formed elements such as red and white blood cells, epithelial cells,
casts, crystals, bacteria, and mucus. Another term used is "urinary sediment."
Microscopic analysis is performed by centrifuging approximately 10 to 15 ml of
urine for about 5 minutes. The resulting sediment is then examined under the
microscope. Microscopic analysis is the most time-consuming component of the
routine urinalysis. It involves both identifying and quantifying the formed elements present.[49]

It should be noted that the Addis count is a variation of the microscopic
urinalysis. For an Addis count, all urine is collected for 12 hours, and then the
nature and quantity of formed elements are determined. This test, which was
once used to follow the progress of acute renal disease, is seldom used today, as
microscopic analysis of a single random sample usually is sufficient.[50]

Red Blood Cells

Red blood cells are too large to pass through the glomerulus; thus, the finding of red blood cells in the urine (hematuria) is considered abnormal. If red
blood cells are present, damage to the glomerular membrane or to the genitourinary tract is indicated. For this test, the number of red blood cells is counted.
The result may indicate the nature and severity of the disorder causing the
hematuria.

Renal and genitourinary disorders associated with the presence of red blood
cells in the urine include glomerulonephritis, lupus nephritis, nephritis associated with drug reactions, tumors of the kidney, kidney stones, infections,
trauma to the kidney, renal vein thrombosis, hydronephrosis, polycystic kidney
disease, acute tubular necrosis (occasionally), and malignant nephrosclerosis
(occasionally).[51]

Red blood cells also may be seen with some nonrenal disorders: acute appendicitis; salpingitis; diverticulitis; tumors involving the colon, rectum, and pelvis; acute systemic febrile and infectious diseases; polyarteritis nodosa; malignant hypertension; and blood dyscrasias. Drugs that may lead to hematuria include salicylates, anticoagulants, sulfonamides, and cyclophosphamide. Strenuous exercise also may cause red blood cells to appear in the urine owing to damage to the mucosa of the bladder.[52] Contamination of the sample with menstrual blood may lead to false-positive results.

White Blood Cells

Normally, only a few white blood cells are found in urine. Increased numbers of leukocytes in the urine generally indicate either renal or genitourinary tract disease. As with red blood cells, white blood cells may enter the urine either through the glomerulus or through damaged genitourinary tissues. In addition, white blood cells may migrate through undamaged tissues to sites of infection or inflammation. Excessive white blood cells in the urine is *pyuria*.[53]

The most frequent cause of pyuria is bacterial infection anywhere in the renal/genitourinary system (e.g., pyelonephritis, cystitis). Noninfectious inflammatory disorders, however, also may lead to pyuria. Such disorders include glomerulonephritis and lupus nephritis. In addition, tumors and renal calculi may cause pyuria because of the resultant inflammatory response.

A higher than normal number of leukocytes may be seen if the sample is contaminated with genital secretions. This is especially true in females. White blood cells disintegrate in dilute, alkaline urine and in samples that are allowed to stand at room temperature for more than 1 to 2 hours.[54]

Epithelial Cells

Epithelial cells found in urine samples derive from three major sources: (1) the linings of the male and female lower urethras and the vagina (squamous epithelial cells), (2) the linings of the renal pelvis, bladder and upper urethra (transitional epithelial cells), and (3) the renal tubules themselves. Because it is normal for old epithelial cells to slough from their respective areas, finding a few epithelial cells in a urine sample is not necessarily abnormal. Large numbers of cells, especially those of renal tubular origin, is considered pathological. When large numbers of renal tubular cells are shed, tubular necrosis is indicated. In addition to acute tubular necrosis (ATN), excessive numbers of tubular epithelial cells may be seen in renal transplant rejection, any ischemic injury to the kidney, glomerulonephritis, pyelonephritis, and damage to the kidney by drugs and toxins.[55]

Renal tubular epithelial cells may contain certain lipids and pigments. Cells that contain lipoproteins, triglycerides, and cholesterol are called *oval fat bodies.* Presence of oval fat bodies occurs in lipid nephrosis and results from lipids leaked through nephrotic glomeruli. Histiocytes are fat-containing cells that are larger than oval fat bodies and that can usually be distinguished from the latter on microscopic examination. Histiocytes may be seen in nephrotic syndrome and in lipid-storage diseases.[56]

Pigments that may be absorbed into renal tubular epithelial cells include hemoglobin that is converted to hemosiderin, melanin, and bilirubin. Hemoglobin and bilirubin have previously been discussed (see pp. 298 to 301). Melanin may be found in tubular epithelial cells in the presence of malignant melanoma that has metastasized to the genitourinary tract.

Finding increased epithelial cells from the lower genitourinary tract is generally not of major clinical significance, with one exception. If excessive numbers of transitional epithelial cells are found in large clumps, or sheets, carcinoma involving any portion of the area from the renal pelvis to the bladder may be indicated.[57]

Casts

Casts are gel-like substances that form in the renal tubules and collecting ducts. They are termed *casts* because they take the shape of the area of the tubule or collecting duct in which they form. Tamm-Horsfall protein, a glycoprotein secreted by the distal renal tubular cells (see p. 294) is the major constituent of casts. This protein forms a framework in which other elements may be trapped (e.g., red and white blood cells, bacteria, fats, urates). Healthy individuals may normally excrete a few casts. This is especially true if there is a low urinary pH, increased protein in the urine, increased excretion of solutes, and decreased rate of urine flow.[58] As noted previously (p. 294), proteinuria may occur after strenuous exercise. This may lead to the formation and excretion of an increased number of casts in healthy individuals. Red blood cells also may be found in casts excreted in response to such exercise. Otherwise, excretion of an excessive number of casts is usually associated with widespread kidney disease that involves the renal tubules.[59]

Casts are classified according to the nature of the substances present in them (Table 6–4). As can be seen in this table, the finding of excessive numbers of casts requires further diagnostic follow-up, as it may indicate serious renal disease.

Crystals

Crystals form in urine owing to the presence of the salts from which they are precipitated. There are numerous types of crystals (Table 6–5), many of which are not of major clinical significance. Also, several factors affect the formation of urinary crystals: (1) pH of the urine, (2) temperature of the urine, and (3) concentration of the substances from which they are formed. Table 6–5 shows the pH of the urine at which the several types of crystals are most likely to be formed. In terms of the temperature of the sample, crystals are most likely to be seen in samples that have stood at room temperature for several hours or have been refrigerated, depending on the type of crystal. The concentration of various substances that lead to the formation of crystals is important in that the greater the concentration, the greater the likelihood of precipitation of the substance into the urine in crystal formation.

In analyzing crystals on microscopic examination, it is important to determine the type of crystal present. The presence of certain crystals may indicate disease states (e.g., liver disease, cystinuria). In addition, drug therapy or use of radiographical dyes may cause precipitation of crystals that may portend renal damage by blocking the tubules.[60]

Other Substances

A number of other substances may be found on microscopic urinalysis: bacteria, yeast, mucus, spermatozoa, and parasites. Bacteria are not normally present but may be seen if urinary tract infection is present or if the sample was contaminated externally. The number of bacteria will increase if the specimen is allowed to stand at room temperature for several hours. Bacteria in the urine are generally not of major significance unless accompanied by excessive numbers of white blood cells, which may indicate an infectious or inflammatory process. Yeast in the urine usually indicates contamination of the sample with vaginal secretions in women with yeast infections such as *Candida albicans*. Yeasts

TABLE 6-4. Summary of Urine Casts

Type	Origin	Clinical Significance
Hyaline	Tubular secretion of Tamm-Horsfall protein	Glomerulonephritis Pyelonephritis Chronic renal disease Congestive heart failure Stress and exercise
Red blood cell	Attachment of red blood cells to Tamm-Horsfall protein matrix	Glomerulonephritis Strenuous exercise Lupus nephritis Subacute bacterial endocarditis Renal infarction Malignant hypertension
White blood cell	Attachment of white blood cells to Tamm-Horsfall protein matrix	Inflammation or infection involving the glomerulus Pyelonephritis Lupus nephritis
Epithelial cell	Tubular cells remaining attached to Tamm-Horsfall protein fibrils	Renal tubular damage
Granular	Disintegration of white cell casts Bacteria Urates Tubular cell lysosomes Protein aggregates	Stasis of urine flow Urinary tract infection Stress and exercise Acute glomerulonephritis Renal transplant rejection Pyelonephritis Lead poisoning
Waxy	Hyaline casts in an advanced stage of development	Stasis of urine flow Renal transplant rejection Renal tubular inflammation and degeneration Chronic renal failure End stage renal disease Nephrotic syndrome
Broad	Formation in collecting ducts (i.e., casts are larger than those formed in the tubules)	Extreme stasis of urine flow Renal failure (severe) Chronic glomerulonephritis
Fatty	Renal tubular cells Oval fat bodies	Nephrotic syndrome
Crystal	Inclusion of urates, calcium oxalate, and sulfonamides in a hyaline cast	Deposition of crystals in the tubules or collecting ducts Sulfonamide therapy Hyperparathyroidism (calcium inclusion)

Adapted from Strasinger, SK: Urinalysis and Body Fluids. FA Davis, Philadelphia, 1985, p 96.

also may be seen in the urine of clients with diabetes. Mucus in urine generally reflects secretions from the genitourinary tract and is usually associated with contamination of the sample with vaginal secretions. Spermatozoa may be found in urine after sexual intercourse or nocturnal emissions. Parasites are frequently of vaginal origin and may indicate vaginitis due to *Trichomonas vaginalis*. A true urinary parasite is *Schistosoma haematobium*. This is seen in the urine of

TABLE 6–5. Major Characteristics and Clinical Significance of Urinary Crystals

Crystal	pH	Color	Clinical Significance	Appearance
Uric Acid	Acid	Yellow-Brown	Gout Leukemias and lymphomas, especially if receiving chemotherapy	
Amorphous urates	Acid	Brick dust or yellow-brown	Not of major clinical significance	
Calcium oxalate	Acid/Neutral (Alkaline)	Colorless (envelopes)	High doses of ascorbic acid Severe chronic renal disease Ethylene glycol toxicity Crohn's disease, hypercalcemia	
Amorphous phosphates	Alkaline Neutral	White-colorless	May be found in urine that has stood at room temperature for several hours	
Calcium phosphate	Alkaline Neutral	Colorless	Not of major clinical significance	
Ammonium biurate	Alkaline	Yellow-brown (thorny apples)	Not of major clinical significance	
Calcium carbonate	Alkaline	Colorless (dumb-bells)	Not of major clinical significance	

Crystal	pH	Color	Comments
Cystine	Acid	Colorless	Cystinuria (inherited metabolic defect that prevents reabsorption of cystine by the proximal tubules)
Cholesterol	Acid	Colorless (Notched Plates)	High serum cholesterol. More likely to be seen in refrigerated specimens
Leucine	Acid/Neutral	Yellow	Severe liver disease
Tyrosine	Acid/Neutral	Colorless-Yellow	Severe liver disease
Sulfonamides	Acid/Neutral	Green	Therapy with sulfonamides
Radiographical dye	Acid	Colorless	Dye excretion
Ampicillin	Acid/Neutral	Colorless	Therapy with ampicillin

Adapted from Strasinger, SK: Urinalysis and Body Fluids. FA Davis, Philadelphia, 1985, pp 100–101.

TABLE 6–6. Laboratory Correlations in Renal Diseases

Disease	Macroscopic Examination	Microscopic Examination	Other Laboratory Findings	Remarks
Acute glomerulonephritis	Macroscopic hematuria Specific gravity ↑ Protein <5 g/day "Smokey" turbidity	RBCs RBC casts Granular casts WBCs	ASO titer ↑ GFR ↓ Sedrate ↑	Microscopic hematuria remains longer than proteinuria
Rapidly progressive (crescentic) glomerulonephritis	Macroscopic hematuria Protein	RBCs WBCs Granular casts	BUN ↑ Creatinine ↑ Fibrin degradation products ↑ GFR ↓	Oliguria
Chronic glomerulonephritis	Macroscopic hematuria Specific gravity 1.010 Protein	RBCs WBCs All types of casts Broad casts	Cryoglobulins ↑ BUN ↑ Creatinine ↑ Serum phosphorus ↑ Serum calcium ↓	Oliguria or anuria Nocturia Anemia
Membranous glomerulonephritis	Blood Protein	RBCs Hyaline casts	Positive ANA Positive HB$_s$Ag	Microscopic hematuria
Membranoproliferative (Mesangioproliferative) glomerulonephritis	Macroscopic hematuria Protein	RBCs RBC casts	BUN ↑ Creatinine ↑ ASO titer ↑ Complement ↓	Hematuria may be microscopic
Focal glomerulonephritis	Blood Protein	RBCs Fat droplets	IgA deposits on membrane	Macroscopic or microscopic hematuria
Minimal change disease	Blood	RBCs Oval fat bodies Fat droplets Hyaline casts Fatty casts	Serum protein ↓ Serum albumin ↓	Hematuria may be absent
Nephrotic syndrome	Protein	Oval fat bodies Fat droplets Generalized casts Waxy casts Fatty casts	Serum lipids ↑ Serum protein ↓ Serum albumin ↓	Heavy proteinuria >5 g/day
Pyelonephritis	Cloudy Protein Nitrite Leukocytes	WBCs WBC casts Bacteria RBCs		Concentrating ability decreased in chronic cases

Adapted from Strasinger, SK: Urinalysis and Body Fluids. FA Davis, Philadelphia, 1985, pp 34–35.

individuals with schistosomiasis, an uncommon disorder in the United States. If pinworms and other intestinal parasites are found, contamination of the sample with fecal material is indicated.[61]

Summary

The routine urinalysis, which consists of macroscopic and microscopic components, yields a great deal of information about the client. All the tests may be performed separately, especially those associated with macroscopic analysis. The most complete picture, however, is obtained by synthesizing the data obtained from all the various tests.

Although a variety of disorders may be indicated by abnormal results on routine urinalysis, the most common disorders indicated are the several types of renal disease. Table 6–6 shows how the results of macroscopic and microscopic analyses are combined to indicate certain types of renal disease. Other types of disorders associated with abnormal urinalysis results are listed in Clinical Applications Data (see further on).

Clinical Applications Data (Background Information, p. 290)

Reference Values

Macroscopic Analysis	
Color	Pale yellow to amber
Appearance	Clear to slightly hazy
Odor	Mildly aromatic
Specific gravity	1.001–1.035 (usual range 1.010–1.025)
pH	4.5–8.0
Protein	Negative
Glucose	Negative
Other sugars	Negative
Ketones	Negative
Blood	Negative
Bilirubin	Negative
Urobilinogen	0.1–1.0 Ehrlich units/dl (1–4 mg/24 hrs)
Nitrite	Negative
Leukocyte esterase	Negative

Microscopic Analysis	
Red blood cells	0–3/high-powered field (HPF)
White blood cells	0–4/HPF
Epithelial cells	Few
Casts	Occasional (hyaline or granular)
Crystals	Occasional (uric acid, urate, phosphate, or calcium oxalate)

Interfering Factors

■ Improper specimen collection such that the sample is contaminated with vaginal secretions or feces
■ Use of collection containers contaminated with bacteria
■ Therapy with medications or ingestion of foods that may alter the color, odor, or pH of the sample
■ Delay in sending unrefrigerated samples to the laboratory within 1 hour of collection, which may lead to
  ☐ Deepening of the color of the sample
  ☐ Increased alkalinity of the sample
  ☐ Increased concentration of glucose, if already present
  ☐ Oxidation of bilirubin, if present, and urobilinogen
  ☐ Deterioration of urinary sediment
  ☐ Multiplication of bacteria, if present
■ Failure to time properly those tests done by dipstick method (e.g., glucose and ketones)

Indications/Purposes for Routine Urinalysis

The routine urinalysis is a screening technique that is an essential component of a complete physical examination, especially when performed upon admission to a health care facility or prior to surgery. It also may be performed when renal or systemic disease is suspected. It should be noted that the components of a routine urinalysis may be performed separately if necessary. This may be done to monitor previously identified conditions. Other indications or purposes for a routine include:

■ Detection of infection involving the urinary tract as indicated by urine with a "fishy" or fetid odor and presence of nitrite, leukocyte esterase, white blood cells, red blood cells (possibly), and bacteria
■ Detection of uncontrolled diabetes mellitus as indicated by the presence of glucose and ketones (seen primarily in insulin-dependent diabetes mellitus), and urine with low specific gravity
■ Detection of gestational diabetes during pregnancy
■ Detection of possible complications of pregnancy as indicated by proteinuria
■ Detection of bleeding within the urinary system, as indicated by positive dipstick test for blood and detection of red blood cells on microscopic examination
■ Detection of various types of renal disease (see Table 6–6, p. 308)
■ Detection of liver disease as indicated by the presence of bilirubin (possibly), excessive urobilinogen, and leucine and/or tyrosine crystals
■ Detection of obstruction within the biliary tree as indicated by presence of bilirubin and absence of urobilinogen
■ Detection of multiple myeloma as indicated by the presence of Bence Jones protein
■ Monitoring the effectiveness of weight reduction diets as indicated by the presence of ketones in the urine
■ Detection of excessive red blood cell hemolysis within the systemic circulation as indicated by the presence of free hemoglobin and elevated urobilinogen levels
■ Detection of extensive injury to muscles as indicated by the presence of myoglobin in the urine.

Nursing Alert

- Improper collection and dispostion of sample for routine urinalysis may lead to spurious results (see "Interfering Factors"). The best samples, in general, are those that are collected first thing in the morning after urine has collected in the bladder overnight. The sample should be received in the laboratory within one hour of collection. If this is not possible, the sample may be refrigerated.
- The time of collection and source of the sample must be noted since this information is important in evaluating the results and in distinguishing normal from abnormal results.
- Since many drugs and foods may alter results, a thorough medication and diet history is necessary for evaluating the data obtained.

Client Preparation

Client Teaching. Explain to the client:

- the purpose of the urinalysis
- that results are most reliable if the specimen is obtained upon arising in the morning, after urine has accumulated overnight in the bladder (exception: serial urine samples for glucose should consist of fresh urine)
- the proper way to collect the sample, if the client is to do this independently (see Appendix II)
- the importance of the sample's being received in the laboratory within 1 hour of collection

Encourage questions and verbalization of concerns appropriate to the client's age and mental status.

Physical Preparation

- Provide the client with the proper specimen container.
- For women, a clean-catch midstream kit should be provided.
- Techniques for collecting samples from children are described in Appendix II.
- For catheterized specimens, a catheterization tray is needed if an indwelling catheter is not already present.

The Procedure

A voided or catheterized sample of approximately 15 ml is collected (see Appendix II).

Aftercare and Nursing Observations

There is no specific aftercare. The nurse should observe the color, clarity, and odor of the sample when it is obtained. Preliminary dipstick tests for glucose, ketones, protein, and blood may be performed by the nurse on separate portions of the sample, if desired.

─────────────── **TESTS OF RENAL FUNCTION** ───────────────

Background Information

Renal function tests are employed to evaluate the excretory, secretory, and osmolar regulation dynamics of the kidney. Broad categories of such tests include (1) clearance tests, (2) tubular function tests, and (3) concentration tests.

CLEARANCE TESTS AND CREATININE CLEARANCE (CLINICAL APPLICATIONS DATA, p. 315)

The term "clearance" refers to the relationship between the renal excretory mechanisms and the circulating blood levels of the materials to be excreted. Clearance reflects the overall efficiency of glomerular functioning.

Substances filtered through the glomerulus are (1) excreted into the urine unaltered by the renal tubules, (2) reabsorbed partially or entirely by the renal tubules, or (3) added to by the renal tubules. For the purpose of clearance tests, substances that pass through the glomerulus and are not altered by the renal tubules are analyzed. The assumption is that all of the substance is cleared from the plasma via the glomerulus and is excreted unchanged into the urine. Substances that may be measured in clearance tests include inulin, urea, para-aminohippuric acid (PAH), and creatinine.[62]

Inulin is an inert sugar that is not metabolized, absorbed, or secreted by the body. To determine renal clearance, inulin must be infused intravenously at a constant rate throughout the testing period. Renal clearance is then calculated by measuring the urinary excretion of inulin in relation to plasma concentration. Because this test involves administration of an exogenous substance, it is not used frequently.[63] *PAH* is similar to inulin in that it also must be administered intravenously for clearance tests.

Urea, an end product of protein metabolism, is formed in the liver and excreted relatively unchanged by the kidneys. Blood urea levels are affected by a variety of factors and, therefore, it is not the ideal substance for renal clearance tests. Blood urea levels may be elevated if shock, trauma, sepsis, or tumors cause increased protein metabolism. A high-protein diet or state of dehydration will also cause elevated blood urea levels. High blood urea levels could result in normal clearance test values even though renal function is depressed.

Creatinine is the ideal substance for determining renal clearance because a fairly constant quantity is produced within the body. As discussed in Chapter 5 (see p. 150), creatinine is the end product of creatine metabolism. Creatine resides almost exclusively in skeletal muscle where it participates in energy-requiring metabolic reactions. In these processes, a small amount of creatine is irreversibly converted to creatinine, which then circulates to the kidneys and is excreted. The amount of creatinine generated in an individual is proportional to the mass of skeletal muscle present and will remain fairly constant unless there is massive muscle damage due to crushing injury or degenerative muscle disease.[64] As muscle mass is usually greater in men than in women, the quantity of creatinine excreted is usually greater in men.

Creatinine clearance is a sensitive indicator of glomerular function because those factors affecting creatinine clearance are primarily due to alterations in renal function. These factors include the number of functioning nephrons, the efficiency with which they function (i.e., if there is decreased functioning of some nephrons, others may function more efficiently to compensate), and the amount of blood entering the nephrons. In general, a 50 percent reduction in functioning nephrons will cause creatinine clearance to be slightly decreased. Loss of two thirds of the nephrons will, however, produce a sharp decrease. It should be noted that creatinine clearance tends to decline with normal aging. Thus, it is important to know the client's age when interpreting test results.[65]

Renal disease is the major cause of reduced creatinine clearance. Other disorders that may result in decreased creatinine clearance include shock, hypovolemia, and exposure to nephrotoxic drugs and chemicals.

The creatinine clearance test is performed by collecting all urine for 24 hours, measuring the creatinine present and calculating clearance according to the basic formula shown further on. As indicated by the formula, it is necessary to determine the dye plasma level of creatinine at some point during the test.

$$C = \frac{UV}{P}$$

where:
 C = creatinine clearance.
 U = amount of creatinine in urine.
 V = volume of urine excreted per 24 hours.
 P = plasma creatinine level.

TUBULAR FUNCTION TESTS AND PSP TEST (CLINICAL APPLICATIONS DATA, p. 316)

Tubular function tests assess the ability of the renal tubules to remove waste products and other substances (e.g., drugs) from the blood and secrete them into the urine. Normal tubular function is dependent on two main factors: (1) adequate renal blood flow and (2) effective tubular function. According to Widmann,[66] while tests of tubular function may provide valuable physiological insight, they provide little diagnostic information in individual clinical situations. More appropriate information may be obtained by measuring blood and urine levels of substances such as glucose and electrolytes, and comparing the results. Elevated serum potassium levels, for example, combined with decreased potassium in the urine indicates impaired tubular secretion of potassium. Failure to excrete an appropriate acidic or alkaline urine in relation to blood pH levels (see p. 294) also indicates disruption of normal tubular secreting mechanisms.

If tubular function tests are to be performed, they are usually carried out by injecting *phenolsulfonphthalein (PSP)* intravenously and then measuring its excretion in serial urine samples. PSP is a dye that binds to albumin in the bloodstream and, therefore, cannot be excreted through the glomerulus. To be excreted, the dye must be secreted by renal tubular cells. In the proximal renal tubules, the dye has greater affinity for the cells lining the tubules than it does for the protein. When it dissociates from the protein, it can be secreted by the tubules.[67] Because it is a dye, PSP imparts a pinkish color to alkaline urine upon excretion. Within 2 hours of injection, 75 percent of the dose is excreted if renal blood flow and tubular function are normal.

Measurement of the dye present is done with a spectrophotometer. Thus, any substances that alter the color of urine (see Table 6–1, p. 292) may also alter test results. The client must be well hydrated so that there is adequate renal perfusion and brisk urine flow. If the urine lacks sufficient alkalinity, substances such as sodium hydroxide may be added to the sample in the laboratory to produce the necessary pH for testing.

After the dye is injected, urine samples are obtained at 15-, 30-, 60-, and

120-minute intervals. As reference values for this test are based on these time intervals, it is critical that the samples be collected exactly on time and that the bladder be completely emptied each time.

Other factors that may alter the results of the PSP test include radiographical dyes and drugs such as salicylates, sulfonamides, and penicillin. These substances compete with the PSP dye for tubular secretion pathways, leading to decreased excretion of PSP and falsely abnormal test results. Similarly, high serum protein levels (e.g., as occur in multiple myeloma) increase PSP binding, leading to decreased PSP excretion. In contrast, increased excretion of PSP dye occurs with severe hypoalbuminemia, excessive albuminuria, or severe liver disease.

It should be noted that the test should not be performed on individuals who have demonstrated a previous allergy to PSP dye.

CONCENTRATION TESTS AND DILUTION TESTS (CLINICAL APPLICATIONS DATA, p. 318)

Concentration tests assess the ability of the renal tubules to appropriately absorb water and essential salts such that the urine is properly concentrated. The glomerular filtrate entering the renal tubules normally has a specific gravity of 1.010. If the renal tubules are damaged such that they cannot effectively reabsorb water and salt, the specific gravity of the excreted urine will remain at 1.010 (see p. 293). Loss of tubular concentrating ability is one of the earliest indicators of renal disease, and may occur before blood levels of urea and creatinine rise. In addition to the various forms of renal disease, other situations in which renal concentrating ability may be impaired include failure to secrete antidiuretic hormone (central diabetes insipidus), lack of renal response to antidiuretic hormone (nephrogenic diabetes insipidus), prolonged overhydration, osmotic diuresis (especially that due to uncontrolled diabetes mellitus), hypokalemia, hypocalcemia, lithium and ethanol use, severe hypoproteinemia, multiple myeloma, amyloidosis, sickle cell disease or trait, and psychogenic polydipsia.

The concentration of urine may be determined by measuring either the *specific gravity* or the *osmolality* of the sample. In some cases, a single early morning specimen will suffice. In other situations, timed tests conducted over 12 to 24 hours may be necessary. Another approach is to measure both the serum and the urine osmolality and to compare the results.

Measuring the osmolality of urine is considered more accurate than determining the specific gravity. As noted previously, both the number and size of particles present influence the specific gravity of urine (see p. 293). In contrast, osmolality is affected only by the number of particles present. Thus, smaller molecules such as sodium and chloride, which are of interest in renal concentration tests, contribute more to urine osmolality measures than they do to specific gravity determinations. In the laboratory, osmolality is reported as milliosmols (mOsm).

Normally, the kidneys can concentrate urine to an osmolality of about 3 to 4 times that of plasma (normal plasma osmolality is 275 to 300 mOsm). If the client is overhydrated, the kidneys will excrete the excess water and produce urine with an osmolality as low as one fourth or less that of plasma.[68] Because factors such as fluid intake, diet (especially protein and salt intake), and exercise influence urine osmolality, it has been difficult to establish exact reference values. The possible range is from 50 to 1400 mOsm, with an average of 850 mOsm. As this is such a wide range, it is considered more reliable to measure serum and urine osmolalities and compare the two in terms of a ratio relationship. The ratio of urine to plasma osmolality after controlled fluid intake, for example, should reach about 3:1.[69]

Timed concentration tests are performed if early morning samples indicate inadequate overnight urine concentrating ability. In the *Fishberg test,* an attempt is made to maximally concentrate urine through fluid restriction. In the standard version of this test, the client consumes no fluid for 24 hours (from breakfast one day to breakfast the next). In the simplified version, fluids are restricted from the evening meal until breakfast the next morning (see Procedure, p. 319).[70] The 24-hour fluid restriction should produce the maximum concentration possible. The 12-hour overnight restriction will increase the concentration to about 75 percent of maximum, partly because of the normal increase in urine concentration that occurs at night.[71]

The *Mosenthal test* also derives from the principle of increased urine concentration at night. In this test, two consecutive 12-hour urine specimens are collected, one from approximately 8 A.M. to 8 P.M. and one from 8 P.M. to 8 A.M. If kidney function is normal, the specific gravity of the night-time collection should be greater than that of the daytime collection.[72]

It should be noted that tests of the kidney's ability to produce *dilute* urine are rarely done. These tests involve overhydrating the client, and then observing for the appearance of dilute urine with low specific gravity and osmolality. The danger is that not all clients can tolerate the fluid load needed to produce the desired results.

Clinical Applications Data

CLEARANCE TESTS AND CREATININE CLEARANCE (BACKROUND INFORMATION, p. 312)

Reference Values

Creatinine Clearance	
Male	85–125 ml/min
	20–26 mg/kg/24 hr
	1.0–2.0 g/24 hr
	0.18–0.23 mmol/kg/24 hr
	8.8–17.6 mmol/24 hr
Female	75–115 ml/min
	14–22 mg/kg/24 hr
	0.8–1.8 g/24 hr
	0.12–0.19 mmol/kg/24 hr
	7.0–15.8 mmol/24 hr

Interfering Factors

■ Incomplete urine collection may yield a falsely lowered value
■ Excessive ketones in urine and presence of substances such as barbiturates, PSP, and Bromsulphalein (BSP) may cause falsely lowered values

Indications/Purposes for Clearance Tests and Creatinine Clearance

■ Determination of the extent of nephron damage in known renal disease (i.e., at least 50 percent of functioning nephrons must be lost before values will be decreased)

■ Monitoring the effectiveness of treatment in renal disease
■ Determination of renal function prior to administering nephrotoxic drugs or drugs that may build up if glomerular filtration is reduced

Client Preparation

Client Teaching. Explain to the Client:

■ the purpose of the test
■ the necessity of collecting all urine for 24 hours
■ how to maintain the sample (e.g., on ice, refrigerated) if being collected at home
■ that a blood sample also will be collected once during the test

Encourage questions and verbalization of any concerns about the test.

Physical Preparation

■ Provide the proper collection container.
■ Provide for proper preservation of the sample.
■ Techniques for collecting a 24-hour sample are described in Appendix II.

The Procedure

Creatinine Clearance. A 24-hour urine sample is collected (see Appendix II). A preservative may be added to the collection container by the laboratory in order to prevent degradation of the creatinine. If this is not available, the urine should be kept on ice or refrigerated throughout the collection period. A blood sample is obtained at some point during the urine collection to determine plasma creatinine level.

Aftercare and Nursing Observations

Special aftercare and nursing observations are not required for this test.

TUBULAR FUNCTION TESTS AND PSP TEST (BACKROUND INFORMATION, p. 313)

Reference Values

PSP Excretion Test	
Adults	15 minutes = 25% of dose excreted
	30 minutes = 50–60% of dose excreted
	60 minutes = 60–70% of dose excreted
	2 hours = 70–80% of dose excreted
Children	5–10% higher than adults at the same time intervals

Interfering Factors

■ Failure to collect the urine samples at the required times (reference values are based on these times)
■ Failure to completely empty the bladder each time a specimen is collected
■ Presence in the urine of any substance that alters the color of urine (see Table 6–1, p. 292), as results are based on dye excretion
■ Inadequately hydrated client such that the kidneys are inadequately perfused or there is decreased urine flow

■ Presence in the blood of radiographical dye, salicylates, sulfonamides, and penicillin that may lead to decreased excretion of the dye
■ High serum protein levels, which may lead to decreased excretion of the dye
■ Severe hypoalbuminemia, excessive albuminuria, or severe liver disease, which may lead to increased excretion of the dye

Indications/Purposes for Tubular Function Tests and PSP Test

■ Assessment of renal blood flow and tubular secreting ability (the PSP test is of limited clinical usefulness)

Nursing Alert

■ The PSP excretion test should not be performed on clients who have demonstrated previous allergy to the dye.

Client Preparation (PSP Excretion Test)

Client Teaching. Explain to the client:

■ the purpose of the test
■ the importance of increased fluid intake prior to the test
■ that foods and drugs that impart color to the urine (e.g., carrots, beets, rhubarb, azo- drugs) should be avoided for 24 hours prior to the test
■ that a dye that circulates through the blood and then is excreted by the kidneys will be injected intravenously
■ that four urine specimens will be obtained at timed intervals (i.e., 15 minutes, 30 minutes, 1 hour, and 2 hours) after injection of the dye
■ the importance of completely emptying the bladder each time a urine sample is obtained

Encourage questions and verbalization of any concerns about the test.

Physical Preparation

■ Ensure to the extent possible that dietary and medication restrictions are followed.
■ Provide sufficient fluids to promote adequate hydration.
■ Obtain four containers for the urine samples.

The Procedure

PSP Excretion Test. PSP dye is injected intravenously, after which a pressure dressing is applied to the injection site. Urine samples are then collected at 15-minute, 30-minute, 1-hour, and 2-hour intervals. Each specimen should consist of at least 50 ml. If the client cannot void at the required time, a Foley catheter may be inserted and the specimen obtained. The catheter is then clamped until the next specimen is due.

Aftercare and Nursing Observations

Any foods and medications withheld for the test should be resumed. The dye injection site should be observed for inflammation and hematoma formation. The client should be observed for signs of allergic response to the drug. If a Foley catheter was inserted for the test, it is removed and the client's postremoval voiding pattern monitored.

CONCENTRATION TESTS AND DILUTION TESTS (BACKGROUND INFORMATION, p. 314)

Reference Values

Concentration Tests

Specific gravity	1.001–1.035 (usual range 1.010–1.025)
Osmolality	50–1400 mOsm (usual range 300–900 mOsm; average 850 mOsm)
Ratio of urine to serum osmolality	1.2:1 to 3:1
Fishberg test (standard)	Specific gravity 1.026 or higher on at least one sample
Fishberg test (simplified)	Specific gravity 1.022 or higher on at least one sample
Mosenthal test	Specific gravity 1.020 or higher with at least a seven-point difference between the specific gravities of the daytime and night-time samples

---

Dilution Tests

Specific gravity <1.003
or
Osmolality <100 mOsm

Interfering Factors

Concentration Tests

■ Failure of the client to follow the fluid restrictions necessary for the Fishberg test
■ Ingestion of a diet with an excessive or inadequate amount of protein or sodium or both
■ Presence of disorders that alter serum protein or sodium levels

Dilution Tests

■ Inability of the client to ingest the required fluids for the test
■ Inability of the client to tolerate the fluid load required for the test

Indications/Purposes for Concentration Tests and Dilution Tests

Concentration Tests

■ Early detection of renal tubular damage (i.e., before serum levels of urea and creatinine are elevated) as indicated by loss of tubular concentrating ability
■ Detection of disorders that impair renal concentrating ability (e.g., diabetes insipidus)

■ Differentiation of psychogenic polydipsia from organic disease as indicated by a normal response to timed concentration tests (e.g., Fishberg test)
■ Detection of excessive or prolonged overhydration

Dilution Tests

■ Evaluation of renal tubular response to high fluid volume as indicated by production of urine with low specific gravity and osmolality

---

Nursing Alert

■ Dilution tests should not be performed on clients who may have difficulty tolerating an increased fluid load (e.g., clients with congestive heart failure).

Client Preparation

Specific Gravity and Urine Osmolality. There is no specific preparation other than reviewing with the client when the specimen is to be obtained (e.g., first voided morning urine) and providing a collection container.

Fishberg Test (Standard Version)
Client Teaching. Explain to the client:

■ the purpose of the test
■ that no fluids are to be taken from after breakfast one morning until the test is completed the next morning
■ that solid (dry) foods are not restricted
■ that client should completely empty the bladder at approximately 10 P.M., before retiring for the night
■ that client should remain in bed during the night (i.e., during the usual hours of sleep)
■ that a urine specimen will be obtained at 8 A.M., after 24 hours without fluids
■ that client should return to bed for 1 hour after the first specimen is collected
■ that a second specimen will be collected at 9 A.M.
■ that client should resume normal acitivty for 1 hour after the second specimen is collected
■ that a third specimen will be collected at 10 A.M.

Encourage questions and verbalization of concerns appropriate to the client's age and mental status.

Physical Preparation

■ Ensure to the extent possible that fluid restrictions are followed.
■ Provide the proper specimen containers.

Fishberg Test (Simplified Version)
Client Teaching. Explain to the client:

■ the purpose of the test
■ that no fluids should be taken from the time of the evening meal until the test is completed
■ that client should completely empty the bladder at approximately 10 P.M. before retiring for the night
■ that urine samples will be collected at 7 A.M., 8 A.M., and 9 A.M. after approximately 12 hours without fluids

Note: Some laboratories require that the evening meal consist of a high-protein, low-salt diet with no more than 200 ml fluid. If this is the case, the client should be so informed.

Physical Preparation

■ Ensure to the extent possible that fluid restrictions are followed.
■ Provide the proper specimen containers.

Mosenthal Test
Client Teaching. Explain to the client:

■ the purpose of the test
■ that two consecutive 12-hour urine collections will be obtained—one from 8 A.M. to 8 P.M. in one container and one from 8 P.M. to 8 A.M. in another container
■ the importance of collecting all urine voided during the time period
■ that there are no diet or fluid restrictions

Encourage questions and verbalization of concerns appropriate to the client's age and mental status.

Physical Preparation
Provide the proper specimen containers.

Dilution Tests
Client Teaching. Explain to the client:

■ the purpose of the test
■ that it will be necessary to drink approximately 3 pints (1500 ml) of water in a half-hour period
■ that hourly urine specimens will be obtained for 4 hours after ingestion of the water
■ that any symptoms of fluid excess (e.g., palpitations, shortness of breath) should be reported immediately

Encourage questions and verbalization of concerns appropriate to the client's age and mental status.

Physical Preparation

■ Ensure to the extent possible that the client consumes or receives the required fluids.
■ Provide the proper specimen containers.

The Procedure

Specific Gravity and Urine Osmolality. A random urine specimen of at least 15 ml is collected, preferably first thing in the morning.

Fishberg Test (Standard Version). The client eats his or her usual breakfast, after which no further fluids are ingested until the test is completed the next morning. Solid (dry) foods are allowed. The client voids at approximately 10 P.M., or before retiring for the night. Urine specimens are collected at 8 A.M., 9 A.M., and 10 A.M. the next morning. The client is to remain in bed between the 8 and 9 A.M. specimens, and to resume normal activities between the 9 and 10 A.M. specimens.

Fishberg Test (Simplified Version). The client eats his or her evening meal, after which no fluids are ingested until the test is completed the next morning. Some laboratories require that the evening meal consist of a high-protein, low-salt diet with no more than 200 ml of fluid. The client voids at approximately

10 P.M. or before retiring for the night. Urine samples are collected at 7 A.M., 8 A.M., and 9 A.M. the next morning.

Mosenthal Test. Two separate but consecutive 12-hour urine collections are obtained, one from 8 A.M. to 8 P.M. and one from 8 P.M. to 8 A.M. the next day.

Dilution Tests. These tests, although rarely done, may be performed upon completion of the Fishberg Tests. The client ingests 1500 ml of water over a half-hour period. An alternative approach is to administer intravenous fluids, with the type and amount determined by the physician ordering the test. Urine samples are collected every hour for 4 hours after ingestion or administration of the fluid.

Aftercare and Nursing Observations

Specific Gravity and Urine Osmolality. Special aftercare and nursing observations are not required.

Fishberg Tests. Resume normal fluid intake and diet.

Mosenthal Test. Special aftercare and nursing observations are not required.

Dilution Tests. The client's response to the fluid load must be carefully monitored. Note especially increased pulse rate or difficulty breathing.

MEASUREMENT OF OTHER SUBSTANCES

Background Information

A variety of substances may be measured in urine in order to detect alterations in physiological function. Among these are electrolytes, pigments, enzymes, hormones and their metabolites, proteins and their metabolites, vitamins, and minerals.

ELECTROLYTES (CLINICAL APPLICATION DATA, p. 333)

One of the major functions of the kidney is the regulation of electrolyte balance. Electrolytes are filtered through the glomerulus and reabsorbed in the renal tubules. Those electrolytes most commonly measured in urine are sodium, chloride, potassium, calcium, phosphorus, and magnesium. Tests for electrolytes in urine usually involve 24-hour urine collections. Serum determinations of electrolyte levels are, therefore, preferred to the more cumbersome urinary determinations (see Chapter 5). An exception is magnesium, which indicates deficiency earlier than does serum assay.

Sodium. Most of the sodium filtered through the glomerulus is reabsorbed in the proximal renal tubule. Additional amounts may be reabsorbed in the distal tubule under the influence of aldosterone, a hormone (mineralocorticoid) released by the adrenal cortex. Aldosterone is released in response to decreased serum sodium, decreased blood volume, and increased serum potassium. Enhanced sodium reabsorption is reflected in decreased amounts being excreted in the urine. This may be seen in situations such as hyperaldosteronism, hemorrhage, shock, congestive heart failure with inadequate renal perfusion, and therapy with adrenal corticosteroids. Increased loss of sodium into the urine is associated with excessive salt intake, diuretic therapy, diabetic ketoacidosis, adrenocortical hypofunction, toxemia of pregnancy, hypokalemia, and excessive licorice ingestion. Renal failure may cause either retention or loss of sodium. In acute renal disease involving the renal tubules (e.g., ATN) there may be excessive loss of sodium into the urine, as the tubules are too impaired to reabsorb sodium normally.

Chlorides. Chlorides are generally reabsorbed passively along with sodium. The kidney may also secrete either chloride or bicarbonate, depending on the acid-base balance of the body. Chloride excretion is directly influenced by chloride intake. It is also influenced by factors that affect sodium excretion. Chloride excretion may be impaired in certain types of renal disease.[73]

Potassium. Like sodium, potassium is filtered through the glomerulus and reabsorbed through the tubules. Adequate excretion of potassium from the body also requires that the distal tubules and collecting ducts secrete potassium into the urine. Aldsoterone also influences potassium excretion in that potassium is excreted in exchange for the sodium that is reabsorbed. Urinary excretion also varies in relation to dietary intake. Causes of excessive potassium loss in the urine include diabetic ketoacidosis, therapy with diuretics, and consumption of large amounts of licorice. The most common cause of decreased potassium in the urine is chronic renal failure, in which tubular secretory activity is impaired.

Calcium. Calcium is the most abundant cation in the body, with bone its major reservoir. Only a small amount of calcium circulates in the blood, and most calcium excretion takes place via the stools. Serum calcium levels are largely regulated by the parathyroid glands and vitamin D. Urinary calcium excretion varies directly with the serum calcium level. If blood levels are high, more calcium is excreted. Blood levels of calcium vary with dietary intake, although they are more influenced by increased intake than by decreased intake. Calcium excretion is highest just after a meal and lowest at night.[74] Although many disorders may alter calcium excretion, determination of urinary calcium is done primarily to evaluate individuals with kidney stones or with suspected parathyroid disorders.

Seventy-five percent of all kidney stones contain calcium compounds. Contrary to popular belief, the most common cause of calcium-containing kidney stones is not excessive calcium intake. The hypercalcemia and increased calcium excretion associated with calcium kidney stones are due to lack of appropriate renal tubular reabsorption of calcium, increased calcium reabsorption in the intestines, loss of calcium from bone, and/or low serum phosphorus levels. A variety of disorders can cause these basic defects,[75] among them hyperparathyroidism; sarcoidosis; renal tubular acidosis; cancers of the lung, breast, and bone; multiple myeloma; and metastatic cancer. Drugs that may lead to excessive calcium excretion include toxic doses of vitamin D, adrenal corticosteroids, and calcitonin.

Decreased calcium in the urine is related to hypoparathyroidism, nephrosis, acute nephritis, chronic renal failure, osteomalacia, steatorrhea, and vitamin D deficiency. Drugs associated with decreased calcium in the urine are thiazides and viomycin.

As noted, a 24-hour urine collection is done to determine the quantity of calcium lost in the urine. Sulkowitch's test, a qualitative measure, may be used to determine the presence of calcium in random urine specimens. If necessary, clients may be taught to perform this test at home.

Phosphorus. As with calcium, serum contains relatively small amounts of phosphorus, with bone serving as the major reservoir. Phosphorus levels also are regulated by the parathyroid glands and vitamin D, with excretion controlled primarily by the kidneys. Causes of increased loss of phosphorus in the urine include hyperparathyroidism and renal tubular acidosis. Causes of decreased loss in the urine are hypoparathyroidism, nephrosis, nephritis, and chronic renal failure. Toxic doses of vitamin D may also result in decreased urinary excretion of phosphorus. Dietary intake of phosphates also influences urinary excretion.

Magnesium. Magnesium is an essential nutrient found in bone, muscle, and red blood cells. Relatively little is found in the serum. Magnesium participates in the control of serum electrolyte levels and increases intestinal absorption of calcium. Signs and symptoms of magnesium imbalance are manifested primarily in the central nervous and neuromuscular systems. Urinary measures of magnesium may be used instead of serum measures because changes in magnesium levels are reflected more quickly in the urine than in the blood and may facilitate prompt diagnosis of the client's problem. Causes of increased magnesium excretion include alcoholism, adrenocortical insufficiency, renal insufficiency, hypothyroidism, hyperparathyroidism, and excessive ingestion of magnesium-containing antacids. Thiazide diuretics and ethacrynic acid also may produce excessive urinary excretion of magnesium. Decreased urinary excretion is associated with malabsorption syndromes, dehydration, hyperaldosteronism, diabetic acidosis, pancreatitis, and advanced chronic renal disease. Increased calcium intake also will result in decreased urinary excretion of magnesium.

PIGMENTS (CLINICAL APPLICATIONS DATA, p. 334)

Pigments that may be found in urine consist primarily of those substances involved in the synthesis and breakdown of hemoglobin. These consist of hemoglobin, hemosiderin, bilirubin, urobilinogen, and porphyrins. Myoglobin, which is related to hemoglobin but found primarily in skeletal muscle, is another type of pigment, as is melanin, which is found in hair and skin. With the exceptions of urobilinogen and the porphyrins, these substances are not normally found in urine.

Hemoglobin, hemosiderin, bilirubin, and urobilinogen were previously discussed (see pp. 298 to 301). Myoglobin is discussed on page 295. Its presence is associated with extensive damage to skeletal muscles. Melanin, which may be incorporated into tubular epithelial cells, is seen in malignant melanoma (see p. 295). The focus of this section, therefore, is on the porphyrins.

Porphyrins. Porphyrins are produced during the synthesis of heme (Fig. 6–2). If heme synthesis is deranged, these precursors accumulate and are excreted in the urine in excessive amounts. Conditions producing increased levels of heme precursors are called *porphyrias.* The two main categories of genetically determined porphyrias are erythropoietic porphyrias, in which major diagnostic abnormalities occur in red cell chemistry, and hepatic porphyrias, in which heme precursors are found in urine and feces. Erythropoietic and hepatic porphyrias are very rare. Acquired porphyrias are characterized by greater accumulation of precursors in urine and feces than in red blood cells. Lead poisoning is the most common cause of acquired porphyria.

Those prophyrins for which urine may be tested include aminolevulinic acid (ALA), porphobilinogen (PBG), uroporphyrin, and coproporphyrin. Knowing the type of porphyrin excreted in excess aids in diagnosing specific disorders. Tests for porphyrins usually involve collection of 24-hour urine samples to determine the quantity of the specific substance present. Screening tests on random specimens to determine the presence of excessive amounts of porphyrins (i.e., qualitative studies) also are available.

The presence of ALA in the urine is associated with lead poisoning. It is also found in liver disease (e.g., hepatic carcinoma and hepatitis) and in acute intermittent and varigate porphyria. PBG is found in the same disorders and also may be seen in clients taking griseofulvin. Rifampin, elevated urobilinogen, and light exposure may falsely elevate values. Uroporphyrin and coproporphyrin

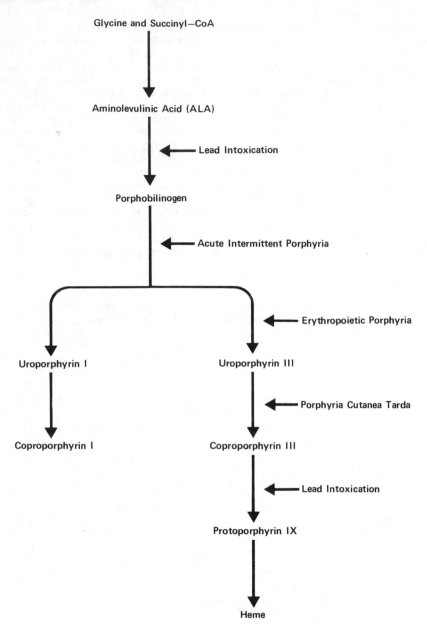

FIGURE 6–2. Pathway of heme formation, including stages affected by the major disorders of porphyrin metabolism. (From Strasinger, SK: Urinalysis and Body Fluids. FA Davis, Philadelphia, 1985, p. 125, with permission.)

also are seen in clients having lead poisoning and liver disease, as well as in those with uroporphyria and porphyria cutanea tarda. Uroporphyrin may be found in hemochromatosis, a disorder of iron metabolism that affects the liver and certain other body organs. Coproporphyrin is associated with obstructive jaundice and exposure to toxic chemicals.

It should be noted that porphyrins are reddish fluorescent compounds.

Depending on the type of porphyrin present, therefore, the urine may be reddish or the color of port wine (see Table 6–1, p. 292). The presence of congenital porphyria may be suspected when an infant's wet diapers show a red discoloration. PBG is excreted as a colorless compound. If a sample containing PBG is acidic and is exposed to air for several hours, however, a color change may occur.[76]

ENZYMES (CLINICAL APPLICATIONS DATA, p. 336)

As noted in Chapter 5, enzymes are catalysts that enhance reactions without directly participating in them. Enzymes are normally intracellular molecules. When the cells and tissues in which they are found are damaged, enzymes are released. Increased levels will be found in the blood and the urine. Because some enzymes are specific to only certain tissues, elevated levels may aid in pinpointing the source of pathophysiological problems.

Although many enzymes may be measured in blood, only a few are analyzed in urine, including amylase, arylsulfatase A (ARS-A), lysozyme (muramidase), and leucine aminopeptidase (LAP). All studies of urinary enzymes involve the collection of 24-hour urine samples, with the exception of amylase, which may be evaluated in timed-specimens over shorter periods of time (e.g., 1 or 2 hours).

Amylase. Amylase is a digestive enzyme that splits starch into disaccharides such as maltose. Although many cells have amylase activity, amylase circulating in serum (and ultimately excreted in the urine) derives from the parotid glands and the pancreas. Unlike many other enzymes, amylase activity is primarily extracellular; it is secreted into saliva and the duodenum where it splits large carbohydrate molecules into smaller units for further digestive action by intestinal enzymes.

Urinary amylase levels are elevated when there is inflammation involving the pancreas or the parotid glands, and generally parallel the levels found in blood. There is, however, a lag time between when blood and urinary levels rise. In acute pancreatitis, for example, urinary levels may not rise for 6 to 10 hours after serum levels rise. Elevated urine levels also return to normal more slowly than blood levels. Whereas blood levels may return to normal 2 to 3 days after an attack of acute pancreatitis, elevated urine levels may persist for 7 to 10 days.[77] This difference between blood and urinary levels of amylase aids in diagnosing and monitoring disorders associated with elevated amylase levels. An individual with signs and symptoms of pancreatitis who did not seek immediate treatment, for example, may show normal serum amylase levels. If the urine is analyzed, however, the elevation may be detected. Similarly, the client's response to treatment may be monitored through urinary amylase levels.

The highest elevations in urinary amylase are seen in acute pancreatitis. Other disorders associated with elevated urinary amylase levels include pancreatic pseudocyst, obstruction of the pancreatic duct (e.g., with gallstones, by tumor), and perforated peptic ulcer. Elevations also may be seen in salivary gland inflammation.

Numerous drugs may cause false elevations in blood and urinary amylase levels. These include morphine, codeine, meperidine, pentazocine, chlorthiazides, aspirin, corticosteroids, oral contraceptives, alcohol, indomethacin, urecholine, secretin, and pancreozymin.

Arylsulfatase A (ARS-A). ARS-A is a lysosomal enzyme found in all body cells except mature red blood cells. Its main sites of activity are in the liver, pancreas, and kidney. Elevated levels are associated with cancers involving the bladder, colon, and rectum. Increases may be seen also in clients having granulocytic leukemia or one of the genetic lysosomal disorders (lipid storage diseases), mucolipidoses II and III. Decreased values are seen in metachromatic leukodystrophy. Levels may be falsely elevated if the client has had recent (i.e., within 1 week) abdominal surgery and if there is mucus, blood, or feces in the sample.

Lysozyme (Muramidase). Lysozyme is a bacteriocidal enzyme present in tears, saliva, mucus, and phagocytic cells. Lysozyme is produced in granulocytes and monocytes, and destruction of such cells (as occurs in granulocytic and monocytic leukemias) will produce elevated urinary levels. In addition, lysozyme is found in renal tissue. Thus, various renal diseases and renal transplant rejection also will lead to elevated levels. It should be noted that bacteria in the sample will falsely lower lysozyme levels, whereas blood or saliva in the specimen will falsely elevate the levels.[78]

Leucine Aminopeptidase (LAP). LAP is an isoenzyme of alkaline phosphatase, an enzyme that cleaves phosphate from compounds and is optimally active at a pH of 9. Although widely distributed in body tissues, LAP is most abundant in hepatobiliary tissues, the pancreas, and the small intestine. Elevated levels are associated with liver disease (cirrhosis, hepatitis, cancer involving the liver), pancreatic disease (pancreatitis, cancer of the pancreas), and biliary obstruction due to gallstones, strictures, and atresia. As with amylase, urinary elevations of LAP lag behind serum elevations. Advanced pregnancy and therapy with drugs containing estrogens and progesterone may falsely elevate LAP levels.

HORMONES AND THEIR METABOLITES (CLINICAL APPLICATIONS DATA, p. 339)

Hormones are chemicals that control the activities of responsive tissues. Some hormones exert their effects in the vicinity of their release; others are released into the extracellular fluids of the body and affect distant tissues. Numerous hormones may be measured in blood (see Chapter 5). Most urinary measures focus on the hormones secreted by the adrenal cortex, the adrenal medulla, the gonads, and the placenta. Either the hormone itself or the metabolites thereof may be measured.

Urinary measures of hormones and their metabolites usually involve collection of 24-hour urine specimens. The advantage of such quantitative measures over single blood level determinations is that overall levels of hormone secretion are reflected. This is important because blood levels of hormones tend to vary depending on time of day.

Cortisol. The adrenal cortex secretes three types of steroids: (1) glucocorticoids, which affect carbohydrate metabolism; (2) mineralocorticoids, which promote potassium excretion and sodium retention by the kidneys; and (3) adrenal androgens, which the liver converts primarily to testosterone. Cortisol is the predominant glucocorticoid. It is produced and secreted in response to adrenocorticotropin (ACTH), which is secreted by the adenohypophysis. Ninety percent of cortisol is bound to cortisol-binding globulin (CBG) and albumin. The "free" (unbound) portion is responsible for its physiological activity and also is the portion excreted into the urine. Cortisol stimulates gluconeogenesis, mobilizes fats and proteins, antagonizes insulin, and suppresses inflammation.

The purpose of urinary measures of cortisol is to detect elevated levels of free cortisol, which may not be apparent in random blood samples. Elevated cortisol levels occur in Cushing's syndrome, in which there is excessive production of adrenal corticosteroids. Cushing's syndrome may be due to pituitary adenoma, adrenal hyperplasia, benign or malignant adrenal tumors, and nonendocrine malignant tumors that secrete ectopic ACTH. Therapy with adrenal corticosteroids also may produce cushingoid signs and symptoms. Elevated cortisol levels are additionally associated with stress, hyperthyroidism, obesity, diabetic ketoacidosis, pregnancy, and excessive exercise. Other drugs that may elevate cortisol levels include estrogens, oral contraceptives, lithium carbonate, methadone, alcohol, phenothiazines, amphetamines, morphine, and reserpine.

Aldosterone. Aldosterone, the predominant mineralocorticoid, is secreted by the zona glomerulosa of the adrenal cortex in response to decreased serum sodium, decreased blood volume, and increased serum potassium. Aldosterone is released in response to direct stimulation by altered serum sodium and potassium levels. In addition, decreased blood volume and altered sodium and potassium levels stimulate the juxtaglomerular apparatus of the kidney to secrete renin. Renin is subsequently converted to angiotensin II, which then stimulates the adrenal cortex to secrete aldosterone. In normal states, adrenocorticotropic hormone (ACTH) does not play a major role in aldosterone secretion. In disease states, however, ACTH also may enhance aldosterone secretion.

Aldosterone increases sodium reabsorption in the renal tubules, gastrointestinal tract, salivary glands, and sweat glands. This subsequently results in increased water retention, blood volume, and blood pressure. Aldosterone also increases potassium excretion by the kidneys in exchange for the sodium ions that are retained.

Excessive aldosterone levels are categorized as primary and secondary hyperaldosteronism. Primary hyperaldosteronism represents inappropriate aldosterone secretion, which is usually due to benign adenomas or bilateral hyperplasia of the aldosterone-secreting zona glomerulosa cells. In primary aldosteronism, aldosterone is secreted independently of the renin-angiotensin system. A hallmark of primary aldosteronism is low plasma renin levels.

Secondary hyperaldosteronism indicates an appropriate response to pathological changes in blood volume and electrolytes. Common causes of secondary hyperaldosteronism include congestive heart failure, cirrhosis, nephrotic syndrome, chronic obstructive pulmonary disease, and renal artery stenosis. Other causes of elevated aldosterone levels are stress, excessive exercise, pregnancy, and several drugs (diuretics, apresoline, diazoxide, and nitroprusside). In secondary hyperaldosteronism, plasma renin levels are elevated.

Decreased aldosterone levels are associated with Addison's disease, hypernatremia, hypokalemia, diabetes mellitus, toxemia of pregnancy, excessive licorice ingestion, and certain drugs (propranolol and fludrocortisone).

17-Hydroxycorticosteroids (17-OHCS). All glucocorticoids are degraded by the liver to metabolites, which as a group are called 17-hydroxycorticosteroids (17-OHCS). These steroid metabolites also are called Porter-Silber chromogens because of the method used to measure them in urine. Because 80 percent of urinary 17-OHCS are metabolites of cortisol, those disorders that are associated with elevated cortisol levels also are associated with elevated 17-OHCS (e.g., Cushing's syndrome). Decreased levels of 17-OHCS are associated with Addison's disease, hypopituitarism and myxedema. As with cortisol, numerous drugs may alter urinary excretion of 17-OHCS. Thus, a thorough medication history is necessary. Some medications may be held prior to and during the test.

When adrenocortical hypofunctioning or hyperfunctioning is suspected, 17-OHCS may be measured in urine as part of the diagnostic process. It should be noted, however, that measurement of urinary cortisol levels will provide more accurate quantification than will 17-OHCS levels in individuals receiving drugs that alter hepatic metabolism of steroids.

17-Ketosteroids (17-KS). 17-Ketosteroids (17-KS) are metabolized from androgenic hormones. In males, two thirds of 17-KS originate in the adrenal cortex and one third derive from the testes. In females, virtually all 17-KS originate in the adrenal cortex. It should be noted that 17-KS does not include testosterone. Components of 17-KS, which may be measured individually, include androsterone, dehydroepiandrosterone, etiocholanolone, 11-hydroxyandrosterone, 11-hydroxyetiocholanolone, 11-ketoandrosterone, 11-ketoetiocholanolone, pregnanediol, pregnanetriol (see p. 328), 5-pregnanetriol, and 11-ketopregnanetriol.

Levels of 17-KS are elevated in clients having adrenogenital syndrome (congenital adrenal hyperplasia), Cushing's syndrome, hormone-secreting tumors of the adrenal glands or gonads, adrenocortical carcinoma, hyperpituitarism, and stressful conditions. Decreased levels of 17-KS are associated with Addison's disease, liver disease, hypopituitarism, hypothyroidism, gout, nephrotic syndrome, and starvation. As with other urinary hormones, drugs may alter the excretion of 17-KS. Thus, a thorough medication history is necessary.

17-Ketogenic Steroids (17-KGS). Cortisol and its many metabolites can be manipulated in the laboratory to form 17-ketosteroids. The substances thus formed are called 17-ketogenic steroids (17-KGS) and may be studied as an index of overall glucocorticoid metabolism. Before urinary 17-KGS can be evaluated, the 17-KS of androgenic origin must be either removed or measured separately.[79] Because such a large array of steroid metabolites are reflected in 17-KGS measures, this test provides for a good overall assessment of adrenal function.

17-KGS levels are elevated in the presence of Cushing's syndrome, adrenogenital syndrome, carcinoma of the adrenal glands, and severe stress. Decreased levels are associated with Addison's disease, hypothyroidism, hypopituitarism, and long-term steroid use. As with other urinary hormone metabolites, drugs may alter 17-KGS levels. Thus, a thorough medication history is necessary.

Pregnanetriol. Pregnanetriol is a metabolite of the cortisone precursor, 17-hydroxyprogesterone. It should not be confused with pregnanediol, which is a metabolite of the hormone progesterone secreted by the corpus luteum and the placenta (see p. 330). Elevated pregnanetriol levels are associated with adrenogenital syndrome. In this disorder, cortisol synthesis is impaired at the point of 17-hydroxyprogesterone conversion. Instead, the substance accumulates and its metabolite, pregnanetriol, is excreted in the urine in increased amounts. Excessive amounts of 17-hydroxyprogesterone, and the resultant pregnanetriol, are produced in response to feedback mechanisms. Because cortisol synthesis is impaired, serum cortisol levels are low. This, in turn, stimulates the adenohypophysis to secrete ACTH, which normally would cause cortisol levels to rise. Since cortisol synthesis is impaired, however, pregnanetriol accumulates instead. Furthermore, the feedback mechanism continues to stimulate ACTH production. It should be noted that excessive 17-hydroxyprogesterone may be converted to androgens. This plus excessive androgen secretion in response to ACTH may result in virilization in females and sexual precocity in boys.

Adrenogenital syndrome is treated with cortisol replacement. Evaluation of urinary pregnanetriol may be used to evaluate response to therapy; that is, if cortisol levels are adequate, ACTH production, as well as pregnanetriol excretion, should be decreased.[80]

Catecholamines. The adrenal medulla, a component of the sympathetic nervous system, secretes epinephrine and norepinephrine, which are collectively known as the catecholamines. A third catecholamine, dopamine, is secreted in the brain, where it functions as a neurotransmitter. Dopamine is a precursor of epinephrine and norepinephrine. Serotonin, an amine related to the catecholamines, is found in platelets and in the argentaffin cells of the intestines.

Epinephrine (adrenalin) and norepinephrine are normally secreted in response to generalized sympathetic nervous system stimulation. Epinephrine increases the metabolic rate of all cells, heart rate, arterial blood pressure, blood glucose, and free fatty acids. Norepinephrine, the predominant catecholamine, decreases heart rate, while increasing peripheral vascular resistance and arterial blood pressure.

The most clinically significant disorder involving the adrenal medulla is the catecholamine-secreting tumor, pheochromocytoma. Pheochromocytomas may release catecholamines—primarily epinephrine—continuously or intermittently. For this reason, urinary measurements are helpful in quantifying overall excretory levels. Since the most common sign of pheochromocytoma is arterial hypertension, measurement of either plasma (see Chapter 5) or urinary catecholamines and their metabolites is indicated in new-onset hypertension of unknown etiology. Elevated catecholamine levels also are associated with neuroblastomas and ganglioneuromas.

Total catecholamines may be measured in either random or 24-hour urine specimens. The individual catecholamines, epinephrine and norepinephrine, may be measured in 24-hour urine collections, as may metanephrine, a metabolite of epinephrine. Numerous drugs may alter blood and urine levels of catecholamines, and stress, smoking, and strenuous exercise may produce elevated levels. Thus, a thorough health history is required prior to testing.

Vanillylmandelic Acid (VMA). Vanillylmandelic acid (VMA) is the predominant catecholamine metabolite found in urine. VMA is easier to detect by laboratory methods than the catecholamines themselves. Therefore, this test is more frequently used when pheochromocytoma is suspected.

A disadvantage of the test is the need for a special diet for 2 days prior to the study as well as on the day the 24-hour urine specimen is collected. The following foods are restricted on a "VMA diet": bananas, nuts, cereals, grains, tea, coffee, gelatin foods, citrus fruits, chocolate, vanilla, cheese, salad dressing, jelly, candy, chewing gum, cough drops, most carbonated beverages, licorice, and foods with artificial flavoring or coloring. Ingestion of such foods will falsely elevate VMA levels. It should be noted, however, that as laboratory methods become more precise, it may be possible to dispense with the VMA diet in urinary measures of VMA.[81] As with other hormones and their metabolites, VMA levels also may be elevated in relation to stress and physical exertion. Numerous drugs also may alter VMA levels.

Homovanillic Acid (HVA). Homovanillic acid (HVA) is a metabolite of dopamine, a major catecholamine itself, as well as a precursor to the catecholamines epinephrine and norepinephrine. HVA is synthesized in the brain, and elevated levels are associated with tumors involving the nervous system (e.g., neuroblastomas and ganglioneuromas). Analysis of urinary levels of HVA also is used to rule out benign pheochromocytoma. In this disorder, epinephrine is the catecholamine in excess (as indicated by elevated urinary VMA levels). Urinary excretion of HVA should be normal. It should be noted, however, that HVA levels will be elevated in malignant pheochromocytoma. As with other metabolites, numerous drugs, stress, and excessive exercise may alter HVA levels.

5-Hydroxyindoleacetic Acid (5-HIAA). 5-Hydroxyindoleacetic acid (5-HIAA) is a metabolite of serotonine, which is normally present only in platelets and the argentaffin cells of the intestines. Elevated 5-HIAA levels are associated with carcinoid tumors (argentaffinomas) of the intestine or appendix, which secrete large amounts of serotonin. Numerous drugs may alter 5-HIAA levels. In addition, foods containing serotonin (e.g., bananas, plums, pineapples, avocados, eggplant, tomatoes, and walnuts) may falsely elevate levels and must be restricted for several days prior to the test.[82]

Estrogens and Estrogen Fractions. Estrogens are secreted in large amounts by the ovaries and, during pregnancy, by the placenta. Minute amounts are secreted by the adrenal glands and, possibly, by the testes. Estrogens induce and maintain the female secondary sex characteristics, promote growth and maturation of the female reproductive organs, influence the pattern of fat deposition that characterizes the female form, and cause early epiphyseal closure. They also promote retention of sodium and water by the kidneys and sensitize the myometrium to oxytocin.

Total estrogens as well as the estrogen fractions (estrone, estradiol, and estriol) may be measured in urine. In blood tests, only the fractions are routinely measured (see Chapter 5). Estrone (E_1) is the immediate precursor of estradiol (E_2), which is the most biologically potent. Estriol (E_3), in addition to ovarian sources, is secreted in large amounts by the placenta during pregnancy. It is also secreted by maternal and fetal adrenal glands. Normally, estriol levels should rise steadily during pregnancy.

In addition to advancing and multiple pregnancy, elevated estrogen levels are associated with ovarian and adrenal tumors as well as estrogen-producing tumors of the testes. Drugs that elevate estrogen levels include estrogen-containing drugs, adrenal corticosteroids, tetracyclines, ampicillin, and phenothiazines.

Decreased estrogen levels are seen with primary and secondary ovarian failure, Turner's syndrome, hypopituitarism, adrenogenital syndrome, Stein-Leventhal syndrome, anorexia nervosa, and menopause. Low or steadily decreasing levels of estriol during pregnancy may indicate placental insufficiency, impending fetal distress, fetal anomalies (e.g., anencephaly), and Rh isoimmunization. Decreased estriol levels are associated also with diabetes and hypertensive disorders and other maternal complications of pregnancy.

It should be noted that in ovulating women, estrogen levels vary in relation to the menstrual cycle. Thus, the date of the last menstrual period should be noted when analysis of urinary estrogens is performed.

Pregnanediol. Pregnanediol is the chief metabolite of progesterone, which is secreted by the corpus luteum and by the placenta during pregnancy. Progesterone also is secreted in minute amounts by the adrenal cortex in both males and females. Progesterone prepares the endometrium for implantation of the fertilized ovum, decreases myometrial excitability, stimulates proliferation of the vaginal epithelium, and stimulates growth of the breasts during pregnancy. During pregnancy, after implantation of the embryo, progesterone production increases, thus sustaining the pregnancy. This increase continues until about the 36th week of pregnancy, after which levels begin to diminish.

Although serum determination of progesterone may be done (see Chapter 5), the study of its metabolite, pregnanediol, in urine reflects overall progesterone levels, which may not be apparent in single blood measures. In addition to pregnancy, elevated pregnanediol levels may be associated with ovarian tumors and cysts, adrenocortical hyperplasia and tumors, precocious puberty, and therapy with adrenocorticosteroids. Biliary tract obstruction also may produce elevated levels.

Decreased levels of pregnanediol are associated with placental insufficiency, fetal abnormalities or demise, threatened abortion, and toxemia of pregnancy. It should be noted, however, that decreased levels may not occur in the event of fetal demise if adequate circulation to the placenta continues. Other causes of decreased levels include panhypopituitarism, ovarian failure, Turner's syndrome, adrenogenital syndrome, and Stein-Leventhal syndrome. Therapy with drugs containing progesterone may also lead to decreased pregnanediol levels.

In ovulating women, pregnanediol levels vary in relation to the menstrual cycle. Thus, the date of the last menstrual period should be noted when analysis of pregnanediol is performed.

Human Chorionic Gonadotropin (hCG). Human chorionic gonadotropin (hCG) is produced only by the developing placenta, and its presence in blood (see Chapter 5) and urine has been used for decades to detect pregnancy. hCG is secreted at increasingly higher levels during the first 2 months of pregnancy, declining during the third and fourth months, and then remaining relatively stable until term. Levels return to normal within 1 to 2 weeks of termination of pregnancy. With the newer testing methods available, hCG can be detected in urine within 8 to 10 days after conception.

In addition to pregnancy, elevated hCG levels are associated with hydatidiform mole, choriocarcinoma and testicular epithelioma. Elevated levels also may be seen in nonendocrine tumors that produce hCG ectopically (e.g., carcinomas of the stomach, liver, pancreas, and breast; multiple myeloma; and malignant melanoma). Decreased levels of hCG are associated with fetal demise, threatened abortion, and incomplete abortion. Drugs that may alter test results include phenothiazines and anticonvulsants.

PROTEINS (CLINICAL APPLICATIONS DATA, p. 344)

Normally, the urine contains only a scant amount of protein. Excessive amounts of protein in the urine are generally associated with renal disease. Thus, part of the screening process in a routine urinalysis is to test the sample for protein (see p. 294). If increased amounts are found, a quantitative 24-hour urine collection is performed. The presence of certain types of proteins in urine also is diagnostic of specific disease states. The presence of Bence Jones protein in the urine, for example, is associated with multiple myeloma (see p. 295).

Protein metabolites such as creatinine and uric acid also may be measured in urine. Creatinine, which is produced at a fairly constant rate within the body, is a sensitive indicator of glomerular function because those factors affecting creatinine clearance are primarily due to alteration in renal function (see p. 312). Creatinine levels may also be measured along with 24-hour measures of other substances in urine (e.g., protein) as an indicator of the accuracy of the collection, as the amount excreted in 24 hours should be fairly constant. Measurement of urinary levels of uric acid are discussed further on. Amino acids also are products of protein metabolism. As will be discussed later, abnormal metabolism and congenital disorders (e.g., phenylketonuria) are associated with excessive levels of certain amino acids.

Uric Acid. Uric acid is an end product of purine metabolism. Purines are constituents of nucleic acids in the body and will appear in the urine in the absence of dietary sources of purines. Dietary sources of purines include organ meats, legumes, and yeasts. Uric acid is filtered, absorbed, and secreted by the kidneys and is a common constituent of urine (see p. 290).

The amount of uric acid produced in the body and the efficiency of renal excretion affect the amount of uric acid found in urine. Excessive amounts of uric acid may be found when there is excessive dietary intake of purines, in massive cell turnover with degradation of nucleic acids, and in disorders of purine metabolism. The body's ability to filter, reabsorb, and secrete uric acid affects the amount of uric acid ultimately found in urine.[83]

Elevated urinary uric acid is commonly associated with neoplastic disorders such as leukemia and lymphosarcoma. It may be found also in individuals with pernicious anemia, sickle cell anemia, and polycythemia. Disorders associated with impaired renal tubular absorption (e.g., Fanconi's syndrome and Wilson's disease) will also lead to elevated uric acid levels in urine.[84]

Drugs used to treat elevated serum uric acid levels frequently work by increasing urinary excretion of the substance. Such drugs include probenecid and sulfinpyrazone. Allopurinol also decreases serum uric acid levels, but without necessarily leading to excessive urinary levels.[85] It should be noted that colchicine, a drug frequently used to treat gout, does not alter urinary levels of uric acid. Other drugs associated with elevated urinary uric acid include aspirin (large doses), adrenal corticosteroids, coumarin anticoagulants, and estrogens.

Although gout is associated with elevated serum uric acid levels (see Chapter 5), decreased amounts of uric acid are often found in urine because of impaired tubular excretion. Decreased amounts of urinary uric acid also are associated with various renal diseases, for the same reason. Decreased urinary uric acid levels are associated with lactic acidosis and ketoacidosis, owing to impaired renal excretion, and also with ingestion of alcohol, aspirin (small doses), and thiazide diuretics.

Amino Acids. Elevated amino acid levels in urine are associated with congenital defects and disorders of amino acid metabolism. The major inherited disorders include phenylketonuria (PKU), tyrosyluria, and alkaptonuria. PKU occurs when the normal conversion of phenylalanine to tyrosine is impaired. This leads to the excretion of increased keto acids such as phenylpyruvate in the urine, which can be detected on screening tests. If undetected and untreated, PKU results in severe mental retardation. Blood tests for PKU also may be performed.

Tyrosyluria occurs due to either inherited disorders or metabolic defects. It is most frequently seen in premature infants owing to underdeveloped liver function but seldom results in permanent damage. Acquired severe liver disease will also lead to tyrosyluria, as well as to the appearance of tyrosine crystals in the urine (see p. 307).

Alkaptonuria represents another defect in the phenylalanine-tyrosine conversion pathway. In this disorder, homogentisic acid accumulates in the urine. Alkaptonuria generally manifests in adulthood and leads to deposition of brown pigment in the body, arthritis, liver disease, and cardiac disorders.[86]

Numerous other disorders are associated with altered metabolism and excretion of amino acids. These include maple syrup urine disease and cystinuria. Amino acid screening tests may also indicate the presence of such disorders.

Urine Hydroxyproline. A special urinary test for a specific amino acid is measurement of urine hydroxyproline, a component of collagen in skin and bone. Elevated levels are seen in disorders associated with rapid bone resorption, including Paget's disease, metastatic bone tumors, and certain endocrine disorders. Foods such as meat, poultry, fish, and any foods containing gelatin will falsely elevate levels and must, therefore, be restricted for at least 24 hours prior to the test. Drugs such as ascorbic acid, vitamin D, glucocorticoids, aspirin, mithramycin, and calcitonin will also elevate levels, as will skin disorders such as burns and psoriasis.[87]

VITAMINS AND MINERALS (CLINICAL APPLICATIONS DATA, p. 346)

The functions and serum assays of vitamins and minerals are discussed in Chapter 5. In general, serum assays are preferred to the more cumbersome urine level determinations, which require 24-hour urine collections.

Vitamins. Fat-soluble vitamins are not readily excreted in the urine, and therefore, urinary determinations focus on water-soluble vitamins B and C. Urinary determinations for vitamins B_1 (thiamine), B_2 (riboflavin), and C may be done in suspected deficiency states. The Schilling test for vitamin B_{12} absorption was discussed in Chapter 1, as it is used to diagnose an abnormality of hematopoiesis.

Minerals. Minerals are essential to normal body metabolism. In urine, three commonly measured minerals include iron (found in hemosiderin, see p. 298), copper, and oxalate. Copper aids in the formation of hemoglobin and is a component of certain enzymes necessary for energy production.[88] Elevated urinary copper levels are associated with Wilson's disease, an inherited disorder of copper metabolism. Oxalate is found in combination with calcium in certain kidney stones. Elevated urinary oxalate levels are seen in hyperoxaluria, a disorder in which oxalate accumulates in soft tissues, especially those of the kidney and bladder.[89] Oxalate levels also may be elevated if there is excessive ingestion of strawberries, tomatoes, rhubarb, or spinach.

Clinical Applications Data

ELECTROLYTES (BACKGROUND INFORMATION, p. 321)
Reference Values

Sodium	30–280 mEq/24 hr
Chloride	110–250 mEq/24 hr
Potassium	40–80 mEq/24 hr
Calcium	
Quantitative	
Men	<275 mg/24 hr
Women	<250 mg/24 hr
Qualitative	
Sulkowitch test	0–+2 turbidity
Phosphorus	0.9–1.3 g/24 hr
	29–42 mmol/24 hr
Magnesium	<150 mg/24 hr
	6.0–8.5 mEq/24 hr
	3.0–4.3 mmol/24 hr

Interfering Factors

- Dietary deficiency or excess of the electrolyte to be measured may lead to spurious results
- Increased calcium intake may result in decreased magnesium excretion
- Increased sodium and magnesium intake may cause increased calcium excretion
- Diuretic therapy with excessive loss of electrolytes into the urine may falsely elevate results
- Therapy with adrenal corticosteroids may lead to decreased sodium loss and increased calcium loss
- Excessive ingestion of magnesium-containing antacids may lead to increased excretion of magnesium

Indications/Purposes for Measurement of Urinary Electrolytes

With the exception of magnesium, electrolytes are more likely to be measured by serum determinations than by urinary measures of the substances. General reasons for analyzing electrolytes in urine are:

- Suspected renal disease
- Suspected endocrine disorder
- History of kidney stones
- Suspected malabsorption problem
- CNS signs and symptoms of unknown etiology, especially if thought to be due to magnesium imbalance, which is detected earlier in urine than in blood

Client Preparation

For quantitative studies (i.e., studies to determine the amount of the electrolyte present), client preparation is the same as that for any test involving collection of a 24-hour urine sample (see Appendix II). For calcium studies, some laboratories require that the client be on a diet with a set amount of calcium for at least 3 days prior to beginning the urine collection. If this is the case, the client should be instructed about the diet. Medications are not usually withheld, but the laboratory should be informed about those taken.

If the Sulkowitch test, a qualitative study, is used for home monitoring of urinary calcium, the client should be instructed in the procedure.

The Procedure

Quantitative Tests. A 24-hour urine collection is obtained (see Appendix II). Check with the laboratory or individual ordering the test to see if the diet is to be modified for calcium studies. The laboratory should be informed of any medications taken by the client that may alter test results (see section on Interfering Factors).

Qualitative Tests (Sulkowitch Test). A random urine specimen is obtained, 5 ml of which is poured into a test tube. Acetic acid (5 ml of a 10 percent solution) is added to the sample, and the mixture is boiled to remove protein. Distilled water is then added to the sample until the original volume is restored. Sulkowitch reagent (5 ml), which contains oxalic acid and ammonium oxalate, is then added. This reagent reacts with the calcium present in the sample and produces turbidity (cloudiness) in the sample. Turbidity is graded on a scale of 0 to +4.[90,91]

Aftercare and Nursing Observations

There are no specific aftercare or nursing observations. If the client's diet was modified for the test, the usual diet may be resumed after specimen collection is completed.

PIGMENTS (BACKGROUND INFORMATION, p. 323)

Reference Values

Hemoglobin	Negative
Hemosiderin	Negative
Bilirubin	Negative
Urobilinogen	
Random specimen	0.1–1.0 Ehrlich units/dl
24-hr urine	1–4 mg/24 hr
Myoglobin	Negative
Melanin	Negative
Porphyrins	
Aminolevulinic acid (ALA)	
Random specimen	
Children	38.1 μmol/L
	<0.5 mg/dl
Adults	7.6–45.8 μmol/L
	0.1–0.6 mg/dl
24-hr urine	11.15–57.2 μmol/24 hr
	1.5–7.5 mg/dl/24 hr
Porphobilinogen (PBG)	
Random specimen	Negative
24-hr urine	0–4.4 μmol/24 hr
	0–1.5 mg/24 hr

Uroporphyrin
    Random specimen   Negative
    24-hr urine $0.012-0.037$ μmol/24 hr
                             $10-30$ μg/24 hr (values may be slightly higher in men than in women)

Coproporphyrin
    Random specimen
        Adults $0.045-0.30$ μmol/L
    24-hr urine
        Children $0-0.12$ μmol/24 hr
                             $0-80$ μg/24 hr
        Adults $0.075-0.24$ μmol/24 hr
                             $50-160$ μg/24 hr (values may be slightly higher in men than in women)

INTERFERING FACTORS

■ For random samples, delay in sending the specimen to the laboratory within 1 hour of collection may lead to oxidation of bilirubin, if present, and of urobilinogen; random samples for porphyrin tests must be fresh and, thus, must be sent to the laboratory immediately upon collection

■ For 24-hour samples, failure to collect the specimen in a dark container, or in a container covered with aluminum foil or a dark plastic bag, may result in invalid results; the specimen must also be refrigerated or kept on ice throughout the collection period, unless a preservative has been added to the container by the laboratory (if the client has a Foley catheter, the drainage bag must be covered with a dark plastic bag and placed in a basin of ice)

■ Therapy with griseofulvin, rifampin, and barbiturates may falsely elevate values in tests for porphyrins

Indications/Purposes for Analysis of Urinary Pigments

■ Detection of liver disease as indicated by the presence of bilirubin (possible), excessive urobilinogen, and elevated porphyrins

■ Diagnosis of the source of obstructive jaundice (i.e., obstruction in the biliary tree) as indicated by presence of bilirubin, absence of urobilinogen, and elevated coproporphyrins

■ Detection of suspected lead poisoning as indicated by elevated porphyrins, especially ALA and PBG

■ Detection of excessive red blood cell hemolysis within the systemic circulation as indicated by the presence of free hemoglobin, elevated urobilinogen levels, and presence of hemosiderin a few days after the acute hemolytic episode

■ Detection of extensive injury to muscles as indicated by the presence of myoglobin in the urine

■ Detection of malignant melanoma as indicated by the presence of melanin in the urine

Client Preparation

For quantitative studies, client preparation is the same as that for any test involving collection of a 24-hour urine sample (see Appendix II). The client should receive the proper container and instructions for maintaining the collection (e.g., refrigerated, protected from light). For studies involving the porphyrins, medications such as griseofulvin, rifampin, and barbiturates may be withheld. This should be confirmed with the person ordering the test.

For random samples, there is no specific preparation other than informing the client that the sample must be protected from light and sent to the laboratory within 1 hour of collection. The proper container should be provided to the client.

The Procedure

Quantitative Tests. A 24-hour urine collection is obtained in a dark container or in one covered with aluminum foil or a dark plastic bag. The sample must be kept refrigerated or on ice throughout the collection period, unless a preservative has been added to the container by the laboratory. If the client has a Foley catheter, the drainage bag must be covered with a dark plastic bag and placed in a basin of ice.

Random Specimens (Qualitative Tests). A random sample is collected and sent promptly (within 1 hour) to the laboratory. The specimen must be protected from excessive exposure to light.

Aftercare and Nursing Observations

There is no specified aftercare. Any medications withheld for the test should be resumed.

ENZYMES (BACKGROUND INFORMATION, p. 325)

Reference Values

Amylase	10–80 amylase units/hr (Mayo clinic)
	35–260 Somogyi units/hr
	6.5–48.1 SI units/hr
Arylsulfatase A (ARS-A)	
Children	>1 U/L
Men	1.4–19.3 U/L
Women	1.4–11 U/L
Lysozyme (Muramidase)	1.3–3.6 mg/24 hr
Leucine aminopeptidase (LAP)	2–18 U/24 hr

Interfering Factors

Incomplete specimen collection and improper specimen maintenance may lead to spurious results.

Amylase

■ Ingestion of drugs that may falsely elevate values (morphine, codeine, meperidine, pentazocine, chlorthiazides, aspirin, corticosteroids, oral contraceptives, alcohol, indomethacin, urecholine, secretin, and pancreozymin)
■ Inadvertant addition of salivary amylase to the sample due to coughing or talking over it may falsely elevate values

ARS-A

■ Contamination of the sample with blood, mucus, and feces may falsely elevate levels
■ Abdominal surgery within 1 week of the collection may falsely elevate levels

Lysozyme (Muramidase)

■ Presence of bacteria in the sample, which will falsely decrease levels
■ Presence of blood and saliva in the sample, which will falsely elevate levels

Leucine Aminopeptidase (LAP)

■ Advanced pregnancy and therapy with drugs containing estrogen and progesterone may falsely elevate levels

Indications/Purposes for Urinary Enzyme Tests

Amylase

■ Retrospective diagnosis of acute pancreatitis when serum amylase levels have returned to normal but urine levels remain elevated
■ Diagnosis of chronic pancreatitis as indicated by persistently elevated urinary amylase levels
■ Monitoring response to treatment for pancreatitis
■ Assist in identifying the cause of "acute abdomen"
■ Differentiation of acute pancreatitis from perforated peptic ulcer (urinary amylase levels are higher in pancreatitis)
■ Diagnosis of macroamylasemia, a disorder seen in alcoholism and malabsorption syndromes, as indicated by elevated serum amylase and normal urinary amylase
■ Confirmation of the diagnosis of salivary gland inflammation

ARS-A

■ Suspected malignancy involving the bladder, colon, or rectum as indicated by elevated levels
■ Suspected granulocytic leukemia as indicated by elevated levels
■ Family history of lipid storage diseases (e.g., mucolipidoses II and III), with support for the diagnosis indicated by elevated levels
■ Suspected metachromatic leukodystrophy as indicated by decreased levels

Lysozyme (Muramidase)

■ Suspected acute granulocytic or monocytic leukemia as indicated by elevated levels
■ Monitoring the extent of destruction of monocytes and granulocytes in known leukemias
■ Suspected renal tubular damage as indicated by elevated levels
■ Monitoring response to renal transplant with rejection indicated by elevated levels

Leucine Aminopeptidase (LAP)

■ Elevated serum alkaline phosphatase or leucine aminopeptidase levels of unknown etiology
■ Suspected liver, pancreatic, and biliary diseases, including malignancies, especially when serum LAP levels are normal (urinary elevations lag behind serum elevations)

Client Preparation

Amylase. Client preparation is the same as that for any study involving a 24-hour or timed urine collection. The proper container and instructions for maintaining the collection (e.g., refrigerated, protected from exposure to salivary secretions) should be provided. Drugs that may alter test results (see section on Interfering Factors) may be withheld during the test, although this should be confirmed with the person ordering the study.

ARS-A. Client preparation is the same as that for any study involving a 24-hour urine collection (see Appendix II). The proper container and instructions for maintaining the collection (e.g., refrigerated, placed on ice) should be provided.

Lysozyme (Muramidase). Client preparation is the same as that for any study involving a 24-hour urine collection. The proper container and instructions for maintaining the collection (e.g., refrigerated, placed on ice) should be provided. The client should be cautioned to avoid touching the inside of the collection container in order to avoid bacterial contamination of the sample. The client also should be cautioned to avoid contaminating the sample with saliva (e.g., coughing over the specimen) or blood.

Leucine Aminopeptidase (LAP). Client preparation is the same as that for any study involving a 24-hour urine collection. The proper container and instructions for maintaining the collection (e.g., refrigerated, placed on ice) should be provided. Because drugs containing estrogens and progesterone may falsely elevate levels, a medication history regarding these types of drugs should be obtained.

The Procedure

Amylase. A timed urine collection is obtained. The collection may be done over 1-, 2-, 6-, 8-, and 24-hour periods. The sample must be kept refrigerated or on ice throughout the collection period unless the laboratory has added a preservative to the container. If the client has a Foley catheter, the drainage bag must be placed in a basin of ice. Care must be taken to avoid adding salivary secretions to the sample by coughing or talking over the specimen. The sample should be sent promptly to the laboratory when the collection is completed.

ARS-A. A 24-hour urine collection is obtained. The sample must be kept refrigerated or on ice throughout the collection period, unless a preservative has been added to the container by the laboratory. If the client has a Foley catheter, the drainage bag must be placed in a basin of ice. Care must be taken not to contaminate the sample with blood, mucus, or feces. The sample should be sent promptly to the laboratory when the collection is completed.

Lysozyme (Muramidase). A 24-hour urine collection is obtained. The sample must be kept refrigerated or on ice throughout the collection period, unless a preservative has been added to the container by the laboratory. If the client has a Foley catheter, the drainage bag must be placed on ice. Care must be taken not to contaminate the sample with bacteria, blood, or saliva. The sample should be sent promptly to the laboratory when the collection is completed.

Leucine Aminopeptidase (LAP). A 24-hour urine collection is obtained. The sample must be kept refrigerated or on ice throughout the collection period, unless a preservative has been added to the container by the laboratory. If the client has a Foley catheter, the drainage bag must be placed on ice. The sample should be sent promptly to the laboratory when the collection is completed.

Aftercare and Nursing Observations

There are no specific aspects of aftercare or nursing observations for these tests. Any medications withheld during the test should be resumed when specimen collection is complete.

HORMONES AND THEIR METABOLITES (BACKGROUND INFORMATION, p. 326)
Reference Values

Cortisol	20–90 μg/24 hr
Aldosterone	2–26 μg/24 hr
17-Hydroxycorticosteroids (17-OHCS)	
Children	1.5–4.0 mg/24 hr (age-related: the younger the child, the less secreted)
Men	5.5–14.4 mg/24 hr
Women	4.9–12.9 mg/24 hr
17-Ketosteroids (17-KS)	
Children	<1–3 mg/24 hr (age-related: the younger the child, the less secreted)
Men	8–25 mg/24 hr
Women	5–15 mg/24 hr
Elderly	4–8 mg/24 hr
17-Ketogenic steroids (17-KGS)	
Children	<2–6 mg/24 hr (age-related: the younger the child, the less secreted)
Men	5–23 mg/24 hr
Women	3–15 mg/24 hr
Elderly	3–12 mg/24 hr
Pregnanetriol	
Children, 6 yr old	Up to 0.2 mg/24 hr
Children, 7–16 yr old	0.3–1.1 mg/24 hr
Adults	<3.5 mg/24 hr
Catecholamines	
Total	
Random urine	0–14 μg/dl
24-hour urine	<100 g/24 hr
Epinephrine	<10 ng/24 hr
Norepinephrine	<100 ng/24 hr
Metanephrines	0.1–1.6 mg/24 hr
Vanillylmandelic acid (VMA)	0.7–6.8 mg/24 hr
Homovanillic acid (HVA)	
Children	
1–2 yr old	0–25 mg/24 hr
2–10 yr old	0.5–10 mg/24 hr
10–15 yr old	0.5–12 mg/24 hr
Adult	<8 mg/24 hr
5-Hydroxyindoleacetic acid (5-HIAA)	2–9 mg/24 hrs
Estrogens	
Total	
Adult males	4–24 μg/24 hr
Nonpregnant females	
Preovulatory phase	5–25 μg/24 hr
Ovulatory phase	24–100 μg/24 hr
Luteal phase	12–80 μg/24 hr
Postmenopausal females	<10 μg/24 hr
Estrone (E_1)	
Children	0.2–1 g/24 hr
Adult males	3.4–8.2 g/24 hr
Nonpregnant females	
Early in cycle	4–7 g/24 hr
Luteal phase	11–31 g/24 hr
Postmenopausal females	0.8–7.1 g/24 hrs

Estradiol (E_2)
Children .... 0–0.2 µg/24 hr
Adult males .... 0–0.4 µg/24 hr
Nonpregnant females
  Early in cycle .... 0–3 µg/24 hr
  Luteal phase .... 4–14 µg/24 hr
Postmenopausal females .... 0–2.3 µg/24 hr
Estriol (E_3)
Children .... 0.3–2.4 µg/24 hr
Adult males .... 0.8–7.5 µg/24 hr
Nonpregnant females
  Early in cycle .... 0–15 µg/24 hr
  Luteal phase .... 13–54 µg/24 hr
Postmenopausal females .... 0.6–6.8 µg/24 hr
Pregnant females .... Up to 28 mg/24 hr (when plotted on a graph, levels should steadily rise during pregnancy)

Pregnanediol
Adult males .... <1.5 mg/24 hr
Nonpregnant females
  Proliferative phase .... 0.5–1.5 mg/24 hr
  Luteal phase .... 2–7 mg/24 hr
Postmenopausal females .... 0.2–1 mg/24 hr
Pregnant females
  16 weeks .... 5–21 mg/24 hr
  20 weeks .... 6–26 mg/24 hr
  24 weeks .... 12–32 mg/24 hr
  28 weeks .... 19–51 mg/24 hr
  32 weeks .... 22–66 mg/24 hr
  36 weeks .... 13–77 mg/24 hr
  40 weeks .... 23–63 mg/24 hr
Human chorionic gonadogropin (hCG)
Random urine .... Negative if not pregnant
24-hour urine
  Adult males .... Not measurable
  Nonpregnant females .... Not measurable
  Pregnant females
    1st trimester .... Up to 500,000 IU/24 hr
    2nd trimester .... 10,000–25,000 IU/24 hr
    3rd trimester .... 5,000–15,000 IU/24 hr

Interfering Factors

■ Improper specimen collection and improper specimen maintenance may lead to spurious results

■ Numerous drugs may alter test results; a thorough medication history should be obtained prior to testing; some medications may be withheld

Cortisol

■ Excessive exercise and stressful situations during the testing period may lead to falsely elevated levels

Aldosterone

■ Ingestion of foods that lower levels (e.g., licorice and excessive sodium intake)

■ Excessive exercise and stressful situations during the testing period may falsely elevate levels

■ Radioactive scans within 1 week of the study, since urinary aldosterone determinations are done by radioimmunoassay method

17-OHCS

■ Excessive exercise and stressful situations during the testing period may falsely elevate levels

17-KS

■ Blood in the specimen may alter test results; the test should be postponed if the female client is menstruating

■ Excessive exercise and stressful situations during the testing period may falsely elevate levels

17-KGS

■ Excessive exercise and stressful situations during the testing period may falsely elevate levels

Pregnanetriol

■ None, except drugs and improper specimen collection and maintenance

Catecholamines

■ Excessive exercise and stressful situations during the testing period may falsely elevate levels

Vanillylmandelic Acid (VMA)

■ Numerous foods may falsely elevate levels (see Background Information, p. 329); the client must follow a special diet for this test

■ Excessive exercise and stressful situations during the testing period may falsely elevate levels

Homovanillic Acid (HVA)

■ Excessive exercise and stressful situations during the testing period may falsely elevate levels

5-HIAA

■ Certain foods (bananas, plums, pineapples, avocados, eggplants, tomatoes, and walnuts) will falsely elevate levels and must be withheld for 4 days prior to the test

■ Severe gastrointestinal disturbance or diarrhea may alter test results

Estrogens and Estrogen Fractions

■ Maternal disorders (e.g., hypertension, diabetes, anemia, malnutrition, hemoglobinopathy, liver disease, intestinal disease) may result in decreased estriol levels during pregnancy

■ Threatened abortion, ectopic pregnancy and early pregnancy may result in falsely decreased estriol levels

Pregnanediol

■ None, except drugs and improper specimen collection

Human Chorionic Gonadotropin (hCG)

■ Proteinuria and hematuria may lead to falsely elevated levels

Indications/Purposes for Measuring Urinary Hormones and Their Metabolites

Cortisol

■ Diagnostic evaluation of signs of Cushing's syndrome without definitive elevation of plasma cortisol levels (adrenal hyperplasia will raise the urinary cortisol level more significantly than the plasma cortisol)
■ Diagnostic evaluation of obesity of undetermined etiology (obesity may raise plasma cortisol levels but does not significantly elevate free cortisol levels in urine)
■ Quantification of cortisol excess, regardless of its source
■ More accurate quantification than 17-hydroxycorticosteroids (17-OHCS) in individuals receiving drugs that alter hepatic metabolism of steroids

Aldosterone

■ Suspected hyperaldosteronism, especially when serum aldosterone levels are not definitive for the diagnosis

17-OHCS

■ Signs and symptoms of adrenal cortical hypofunctioning or hyperfunctioning
■ Suspected Cushing's syndrome as indicated by elevated levels
■ Suspected Addison's disease as indicated by decreased levels

17-KS

■ Suspected adrenocortical dysfunction, especially if urinary levels of 17-OHCS are normal
■ Suspected Cushing's syndrome as indicated by elevated levels
■ Suspected adrenogenital syndrome, as indicated by elevated levels
■ Monitoring response to therapy for adrenogenital syndrome

17-KGS

■ Suspected adrenal hypofunctioning or hyperfunctioning (the test provides a good overall assessment of adrenal function)
■ Suspected Cushing's syndrome as indicated by elevated levels
■ Suspected Addison's disease as indicated by decreased levels
■ Monitoring response to therapy with corticosteroid drugs or other drugs that alter adrenal function

Pregnanetriol

■ Suspected adrenogenital syndrome (virilization in females, precocious sexual development in males) as indicated by elevated levels
■ Family history of adrenogenital syndrome
■ Monitoring response to cortisol therapy for adrenogenital syndrome
■ Suspected testicular tumors as indicated by elevated levels
■ Suspected Stein-Leventhal syndrome as indicated by elevated levels

Catecholamines

■ Hypertension of unknown etiology
■ Suspected pheochromocytoma as indicated by elevated levels
■ Acute hypertensive episode (a random sample is collected in such cases)
■ Suspected neuroblastoma or ganglioneuroma as indicated by elevated levels

Vanillylmandelic Acid (VMA)

■ Hypertension of unknown etiology
■ Suspected pheochromocytoma as indicated by elevated levels
■ Suspected neuroblastoma or ganglioneuroma as indicated by elevated levels

Homovanillic Acid (HVA)

■ Suspected neuroblastoma or ganglioneuroma as indicated by elevated levels
■ Diagnosis of benign pheochromocytoma as indicated by normal HVA levels with elevated VMA levels
■ Diagnosis of malignant pheochromocytoma as indicated by elevated HVA and VMA levels

5-HIAA

■ Detection of early carcinoid tumors of the intestine as indicated by elevated levels

Estrogens and Estrogen Fractions

■ Suspected tumor of the ovary, testicle, or adrenal gland as indicated by elevated total estrogens and fractions
■ Suspected ovarian failure as indicated by decreased total estrogens and fractions
■ Detection of placental and fetal problems as indicated by estriol levels that fail to show a steady increase over several days or weeks (a sharp decline over several days indicates impending fetal demise; consistently low levels may indicate fetal anomalies)
■ Detection of maternal disorders of pregnancy as indicated by estriol levels that fail to show a steady increase over several days or weeks

Pregnanediol

■ Verification of ovulation in planning pregnancy or in determining the cause of infertility as indicated by normal values in relation to the menstrual cycle
■ Diagnosis of placental dysfunction, as indicated by either low levels or failure of levels to progressively increase, and identification of the need for progesterone therapy to sustain the pregnancy
■ Detection of fetal demise as indicated by decreased levels, although levels may remain within normal limits if placental circulation is adequate

Human Chorionic Gonadotropin (hCG)

■ Confirmation of pregnancy within 8 to 10 days after conception, especially in women with a history of infertility or habitual abortion, or in women who may desire a therapeutic abortion
■ Suspected hydatidiform mole as indicated by elevated levels
■ Suspected choriocarcinoma or testicular tumor as indicated by elevated levels
■ Suspected nonendocrine tumor that produces hCG ectopically as indicated by elevated levels
■ Threatened abortion as indicated by decreased levels

Client Preparation

All urine studies for hormones and their metabolites involve collecting 24-hour urine samples (see Appendix II); exceptions are catecholamines and human chorionic gonadotropin, which also may be analyzed in random samples. The client should, therefore, be instructed on how to collect the sample. The proper container and instructions for maintaining the collection (e.g., refrigerated or on ice) should be provided. Drugs that may alter test results may be withheld during the test, although this should be confirmed with the person ordering the study.

The client should be cautioned to avoid excessive exercise and stress during the following studies: cortisol, aldosterone, 17-OHCS, 17-KS, 17-KGS, catecholamines, VMA, and HVA. The client also should be instructed on the following dietary restrictions in relation to specific tests: (1) aldosterone—maintain a normal salt intake; (2) VMA—maintain a "VMA diet" (see p. 329) for 2 days prior to the test and for the day of the test; and (3) 5-HIAA—maintain a diet low in serotonin (see p. 329) for 4 days prior to the test.

For gonadal and placental hormone studies, the date of the last menstrual period should be noted.

The Procedure

All urine studies for hormones and their metabolites involve collecting 24-hour urine specimens; exceptions are catecholamines and human chorionic gonadotropin, which also may be analyzed in random samples. For the 24-hour collections, an acidifying preservative is added to the container by the laboratory. In addition, some laboratories require that the sample be refrigerated or placed on ice throughout the collection period. Special diets may be required prior to collection of 24-hour urines for VMA and 5-HIAA (see Client Preparation, above).

Random samples for catecholamines may be collected at any time but frequently are obtained after a hypertensive episode. Random samples for hCG are more reliable if collected first thing in the morning because dilute urine may lead to false-negative results.

All specimens should be sent promptly to the laboratory when the collection is completed.

Aftercare and Nursing Observations

There are no specific aspects of aftercare or nursing observations for these tests. If the client's usual diet, drugs, or activities were altered for the test, they should be resumed upon its completion.

PROTEINS (BACKROUND INFORMATION, p. 331)
Reference Values

Protein	0–150 mg/24 hr
Creatinine	
Men	1–1.9 g/24 hr
Women	0.8–1.7 g/24 hr
Bence Jones protein	Negative
Uric acid	250–750 mg/24 hr
Amino acids	
Screening tests	Negative
(e.g., for PKU, tyrosyluria, alkaptonuria, cystinuria, maple syrup urine disease)	
Urine hydroxyproline	
2-hour sample	
Men	0.4–5 mg/2 hr
Women	0.4–2.9 mg/2 hr
24-hour sample	
Adults	14–45 mg/24 hr

Note: Values are higher in children and during the 3rd trimester of pregnancy.

Interfering Factors

■ Improper specimen collection and improper specimen maintenance
■ Ingestion of foods and drugs that may alter test results (see Background Information, p. 331), or failure to ingest certain foods (e.g., a low purine diet will lead to decreased levels of urinary uric acid; lack of protein intake in the infant may lead to false-negative PKU test results in infants)
■ Skin disorders such as psoriasis and burns may falsely elevate urine hydroxyproline levels

Indications/Purposes for Measurement of Urinary Proteins

Protein

■ Detection of various types of renal disease as indicated by elevated levels
■ Detection of possible complications of pregnancy as indicated by elevated levels

Bence Jones Protein

■ Detection of multiple myeloma

Creatinine

■ Assessment of glomerular function with decreased levels indicating impairment (see also Clinical Applications Data, p. 315)
■ Assessment of the accuracy of 24-hour urine collections for other substances

Uric Acid

■ Monitoring urinary effects of disorders that cause hyperuricemia (see p. 331)
■ Monitoring response to therapy with uricosuric drugs
■ Comparison of urine levels with serum uric acid levels to provide for an index of renal function

Amino Acid Screening Tests

■ Detection of inherited and metabolic disorders such as PKU, tyrosyluria, alkaptonuria, cystinuria, and maple syrup urine disease

Urine Hydroxyproline

■ Detection of disorders associated with increased bone resorption (e.g., Paget's disease, metastatic bone tumors, and certain endocrine disorders)
■ Monitoring treatment for Paget's disease

Client Preparation

The client should be instructed in the method to be used for obtaining the sample (e.g., 24-hour urine, 2-hour urine, clean-catch midstream sample). A medication history should be obtained. Drugs that may alter test results may be withheld during the test, although this should be confirmed with the person ordering the study. The client also must be instructed in any dietary modifications needed for the test. Such dietary modifications may be necessary in uric acid and urine hydroxyproline tests.

The Procedure

Protein, Creatinine, and Uric Acid. A 24-hour urine specimen is collected. For creatinine measures, a preservative is usually added to the collection container by the laboratory. It may be necessary also to refrigerate the sample.

Bence Jones Protein. An early morning sample of at least 60 ml is collected. The sample should be sent promptly to the laboratory. It is recommended that the sample be collected using the clean-catch midstream technique (see Appendix II) to avoid contaminating the sample with other proteins from bodily secretions.

Amino Acid Screening Tests. A random urine specimen of at least 20 ml is collected. In infants, this involves application of a urine-collecting device. The specimen should be sent immediately to the laboratory.

Urine Hydroxyproline. A 2- or 24-hour urine specimen is collected in a container to which preservative has been added. It also may be necessary to refrigerate the sample.

Aftercare and Nursing Observations

There are no specific aspects of aftercare or nursing observations for these tests. Any medications withheld for the test should be resumed. The usual diet, if modified for the test, also should be resumed upon completion of the collection.

VITAMINS AND MINERALS (BACKGROUND INFORMATION, p. 332)
Reference Values

Vitamins	
B$_1$ (thiamine)	100–200 μg/24 hr
B$_2$ (riboflavin)	
Men	0.51 mg/24 hr
Women	0.39 mg/24 hr
C (ascorbic acid)	30 mg/24 hr
Minerals	
Copper	15–60 μg/24 hr
Oxalate	<40 mg/24 hr

Interfering Factors

■ Improper specimen collection and maintenance
■ Ingestion of strawberries, tomatoes, rhubarb, or spinach may falsely elevate oxalate levels

Indications/Purposes for Urinary Measures of Vitamins and Minerals

■ Detection of vitamin deficiency states
■ Screening for and detection of Wilson's disease as indicated by elevated urinary copper levels
■ Detection of hyperoxaluria as indicated by elevated oxalate levels

Client Preparation

The client should be instructed in the method of obtaining the sample (i.e., usually a 24-hour urine collection).

The Procedure

A 24-hour urine specimen is collected. Samples for oxalate should be collected in containers to which hydrochloric acid has been added and which are protected from light

Aftercare and Nursing Observations

There are no specific aspects of aftercare or nursing observations for these tests.

Microbiological Examination of Urine

BACKGROUND INFORMATION

Urine tests for culture and sensitivity indicate the type and number of organisms present in the specimen (culture) and the antibiotics to which the organisms are susceptible (sensitivity). In urine, it is common to culture out only one organism, although polymicrobial infections may be seen in individuals with Foley catheters. Most organisms infecting the urinary tract derive from fecal flora that have ascended the urethra. Organisms commonly found in urine include *Escherichia coli,* enterococci, *Klebsiella, Proteus,* and *Pseudomonas.*[92]

After treatment with the appropriate antibiotic, as indicated by sensitivity tests, follow-up urine cultures may be done to determine the effectiveness of treatment.

CLINICAL APPLICATIONS DATA

Reference Values

Negative for pathological organisms.

Interfering Factors

- Improper specimen collection such that the sample is contaminated with nonurinary organisms
- Delay in sending the specimen to the laboratory (bacteria may multiply in nonrefrigerated samples)

Indications/Purposes for Microbiological Examination of Urine

- Suspected urinary tract infection
- Identification of antibiotics to which the cultured organism is sensitive
- Monitoring response to treatment for urinary tract infections

Client Preparation

Client preparation is the same as that for any test involving collection of either a clean-catch midstream urine specimen, a catheterized specimen, or a suprapubic aspiration (see Appendix II).

The Procedure

A sample of at least 5 to 10 ml is obtained either by clean catch technique, catheterization, or suprapubic aspiration. The sample is placed in a sterile container and is transported to the laboratory immediately.

Aftercare and Nursing Observations

There are no specific aspects of aftercare or nursing observations, unless the sample was obtained by suprapubic aspiration. In this case, the aspiration site should be observed for signs of inflammation and should be kept covered with a sterile dressing.

Cytological Examination of Urine

BACKGROUND INFORMATION

Cytology is the study of the origin, structure, function, and pathology of cells. In clinical practice, cytological examinations are generally performed to detect cell changes due to malignancies or inflammatory conditions.

Cytological examination of urine is done when cancer or inflammatory disorders of the urinary tract are suspected. It is especially indicated to detect cancer of the bladder and cytomegalic inclusion disease.[93] In these disorders, abnormal cells are shed into the urine and can be detected upon examination of the sample.

CLINICAL APPLICATIONS DATA

Reference Values

Negative for abnormal cells and inclusions.

Interfering Factors

- Improper specimen collection such that the sample is contaminated with extraneous cells
- Delay in sending the sample to the laboratory (cells may begin to disintegrate)

Indications/Purposes for Cytological Examination of Urine

- Suspected cancer of the bladder or other urinary tract structure, especially in individuals exposed to environmental carcinogens
- Suspected infection with cytomegalovirus

Client Preparation

Client preparation is the same as that for any test involving collection of a clean-catch midstream urine specimen, a catheterized specimen, or a suprapubic aspiration (see Appendix II).

The Procedure

A sample of at least 180 ml in adults and 10 ml in children is obtained either by clean-catch technique, catheterization, or suprapubic aspiration. Depending on the laboratory, a special container and/or preservative may be needed. The sample must be transported to the laboratory immediately.

Aftercare and Nursing Observations

There are no specific aspects of aftercare or nursing observations unless the sample was obtained by suprapubic aspiration. In this case, the aspiration site should be observed for signs of inflammation and should be kept covered with a sterile dressing.

REFERENCES

1. Strasinger, SK: Urinalysis and Body Fluids. FA Davis, Philadelphia, 1985, pp 1–2.
2. *Ibid*, pp 2–3.
3. Bullock, BL and Rosendahl, PP: Pathophysiology: Adaptations and Alterations in Function. Little, Brown & Co, Boston, 1984.
4. Strasinger, *op cit*, p 2.
5. *Ibid*, p 7.
6. Widmann, FK: Clinical Interpretation of Laboratory Tests, ed 9. FA Davis, Philadelphia, 1983, p 504.
7. *Ibid.*
8. Strasinger, *op cit*, p 43.
9. Bradley, M and Schumann, GB: Examination of Urine. In Henry, JB: Clinical Diagnosis and Management by Laboratory Methods, ed 17. WB Saunders, Philadelphia, 1984, p 390.
10. Strasinger, *op cit*, p 43.
11. *Ibid.*, pp 43, 45.
12. Strasinger, *op cit*, pp 45–46.
13. Bradley and Schumann, *op cit*, p 390.
14. *Ibid*, p 392.
15. Strasinger, *op cit*, p 50.
16. *Ibid*, pp 46–47.
17. *Ibid*, p 50.
18. Bradley and Schumann, *op cit*, p 395.
19. Strasinger, *op cit*, p 61.
20. Bradley and Schumann, *op cit*, p 395.
21. *Ibid.*
22. *Ibid*, p 413.
23. *Ibid.*
24. *Ibid*, pp 414–415.
25. Strasinger, *op cit*, p 62.
26. Bradley and Schumann, *op cit*, pp 414, 418.
27. Strasinger, *op cit*, p 62.
28. Hole, JW: Human Anatomy and Physiology, ed 4. William C. Brown, Dubuque, IA, 1987, p 760.
29. Bradley and Schumann, *op cit*, p 412.
30. *Ibid*, pp 402–403.
31. Strasinger, *op cit*, p 67.
32. *Ibid*, p 69.
33. Bradley and Schumann, *op cit*, p 417.
34. *Ibid.*
35. *Ibid.*

350 STUDIES OF URINE

350 STUDIES OF URINE

36. Strasinger, op cit, p 69.
37. Bradley and Schumann, op cit, p 417.
38. Ibid.
39. Strasinger, op cit, p 71.
40. Ibid, p 74.
41. Bradley and Schumann, op cit, p 417.
42. Ibid, pp 416–417.
43. Strasinger, op cit, pp 74–76.
44. Ibid, p 77.
45. Bradley and Schumann, op cit, p 419.
46. Strasinger, op cit, pp 78–79.
47. Bradley and Schumann, op cit, p 419.
48. Strasinger, op cit, p 79.
49. Ibid, pp 88–89.
50. Bradley and Schumann, op cit, p 420.
51. Strasinger, op cit, p 93.
52. Bradley and Schumann, op cit, p 422.
53. Strasinger, op cit, p 94.
54. Bradley and Schumann, op cit, p 423.
55. Ibid, p 424.
56. Ibid.
57. Ibid.
58. Strasinger, op cit, p 95.
59. Bradley and Schumann, op cit, p 425.
60. Strasinger, op cit, p 99.
61. Ibid, p 98.
62. Widmann, op cit, pp 510–511.
63. Strasinger, op cit, pp 22–23.
64. Widmann, op cit, p 249.
65. Ibid, pp 514–517.
66. Ibid, p 518.
67. Strasinger, op cit, p 30.
68. Widmann, op cit, p 519.
69. Strasinger, op cit, p 29.
70. Ibid, p 27.
71. Widmann, op cit, p 521.
72. Strasinger, op cit, p 27.
73. Corbett, JV: Laboratory Tests and Diagnostic Procedures with Nursing Diagnoses, ed 2. Appleton & Lange, Norwalk, CT, 1987, p. 118.
74. Widmann, op cit, p 527.
75. Bradley and Schumann, op cit, p 437.
76. Strasinger, op cit, p 125.
77. Diagnostics, ed 2. Springhouse Corp, Springhouse, PA, 1986, p 374.
78. Ibid, pp 376, 377.
79. Widmann, op cit, p 408.
80. Diagnostics, op cit, pp 394–396.
81. Widmann, op cit, p 425.
82. Diagnostics, op cit, pp 403–404.
83. Widmann, op cit, p 250.
84. Diagnostics, op cit, p 423.
85. Widmann, op cit, p 251.
86. Strasinger, op cit, pp 116–120.
87. Diagnostics, op cit, pp 418–419.
88. Ibid, p 451.
89. Ibid, pp 464–465.
90. Ibid, p 459.
91. Strasinger, op cit, p 127.
92. Widmann, op cit, p 352.
93. Fischbach, FT: A Manual of Laboratory Diagnostics Tests, ed 3. JB Lippincott, Philadelphia, 1988, p 662.

BIBLIOGRAPHY

Beare, PG, Rahr, VA and Ronshausen, CA: Nursing Implications of Diagnostic Tests, ed 2. JB Lippincott, Philadelphia, 1985.

Byrne, CJ, Saxton, DF, Pelikan, PK and Nugent, PM: Laboratory Tests: Implications For Nursing Care. Addison-Wesley, Menlo Park, CA, 1986.

Harvey, AM, Johns, RJ, Owens, AH and Ross, RS: The Principles and Practice of Medicine, ed 19. Appleton-Century-Crofts, New York, 1976.

Lamb, JO: Laboratory Tests for Clinical Nursing. Robert J. Brady Co, Bowie, MD, 1984.

Luckmann, J and Sorensen, KC: Medical-Surgical Nursing: A Psychophysiologic Approach, ed 3. WB Saunders, Philadelphia, 1987.

Michaels, D: Diagnostic Procedures: The Patient and the Health Care Team. John Wiley & Sons, New York, 1983.

Pagana, KD and Pagana, TJ: Diagnostic Testing and Nursing Implications: A Case Study Approach, ed 2. CV Mosby, St Louis, 1986.

Tilkian, SM, Conover, MB and Tilkian AG: Clinical Implications of Laboratory Tests, ed 4. CV Mosby, St Louis, 1987.

Williams, SR: Nutrition and Diet Therapy, ed 4. CV Mosby, St. Louis, 1981.

Widmann, FK: Pathobiology: How Diseases Happen. Little, Brown & Company, Boston, 1978.

7

SPUTUM ANALYSIS

OVERVIEW OF SPUTUM PRODUCTION AND ANALYSIS

Sputum is the material secreted by the tracheobronchial tree and, by definition, brought up by coughing. The submucosal glands and secretory cells of the tracheobronchial mucosa normally secrete up to 100 ml of mucus per day as part of bronchopulmonary cleansing. The secretions form a thin layer over the ciliated epithelial cells and travel upward toward the oropharynx, carrying inhaled particles away from the bronchioles. From the oropharynx the secretions are swallowed; therefore, the healthy person does not produce sputum.

In addition to its mechanical cleansing action, mucus attacks inhaled bacteria directly. This antibacterial effect is due primarily to antibodies, which are predominantly IgA, but also to lysozymes and a slightly acid pH. Normally, the contents of the lower respiratory tract are sterile.

Environmental factors, drugs, and respiratory tract disease alter tracheobronchial secretions and may lead to sputum production. Tobacco smoke, cold air, alcohol, and sedatives depress ciliary action and may cause stasis of secretions. Respiratory infections cause an increase in secretions and may lead to a more acidic pH and changes in the chemical composition. A pH below 6.5 inhibits ciliary action, as does increased sputum viscosity. Leukocytes present in respiratory secretions also rise during infection and membrane permeability increases due to the normal inflammatory response. Thus, antibiotics and other elements normally found in the blood may be present in the sputum. The quantity of sputum produced in pathological states is roughly parallel to the severity

352

of the problem. Specific characteristics and constituents of sputum help to determine the nature of the disorder.[1]

The most common laboratory tests performed on sputum are (1) Gram stain and other staining tests; (2) culture and sensitivity; (3) examination for acid-fast bacillus (AFB); and (4) cytological examination. The gross appearance of the specimen should, however, be observed and documented prior to sending the sample to the laboratory. Respiratory secretions are normally clear, colorless, odorless, and slightly watery.

Abnormal sputum may be described as mucoid (consisting of mucus), mucopurulent (consisting of mucus and pus), and purulent (consisting of pus). Expectoration of mucoid sputum is seen in chronic bronchitis and asthma. A change from mucoid to mucopurulent sputum indicates infection superimposed on the chronic inflammatory condition.[2] Purulent sputum may indicate acute bacterial pneumonia, bronchiectasis, or rupture of a pulmonary abscess. Foul-smelling sputum is associated also with bronchiectasis and lung abscess, as well as with cystic fibrosis. Viscous (tenacious) secretions are seen in clients with cystic fibrosis, *Klebsiella* pneumonia, and dehydration.

Purulent sputum is yellow to green. Gray sputum may indicate inhaled dust; grayish-black sputum is seen following smoke inhalation. Frothy pink or rusty-colored sputum is associated with congestive heart failure. It is abnormal to expectorate blood (hemoptysis), whether the quantity involves only a few scant streaks or a life-threatening hemorrhage. In addition to being associated with congestive heart failure, rusty-colored sputum may be seen also in pneumococcal pneumonia, whereas bright streaks of blood are associated with *Klebsiella* pneumonia. Dark blood in small amounts is associated with tuberculosis, tumors, and trauma due to instrumentation. Bright blood in moderate to large amounts is associated with cavitary tuberculosis, broncholithiasis, and pulmonary thrombosis.

SPUTUM TESTS

Background Information

GRAM STAIN AND OTHER STAINS (Clinical Applications Data, p. 355)

Gram staining is one of the oldest and most useful microbiological staining techniques. It involves smearing a small amount of sputum on a slide and then exposing it to gentian or crystal violet, iodine, alcohol, and safranine, a red dye. This technique allows for morphological examination of the cells contained in the specimen and differentiates any bacteria present into either gram-positive organisms, which retain the iodine stain, or gram-negative organisms, which do not retain the iodine stain but can be counterstained with safranine.

Gram staining may be used to differentiate true sputum from saliva and upper respiratory tract secretions. True sputum contains polymorphonuclear leukocytes and alveolar macrophages. It should also contain a few squamous epithelial cells. Excessive squamous cells or absence of polymorphonuclear leukocytes usually indicates that the specimen is not true sputum.

Gram staining also may provide a tentative determination of the types of leukocytes contained in the specimen. Neutrophils, which are found in infection, may be differentiated from eosinophils, characteristic of asthmatic attacks. Use of other stains such as Wright's stain can provide conclusive distinctions among types of leukocytes.

As noted, Gram staining aids in differentiating gram-positive from gram-negative bacteria. Gram staining may be used also to identify Curschmann's spirals, which are coiled mucous filaments seen in disorders characterized by excessive mucus production accompanied by bronchial obstruction. Curschmann's spirals are most commonly seen in asthmatic attacks, acute bronchitis, and bronchopneumonia but may also be found in sputum arising from small bronchi adjacent to lung carcinoma.[3] Fungi and other microbial parasites also may be identified by Gram staining.

Other stains employed in sputum examinations include periodic acid–Schiff (PAS) and silver stains. PAS stain is used whem pulmonary alveolar proteinosis or *Pneumocystis carinii* pneumonia is suspected. A characteristic of pulmonary alveolar proteinosis is compacted protein, which may be found either inside mononuclear cells, free in round or laminated clumps, or in aggregates with cleftlike spaces. The round and laminated clumps may resemble the cysts of *Pneumocystic carinii*. Although both the protein clumps and the cysts stain PAS-positive, only *Pneumocystis* takes the silver stain.[4]

CULTURE AND SENSITIVITY (C&S) (Clinical Applications Data, p. 358)

Sputum tests for culture and sensitivity indicate the type and number of organisms present in the specimen (culture) and the antibiotics to which the organisms are susceptible (sensitivity). Although examination of the organisms found in sputum by microscopy or stain may lend support to diagnosing suspected infectious disorders, growth of a pathogen in culture is more definitively diagnostic.

The pathogenic organisms most often cultured from the sputum of individuals with bacterial pneumonia are *Streptococcus penumoniae*, *Hemophilus influenzae*, staphylococci, and gram-negative bacilli. Other pathogens that may be identified in sputum cultures include *Klebsiella* pneumonia, *Mycobacterium* tuberculosis, fungi such as *Candida* and *Aspergillus*, *Corynebacterium diphtheriae*, and *Hemophilus* pertussis. In contrast, other organisms that may cause pneumonia such as mycoplasmas, respiratory viruses, and rickettsiae, will not be detected on routine culture.[5] Sputum collected by expectoration or suctioning with catheters and by bronchoscopy cannot be cultured for anaerobic organisms. Instead, transtracheal aspiration or lung biopsy must be used.[6]

Interpretation of the results of sputum cultures requires knowledge of the client's symptomatology and the nature of the pathogen cultured. Pathogens may be identified in the sputum of individuals who do not have pneumonia or whose pneumonia is actually due to an organism not identified on culture. Similarly, a person may be diagnosed as having pneumonia on the basis of sputum cultures, when the infection is due to an obstruction by tumors or foreign bodies, pulmonary infarction, or pulmonary hemorrhage. If *Candida* or *Aspergillus* are found on culture, the client must be further evaluated, as these environmental contaminants may be the cause of serious pulmonary disease.[7] In legionnaires' disease, sputum cultures and Gram staining are negative, despite clinical signs of severe pneumonia. When this disease is suspected, confirmation must be obtained through immunological blood tests (see Chapter 3).[8]

Rapidity of results from sputum cultures varies according to the rate of growth of the organisms. Routine cultures of *Mycobacterium* tuberculosis, for example, may take weeks to become positive. In order to provide more rapid and reliable diagnostic information, some laboratories employ immunological methods such as counterimmunoelectrophoresis (CIEP) to identify microbial pathogens. In CIEP, antibodies specific to the suspected organisms are used, and rapid confirmation of significant tissue involvement is possible.[9] Radioimmunoassay techniques have been used in diagnosing tuberculosis because antigens produced by the organisms can be detected in cultures grown under suitable conditions before recognizable colonies of the organisms appear. This method can significantly reduce delays in diagnosis.

ACID-FAST BACILLUS (AFB) SMEAR AND CULTURE (Clinical Applications Data, p. 358)

The acid-fast staining method is used primarily to identify tubercle bacilli (*Mycobacterium* tuberculosis). Acid-fast bacilli have a cell wall that resists decolorization by acid treatment;[10] that is, they will retain the stain applied to the specimen, a small portion of which is smeared on a slide, even after treatment with an acid-alcohol solution.

Since the tubercle bacillus is slow growing and culture results may take weeks, an acid-fast bacillus (AFB) smear aids in early detection of the organism and timely initiation of antituberculosis therapy. In addition to organisms of the *Mycobacterium* genus, *Nocardia* and *Actinomyces* species may also be identified by acid-fast techniques.

AFB cultures are used to confirm both positive and negative results of AFB smears. By specifying that AFB is the organism to be detected on culture, the laboratory is alerted to the fact that several weeks may be needed for conclusive results. As noted, immunological methods also may be employed in diagnosing tuberculosis by sputum analysis.

CYTOLOGICAL EXAMINATION (Clinical Applications Data, p. 359)

Cytology is the study of the origin, structure, function, and pathology of cells. In clinical practice, cytological examinations are generally performed to detect cell changes due to malignancies or inflammatory conditions. Curschmann's spirals, which may also be demonstrated by Gram staining (see p. 354), may be identified on cytological examination, as may cellular changes due to viral infections and diseases of the lung. In addition, fungi, ova, and parasites may be detected, indicating infection with these organisms. Lipid droplets contained in macrophages may be found on cytological examination and may indicate lipoid or aspiration pneumonia.[11]

Sputum specimens for cytological examination may be collected by expectoration alone, during bronchoscopy, or by expectoration following bronchoscopy. The method of reporting results of cytological examinations varies according to the laboratory performing the test. Terms used to report results include negative (no abnormal cells), inflammatory, benign atypical, suspect for malignancy, and positive for malignancy.

Clinical Applications Data

GRAM STAIN AND OTHER STAINS (Background Information, p. 353)
Reference Values

Normal sputum contains polymorphonuclear leukocytes, alveolar macrophages, and a few squamous epithelial cells.

Interfering Factors

- Improper specimen collection
- Delay in sending specimen to the laboratory

Indications/Purposes for Gram Stain and Other Stains

Gram Stain

■ Differentiation of sputum from upper respiratory tract secretions, the latter being indicated by excessive squamous cells or absence of polymorphonuclear leukocytes
■ Determination of types of leukocytes present in sputum (e.g., neutrophils indicating infection and eosinphils seen in asthma)
■ Differentiation of gram-positive from gram-negative bacteria in respiratory infections
■ Identification of Curschmann's spirals, which are associated with asthma, acute bronchitis, bronchopneumonia, and lung cancer

Wright's Stain

■ Confirmation of the types of leukocytes present in sputum

Periodic Acid–Schiff (PAS) Stain

■ Identification of compacted proteins associated with pulmonary alveolar proteinosis
■ Identification of cysts associated with *Pneumocystis carinii* infections

Silver Stains

■ Confirmation of the presence of cysts associated with *Pneumocystis carinii* infections

Client Preparation

Client Teaching. Explain to the client:

■ the purpose of the sputum examination
■ that results are most reliable if the specimen is obtained upon arising in the morning, after secretions have accumulated overnight
■ that a sample of secretions from deep in the respiratory tract, not saliva or postnasal drainage, is needed
■ the methods by which the specimen will be obtained (i.e., by coughing or by tracheal suctioning)
■ that increasing fluid intake before retiring for the night aids in liquifying secretions and may make them easier to expectorate
■ that humidifying inspired air also helps to liquify secretions
■ that, if feasible, the client should brush the teeth or rinse the mouth prior to obtaining the specimen, to avoid excessive contamination of the specimen with organisms normally found in the mouth
■ proper handling of the container and specimen, if the client is to obtain the specimen independently
■ the number of samples to be obtained, as it may be necessary to analyze more than one sample for accurate diagnosis

Encourage questions and verbalization of concerns appropriate to the client's age and mental status.

Physical Preparation

■ Assist in providing extra fluids, unless contraindicated, and proper humidification
■ Assist with mouth care as needed
■ Provide sputum collection container(s)
■ If the specimen is to be obtained by tracheal suctioning, it is recommended that oxygen be administered for 20 to 30 minutes prior to the procedure

The Procedure

The procedure varies with the method for obtaining the sputum specimen. It should be noted that the nurse should wear gloves, a face mask, and possibly glasses or goggles when obtaining the sputum sample.

Expectorated Specimen. The client should sit upright, with assistance and support (e.g., with an overbed table) as needed. The client should then take two or three deep breaths and cough deeply. Any sputum raised should be expectorated directly into a sterile container. The client should not touch the lip or inside of the container with the hands or mouth. A 10 to 15 ml specimen is adequate.

If the client is unable to produce the desired amount of sputum, several strategies may be attempted. One approach is to have the client drink two glasses of water and then assume the positions for postural drainage of the upper and middle lung segments. Support for effective coughing may be provided by placing the hands or a pillow over the diaphragmatic area and applying slight pressure. Another approach is to place a vaporizer or other humidifying device at the bedside. After sufficient exposure to adequate humidification, postural drainage of the upper and middle lung segments may be repeated before attempting to obtain the specimen.

It may also be helpful to obtain an order for an expectorant and administer it along with additional water approximately 2 hours before attempting to obtain the specimen. In addition, chest percussion and postural drainage of all lung segments may be employed. If the client still is unable to raise sputum, the use of an ultrasonic nebulizer ("induced sputum") may be necessary. This is usually done by a respiratory therapist.

Tracheal Suctioning. Suction equipment, a suction kit, and a Lukens tube or in-line trap are obtained. The client is positioned with head elevated as high as tolerated. Sterile gloves are applied, with the dominant hand maintained as "sterile" and the nondominant hand as "clean." Using the "sterile" hand, the suction catheter is attached to the rubber tubing of the Lukens tube or in-line trap. The suction tubing is then attached to the male adaptor of the trap with the "clean" hand. The suction catheter is lubricated with sterile saline.

Nonintubated clients should be instructed, if feasible, to protrude the tongue and take a deep breath as the suction catheter is passed through the nostril. When the catheter enters the trachea, a reflex cough will be stimulated; the catheter is immediately advanced into the trachea and suction is applied.

Suction should be maintained for approximately 10 seconds and never for more than 15 seconds. The catheter is then withdrawn without applying suction. The suction catheter and suction tubing are separated from the trap, and the rubber tubing is placed over the male adaptor to seal the unit. The specimen is labeled and sent to the laboratory immediately.

For clients who are intubated or have a tracheostomy, the aforementioned procedure is followed, except that the suction catheter is passed through the existing endotracheal or tracheostomy tube rather than through the nostril. The client should be hyperoxygenated before and after the procedure in accordance with usual protocols for suctioning such clients.

Aftercare and Nursing Observations

For specimens obtained by expectoration or nasotracheal suctioning, mouth care should be offered or provided after the specimen has been obtained. A cool beverage also may aid in relieving throat irritation due to coughing and suctioning. The client's color and respiratory rate also should be observed, and supplemental oxygen administered as necessary.

For specimens obtained by endotracheal tube or tracheostomy, the client should be hyperoxygenated after the procedure according to usual protocols. Additional suctioning may be necessary to clear secretions raised during suctioning to obtain the specimen.

The characteristics (e.g., color, consistency, volume) of the sample should be noted and documented.

CULTURE AND SENSITIVITY (C&S) (Background Information, p. 354)

Reference Values

Normal respiratory flora include *Neisseria catarrhalis*, *Candida albicans*, diphtheroids, alpha-hemolytic streptococci, and some staphylococci.

Interfering Factors

- Improper specimen collection
- Delay in sending specimen to the laboratory

Indications/Purposes for Culture and Sensitivity

- Support for diagnosing the cause of respiratory infection as indicated by presence or absence (e.g., viral infections, legionnaires' disease) of organisms in culture
- Confirmatory diagnosis of tuberculosis (see also AFB smear and culture)
- Monitoring response to treatment for respiratory infections, especially tuberculosis
- Identification of antibiotics to which the cultured organism is sensitive

Client Preparation

Client preparation is the same as that for any test involving collection of sputum or lower respiratory secretions (see p. 356).

The Procedure

The procedures for obtaining the specimen are the same as those described on page 357.

Aftercare and Nursing Observations

Care and assessment following the procedure are the same as those for any test involving collection of sputum or lower respiratory secretions. Depending on the nature of the suspected or confirmed infection, respiratory isolation or drainage/secretion precautions may be employed, although these infection control protocols may have been implemented already, prior to obtaining sputum cultures.

ACID-FAST BACILLUS (AFB) SMEAR AND CULTURE (Background Information, p. 355)

Reference Values

Negative for AFB.

Interfering Factors

■ Improper specimen collection
■ Delay in sending specimen to the laboratory

Indications/Purposes for Acid-Fast Bacillus Smear and Culture

■ Suspected pulmonary tuberculosis
■ Monitoring response to treatment for pulmonary tuberculosis

Client Preparation

Client preparation is the same as that for any test involving collection of sputum or lower respiratory secretions (see p. 356). The client should be informed that it may be several weeks before culture results are available.

The Procedure

The procedures for obtaining the specimen are the same as those described on page 357.

Aftercare and Nursing Observations

Care and assessment following the procedure are the same as those for any test involving collection of sputum or lower respiratory secretions. If tuberculosis is suspected, the client may be placed on AFB or respiratory isolation, pending AFB smear results.

CYTOLOGICAL EXAMINATION (Background Information, p. 355)

Reference Values

Negative for abnormal cells, Curschmann's spirals, fungi, ova and parasites.

Interfering Factors

■ Improper specimen collection
■ Delay in sending specimen to the laboratory

Indications/Purposes for Cytologic Examination

■ Suspected lung cancer
■ History of cigarette smoking, which may lead to metaplastic (nonmalignant) cellular changes
■ History of acute or chronic inflammatory or infectious lung disorders, which may lead to benign atypical or metaplastic cellular changes
■ Known or suspected viral disease involving the lung
■ Known or suspected fungal or parasitic infection involving the lung

Client Preparation

Client preparation is the same as that for any test involving collection of sputum or lower respiratory secretions (see p. 356)

The Procedure

The procedures for obtaining the specimen are the same as those described on page 357. It is common practice to collect three sputum specimens for cytological examination, usually on three separate mornings. Following bronchoscopy, however, serial specimens may be obtained from sputum expectorated within 12 to 24 hours of the procedure. Specimens are collected either in sterile containers or sterile containers to which 50 percent alcohol has been added, depending on specific laboratory procedures.

Aftercare and Nursing Observations

Care and assessment following the procedure are the same as that for any test involving collection of sputum or lower respiratory secretions.

REFERENCES

1. Widmann, FK: Clinical Interpretation of Laboratory Tests, ed 9. FA Davis, Philadelphia, 1983, pp 565–566.
2. *Ibid,* p 567.
3. *Ibid,* p 570.
4. *Ibid,* pp 569–570.
5. *Ibid,* p 569.
6. *Ibid,* p 350.
7. *Ibid,* pp 568–569.
8. *Ibid,* p 351.
9. *Ibid,* p 569.
10. *Ibid,* p 343.
11. *Ibid,* p 570.

BIBLIOGRAPHY

Beare, PG, Rahr, VA and Ronshausen, CA: Nursing Implications of Diagnostic Tests, ed 2. JB Lippincott, Philadelphia, 1985.
Braunstein, H: Outlines of Pathology. CV Mosby, St Louis, 1982.
Byrne, CJ, Saxton, DF, Pelikan, PK and Nugent, PM: Laboratory Tests: Implications for Nursing Care. Addison-Wesley, Menlo Park, CA, 1986.
Diagnostics, ed 2. Springhouse Corp, Springhouse, PA, 1986.
Fischbach, FT: A Manual of Laboratory Diagnostic Tests, ed 3. JB Lippincott, Philadelphia, 1988.
Groer, MW and Shekleton, ME: Basic Pathophysiology: A Conceptual Approach, ed 2. CV Mosby, St Louis, 1983.
Guyton, AC: Textbook of Medical Physiology, ed 6. WB Saunders, Philadelphia, 1981.
Harvey, AM, Johns, RJ, Owens, AH and Ross, RS: The Principles and Practice of Medicine, ed 19. Appleton-Century-Crofts, New York, 1976.
Lamb, JO: Laboratory Tests for Clinical Nursing. Robert J Brady, Bowie, MD, 1984.
Luckmann, J and Sorensen, KC: Medical-Surgical Nursing: A Psychophysiologic Approach, ed 3. WB Saunders, Philadelphia, 1987.
Michaels, D: Diagnostic Procedures: The Patient and the Health Care Team. John Wiley & Sons, New York, 1983.
Price, SA and Wilson, LM: Pathophysiology: Clinical Concepts of Disease Processes, ed 3. McGraw-Hill, New York, 1986.
Selkurt, EE: Basic Physiology for the Health Sciences, ed 2. Little, Brown & Co, Boston, 1982.
Widmann, FK: Pathobiology: How Diseases Happen. Little, Brown & Co, Boston, 1978.

8

CEREBROSPINAL FLUID ANALYSIS

OVERVIEW OF CEREBROSPINAL FLUID FORMATION AND ANALYSIS

Cerebrospinal fluid (CSF) is secreted into the ventricles of the brain by specialized capillaries called choroid plexuses. Most of the cerebral spinal fluid arises in the lateral ventricles, although additional amounts are secreted in the third and fourth ventricles. CSF formed in the ventricles circulates into the central canal of the spinal cord and also enters the subarachnoid space through an opening in the wall of the fourth ventricle near the cerebellum, after which it circulates around the brain and spinal cord. Although 500 to 800 ml of CSF are formed daily, only 125 to 140 ml are normally present. Thus, almost all of the CSF formed is reabsorbed via arachnoid granulations, which project from the subarachnoid space into the venous sinuses, and is subsequently returned to the venous circulation. The functions of CSF include cushioning the brain against shocks and blows, maintaining a stable concentration of ions in the central nervous system (CNS), and providing for removal of wastes.[1,2]

CSF is produced by the processes of filtration, diffusion, osmosis, and active transport. Initially, sodium is actively transported into the CSF; then water follows passively by osmosis. Facilitated diffusion allows glucose to move between the blood and CSF. Although similar in composition to plasma, CSF generally contains more sodium and chloride and less potassium, calcium, and glucose.

Most constituents of CSF will, however, parallel those found in plasma and are found in amounts equal to or slightly less than those in the blood.[3,4]

In addition to entering CSF via the choroid plexuses, substances may pass into CSF from the blood through capillaries in the parenchyma and meninges of the brain and spinal cord. "Barriers" exist between the blood and the CSF and between the brain and the CSF. That is, substances do not pass as readily into the CSF as they would pass into extracellular fluid through other capillary beds. Water, carbon dioxide, oxygen, glucose, small molecules, lipid-soluble substances, nonionized substances, and some drugs (e.g., erythromycin and sulfadiazine) pass rapidly into CSF, whereas large molecules, ionized substances, various toxins, and certain other drugs (e.g., chlortetracyclines and penicillins) do not pass readily into CSF.[5]

Under pathological conditions, elements normally held back by the "blood-brain barrier" may enter CSF. Red cells and white cells can enter the CSF either from rupture of vessels or from meningeal reaction to irritation. Unconjugated (prehepatic) bilirubin may be found after intracranial hemorrhage, while conjugated bilirubin may be found if the circulating plasma contains large amounts. Fibrinogen, which is normally absent from CSF, may be found along with albumin and globulins when inflammatory disorders cause increased permeability of the blood-brain barrier. Urea, lactic acid, and glutamine levels in CSF will rise if plasma levels of these or related substances are elevated. Bacteria and fungi found in CSF indicate infection with these organsims.[6]

Samples of CSF are obtained by lumbar puncture (spinal tap) but may be obtained by cisternal or ventricular puncture if lumbar puncture is contraindicated or hazardous because of bony abnormalities or infection at the lumbar area or, in cases of increased intracranial pressure, when a lumbar puncture may predispose to brainstem herniation. All methods of obtaining CSF samples should be performed with extreme caution, if at all, in clients with bleeding disorders.

As a general rule, at least three tubes of 3 to 10 ml of CSF are withdrawn for analysis and are labeled according to the order in which each is obtained. Routine CSF analysis includes a cell count and differential, as well as determinations of protein and glucose levels. In addition, CSF may be analyzed for electrolytes, lactic acid, urea, glutamine, and enzymes. Microbiological studies of CSF include culture and sensitivity, Gram stain and other stains, acid-fast bacillus (AFB) smear and culture, and the Limulus assay for gram-negative bacteria. Cytological examination for malignant cells, as well as serological tests for syphilis, may be performed on CSF.

The gross appearance, opening pressure, and closing pressure should be noted during the procedure and documented. The pH of the sample also may be noted. CSF is normally clear, colorless, and the consistency of water. Turbidity indicates the presence of a significant number of leukocytes (i.e., greater than 200 to 500 white cells per mm^3). Yellowish discoloration of CSF (xanthochromia) usually indicates previous bleeding but may also be seen when CSF protein levels are greatly elevated. Fresh blood in the specimen may be due to traumatic spinal tap, although clearing should be noted as the second and third tubes are withdrawn if this is the case. Bleeding from a traumatic tap adds approximately 1 to 2 white cells and 1 mg/dl of protein for every 1000 red cells per mm^3 contained in the sample. If blood does not clear as subsequent samples are obtained, bleeding due to a subarachnoid hemorrhage is usually indicated. Brown CSF generally indicates a chronic subdural hematoma with CSF stained from methemalbumin.[7]

As fibrinogen is normally absent from CSF, the sample should not clot. Clotting may occur, however, when the protein content of the sample is elevated. In conditions involving spinal subarachnoid block, CSF may be yellow and have a tendency toward rapid spontaneous clotting. The pH of CSF is normally slightly lower than that of blood, with a range of 7.32 to 7.35 when arterial blood pH is within normal limits.[8]

It should be noted that CSF specimens must be transported to the laboratory immediately. Within 1 hour of collection, any red cells contained in the sample begin to lyze and may cause spurious coloration of the specimen. Neutrophils and malignant cells also may disintegrate in a short time. Bacteria and other cells will continue to metabolize glucose, such that delays in analysis may alter chemical values.[9]

CSF pressure in the lumbar area ranges from 75 to 200 mm of water in adults, with an average of 120 mm, and from 50 to 100 mm of water in children. The opening pressure (OP) is measured after the spinal needle is determined to be in the subarachnoid space. CSF pressure may be elevated if clients are anxious and hold their breath or tense their muscles. It also may be elevated if there is venous compression such as may occur if the client's knees are flexed too firmly against the abdomen. Significant elevations in CSF pressure may occur with intracranial tumors and with purulent or tuberculous meningitis. Less marked increases (i.e., 250 to 500 mm of water) are associated with low-grade inflammatory processes, encephalitis, or neurosyphilis. Decreases in CSF pressure are rare but may occur with dehydration, high obstruction to CSF flow, or previous aspiration of spinal fluid.[10]

The closing pressure (CP) is recorded prior to removal of the spinal needle from the subarachnoid space. Normally, CSF pressure will decrease 5 to 10 mm of water for every milliliter of CSF withdrawn. The expected decrease in CSF pressure will not occur in disorders in which the total quantity of CSF is increased (e.g., hydrocephalus). In contrast, a large drop in pressure indicates a small CSF pool and is seen in tumors or spinal block.[11]

CEREBROSPINAL FLUID TESTS

Background Information

ROUTINE CEREBROSPINAL FLUID (CSF) ANALYSIS (Clinical Applications Data, p. 367)

Routine CSF analysis includes a cell count and differential, as well as determinations of protein and glucose levels. CSF also may be analyzed for electrolytes, lactic acid, urea, glutamine, and enzymes.

Cell Count and Differential

Normal spinal fluid is free of cells, although five small lymphocytes per mm^3 may normally be found in adults, with as many as 20 small lymphocytes per mm^3 in children. Granulocytes, large mononuclear cells and red blood cells should not be present. When cells are found in CSF, they should be identified as to type. A cell count of 10 to 200 that consists mostly of lymphocytes indicates viral meningitis, late neurosyphilis, multiple sclerosis, tumor, or cerebral thrombosis. A cell count of 200 to 500 consisting mostly of lymphocytes, or of lymphocytes and granulocytes, indicates tuberculous meningitis, choriomeningitis, herpes infection of the CNS, or acute syphilitic meningitis. If a large number of blast cells are found, CNS leukemia is indicated. A cell count of more than

500 that is composed largely of granulocytes indicates acute bacterial meningitis.[12] It should be noted that cryptococcal organisms in the sample may be mistaken for small lymphocytes.

Proteins

CSF normally contains very little protein because most proteins cannot cross the blood-brain barrier. In addition to determining the amount of protein present in CSF, levels of certain types of protein also may be measured. Albumin, for example, is a relatively small molecule and may pass more easily into CSF. For this reason, the albumin/globulin (A/G) ratio is normally higher in CSF than in serum. Protein electrophoresis also may be performed on CSF samples.

The protein concentration in CSF may rise as a result of increased permeability of the blood-barrier due to inflammation and infection. Slight elevations of CSF protein (i.e., less than 100 mg/dl) may be seen in multiple sclerosis. Mild elevations in CSF protein (up to 300 mg/dl) may be seen in viral meningitis, neurosyphilis, subdural hematoma, cerebral thrombosis, and brain tumor. Moderate or pronounced elevations are associated with acute bacterial meningitis, tuberculous meningitis, spinal cord tumor, cerebral hemorrhage, intracranial tumor (e.g., acoustic neuroma and meningioma), and Guillain-Barré syndrome (ascending polyneuritis). Elevation in CSF protein levels without an increase in cell count is associated with degenerative diseases of the CNS such as multiple sclerosis and neurosyphilis. In these disorders, the globulin and IgG content of CSF also may be elevated. CSF protein levels also may be elevated in clients with diabetes mellitus and cardiovascular disease owing to increased permeability of the blood-brain barrier.[13]

Glucose

The glucose concentration of CSF is normally 50 to 80 percent of the blood glucose level obtained 30 to 60 minutes before the CSF sample is withdrawn. Because all types of organisms consume glucose, levels will be decreased if the CSF contains bacteria, fungi, protozoa, or tubercle bacilli. It should be noted, however, that this decrease is not as pronounced or may not be seen at all in viral meningitis.

In addition to findings in viral meningitis, CSF glucose levels may be relatively unchanged in neurosyphilis, brain or cord tumors, cerebral thrombosis, multiple sclerosis and polyneuritis. Moderate reductions in CSF glucose are associated with CNS leukemia, cancer involving the meninges, subarachnoid hemorrhage, and partially treated bacterial or fungal meningitis. Pronounced decreases, sometimes as low as zero, are seen in bacterial, tuberculous, and fungal meningitis. As noted on page 363, bacterial and other cells present in CSF will continue to metabolize glucose even after the sample has been collected. Thus, spuriously low glucose levels may be found in CSF if analysis is delayed.

Other Substances

Other substances for which CSF may be analyzed include electrolytes, lactic acid, urea, glutamine, and enzymes. The electrolyte levels found in CSF are similar to those of plasma, with the exceptions of sodium and chloride, which are higher, and potassium and calcium, which are lower. The significance of electrolyte levels in CSF is questionable. Some writers, for example, indicate that chlorides are decreased in tuberculosis and bacterial meningitis.[14,15] Others state that chloride levels provide no specific diagnostic information.[16] The calcium found in CSF is that fraction not bound by protein and is about half that of serum levels. Calcium levels rise with CSF protein levels; however, it is more important to determine the protein level in such cases than to measure calcium.[17]

Lactic acid in CSF reflects local glycolytic activity and adds to diagnostic information when results of other analyses are inconclusive. Severe systemic lactic acidosis will cause CSF lactate to rise accordingly. Elevated CSF lactate without a parallel elevation in serum level, indicates increased CSF glucose metabolism, which is usually due to bacterial or fungal meningitis. In early or partially treated bacterial or fungal meningitis, CSF cell count and glucose levels may be similar to those found in viral meningitis or noninfectious conditions. Lactate levels above 35 mg/dl rarely occur, however, unless the client has bacterial or fungal meningitis. Lactate levels will remain elevated until the individual has received effective antiobiotic therapy for several days. Persistent elevation of CSF lactate levels indicates inadequate treatment of meningitis.[18]

Urea levels in CSF and blood are approximately equal; thus, CSF urea levels will rise when blood levels are elevated, as in uremia. Urea is sometimes administered intravenously to lower intracranial pressure. In such cases, the subsequent elevation in CSF urea levels causes fluid to shift from the brain to the CSF. CSF urea levels may remain elevated for 24 to 48 hours after intravenous administration of urea. Glutamine is synthesized in the CNS from ammonia and glutamic acid. CSF glutamine levels rise when blood ammonia levels are high, a situation seen in cirrhosis with altered hepatic blood flow and encephalopathy. It has been found that glutamine levels in CSF correlate as well or better than blood ammonia levels with the degree of hepatic encephalopathy. Enzymes that have been measured in CSF include lactic dehydrogenase (LDH), alanine aminotransferase (ALT, SGPT), and aspartate aminotransferase (AST, SGOT). Levels of these enzymes are normally lower than those found in the blood. CSF enzymes may rise in inflammatory, hemorrhagic, or degenerative diseases of the CNS. CSF enzyme levels, however, are not measured under routine conditions and may not add to the diagnostic information obtained from more routinely available tests.[19]

MICROBIOLOGICAL EXAMINATION OF CSF (Clinical Applications Data, p. 370)

Microbiological studies of CSF include culture and sensitivity, Gram stain and other stains, acid-fast bacillus (AFB) smear and culture, and the Limulus assay for gram-negative bacteria.

Numerous microorganisms may cause meningitis, encephalitis, and brain abscess. Thus, whenever central nervous system (CNS) infection is suspected, CSF should be cultured for the presence of bacteria, fungi, protozoa, and tubercle bacilli, as it is possible that more than one organism is present.[20] CSF rarely contains abundant organisms, so specimens for microbiological examination must be collected and handled with strict aseptic technique. The usual laboratory procedure is to centrifuge a few milliliters of CSF to concentrate any organisms present. After culture plates with several different media are inoculated, the remaining CSF sediment is examined with Gram staining and AFB staining techniques (see Chapter 7).[21]

Failure to isolate organisms on stained smear does not necessarily mean that organisms are absent from the CSF sample. Reliably positive results are obtained only when at least 10^5 bacteria per milliliter are present. Gram stains, for example, are positive in only 80 to 90 percent of individuals with untreated meningitis. CSF is almost routinely examined and cultured for AFB in situations when the cause of the CNS disorder is unknown, since tuberculous meningitis can develop insidiously and presents with few clear diagnostic indicators.[22]

When infection with the fungus *Cryptococcus* is suspected, the specimen may be examined by adding India ink to the specimen or by suspending a portion of the sample in the nonparticulate product, nigrosin. Both substances aid in visualizing the round, transparent, encapsulated yeasts characteristic of such cryptococcal infections. It should be noted that India ink and nigrosin examinations may be negative in up to 50 percent of cases of cryptococcal meningitis. A newer and more reliable approach involves testing for cryptococcal antigen.[23] The cryptococcal antigen test, in which a strong anticryptococcal antibody is employed, may elicit antigenic elements even when cryptococcal organisms are undetected by other methods.[24]

Amebae also may cause meningitis, especially in individuals who swim in lakes or indoor swimming pools. A wet-mount preparation of CSF is examined for motile cells when such an infection is suspected.[25]

As noted, spinal fluid is normally cultured on several different media. The meningococcus *(Neisseria meningitidis)*, for example, prefers to grow in a medium with a high carbon dioxide atmosphere. Sometimes a portion of the original sample is incubated at normal body temperature for 24 hours to allow any organisms present to multiply. A second set of cultures is then prepared. Counterimmunoelectrophoresis also may be used to detect bacterial antigens when usual techniques fail to demonstrate bacteria in CSF.[26]

The presence of gram-negative organisms in CSF may be demonstrated rapidly with the Limulus assay. This test uses the bloodlike fluid of the horseshoe crab of the genus *Limulus,* which is coagulated by gram-negative endotoxins. This test, therefore, provides a quick means of diagnosing gram-negative infections of the CNS and gram-negative endotoxemia. The test is more reliable when performed on CSF than when performed on blood.[27]

Acute bacterial meningitis occurs most commonly in children younger than age 5 and in adults who have experienced head trauma. Gram-negative bacilli *(Escherichia coli)* are the usual etiological agents of meningitis in premature infants and newborns. In young children, meningitis is most frequently caused by gram-positive cocci (streptococci and staphylococci), gram-negative cocci (meningococci), and gram-negative bacilli *(Hemophilus influenzae).* In adults, meningitis also may be caused by pneumococcus. Viral infections, tuberculous meningitis, and fungal and protozoal infections may occur at any age and often present as insidious or misleading syndromes.[28]

CYTOLOGICAL EXAMINATION OF CSF (Clinical Applications Data, p. 371)

Cytological examination of CSF is performed primarily to detect malignancies involving the central nervous system (CNS). Cellular changes due to malignancies whose primary site is the CNS (e.g., brain tumors) or malignancies that have metastasized to the CNS from other sites (e.g., breast and lung) may be detected. Abnormal cells due to acute leukemia involving the CNS also may be seen.

SEROLOGICAL TESTS FOR NEUROSYPHILIS (Clinical Applications Data, p. 372)

When syphilis involving the CNS (neurosyphilis) is suspected, serological tests are performed on samples of CSF. Blood tests for syphilis (see Chapter 3) consist of two main types: (1) nonspecific tests that demonstrate syphilitic reagin and (2) specific tests that demonstrate antitreponemal antibodies. Reagin tests include the Wasserman and Reiter complement fixation tests, and the

Venereal Disease Research Laboratory (VDRL) and rapid plasma reagin (RPR) flocculation tests. The best specific test is the fluorescent treponemal antibody (FTA) test.

Nonspecific reagin tests are usually used for routine testing of CSF, as they are cheaper and more readily available. The false-positive results that may occur when blood is tested with reagin tests occur fairly rarely in CSF specimens. Nonspecific tests are, however, less sensitive than the FTA test. Thus, if neurosyphilis is a serious diagnostic consideration, the FTA is the test of choice.[29]

Clinical Applications Data

ROUTINE CEREBROSPINAL FLUID (CSF) ANALYSIS (Background Information, p. 363)

Reference Values

Cell Count and Differential	
Children	Up to 20 small lymphocytes/mm^3
Adults	Up to 5 small lymphocytes/mm^3
Protein	
Total Proteins	15–45 mg/dl (lumbar area) or less than 1% of serum levels
Albumin/Globulin (A/G) Ratio	8:1
IgG	3–12% of total protein
Glucose	40–80 mg/dl or less than 50–80% of blood glucose level 30 to 60 min earlier
Electrolytes	
Chloride	118–132 mEq/l
Calcium	2.1–2.7 mEq/l
Sodium	144–154 mEq/l
Potassium	2.4–3.1 mEq/l
Lactic acid	10–20 mg/dl
Urea	10–15 mg/dl
Glutamine	Less than 20 mg/dl
Lactic dehydrogenase (LDH)	$\frac{1}{10}$ that of serum level

Interfering Factors

■ Delay in transporting sample to the laboratory (may cause spurious discoloration due to lysis of any red cells present, disintegration of any neutrophils present, and false decrease in glucose due to continued utilization by cells in the sample)

■ Blood in the sample due to traumatic tap (adds 1 to 2 white cells and 1 mg/dl of protein for every 1000 red cells/mm^3 contained in the sample)

Indications/Purposes for Routine CSF Analysis

■ Suspected viral meningitis, cerebral thrombosis, or brain tumor as indicated by a cell count of 10 to 200/mm^3, consisting mostly of lymphocytes, a mild elevation (to 300 mg/dl) in total proteins, and normal or slightly decreased glucose level

■ Suspected multiple sclerosis or neurosyphilis as indicated by a normal or

slightly elevated cell count, consisting mostly of lymphocytes, slightly elevated protein, slightly elevated globulins, elevated IgG on protein electrophoresis, and a normal or slightly decreased glucose level
■ Suspected acute bacterial meningitis as indicated by a cell count of greater than 500/mm^3, consisting largely of granulocytes, moderately or pronounced elevation in protein (greater than 300 mg/dl), pronounced decrease in glucose, and decreased chloride
■ Suspected tuberculous meningitis as indicated by a cell count of 200 to 500/mm^3, consisting of lymphocytes or mixed lymphocytes and granulocytes, moderate or pronounced elevation in proteins, pronounced reduction in glucose, and decreased chloride
■ Suspected early bacterial or fungal meningitis as indicated by CSF lactate level above 35 mg/dl, even when cell count and glucose level are only slightly altered
■ Evaluation of effectiveness of treatment for bacterial or fungal meningitis, with effective treatment indicated by decreasing lactate levels after several days of antimicrobial therapy
■ Suspected CNS leukemia as indicated by a cell count of 200 to 500/mm^3, consisting mainly of blast cells, and a moderate reduction in glucose
■ Suspected spinal cord tumor as indicated by a cell count of 10 to 200/mm^3, moderate or pronounced elevation in protein, and normal or slightly decreased glucose
■ Support for diagnosing subarachnoid hemorrhage as indicated by the presence of red blood cells, elevated proteins, and a moderate reduction in glucose
■ Support for diagnosing hepatic encephalopathy as indicated by elevated glutamine levels
■ Support for diagnosing Guillain-Barré syndrome (ascending polyneuritis) as indicated by pronounced elevation in proteins

Client Preparation

Client Teaching. Explain to the client:

■ the purpose of the test
■ that it will be done by a physician and will require 20 to 30 minutes
■ the positioning used for the procedure and the necessity of remaining still during it
■ that a local anesthetic will be injected at the needle insertion site
■ that the needle is inserted below the area where the spinal cord ends (for lumbar punctures)
■ that a sensation of pressure may be felt when the needle is inserted
■ the necessity of remaining flat in bed for 6 to 8 hours after the procedure (for lumbar punctures), and that turning from side to side is permitted as long as the head is not raised
■ that taking fluids following the procedure will aid in returning the CSF volume to normal (provided that this is not contraindicated for the particular client)

Encourage questions and verbalization of concerns appropriate to the client's age and mental status. Ensure that a signed consent for the procedure has been obtained.

Physical Preparation

■ Have the client void
■ Provide a hospital gown
■ Take and record vital signs

The Procedure

The necessary equipment is assembled (e.g., lumbar puncture tray). The client is assisted to a sidelying position, with the head flexed as far as comfortable and the knees drawn up toward, but not pressing on, the abdomen. Support in maintaining this position may be provided by placing one hand on the back of the client's neck and the other behind the knees. Lumbar punctures also may be performed with the client seated, while leaning forward with arms resting on an overbed table or other support.

The lumbar area is cleansed with an antiseptic and protected with sterile drapes. The skin is infiltrated with a local anesthetic and the spinal needle with stylet is inserted into a vertebral interspace between L2 to S1, usually L3–L4 or L4–L5. The stylet is then removed, and if the needle is properly positioned in the subarachnoid space, spinal fluid will drip from the needle. A sterile stopcock and manometer are then attached to the needle. The opening pressure is read (see p. 363), and if indicated, the Queckenstedt test is performed. It should be noted that when the needle and manometer are properly positioned, the CSF level should fluctuate several millimeters with respiration.[30]

The Queckenstedt test is based on the principle that a change in pressure in one area of the closed system—composed of the ventricular spaces, intracranial subarachnoid space, and vertebral subarachnoid space—will be reflected in other areas of the system as well. The test is indicated when total or partial spinal block (e.g., due to tumor) is suspected and is performed by compressing both jugular veins while monitoring lumbar CSF pressure. Temporary occlusion of the jugular veins impairs the absorption of intracranial fluid and produces an acute rise in CSF pressure. If CSF flow is unimpeded, the pressure elevation will be transmitted to the lumbar area, and the fluid level in the manometer will rise. Total or partial spinal block is diagnosed if the CSF pressure fails to rise or if more than 20 seconds are required for the pressure to return to the pretest level after pressure on the jugular veins is released. The Queckenstedt test is risky in clients with increased intracranial pressure of highly reactive carotid body receptors. Radiological examinations such as myelograms and CAT scans may give more information and carry less risk.[31]

The manometer is then removed and CSF is allowed to drip into three sterile test tubes, 3 to 10 ml per tube. The tubes are numbered in order of filling, labeled with the client's name, and sent to the laboratory immediately. The manometer may then be reattached and the closing pressure recorded. The spinal needle is removed, and pressure is applied to the site. If no excessive bleeding or CSF leakage are noted, an adhesive bandage is applied to the site and the client is assisted to a recumbent position.

Alternatives to the lumbar puncture include cisternal and ventricular punctures. These procedures may be employed when lumbar puncture is not feasible because of bony abnormalities or infection at the lumbar area. For a cisternal puncture, the client is assisted to a sidelying position with the neck flexed and the head resting on the chest. The back of the neck may need to be shaved prior to the procedure. After the skin is infiltrated with local anesthetic, the needle is inserted at the base of the occiput, between the first cervical vertebra and the foramen magnum. CSF samples are then obtained in the same manner as for lumbar punctures. Cisternal punctures are considered somewhat hazardous, as the needle is inserted close to the brainstem; however, clients are said to be less likely to experience postprocedure headaches and may resume usual activities within a few hours of the procedure.[32,33]

Ventricular punctures are surgical procedures (i.e., usually performed in an operating room) in which CSF samples are obtained directly from one of the lateral ventricles in the brain. For this procedure, a scalp incision is made and a burr hole is drilled in the occipital area of the skull. The needle is then inserted through the hole and into the lateral ventricle, and CSF samples are obtained. This procedure is rarely performed.[34]

It should be noted that the cell count and protein content of CSF samples obtained by cisternal or ventricular punctures are normally lower than those found in lumbar samples. The higher levels of cells and protein found in CSF from lumbar punctures are thought to be due to stagnation of CSF, which occurs in the lumbar sac.[35]

Aftercare

The client is assisted to a recumbent position and should remain flat for 6 to 8 hours following the procedure to prevent the occurrence of a headache. The client should be reminded that turning from side to side is permitted, so long as the head is not raised. The client should be assisted to take liberal amounts of fluids, unless otherwise contraindicated. Assistance with eating and elimination also should be provided.

Care following cisternal and ventricular punctures is essentially the same as that for lumbar punctures. For cisternal punctures, bed rest is necessary for only 2 to 4 hours, after which usual activities may be resumed. For ventricular punctures, bed rest usually is required for 24 hours.

Nursing Observations

Pretest

■ Assess the client's response to explanations provided; if the client is extremely anxious or verbalizes complaints related to previous lumbar punctures, the physician performing the procedure should be so informed
■ Take and record vital signs
■ Assess level of consciousness

During the Test

■ Note any distress, especially dyspnea, that may be caused by positioning
■ Observe for signs of brainstem herniation such as decreased level of consciousness, irregular respirations, and a unilaterally dilating pupil (uncal herniation)

Post-Test

■ Take and record vital signs every hour for the first 4 hours and then every 4 hours for 24 hours (for hospitalized clients)
■ Perform a neurological check each time vital signs are taken
■ Assess the puncture site for bleeding, CSF drainage, and inflammation each time vital signs are taken during the first 24 hours, and daily thereafter for several days (family members or support persons should be instructed to do this for nonhospitalized clients)
■ Observe for signs of meningeal irritation such as fever, nuchal rigidity, and irritability
■ Assess the client's comfort level, noting presence or absence of headache

MICROBIOLOGICAL EXAMINATION OF CSF (Background Information, p. 365)

Reference Values

Organisms are not normally present in CSF.

Interfering Factors

■ Delay in transporting the sample to the laboratory (organisms may disintegrate if the sample is held at room temperature for more than 1 hour)
■ Contamination of the sample with normal skin flora or other organisms due to improper collection or handling of the sample

Indications/Purposes for Microbiological Examination of CSF

■ Suspected meningitis, encephalitis, or brain abscess
■ CNS disorder of unknown etiology without clear diagnostic indicators
■ Head trauma with possible resultant CNS infection

Client Preparation

Client preparation is the same as that for any test involving collection of CSF samples (see p. 368).

The Procedure

The procedures for obtaining the specimen are the same as those described on pages 369 to 370. Extreme care must be used in obtaining and collecting the sample, so as not to contaminate the sample or introduce organisms into the CNS.

Aftercare and Nursing Observations

Care and assessment following the procedure are the same as those for any test involving collection of a CSF sample (see p. 370). Depending on the nature of the suspected or confirmed infection, infectious disease precautions may be implemented.

CYTOLOGICAL EXAMINATION OF CSF (Background Information, p. 366)

Reference Values

No abnormal cells.

Interfering Factors

■ Delay in transporting the sample to the laboratory (cells may disintegrate if the sample is held at room temperature for more than 1 hour)
■ Contamination of the sample with skin cells

Indications/Purposes for Cytological Examination of CSF

■ Suspected malignancy with primary site in the CNS
■ Suspected metastasis of malignancies to the CNS
■ Suspected CNS involvement in acute leukemia

Client Preparation

Client preparation is the same as that for any test involving collection of CSF samples (see p. 368).

The Procedure

The procedures for obtaining the specimen are the same as those described on pages 369 to 370. Care must be taken not to contaminate the sample with skin cells.

Aftercare and Nursing Observations

Care and assessment following the procedure are the same as those for any test involving collection of a CSF sample (see p. 370).

SEROLOGICAL TESTS FOR NEUROSYPHILIS (Background Information, p. 366)

Reference Values

Negative.

Interfering Factors

■ Delay in transporting the sample to the laboratory (organisms may disintegrate if the sample is held at room temperature for more than 1 hour)

Indications/Purpose for Serological Tests

■ Suspected neurosyphilis

Client Preparation

Client preparation is the same as that for any test involving collection of CSF samples (see p. 368).

The Procedure

The procedures for obtaining the specimen are the same as those described on pages 369 to 370.

Aftercare and Nursing Observations

Care and assessment following the procedure are the same as those for any test involving collection of a CSF sample (see p. 370).

REFERENCES

1. Hole, JW: Human Anatomy and Physiology, ed 4. Wm C Brown, Dubuque, IA, 1987, p 366.
2. Bullock, BL and Rosendahl, PP: Pathophysiology: Adaptations and Alterations in Function. Little, Brown & Co, Boston, 1984, pp 647–650.
3. *Ibid*, p 647.
4. Widmann, FK: Clinical Interpretation of Laboratory Tests, ed 9. FA Davis, Philadelphia, 1983, p 537.
5. Bullock and Rosendahl, *op cit*, pp 651–652.
6. Widmann, *op cit*, pp 537–538, 541, 543–544, 547.

7. *Ibid*, p 540.
8. *Ibid*, pp 539–541.
9. *Ibid*, p 550.
10. *Ibid*, p 541.
11. *Ibid*, p 542.
12. *Ibid*, pp 542–543.
13. *Ibid*, pp 543–544.
14. Fischbach, FT: A Manual of Laboratory Diagnostic Tests, ed 3. JB Lippincott, Philadelphia, 1988, p 227.
15. Diagnostics, ed 2. Springhouse Corp, Springhouse, PA, 1986, p 776.
16. Widmann, *op cit*, p 546.
17. *Ibid*.
18. *Ibid*, p 545.
19. *Ibid*, pp 545–546.
20. *Ibid*, p 547.
21. *Ibid*, p 348.
22. *Ibid*, p. 547.
23. *Ibid*, p 349.
24. *Ibid*, p 547.
25. *Ibid*, p 349.
26. *Ibid*, p 547.
27. *Ibid*, pp 547–548.
28. *Ibid*, p 348.
29. *Ibid*, pp 389–391, 548.
30. *Ibid*, p 549.
31. *Ibid*, p 541.
32. Diagnostics, *op cit*, p 779.
33. Pagana, KD and Pagana, TJ: Diagnostic Testing and Nursing Implications: A Case Study Approach, ed 2. CV Mosby, St Louis, 1986, p 175.
34. Diagnostics, *op cit*, p 779.
35. Widmann, *op cit*, p 538.

BIBLIOGRAPHY

Beare, PG, Rahr, VA and Ronshausen, CA: Nursing Implications of Diagnostic Tests, ed 2. JB Lippincott, Philadelphia, 1985.
Braunstein, H: Outlines of Pathology. CV Mosby, St Louis, 1982.
Byrne, CJ, Saxton, DF, Pelikan, PK and Nugent, PM: Laboratory Tests: Implications for Nursing Care. Addison-Wesley, Menlo Park, CA, 1986.
Carpenito, LJ: Nursing Diagnosis: Application to Clinical Practice. JB Lippincott, Philadelphia, 1983
Groer, MW and Shekleton, ME: Basic Pathophysiology: A Conceptual Approach, ed 2. CV Mosby, St Louis, 1983.
Jacob, SW, Francone, CA and Lossow, WJ: Structure and Function in Man, ed 5. WB Saunders, Philadelphia, 1982.
Kee, JL: Laboratory and Diagnostic Tests With Nursing Implications, ed 2. Appleton & Lange, Norwalk, CT, 1987.
Lamb, JO: Laboratory Tests for Clinical Nursing. Robert J Brady, Bowie, MD, 1984.
Luckmann, J and Sorensen, KC: Medical-Surgical Nursing: A Psychophysiologic Approach, ed 3. WB Saunders, Philadelphia, 1987.
Metheny, NM and Snively, WD: Nurse's Handbood of Fluid Balance, ed 4. JB Lippincott, Philadelphia, 1983.
Michaels, D: Diagnostic Procedures: The Patient and the Health Care Team. John Wiley & Sons, New York, 1983.
Selkurt, EE: Basic Physiology for the Health Sciences, ed 2. Little, Brown & Co, Boston, 1982.

Skydell, B and Crowder, AS: Diagnostic Procedures. Little, Brown & Co, Boston, 1975.

Tilkian, SM, Conover, MB and Tilkian, AG: Clinical Implications of Laboratory Tests, ed 4. CV Mosby, St Louis, 1987.

Wallach, J: Interpretation of Diagnostic Tests: A Handbook Synopsis of Laboratory Medicine, ed 4. Little, Brown & Co, Boston, 1978.

Widmann, FK: Pathobiology: How Diseases Happen. Little, Brown & Co, Boston, 1978.

ANALYSIS OF EFFUSIONS

OVERVIEW OF EFFUSIONS

Effusions are excessive accumulations of fluid in body cavities lined with serous or synovial membranes. Such cavities normally contain only small amounts of fluid (i.e., less than 50 ml). Serous membranes line the closed cavities of the thorax and abdomen and cover the organs within them. Those membranes lining cavities are termed parietal membranes; those covering organs are called visceral membranes. Serous membranes consist of a layer of simple squamous epithelium (mesothelium) that covers a thin layer of connective tissue.[1] Serous membranes secrete a small amount of watery fluid into the potential space between the parietal and visceral membranes. Serous fluid serves as a lubricant, allowing the internal organs to move without excessive friction. Although there is no actual space between visceral and parietal serous membranes, the potential space between them is called a cavity. In certain disease states, these cavities may contain large amounts of fluid (i.e., effusions). Three such serous cavities are the pericardial cavity, the pleural cavity, and the peritoneal cavity.

Synovial membranes line the cavities of most joints, the bursae, and the synovial tendon sheaths. These membranes consist of fibrous connective tissue, which overlies loose connective tissue and adipose tissue.[2] Synovial cells are found in layers one to three cells thick; wide gaps are often found between adja-

375

cent synovial cells. Synovial membranes secrete a thick colorless fluid with a high mucin content. As with serous fluid, synovial fluid acts as a lubricant in joint cavities. It also provides nourishment to articular cartilage.[3]

Serous fluid is formed by diffusion from adjacent capillaries via interstitial fluid and may be described as an ultrafiltrate of plasma. Thus, substances that normally diffuse from capillaries (e.g., water, electrolytes, glucose) will diffuse into serous fluid. Similarly, substances can diffuse from serous fluid back into the capillaries. Protein also may collect in serous cavities due to capillary leakage. Protein and excess fluids are normally removed from these cavities by the surrounding lymphatics.

Synovial fluid is formed in a manner similar to that of serous fluid, but additionally contains a hyaluronate-protein complex (i.e., a mucopolysaccharide containing hyaluronic acid and a small amount of protein) which is secreted by the connective tissue cells of the synovial membrane.[4] As with serous cavities, excess proteins and fluids are normally drained from synovial cavities by the lymphatics.

Changes in fluid production and drainage may lead to the development of effusions in serous and synovial cavities. Mechanical factors that may cause effusions include increased capillary permeability, increased capillary hydrostatic pressure, decreased capillary colloidal osmotic pressure, increased venous pressure, and blockage of the lymphatic vessels. Damage to the serous and synovial membranes (e.g., due to inflammation or infection) also may cause excessive fluid build-up.

Effusions involving serous cavities may be differentiated as transudates or exudates. Transudates occur due to abnormal mechanical factors and are generally characterized by low-protein, cell-free fluids. Exudates are caused by infection or inflammation and contain cells and excessive amounts of protein. Pleural and peritoneal effusions may be either transudates or exudates; however, pericardial effusions are almost always exudates.[5] Chylous effusions due to the escape of chyle from the thoracic lymphatic duct may form in the pleural and peritoneal cavities. Accumulation of large amounts of fluid in the peritoneal cavity is termed ascites.

Samples of effusions for laboratory analysis are obtained by needle aspiration. "Centesis" is a suffix denoting "puncture and aspiration of."[6] Thus, aspiration of pericardial fluid is called pericardiocentesis, aspiration of pleural fluid is called thoracentesis, aspiration of peritoneal fluid is called paracentesis, and aspiration of synovial fluid is called arthrocentesis.

Serous fluids are normally clear and pale yellow, occurring in amounts of 50 ml or less in pericardial and peritoneal cavities and of 20 ml or less in the pleural cavity. Cloudy (turbid) fluid suggests an inflammatory process that may be due to infection. Milky fluid is associated with chylous effusions or chronic serous effusions (pseudochylous effusions). Bloody fluid may indicate a hemorrhagic process or a traumatic tap. Bloody pericardial fluid is associated with a number of disorders including hemorrhagic and bacterial pericarditis, postmyocardial infarction and postpericardiectomy syndromes, metastatic cancer, aneurysms, tuberculosis, systemic lupus erythematosus (SLE), and rheumatoid arthritis. Bloody pleural effusions are most often due to malignancies involving the lung, but also may be seen in pneumonia, pulmonary infarction, chest trauma, pancreatitis, and postmyocardial infarction syndrome. Bloody pleural transudates also have been noted to occur with congestive heart failure (CHF) and cirrhosis of the liver. Bloody peritoneal fluid is associated primarily with malignant processes and abdominal trauma. Greenish peritoneal fluid is seen with perforated duodenal ulcers, intestines, and gallbladders, as well as with cholecystitis and acute pancreatitis.[7]

As with serous fluid, synovial fluid is normally clear and pale yellow, occuring in amounts of approximately 3 ml or less per joint cavity. Synovial fluid is more viscous than serous fluid because of the presence of the hyaluronate-protein complex secreted by the synovial cells. Arthritis and other inflammatory conditions involving the joints may affect the production of hyaluronate and lead to decreased viscosity of synovial fluid. The mucin clot test (Ropes test), in which synovial fluid is added to a 2 to 5 percent acetic acid solution, may be used to assess the viscosity of synovial fluid in relation to the type of clot formed (e.g., solid, soft, friable, or none).[8] This test is not as accurate, however, as specific synovial fluid cell counts and other analyses.[9]

Cloudy synovial fluid suggests an inflammatory process. Substances such as crystals, fibrin, amyloid, and cartilage fragments may also result in cloudy synovial fluid. Milky synovial fluid is associated with various types of arthritis as well as with SLE. Purulent fluid may be seen in acute septic arthritis, while greenish fluid may occur in *Hemophilus influenzae* septic arthritis, chronic rheumatoid arthritis, and acute synovitis due to gout. Bloody synovial fluid may be due to a traumatic tap but is most commonly associated with fractures or tumors involving the joint and traumatic or hemophilic arthritis.[10]

Tests of serous and synovial effusions include cell count and differential, measurement of substances normally found in the fluid (e.g., glucose), culture and sensitivity testing, and cytological examination. These tests are discussed subsequently in relation to the cavity from which the fluid is obtained.

TESTS OF EFFUSIONS

Background Information

PERICARDIAL FLUID ANALYSIS (CLINICAL APPLICATIONS DATA, p. 384)

Pericardial effusions are most commonly due to pericarditis, malignancy, or metabolic damage. As noted previously, most pericardial effusions are exudates. Tests commonly performed on pericardial fluid include red cell count, white cell count and differential, determination of glucose level, and cytological examination. Gram stains and cultures of pericardial fluid are not routinely performed unless bacterial endocarditis is suspected.[11]

Red cells are not normally found in pericardial fluid. Their presence, however, is indicative of a number of disorders (see p. 376). Chest trauma and anticoagulant therapy also may cause bloody pericardial effusions. Bleeding due to a traumatic pericardiocentesis is indicated by gradual clearing of the aspirate as additional amounts are withdrawn.

Fewer than 1,000 white blood cells per mm^3 are normally present in pericardial fluid. An elevated white count indicates inflammation or infection. The predominant type of white cell present may aid in diagnosis. Increased leukocytes with neutrophils predominating may be seen in bacterial or viral pericarditis and in postmyocardial infarction syndrome (Dressler's syndrome). A predominance of lymphocytes is associated with tuberculous or fungal pericarditis.

The glucose level in pericardial fluid is approximately equal to that of whole blood. Changes in blood glucose levels are reflected in pericardial fluid 2 to 4 hours later. Systemic hypoglycemia or hyperglycemia may lead to spurious changes in pericardial fluid glucose levels. A true decrease is associated with bacterial pericarditis and with noninfectious inflammation due to rheumatoid disease or malignancy.

Cytological examination of pericardial fluid is done to detect malignant cells. Gram stain and culture will reveal the causative agent when infection is suspected.

PLEURAL FLUID ANALYSIS (CLINICAL APPLICATIONS DATA, p. 386)

Pleural effusions are most commonly due to congestive heart failure, hypoalbuminemia (e.g., due to cirrhosis of the liver), hypoproteinemia (e.g., due to nephrotic syndrome), neoplasms, and pulmonary infections (e.g., pneumonia, tuberculosis). Other causes include trauma and pulmonary infarctions, both of which are associated with hemorrhagic effusions, rheumatoid disease, SLE, pancreatitis, and ruptured esophagus. Chylous pleural effusions occur when there is damage or obstruction to the thoracic lymphatic duct. Pleural effusions may be either transudates or exudates.

Tests commonly performed on pleural fluid include red cell count, white cell count and differential, Gram stain, culture and sensitivity, and cytological examination. The pH of the sample is usually determined and the fluid is tested for levels of glucose, protein, lactic dehydrogenase (LDH), and amylase. Triglycerides and cholesterol also may be measured when chylous effusion is suspected.

Red cells are not normally found in pleural effusions. When present in significant amounts (e.g., over 5,000/mm^3), they are most likely due to trauma, pulmonary infarction, tuberculosis, carcinoma, or pancreatitis. As with other aspirates, bleeding due to a traumatic thoracentesis is indicated by gradual clearing of the fluid as additional amounts are withdrawn.

Bloody effusions due to hemothorax (i.e., traumatic injury) may be differentiated from hemorrhagic exudates by performing a hematocrit on the sample. Blood from a hemothorax should have a hematocrit similar to that found in whole blood. Blood due to an exudative effusion will have a lower hematocrit, as the blood is mixed with excess pleural fluid characteristic of an exudate.[12]

Fewer than 1,000 white blood cells per mm^3 are normally present in pleural fluid. An elevated white count indicates inflammation or infection, and in most cases is associated with an exudate. The magnitude of the elevation and the predominant type of white cell present aid in diagnosing specific disorders. A white cell count of 5,000 to 10,000/mm^3 consisting mostly of lymphocytes is associated with tuberculosis, carcinoma, lymphoma, and chronic lymphocytic leukemia. A white cell count of 5,000 to 25,000/mm^3 consisting mostly of neutrophils is associated with pneumonia, pulmonary infarctions, and pancreatitis. A white cell count of 25,000 to 100,000/mm^3 consisting mostly of neutrophils is associated with empyemas, including those due to tuberculosis. The white cell count in effusions due to rheumatoid disease may be elevated to 20,000/mm^3, with either lymphocytes or neutrophils predominating.[13]

The presence of eosinophils in pleural fluid is associated with injury to the pleura and may be seen with pneumothorax, following pneumonia, in parasitic and hypersensitivity syndromes, after surgery involving the pleura, and with pulmonary infarctions, congestive heart failure, and neoplasms.[14] The sample also may be analyzed for the presence of mesothelial cells, which are shed from serous membranes in certain disorders. Mesothelial cells are seen with nonseptic inflammations but are uncommon in bacterial or tuberculous infections.[15]

Gram stain and culture and sensitivity tests are generally performed when infection is suspected, in order to identify the causative organism. Cytological examination is done to detect malignant cells.

The pH of pleural fluid is essentially the same as that of blood (i.e., 7.37 to 7.43). Measuring the pH of pleural effusions aids in determining the nature of the effusion and the causative disorder. Transudates usually have a pH of 7.40 or higher, while the pH of exudates tends to be somewhat lower. A pH of less than 7.30 is associated with exudates due to empyema, pneumonia, tuberculosis, and rheumatoid disease. If the pH is less than 7.20 in exudates due to infection, it may be necessary to insert a chest drainage tube to remove the relatively acidic fluid.[16] A pH as low as 6.0 indicates esophageal rupture.[17]

Because pleural fluid is an ultrafiltrate of plasma, its chemistry values should parallel plasma levels of the substances measured. Decreased glucose levels (i.e., below 60 mg/dl, or 40 mg/dl less than plasma glucose) are associated with rheumatoid effusions but not with effusions due to SLE. Decreased glucose levels are occasionally seen with tuberculous or bacterial exudates and with neoplasms but are rarely seen with transudates.

Protein and lactic dehydrogenase (LDH) levels are used primarily to differentiate between transudates and exudates. The normal protein level of pleural fluid is 3.0 g/dl. The protein level of transudates is usually lower than normal, whereas that of exudates is generally higher. The ratio of the protein level in pleural fluid to that in serum also is used to identify exudates. A ratio of less than 0.5 indicates a transudate; a ratio of greater than 0.5 an exudate.[18]

LDH levels in pleural fluid parallel those of serum (i.e., 71 to 207 IU/l). LDH levels less than 200 IU indicate a transudate. Elevated LDH levels (i.e., greater than 200 IU/l) indicate an inflammatory damage to the pleural membranes with enzyme release, and thus, an exudate. As with protein, the ratio of the LDH level in pleural fluid to that in serum also may be used to identify exudates. A ratio of less than 0.6 indicates a transudate, whereas a ratio of greater than 0.6 indicates an exudate.

Measurement of amylase levels in pleural effusions is indicated when either esophageal perforation or pancreatitis is suspected. In both situations, amylase levels are elevated. The normal amylase level in pleural fluid parallels that of serum (i.e., 80 to 180 Somogyi U/dl or 45 to 200 dye U/dl). Amylase in pleural fluid is considered elevated when the level is higher than the upper limit of normal for serum.[19]

Hyaluronate is occasionally measured in pleural fluid if a pleural mesothelioma is suspected. Measurement of cholesterol and triglyceride levels in pleural aspirates is used to differentiate chylous effusions due to leakage of thoracic lymphatic duct contents from pseudochylous (chronic serous) effusions in which there is breakdown of cellular lipids. In chylous effusions, the triglyceride level may be two to three times that of serum, while the cholesterol level is lower than that of serum. In pseudochylous effusions, the triglyceride level is lower than that for serum, while the cholesterol level may be higher. If the pleural fluid aspirate is subjected to lipoprotein electrophoresis, chylous effusions will show markedly elevated chylomicrons (minute fat droplets), whereas only scant amounts, if any, will be present in pseudochylous effusions.[20]

Pleural effusions also may be tested for levels of immunoglobulins, complement components, and carcinoembryonic antigen (CEA) (see Chapter 3) when disorders of immunological and malignant origin are suspected. Elevated immunoglobulins and CEA and/or decreased complement levels are seen in inflammatory or neoplastic reactions involving the pleural membranes.[21]

PERITONEAL FLUID ANALYSIS (CLINICAL APPLICATIONS DATA, p. 390)

Peritoneal transudates are most commonly due to congestive heart failure, cirrhosis of the liver, and nephrotic syndrome. Peritoneal exudates occur with neoplasms including metastatic carcinoma, infections (e.g., tuberculosis, bacterial peritonitis), trauma, pancreatitis, and bile peritonitis. Chylous peritoneal effusions occur when there is damage or obstruction to the thoracic lymphatic duct. Accumulation of large amounts of fluid in the peritoneal cavity is termed ascites, and the peritoneal fluid is referred to as ascitic fluid.

Peritoneal fluid is removed by paracentesis or by paracentesis and lavage with normal saline or Ringer's lactate. Lavage involves instilling the desired solution over 15 to 20 minutes, then removing it and analyzing it for cells and other constituents.

Tests commonly performed on peritoneal or ascitic fluid include red cell count, white cell count and differential, Gram stain, culture and sensitivity, acid-fast bacillus (AFB) smear and culture, and cytological examination. The fluid also may be tested for glucose, amylase, ammonia, alkaline phosphatase, and carcinoembryonic antigen (CEA). Urea and creatinine may be measured if there is suspicion of ruptured or punctured urinary bladder.

The red cell count in peritoneal fluid is normally less than $100,000/mm^3$. Elevated counts usually indicate either hemorrhage due to trauma or a malignant process. In peritoneal lavage, counts greater than $100,000/mm^3$ are considered positive for bleeding, whereas counts in the range of 50,000 to $100,000/mm^3$ are called borderline. It should be noted that blood may not be evident in the initial aspirate and may only be apparent after lavage has been performed.[22]

Fewer than 300 white blood cells per mm^3 are normally present in undiluted peritoneal or ascitic fluid, while less than $500/mm^3$ should be found in fluid obtained by lavage. Elevated white cell counts are associated with bacterial peritonitis but may also be seen in cirrhosis without infection. Normally, less than 25 percent of the white blood cells are neutrophils. Elevated neutrophil counts are associated with bacterial peritonitis and ascites due to cirrhosis. In the latter disorder, however, the neutrophil count rarely rises above 50 percent. Bacterial peritonitis also may be differentiated from sterile ascites due to cirrhosis by performing an absolute granulocyte count. If this count is greater than $250/mm^3$, bacterial peritonitis is indicated.[23]

Lymphocytes have been found to be elevated in tuberculous peritonitis and in chylous ascites. Elevated eosinophil counts are rare but may accompany ascites due to congestive heart failure, chronic peritoneal dialysis, abdominal lymphoma, hypereosinophilic syndrome, eosinophilic gastroenteritis, and ruptured hydatid cyst.[24]

Gram stain and culture and sensitivity tests are generally performed when infection is suspected, in order to identify the causative organism. If tuberculous effusion is suspected, an acid-fast bacillus (AFB) smear and culture may be performed, although positive results are seen in only 25 to 50 percent of cases.[25] Cytological examination is used to detect malignant cells.

Since peritoneal fluid is normally an ultrafiltrate of plasma, chemistry values parallel plasma levels of the substances measured. Glucose levels may be decreased below 60 mg/dl in about 50 percent of individuals with tuberculous peritonitis and abdominal malignancy. Elevated amylase is usually associated with acute pancreatitis, pancreatic trauma, or pancreatitic pseudocyst. Amylase levels also may be elevated, however, in gastrointestinal perforation and in intestinal strangulation and necrosis. Ammonia and alkaline phosphatase levels have been elevated also in gastrointestinal perforation and strangulation.

In situations involving rupture or puncture of the urinary bladder with extravasation of urine into the peritoneal cavity, ammonia, creatinine, and urea levels in peritoneal fluid are usually elevated. Elevated carcinoembryonic antigen (CEA) levels are associated with abdominal malignancy.

SYNOVIAL FLUID ANALYSIS (CLINICAL APPLICATIONS DATA, p. 393)

Synovial fluid is a clear, pale yellow, and viscous liquid formed by plasma ultrafiltration and by secretion of a hyaluronate-protein complex by synovial cells (see pp. 376 and 377). It is secreted in small amounts (i.e., 3 ml or less) into the cavities of most joints. Synovial effusions are associated with disorders or injuries involving the joints. Samples for analysis are obtained by aspirating joint cavities. The most commonly aspirated joint is the knee, although samples also may be obtained from the shoulder, hip, elbow, wrist, and ankle if clinically indicated.

Synovial fluid analysis is used primarily to determine the type or etiology of joint disorders. Joint disorders may be classified according to five categories based on synovial fluid findings: (1) noninflammatory (e.g., degenerative joint disease); (2) inflammatory (e.g., rheumatoid arthritis, systemic lupus erythematosus); (3) septic (e.g., acute bacterial or tuberculous arthritis); (4) crystal-induced (e.g., gout or pseudogout); and (5) hemorrhagic (e.g., traumatic arthritis or hemophilic arthritis).[26]

Tests commonly performed on synovial fluid include red cell count, white cell count and differential, white cell morphology, microscopic examination for crystals, Gram stain, and culture and sensitivity. Determination of protein, glucose, and uric acid levels also aids in diagnosis. Various immunological tests such as determination of complement, rheumatoid factor, and antinuclear antibodies also have been employed in synovial fluid analysis. In the recent past, the Mucin clot test (see p. 377) has been used in analyzing synovial fluid, but this test is not considered as reliable as specific cell counts and other measurements of synovial fluid constituents. Lactate and pH measurements may be used as nonspecific indicators of inflammation and to differentiate between infection and inflammation.[27]

The red cell count in synovial fluid is normally less than $2,000/mm^3$. Elevated counts are associated with trauma, tumors involving the joint, and hemophilic arthritis. A traumatic tap also may produce an elevated red cell count. Fewer than 200 white blood cells per mm^3 are normally present in synovial fluid. White cell counts of less than $5,000/mm^3$ are associated with noninflammatory joint disorders, while counts of $2,000$ to $100,000/mm^3$ are seen with inflammatory disorders. In septic and crystal-induced disorders, the white count may rise to as high as $200,000/mm^3$.

The differential white cell count aids in determining the specific cause of the joint disorder. Mononuclear cells (e.g., lymphocytes, monocytes, macrophages, and synovial tissue cells) are the main cells seen in synovial fluid. Neutrophils normally comprise less than 25 percent of the differential white cell count.[28] In the routine differential count, only the percentage of neutrophils may be reported.[29] An elevated neutrophil count indicates sepsis, while an elevated white count consisting mostly of lymphocytes indicates nonseptic inflammation. Neutrophil levels as high as 90 percent are seen in acute bacterial arthritis. Moderately elevated neutrophil counts may be seen in rheumatic fever, rheumatoid arthritis, gout, pseudogout, and tuberculous arthritis. The structure and form of the white cells also is examined. Table 9–1 lists the various types of white blood cells and inclusions seen in synovial fluid along with the disorders with which the presence of such cells is associated.

Examination of synovial fluid for crystals is used in diagnosing crystal-induced arthritis. The several types of crystals that may be identified are listed in Table 9–2. Monosodium urate (MSU) crystals are associated with arthritis due to gout, while calcium pyrophosphate (CPP) crystals are seen in pseudogout. Cholesterol crystals are associated with chronic joint effusions, which may be due to tuberculous or rheumatoid arthritis. Arthritis associated with the presence of apatite crystals is commonly recognized as a cause of synovitis. Corticosteroid crystals may be seen for a month or more after intra-articular injections of steroids and may induce acute synovitis. Although usually of a rhomboid shape, corticosteroid crystals are sometimes needle-shaped and may be confused with MSU or CPP crystals. Not shown in Table 9–2 are talcum crystals. These crystals, which are shaped like Maltese crosses, are most commonly

TABLE 9-1. **White Blood Cells and Inclusions Seen in Synovial Fluid**

Cell/ Inclusion	Description	Significance
Neutrophil	Polymorphonuclear leukocyte	Bacterial sepsis Crystal-induced inflammation
Lymphocyte	Mononuclear leukocyte	Nonseptic inflammation
Macrophage (Monocyte)	Large mononuclear leukocyte, may be vacuolated	Normal Viral infections
Synovial Lining Cell	Similar to macrophage, but may be multinucleated, resembling a mesothelial cell	Normal
LE Cell	Neutrophil containing characteristic ingested "round body"	Lupus erythematosus
Reiter Cell	Vacuolated macrophage with ingested neutrophils	Reiter's syndrome Nonspecific inflammation
RA Cell (Ragocyte)	Neutrophil with dark cytoplasmic granules containing immune complexes	Rheumatoid arthritis Immunologic inflammations
Cartilage Cells	Large, multinucleated cells	Osteoarthritis
Rice Bodies	Macroscopically resemble polished rice Microscopically show collagen and fibrin	Tuberculosis, septic, and rheumatoid arthritis
Fat Droplets	Refractile intracellular and extracellular globules Stain with Sudan dyes	Traumatic injury
Hemosiderin	Inclusions within synovial cells	Pigmented villonodular synovitis

From Strasinger, SK: Urinalysis and Body Fluids. FA Davis, 1985, p. 166, with permission.

seen after joint surgery and reflect contamination of the joint with talcum powder from surgical gloves.[30]

Gram stain and culture and sensitivity tests are used when infection is suspected, to identify the causative organisms. The Gram stain is positive in about 50 percent of clients with septic arthritis, and cultures are positive in about 30 to 80 percent of individuals with the disorder. It should be noted that septic arthritis may coexist with other forms of arthritis. Acid-fast bacillus (AFB) smear and culture may be performed when tuberculous arthritis is suspected, but results are frequently negative. When the results of microbiological tests of synovial fluid are inconclusive, synovial biopsy may be necessary to establish the diagnosis.[31]

Because synovial fluid is mainly an ultrafiltrate of plasma, chemistry values parallel plasma levels of the substances measured. The normal amount of protein present in synovial fluid is less than 3 g/dl. Elevated protein levels are associated with inflammatory and hemorrhagic joint disorders. As with pleural fluid, the ratio of the protein level in synovial fluid to that of plasma may be reported (see p. 379). The glucose level in synovial fluid is normally not more than 10 mg/dl lower than that of blood. Markedly decreased glucose levels are associated

TABLE 9-2. Synovial Fluid Crystals

Crystal	Shape	
Monosodium urate	Needles	
Calcium pyrophosphate	Rods Needles Rhombics	
Cholesterol	Notched rhombic plates	
Apatite	Small needles	
Corticosteroid	Flat, variable-shaped plates	

Adapted from Strasinger, SK: Urinalysis and Body Fluids. FA Davis, 1985, p. 167.

with inflammatory or septic joint disorders. If the client's blood glucose is not available for comparison with the level in synovial fluid, then a synovial fluid level of less than 40 mg/dl is interpreted as abnormally decreased.

Uric acid levels in synovial fluid may be measured when gout is suspected. Since the uric acid content of synovial fluid is essentially the same as that found in serum, the data obtained may not contribute much to diagnostic determination. If urate crystals cannot be identified in cases of suspected gout, however, then it may be worthwhile to determine the uric acid level in the synovial fluid sample.[32,33]

Measurement of synovial fluid lactate levels is used to differentiate between inflammatory and septic arthritis, and does not require comparison with serum levels. Lactate levels greater than 2 mmol/l (20 mg/dl) are considered elevated. Lactate levels greater than 2 mmol/l but less than 7.5 mmol/l are associated with inflammatory joint problems; lactate levels greater than 7.5 mmol/l are consistently found with septic arthritis, but also may be seen in rheumatoid arthritis.[34] When lactate levels are elevated, the pH of synovial fluid decreases. Thus, a pH of less than 7.3 is associated with the same disorders that produce elevated lactate levels (i.e., inflammatory and septic joint disorders).

The need to perform immunological tests of synovial fluid is indicative of the association of the immune system with inflammatory joint disorders. Substances measured include rheumatoid factor (RF), antinuclear antibodies (ANA), and complement, all of which also may be measured in serum (see Chapter 3). In rheumatoid arthritis, for example, about 80 percent of affected individuals have rheumatoid factor in the serum, whereas 60 percent show rheumatoid factor in synovial fluid. Similarly, although 70 percent of individuals with SLE have antinuclear antibodies in the serum, only about 20 percent manifest them in synovial fluid.

Determination of complement levels in synovial fluid aids in differentiating arthritis of immunological origin from that due to nonimmunological causes. Decreased synovial fluid complement levels are seen in approximately 60 to 80 percent of individuals with rheumatoid arthritis and SLE. Decreased complement levels are occasionally seen in rheumatic fever, gout, pseudogout, and bacterial arthritis; however, synovial complement levels may be high in these disorders if serum levels also are elevated.[35] Complement levels in synovial fluid may be measured as total complement (CH_{50}) or as individual components (C1q, C4, C2, and C3). Since synovial fluid complement levels parallel synovial fluid protein levels, complement levels may be expressed as ratios in relation to the protein levels in order to ensure that abnormal findings are not due to changes in synovial fluid membrane filtration.[36,37]

Clinical Applications Data

PERICARDIAL FLUID ANALYSIS (BACKGROUND INFORMATION, p. 377)
Reference Values

Red blood cells	None normally present
White blood cells	$<1000/mm^3$
Glucose	80–100 mg/dl or essentially the same as the blood glucose level drawn 2 to 4 hours earlier
Cytological examination	No abnormal cells
Gram strain and culture	No organisms present

Interfering Factors

■ Blood in the sample due to a traumatic pericardiocentesis
■ Undetected hypoglycemia or hyperglycemia
■ Contamination of the sample with skin cells and pathogens

Indications/Purposes for Pericardial Fluid Analysis

■ Pericardial effusion of unknown etiology
■ Suspected hemorrhagic pericarditis as indicated by the presence of red cells and an elevated white cell count
■ Suspected bacterial pericarditis as indicated by the presence of red cells, elevated white count with a predominance of neutrophils, and decreased glucose
■ Suspected postmyocardial infarction syndrome (Dressler's syndrome) as indicated by the presence of red cells and elevated white count with a predominance of neutrophils
■ Suspected tuberculous or fungal pericarditis as indicated by the presence of red cells and an elevated white count with a predominance of lymphocytes
■ Suspected viral pericarditis as indicated by the presence of red cells and an elevated white count with neutrophils predominating
■ Suspected rheumatoid disease or SLE as indicated by the presence of red cells, an elevated white count, and decreased glucose levels
■ Suspected malignancy as indicated by the presence of red cells, decreased glucose, and presence of abnormal cells on cytological examination

Client Preparation

Client Teaching. Explain to the client:

- the purpose of the test
- that it will be done by a physician and will require approximately 20 minutes
- where the test will be performed (i.e., it is sometimes performed in the cardiac laboratory)
- any dietary restrictions (fasting for 6 to 8 hours prior to the test may be required)
- that an intravenous infusion will be started prior to the procedure and will be discontinued afterward
- that a sedative may be administered prior to the procedure
- that the skin will be injected with a local anesthetic at the chest needle insertion site and that this may cause a stinging sensation
- that, after the skin has been anesthetized, a needle will be inserted through the chest wall below and slightly to the left of the breast bone into the fluid-filled sac around the heart
- that a sensation of pressure may be felt when the needle is inserted to obtain the pericardial fluid
- that heart rate and rhythm will be monitored during the procedure
- the importance of remaining still during the procedure
- any activity restrictions following the test (usually a few hours of bedrest)

Encourage questions and verbalization of concerns appropriate to the client's age and mental status.
Ensure that a signed consent for the procedure has been obtained.

Physical Preparation

- Ensure to the extent possible that any dietary restrictions are followed
- Withhold anticoagulant medications and aspirin as ordered
- Have the client void
- Provide a hospital gown
- Take and record vital signs
- Administer premedication as ordered

The Procedure (Pericardiocentesis)

The necessary equipment is assembled. This includes a pericardiocentesis tray with solution for skin preparation, local anesthetic, a 50 ml syringe, needles of various sizes including a cardiac needle, sterile drapes, and sterile gloves. Sterile test tubes (same as those used for collecting blood samples) also are needed; at least one red-topped, one green-topped, and one lavender-topped tube should be available. Containers for culture and cytological analysis of pericardial fluid samples also may be needed. Cardiac monitoring equipment should be obtained, along with an alligator clip for attaching a precordial (V) lead to the cardiac needle.

The client is assisted to a supine position with the head elevated 45 to 60 degrees. The limb leads for the cardiac monitor are attached to the client and the intravenous infusion started. The skin is cleansed with an antiseptic solution and protected with sterile drapes. The skin at the needle insertion site is then infiltrated with local anesthetic.

The precordial (V) cardiac lead wire is attached to the hub to the cardiac needle with the alligator clip. The needle is then inserted just below and slightly to the left of the xiphoid process. Gentle traction is sustained on the plunger of the 50 ml syringe until fluid appears, indicating that the needle has entered the pericardial sac. Fluid samples are then withdrawn and placed in appropriate tubes. The samples are labeled and sent promptly to the laboratory.

When the desired samples have been obtained, the cardiac needle is withdrawn. Pressure is applied to the site for 5 minutes. If there is no evidence of bleeding or other drainage, a sterile bandage is applied. If the client's cardiac rhythm is stable, cardiac monitoring is discontinued.

Aftercare

The client is assisted to a position of comfort and is reminded of any activity restrictions following the procedure. Any foods or fluids withheld prior to the test are resumed, as are any medications withheld upon the physician's order. Intravenous fluids may be continued until vital signs are stable and the client is able to resume normal fluid intake.

Nursing Observations

Pretest

- Determine if the client is currently taking any anticoagulant medications or aspirin-containing drugs
- Assess the client's response to explanations provided (if the client appears unduly anxious about the procedure or unable to cooperate during it, the physician performing the pericardiocentesis should be so informed)
- Take and record vital signs and compare to the client's usual baseline

During the Test

- Observe the client for respiratory or cardiac distress; possible complications of a pericardiocentesis include cardiac dysrhythmias, laceration of the pleura, laceration of the cardiac atrium or coronary vessels, injection of air into a cardiac chamber, and contamination of pleural spaces with infected pericardial fluid

Post-Test

- Take and record vital signs as for a postoperative client (i.e., every 15 minutes times four, every 30 minutes times four, every hour times four, and then every 4 hours for 24 hours)
- Assess the puncture site for bleeding, hematoma formation, and inflammation each time the vital signs are taken and daily thereafter for several days
- Observe the client for any cardiac or respiratory distress

PLEURAL FLUID ANALYSIS (BACKGROUND INFORMATION, p. 378)

Reference Values

Red blood cells	$0-<1000/mm^3$
White blood cells	$0-<1000/mm^3$ consisting mainly of lymphocytes
Gram stain and culture	No organisms present
Cytological examination	No abnormal cells
pH	7.37–7.43 (usually >7.40)
Glucose	Parallels serum levels
Protein	3.0 g/dl
Pleural fluid: serum protein ratio	0.5 or less
Lactic dehydrogenase (LDH)	71–207 IU/l
Pleural fluid: serum LDH ratio	0.6 or less

Amylase   <180 Somogyi U/dl or <200 dye U/dl
Triglycerides
Cholesterol
Immunoglobulins   }   Parallel serum levels
Carcinoembryonic antigen (CEA)
Complement

Interfering Factors

■ Blood in the sample due to traumatic thoracentesis
■ Undetected hypoglycemia or hyperglycemia
■ Contamination of the sample with skin cells and pathogens

Indications/Purposes for Pleural Fluid Analysis

■ Pleural effusion of unknown etiology
■ Differentiation of pleural transudates from exudates (Table 9–3)
■ Suspected traumatic hemothorax as indicated by bloody pleural fluid, elevated red cell count, and hematocrit similar to that found in whole blood
■ Suspected pleural effusion due to pulmonary tuberculosis as indicated by presence of red blood cells (less than $10,000/mm^3$), white cell count of 5,000 to $10,000/mm^3$ consisting mostly of lymphocytes, presence of acid fast bacilli (AFB) on smear and culture, pH of less than 7.30, decreased glucose (sometimes), and elevated protein, pleural fluid:serum protein ratio, LDH, and pleural fluid:serum LDH ratio
■ Suspected pleural effusion due to pneumonia (parapneumonic) effusion as indicated by presence of red blood cells ($<5,000/mm^3$), white cell count of 5,000 to $25,000/mm^3$ consisting mainly of neutrophils and sometimes

TABLE 9–3. **Differentiation of Plueral Transudates From Exudates**

	Transudates	Exudates
Appearance	Clear	Cloudy; may be bloody
Red blood cells	$<1,000/mm^3$	$>1,000/mm^3$ (usually)
White blood cells	$<1,000/mm^3$	$>1,000/mm^3$
pH	7.40 or higher	<7.40
Glucose	Parallels serum level	May be less than serum level
Protein	<3.0 g/dl	>3.0 g/dl
Pleural fluid: serum protein ratio	<0.5	>0.5
LDH	<200 IU/l	>200 IU/l
Pleural fluid: serum LDH ratio	<0.6	>0.6
Common causes	Congestive heart failure Cirrhosis Nephrotic syndrome	Pneumonia Tuberculosis Empyema Pulmonary infarction Rheumatoid disease Systemic lupus erythematosus Carcinoma Pancreatitis

including eosinophils, pH less than 7.40, and elevated protein, pleural fluid: serum protein ratio, LDH, and pleural fluid:serum LDH ratio. If the pneumonia is of bacterial origin, the organism may be demonstrated on culture and the pleural fluid glucose level may be decreased.

■ Suspected bacterial or tuberculous empyema as indicated by red cell count of less than 5,000/mm³, white cell count of 25,000 to 100,000/mm³ consisting mostly of neutrophils, pH less than 7.30, decreased glucose, and increased protein, LDH, and related ratios

■ Suspected pleural effusion due to carcinoma as indicated by presence of red blood cells (1,000 to more than 100,000/mm³); white cell count of 5,000 to 10,000/mm³ consisting mostly of lymphocytes and sometimes including eosinophils: detection of malignant cells on cytological examination; pH less than or greater than 7.30; decreased glucose (sometimes); increased protein, LDH, and related ratios; elevated CEA and immunoglobulins; and decreased complement

■ Suspected pleural effusion due to pulmonary infarction as indicated by red cell count of 1,000 to 100,000/mm³, white cell count of 5,000 to 15,000/mm³ consisting mainly of neutrophils and sometimes including eosinophils, pH greater than 7.30, normal glucose, and elevated protein, LDH, and related ratios

■ Suspected pleural effusion due to rheumatoid disease as indicated by a normal red cell count; a white cell count of 1,000 to 20,000/mm³ with either lymphocytes or neutrophils predominating; pH less than 7.30; decreased glucose; elevated protein, LDH, and related ratios; and elevated immunoglobulins

■ Suspected pleural effusion due to SLE as indicated by findings similar to those in rheumatoid disease, except that glucose is not usually decreased

■ Suspected pleural effusion due to pancreatitis as indicated by red cell count of 1,000 to 10,000/mm³; white cell count of 5,000 to 20,000/mm³ consisting mostly of neutrophils; pH greater than 7.30; normal glucose; elevated protein, LDH, and related ratios; and elevated amylase

■ Suspected pleural effusion due to esophageal rupture as indicated primarily by a pH as low as 6.0 and elevated amylase

■ Differentation of chylous pleural effusions due to thoracic lymphatic duct blockage from pseudochylous (chronic serous) effusions, with chylous effusions indicated primarily by a triglyceride level two to three times that of serum, decreased cholesterol, and markedly elevated chylomicrons

Client Preparation

Client Teaching. Explain to the client:

■ the purpose of the test
■ that it will be done by a physician and will require approximately 20 minutes
■ that there are no food or fluid restrictions prior to the test
■ that a sedative usually is not given prior to the procedure, although a cough supressant may be given to prevent coughing
■ the positioning used for the procedure (supported sitting or sidelying)
■ that the skin will be injected with a local anesthetic at the chest needle insertion site and that this may cause a stinging sensation
■ that, after the skin has been anesthetized, a needle will be inserted through the posterior chest into the space near the lungs where excessive fluid has accumulated
■ that a sensation of pressure may be felt when the needle is inserted

■ the importance of remaining still during the procedure and the need to control breathing, coughing, and movement
■ any activity restrictions following the test (usually an hour of bed rest)

Encourage questions and verbalization of concerns appropriate to the client's age and mental status.
Ensure that a signed consent for the procedure has been obtained.

Physical Preparation

■ Withhold anticoagulant medications and aspirin as ordered
■ Have the client void
■ Provide a hospital gown
■ Take and record vital signs
■ Administer cough supressant, if ordered

The Procedure (Thoracentesis)

The necessary equipment is assembled. This includes a thoracentesis tray with solution for skin preparation, local anesthetic, a 50 ml syringe, needles of various sizes including a thoracentesis needle, sterile drapes, and sterile gloves. Sterile collection bottles and containers for culture and cytological examination also are needed.

The client is assisted to the position that will be used for the test. The usual position is sitting on the side of a bed or treatment table, leaning slightly forward to spread the intercostal spaces, with arms supported on an overbed table with several pillows. Alternatively, the client may sit on the bed or table with legs extended on it and arms supported as described earlier. If the client cannot assume either sitting position, the sidelying position is used. In such situations, the client lies on the unaffected side.

The skin is cleansed with an antiseptic solution and protected with sterile drapes. The skin at the needle insertion site is then infiltrated with local anesthetic. The thoracentesis needle is inserted. When fluid appears, a stopcock and 50 ml syringe are attached to the needle, and the fluid is aspirated. The pleural fluid samples are placed in appropriate containers, labeled, and sent promptly to the laboratory.

If the thoracentesis is being performed for therapeutic as well as diagnostic reasons, additional pleural fluid may be withdrawn. When the desired amount of fluid has been removed, the needle is withdrawn, and slight pressure is applied to the site for a few minutes. If there is no evidence of bleeding or other drainage, a sterile bandage is applied to the site.

Aftercare

The client is assisted to lie on the unaffected side and is reminded that this position should be maintained for approximately 1 hour. The head may be elevated for client comfort. A post-thoracentesis chest x-ray examination may be ordered to ensure that a pneumothorax due to the tap has not occurred.

Nursing Observations

Pretest

■ Determine if the client is currently taking any anticoagulant medications or aspirin-containing drugs.
■ Assess the client's response to explanations provided (if the client appears

unduly anxious about the procedure or unable to cooperate during it, the physician performing the thoracentesis should be so informed)
■ Take and record vital signs and compare with the client's usual baseline
■ Auscultate the client's lungs to provide a baseline for post-thoracentesis assessment
■ Determine if the client has a persistent or uncontrollable cough for which a cough supressant may be necessary prior to the test

During the Test

■ Observe the client for signs of respiratory distress or pneumothorax (e.g., anxiety, restlessness, dyspnea, cyanosis, tachycardia, and chest pain); possible complications of a thoracentesis include pneumothorax, mediastinal shift, and excessive reaccumulation of pleural fluid

Post-Test

■ Take and record vital signs as ordered (e.g., every 15 minutes times two, every 30 minutes times two, and then every 4 hours for 24 hours or until stable)
■ Observe the client for respiratory distress
■ Auscultate breath sounds; absent or diminished breath sounds on the side used for the thoracentesis may indicate pneumothorax
■ Assess the puncture site for bleeding, hematoma formation, and inflammation each time vital signs are taken and daily thereafter for several days

PERITONEAL FLUID ANALYSIS (BACKGROUND INFORMATION, p. 379)

Reference Values

Red blood cells	$<100,000/mm^3$
White blood cells	$<300/mm^3$ (undiluted peritoneal fluid)
	$<500/mm^3$ (lavage fluid)
Neutrophils	<25 percent
Absolute granulocyte count	$<250/mm^3$
Gram stain and culture	No organisms present
AFB smear and culture	No acid-fast bacilli present
Cytological examination	No abnormal cells present
Glucose	
Amylase	
Ammonia	
Alkaline phosphatase	Parallel serum levels
Creatinine	
Urea	
Carcinoembryonic antigen (CEA)	

Interfering Factors

■ Blood in the sample due to traumatic paracentesis
■ Undetected hypoglycemia or hyperglycemia
■ Contamination of the sample with skin cells and pathogens

Indications/Purposes for Peritoneal/Fluid Analysis

■ Ascites of unknown etiology
■ Suspected peritoneal effusion due to abdominal malignancy as indicated by

elevated red cell count, decreased glucose, elevated CEA, and detection of malignant cells on cytological examination

■ Suspected abdominal trauma as indicated by elevated red cell count

■ Suspected ascites due to cirrhosis of the liver as indicated by elevated white cell count, neutrophil count of greater than 25 percent but less than 50 percent, and an absolute granulocyte count of less than $250/mm^3$

■ Suspected bacterial peritonitis as indicated by elevated white cell count, neutrophil count greater than 50 percent, and an absolute granulocyte count of greater than $250/mm^3$

■ Suspected tuberculous peritoneal effusion as indicated by elevated lymphocyte count, positive AFB smear and culture in about 25 to 50 percent of cases, and decreased glucose

■ Suspected peritoneal effusion due to pancreatitis, pancreatic trauma, or pancreatic pseudocyst as indicated by elevated amylase levels

■ Suspected peritoneal effusion due to gastrointestinal perforation, strangulation, or necrosis as indicated by elevated amylase, ammonia, and alkaline phosphatase levels

■ Suspected rupture or perforation of the urinary bladder as indicated by elevated ammonia, creatinine, and urea levels

Client Preparation

Client Teaching. Explain to the client:

■ the purpose of the test
■ that it will be performed by a physician and will take approximately 30 minutes
■ that there are no food or fluid restrictions prior to the test
■ the positioning used for the procedure (seated or in high Fowler's position)
■ that the skin will be injected with a local anesthetic at the abdominal needle insertion site and that this may cause a stinging sensation
■ that, after the skin has been anesthetized, a large needle will be inserted through the abdominal wall
■ that a "popping" sensation may be experienced as the needle penetrates the peritoneum
■ the importance of remaining still during the procedure
■ any activity restrictions following the test (usually an hour or more of bed rest)

Encourage questions and verbalization of concerns appropriate to the client's age and mental status.

Ensure that a signed consent for the procedure has been obtained.

Physical Preparation

■ Withhold anticoagulant medications and aspirin as ordered
■ Have the client void
■ Provide a hospital gown and have the client put it on with the opening in the front
■ Take and record vital signs
■ If the client has ascites, obtain weight and measure abdominal girth
■ If the abdominen is hirsute, it may be necessary to shave the area where the puncture is to be made

The Procedure (Paracentesis)

The necessary equipment is assembled. This includes a paracentesis tray with solution for skin preparation, local anesthetic, a 50 ml syringe, needles of various sizes including a large bore paracentesis needle or a trocar and cannula, sterile drapes, and sterile gloves. Specimen collection tubes and bottles for the tests to be performed also are needed.

The client is assisted to the position that will be used for the test. The usual position is sitting on the side of a bed or treatment table, with the feet and back supported. An alternate approach is to place the client in bed in a high Fowler's position.

The skin is cleansed with an antiseptic solution and protected with sterile drapes. The skin at the needle or trocar insertion site is then infiltrated with local anesthetic. The paracentesis needle is inserted approximately 1 to 2 inches below the umbilicus. If a trocar with cannula is to be used, a small skin incision may be made to facilitate insertion. The 50 ml syringe with stopcock is attached to the needle or cannula after the trocar has been removed. Gentle suction may be applied with the syringe to remove fluid. For peritoneal lavage, sterile normal saline or Ringer's lactate may be infused via the needle or cannula over 15 to 20 minutes. The client is then turned from side to side before the lavage fluid is removed.

Samples of peritoneal or ascitic fluid are obtained, placed in appropriate containers, labeled, and sent promptly to the laboratory. If the paracentesis is being performed for therapeutic as well as diagnostic reasons, additional fluid is removed. No more than 1,000 to 1,500 ml of fluid should be removed at any one time, in order to avoid complications such as hypovolemia and shock due to abdominal pressure changes and massive fluid shifts into the space which has been drained by paracentesis.

When the desired amount of fluid has been removed, the needle or cannula is withdrawn, and slight pressure applied to the site for a few minutes. If there is no evidence of bleeding or other drainage, a sterile dressing is applied to the site.

Aftercare

The client is assisted to a position of comfort and is reminded of any activity restrictions. If there is excessive drainage, the puncture site should be redressed using sterile technique.

Nursing Observations

Pretest

- Determine if the client is currently taking any anticoagulant medications or aspirin-containing drugs
- Assess the client's response to explanations provided (if the client appears unduly anxious about the procedure or unable to cooperate during it, the physician performing the paracentesis should be so informed)
- Take and record vital signs and compare with the client's usual baseline
- If the client has ascites, obtain weight and measure abdominal girth

During the Test

- If feasible, check the client's vital signs every 15 minutes during the procedure
- Observe the client for pallor, diaphoresis, vertigo, hypotension, tachycardia, pain, or anxiety; rapid removal of fluid may precipitate hypovolemia and shock

Post-Test

■ Take and record vital signs as for a postoperative client (i.e., every 15 minutes times four, every 30 minutes times four, every hour times four, and then every 4 hours for 24 hours
■ Assess the puncture site for bleeding, excessive drainage, and signs of inflammation each time the vital signs are taken and daily thereafter for several days
■ Continue to observe the client for pallor, vertigo, hypotension, tachycardia, pain, or anxiety for at least 24 hours following the procedure
■ If a large amount of fluid was removed, measure abdominal girth and weigh the client

SYNOVIAL FLUID ANALYSIS (BACKGROUND INFORMATION, p. 380)

Reference Values

Red blood cells	$<2000/mm^3$
White blood cells	$<200/mm^3$
Neutrophils	<25 percent
White cell morphology	No abnormal cells or inclusions (see Table 9–1)
Crystals	None present (see Table 9–2)
Gram stain and culture	No organisms present
AFB smear and culture	No acid-fast bacilli present
Protein	<3 g/dl
Glucose	Not <10 mg/dl of blood level or Not <40 mg/dl
Uric acid	Parallels serum level
Lactate	0.6–2.0 mmol/l or 5–20 mg/dl
Antinuclear antibodies (ANA) } Rheumatoid factor (RF) } Complement }	Parallel serum levels

Interfering Factors

■ Blood in the sample due to traumatic arthrocentesis
■ Undetected hypoglycemia or hyperglycemia and/or failure to comply with dietary restrictions prior to the test
■ Contamination of the sample with pathogens
■ Improper handling of the specimen (refrigeration of the sample may result in an increase in monosodium urate [MSU] crystals due to decreased solubility of uric acid; exposure of the sample to room air with a resultant loss of carbon dioxide and rise in pH encourages the formation of calcium pyrophosphate [CPP] crystals)[38]

Indications/Purposes for Synovial Fluid Analysis

■ Joint effusion of unknown etiology
■ Suspected trauma, tumors involving the joint, or hemophilic arthritis as indicated by an elevated red cell count, elevated protein level, and possibly fat droplets if trauma is involved (see Table 9–1, p. 382)
■ Suspected joint effusion due to noninflammatory disorders (e.g., osteoarthritis, degenerative joint disease) as indicated by a white cell count of less than 5,000/mm³ with a normal differential and the presence of cartilage cells (see Table 9–1)

■ Suspected rheumatoid arthritis as indicated by a white cell count of 2,000 to 100,000/mm^3 with an elevated neutrophil count (i.e., 30 to 50 percent), presence of RA cells and possibly Rice bodies (see Table 9–1), cholesterol crystals if effusion is chronic, elevated protein level, decreased glucose level, moderately elevated lactate level (i.e., 2 to 7.5 mmol/l), decreased pH, presence of rheumatoid factor (60 percent of cases), and decreased complement

■ Suspected systemic lupus erythematosus involving the joints as indicated by a white cell count of 2,000 to 100,000/mm^3 with an elevated neutrophil count (i.e., 30 to 40 percent), presence of LE cells (see Table 9–1), elevated protein level, decreased glucose level (i.e., 2 to 7.5 mmol/l), decreased pH, presence of antinuclear antibodies (20 percent of cases), and decreased complement

■ Suspected acute bacterial arthritis as indicated by a white cell count of 10,000 to 200,000/mm^3 with a markedly elevated neutrophil count (i.e., as high as 90 percent), positive Gram stain (50 percent of cases), positive cultures (30 to 80 percent of cases), possibly presence of Rice bodies (see Table 9–1), decreased glucose, lactate level greater than 7.5 mmol/l, pH less than 7.3, and complement levels paralleling those found in serum (i.e., may be elevated or decreased)

■ Suspected tuberculous arthritis as indicated by a white cell count of 2,000 to 100,000/mm^3 with an elevated neutrophil count (i.e., 30 to 60 percent), possibly presence of Rice bodies (see Table 9–1), cholesterol crystals if effusion is chronic, positive AFB smear and culture in some cases (results are frequently negative), decreased glucose, elevated lactate levels, and decreased pH

■ Suspected joint effusion due to gout as indicated by a white cell count of 500 to 200,000/mm^3 with an elevated neutrophil count (i.e., approximately 70 percent), presence of MSU crystals (see Table 9–2, p. 383), decreased glucose, elevated uric acid levels, and complement levels paralleling those of serum (may be elevated or decreased)

■ Differentiation of gout from pseudogout as indicated primarily by finding CPP crystals (see Table 9–2), which are associated with pseudogout (other findings in pseudogout are similar to those of gout except that the white cell count may not be as high)

Client Preparation

Client Teaching. Explain to the client:

■ the purpose of the test
■ that it will be done by a physician and will require approximately 20 minutes
■ any dietary restrictions (fasting for 6 to 12 hours prior to the test is recommended if the synovial fluid is to be tested for glucose)
■ the positioning to be used (seated or supine for knee, shoulder, elbow, wrist, or ankle aspiration; supine for hip joint aspiration)
■ that the skin at the site to be used will be injected with a local anesthetic and that this may cause a stinging sensation
■ that, after the skin has been anesthetized, a large needle will be inserted into the joint capsule
■ that discomfort may be experienced as the joint capsule is penetrated
■ the importance of remaining still during the procedure
■ any activity restrictions following the test (the client usually is advised to avoid excessive use of the joint for several days following the procedure in order to prevent pain and swelling)
■ that ice packs and/or analgesics may be prescribed following the procedure in order to prevent swelling and alleviate discomfort

Encourage questions and verbalization of concerns appropriate to the client's age and mental status.

Ensure that a signed consent for the procedure has been obtained.

Physical Preparation

■ Withhold anticoagulant medications and aspirin as ordered
■ Ensure to the extent possible that any dietary restrictions are followed
■ Have the client void
■ Provide a hospital gown if necessary to allow access to the site without unduly exposing the client
■ Take and record vital signs
■ If the client is extremely hirsute, it may be necessary to shave the area where the puncture is to be made

The Procedure (Arthrocentesis)

The necessary equipment is assembled. This includes an arthrocentesis tray with solution for skin preparation, local anesthetic, a 20 ml syringe, needles of various sizes, sterile drapes, and sterile gloves. Specimen collection tubes and containers for the tests to be performed also are obtained. For cell counts and differential, lavender-topped tubes containing ethylenediaminetetraacetate (EDTA) are used. Green-topped tubes containing heparin are used for certain immunological and chemistry tests, while samples for glucose are collected in either plain red-topped tubes or gray-topped tubes containing potassium oxalate. Plain sterile tubes (e.g., red-topped tubes) are recommended for microbiological testing and crystal examination.[39]

The client is assisted to the position that will be used for the test (sitting or supine). The skin is cleansed with antiseptic solution, protected with sterile drapes, and infiltrated with local anesthetic. The aspirating needle is inserted into the joint space and as much fluid as possible is withdrawn. The specimen should contain at least 10 ml of synovial fluid, but more may be removed to reduce swelling. Manual pressure may be applied to facilitate fluid removal.

If medication is to be injected into the joint, the syringe containing the sample is detached from the needle and replaced with the one containing the drug. The medication is injected with gentle pressure. The needle is then withdrawn and digital pressure is applied to the site for a few minutes. If there is no evidence of bleeding, a sterile dressing is applied to the site. An elastic bandage also may be applied to the joint.

The samples of synovial fluid are placed in the appropriate containers, labeled, and sent to the laboratory immediately.

Aftercare

The client is assisted to a position of comfort. An ice pack may be applied to the site and analgesics administered as needed. Any foods or fluids withheld prior to the test may be resumed, as are any medications withheld upon the physician's order. The client is reminded of any activity restrictions and, if indicated, site care requirements.

Nursing Observations

Pretest

■ Determine if the client is currently taking any anticoagulant medications or aspirin-containing drugs
■ Assess the client's response to explanations provided (if the client appears

unduly anxious about the procedure or unable to cooperate during it, the physician performing the arthrocentesis should be so informed)
■ Take and record vital signs and compare with the client's usual baseline

During the Test

■ Observe the client's response to the procedure, including degree of discomfort experienced

Post-Test

■ Take and record vital signs
■ Assess comfort level and response to measures such as ice packs and analgesics
■ Assess the puncture site for bleeding, bruising, inflammation, and excessive drainage of synovial fluid approximately every 4 hours for 24 hours and then daily there after for several days

REFERENCES

1. Hole, JW: Human Anatomy and Physiology, ed 4. Wm C Brown, Dubuque, IA, 1987, p 158.
2. *Ibid.*
3. Kjeldsberg, CR and Krieg, AF: Cerebrospinal Fluid and Other Body Fluids. In Henry, JB: Clinical Diagnosis and Management by Laboratory Methods, ed 17. WB Saunders, Philadelphia, 1984, p 475.
4. Strasinger, SK: Urinalysis and Body Fluids. FA Davis, Philadelphia, 1985, p 163.
5. Kjeldsberg and Krieg, *op cit*, p 483.
6. Miller, BF and Keane, CB: Encyclopedia and Dictionary of Medicine, Nursing and Allied Health, ed 4. WB Saunders, Philadelphia, 1987, p 226.
7. Kjeldsberg and Krieg, *op cit*, p 485.
8. Strasinger, *op cit*, p 165.
9. Kjeldsberg and Krieg, *op cit*, p 477.
10. *Ibid*, p 476.
11. Strasinger, *op cit*, pp 174–175.
12. *Ibid*, p 174.
13. *Ibid*, p 173.
14. Kjeldsberg and Krieg, *op cit*, pp 486–487.
15. Strasinger, *op cit*, p 174.
16. Kjeldsberg and Krieg, *op cit*, p 488.
17. Strasinger, *op cit*, p 174.
18. Kjeldsberg and Krieg, *op cit*, p 483.
19. *Ibid*, p 488.
20. *Ibid*, pp 484–485.
21. Strasinger, *op cit*, p 174.
22. Kjeldsberg and Krieg, *op cit*, p 485.
23. Strasinger, *op cit*, p 175.
24. Kjeldsberg and Krieg, *op cit*, p 487.
25. *Ibid.*
26. Strasinger, *op cit*, pp 163–164.
27. Kjeldsberg and Krieg, *op cit*, p 480.
28. Strasinger, *op cit*, p 165.
29. Kjeldsberg and Krieg, *op cit*, p 478.
30. *Ibid*, pp 478–479.
31. *Ibid*, p 478.
32. *Ibid*, p 480.
33. Strasinger, *op cit*, p 169.
34. *Ibid.*

35. Kjeldsberg and Krieg, *op cit*, pp 480–481.
36. *Ibid.*
37. Strasinger, *op cit*, p 169.
38. *Ibid*, p 166.
39. *Ibid*, p 163.

BIBLIOGRAPHY

Beare, PG, Rahr, VA and Ronshausen, CA: Nursing Implications of Diagnostic Tests, ed 2. JB Lippincott, Philadelphia, 1985.
Braunstein, H: Outlines of Pathology. CV Mosby, St Louis, 1982.
Diagnostics, ed 2. Springhouse Corp, Springhouse, PA, 1986.
Fischbach, FT: A Manual of Laboratory Diagnostic Tests, ed 3. JB Lippincott, Philadelphia, 1988.
Harvey, AM, Johns, RJ, Owens, AH and Ross, RS: The Principles and Practice of Medicine, ed 19. Appleton-Century-Crofts, New York, 1976.
Jacob, SW, Francone, CA and Lossow, WJ: Structure and Function in Man, ed 5. WB Saunders, Philadelphia, 1982.
Lamb, JO: Laboratory Tests for Clinical Nursing. Robert J Brady, Bowie, MD, 1984.
Luce, JM, Tyler, ML and Pierson, DJ: Intensive Respiratory Care. WB Saunders, Philadelphia, 1984.
Metheny, NM and Snively, WD: Nurse's Handbook of Fluid Balance, ed 4. JB Lippincott, Philadelphia, 1983.
Michaels, D: Diagnostic Procedures: The Patient and the Health Care Team. John Wiley & Sons, New York, 1983.
Nealon, TF: Fundamental Skills in Surgery, ed 2. WB Saunders, Philadelphia, 1971.
Skydell, B and Crowder, AS: Diagnostic Procedures. Little, Brown & Co, Boston, 1975.
Sokoloff, L (ed): The Joints and Synovial Fluid, Vol 1. Academic Press, New York, 1978.
Tilkian, SM, Conover, MB and Tilkian, AG: Clinical Implications of Laboratory Tests, ed 4. CV Mosby, St Louis, 1987.
Widmann, FK: Pathobiology: How Diseases Happen. Little, Brown & Co, Boston, 1978.

10

AMNIOTIC FLUID ANALYSIS

OVERVIEW OF AMNIOTIC FLUID FORMATION AND ANALYSIS

Amniotic fluid is produced in the membranous sac that surrounds the developing fetus. This sac appears during the second week of gestation and arises from a membrane called the amnion. Amniotic fluid is derived from the exchange of water from maternal blood across fetal membranes, from fetal cellular metabolism, and later in pregnancy from fetal urine. Amniotic fluid serves several purposes. It prevents the amniotic membranes from adhering to the embryo and protects the fetus from shocks and blows. It also aids in controlling the embryo's body temperature and permits the fetus to move freely, thus aiding in normal growth and development.[1] Amniotic fluid may be thought of as an extension of the fetus's extracellular fluid space.[2] Testing samples of amniotic fluid for various constituents and substances may, therefore, be used to assess fetal well-being and maturation. Specifically, amniotic fluid analysis is used to test for various inherited disorders, anatomical abnormalities such as neural tube defects, hemolytic disease of the newborn, and fetal maturity.

Amniotic fluid is normally clear and colorless in early pregnancy. Later in pregnancy, it may appear slightly opalescent due to the presence of particles of vernix caseosa and may be pale yellow due to fetal urine. The presence of meconium in amniotic fluid is normal in breech presentations but abnormal in vertex presentations, and indicates relaxation of the anal sphincter due to hypoxia.

398

Amniotic fluid stained the color of port wine generally indicates abruptio placenta.

As the fetus begins to produce urine, it also swallows amniotic fluid in amounts that nearly equal urinary output (i.e., 400 to 500 ml per day).[3] Failure to swallow sufficient amounts of amniotic fluid results in excessive accumulation of fluid in the amniotic sac (polyhydramnios). This is commonly associated with anencephaly and esophageal atresia, but also may occur in the presence of maternal diabetes and hypertensive disorders of pregnancy. Excessive amounts of amniotic fluid also are seen with fetal edema, which is associated with fetal heart failure, hydrops fetalis, and recipient-twin transfusion syndrome. Excessive swallowing of amniotic fluid results in decreased volume (oligohydramnios) and is associated with chronic illness of the fetus, placental insufficiency, fetal urinary tract malformations, and donor-twin transfusion syndrome.[4] By the 14th to 16th weeks of pregnancy, the amniotic sac normally contains at least 50 ml of fluid; at term, the sac contains 500 to 2,500 ml of amniotic fluid, with an average volume of 1,000 ml.

Samples of amniotic fluid are obtained by needle aspiration. As noted in Chapter 9, "centesis" is a suffix denoting puncture and aspiration of; thus, aspiration of fluid from the amniotic sac is called amniocentesis. For suspected genetic and neural tube defects, amniocentesis is generally performed early in the second trimester of pregnancy (i.e., 14th to 16th weeks) when there is sufficient amniotic fluid for sampling, yet enough time for safe abortion if desired. For hemolytic disease of the newborn, a series of amniocenteses may be performed beginning with the 26th week, while tests for fetal maturity usually are not done until at least the 35th week of gestation.

--- **TESTS OF AMNIOTIC FLUID** ---

Background Information (Clinical Applications Data, p. 404)

Tests of amniotic fluid are discussed hereafter in relation to the three general purposes for which they are performed: (1) to detect genetic and neural tube defects; (2) to test for hemolytic disease of the newborn; and (3) to assess fetal maturity.

TESTS FOR GENETIC AND NEURAL TUBE DEFECTS

Tests for genetic and neural tube defects include sex determination, chromosome analysis, and measurement of alpha-fetoprotein (AFP) and acetylcholinesterase levels. Determining the sex of the fetus is indicated when sex-linked inherited disorders are suspected (e.g., hemophilia, Duchennne's muscular dystrophy). In such disorders, the abnormal gene is carried by females while the disorder itself is inherited only by male offspring. Although no specific tests for these disorders are currently available, knowing the sex of the fetus may aid in deciding whether or not to continue the pregnancy. Some couples carrying these disorders, for example, choose to abort all male fetuses, even though some would have been normal.[5]

Determining the fetus' chromosomal make-up (karyotype) also may assist in the prenatal diagnosis of disorders such as Down's syndrome (trisomy 21) and Tay-Sachs disease. Karyotyping, especially when augmented by staining

TABLE 10–1. **Conditions Associated with Increases in Maternal Serum AFP**

Gestational age underestimated	Hydrocephaly
Open neural tube defects	Hydrops fetalis
Fetomaternal hemorrhage	Twin pregnancy
Omphalocele	Turner's syndrome
Congenital proteinuric nephropathies	Cystic hygroma
Sacrococcygeal teratoma	Cyclopia
Duodenal atresia	Microcephaly
Intrauterine death	Gastroschisis
Esophageal atresia	Maternal malignancy producing AFP
Tetralogy of Fallot	

From: Wenk et al,[8] p. 512, with permission.

techniques, includes determination of the number of chromosomes as well as specific morphological changes in the chromosomes that may indicate various genetic disorders. Karyotyping is performed by culturing fetal cells and then photographing individual chromosomes during the metaphase of mitosis.[6] Among the disorders that may be detected are alterations in carbohydrate, lipid, and amino acid metabolism. It should be noted that karyotyping may take from 2 to 4 weeks before results are available to the client. Specimens for chromosomal analysis must be delivered promptly to the laboratory performing the test. If immediate culturing is not possible, the sample must be incubated at normal body temperature for no longer than 2 days.[7]

Neural tube and other anatomical defects in the fetus may be determined by measuring levels of AFP and acetylcholinesterase in amniotic fluid. In the embryo, the central nervous system develops from the neural tube, which begins to form at about 22 days of gestation. Failure of the neural tube to close properly may result in disorders such as anencephaly, spina bifida, and myelomeningocele. During gestation, the major fetal serum protein is AFP. Similar to albumin, this protein is manufactured in large quantities by the fetal liver until the 32nd week of gestation, with peak production occurring at 13 weeks (see Chapter 3). When there is a severe neural tube defect, higher than normal amounts of AFP escape into the aminotic fluid as well as into the maternal circulation. Routine prenatal screening includes determination of the mother's serum AFP level at 13 to 16 weeks of pregnancy. Causes of elevated maternal AFP levels are listed in Table 10–1. If maternal levels are elevated on two samples obtained 1 week apart, an ultrasound is performed to determine gestational age and to check for twins or gross fetal anomalies. If the ultrasound is normal, amniotic fluid samples are obtained and analyzed for AFP levels.[8,9] If AFP levels are elevated in amniotic fluid, the presence of acetylcholinesterase in the fluid may be determined to confirm the presence of a neural tube defect. Using electrophoretic methods, the isoenzyme of acetylcholinesterase, which originates in fetal spinal fluid, also may be demonstrated and is more specific to the diagnosis of neural tube defect.[10] It should be noted that AFP and acetylcholinesterase may be falsely elevated if the sample is contaminated with fetal blood. The level of the fetal spinal fluid isoenzyme of acetylcholinesterase is not, however, so affected.

TESTS FOR HEMOLYTIC DISEASE OF THE NEWBORN

One of the oldest uses of amniotic fluid analysis is in evaluating suspected hemolytic disease of the newborn, in which the mother builds antibodies against fetal red blood cell antigens (isoimmunization). The result is hemolysis of fetal erythrocytes with release of bilirubin into the amniotic fluid. The most common causes are ABO and Rh incompatibilities (e.g., an Rh-negative mother carrying an Rh-positive fetus), although other red cell antibodies also may be involved. Maternal IgG antibodies may cross the placenta to react with fetal red blood cells as early as the 16th week of pregnancy. As fetal red blood cells are broken down, bilirubin is released and can be detected in the amniotic fluid.[11]

Normally, the bilirubin level in amniotic fluid is highest between the 16th and 30th weeks of gestation. Much of this bilirubin is in the unconjugated form and can be excreted by the placenta. As the fetal liver matures, it begins to conjugate the bilirubin; this may occur as early as 28 weeks of gestation. The conjugated bilirubin is not, however, cleared by the placenta; instead, it is excreted by the fetal biliary tract and absorbed by the intestine. After the 30th week of gestation, the bilirubin level in amniotic fluid normally decreases as pregnancy progresses. This is partly due to dilution of any bilirubin present by the normal increase in amniotic fluid volume. At term, bilirubin is nearly absent from amniotic fluid.[12]

In hemolytic disease of the newborn, fetal red cell destruction leads to excessive bilirubin levels, which overwhelm both placental and fetal liver mechanisms for its clearance. Bilirubin levels in amniotic fluid continue to rise throughout the pregnancy and consist primarily of unconjugated bilirubin.[13] The amount of bilirubin present in the amniotic fluid indicates the degree of fetal red hemolysis and, indirectly, the degree of fetal anemia.

When hemolytic disease of the newborn is suspected or if maternal IgG levels are elevated, or both, serial amniocenteses for bilirubin determinations are performed beginning at approximately the 26th week of pregnancy. Bilirubin measurement in amniotic fluid is performed by spectrophotometric analysis, with the optical density (OD) of the fluid measured at wavelength intervals between 365 mμ and 550 mμ. When excessive bilirubin is present, a rise in OD at 450 mμ, the wavelength of maximum bilirubin absorption, will be seen.[14] The results of spectrophotometric analysis may be compared with the Liley graph (Fig. 10–1) or the Freda Management Table (Table 10–2) to predict fetal outcome or to plan medical management of the problem.

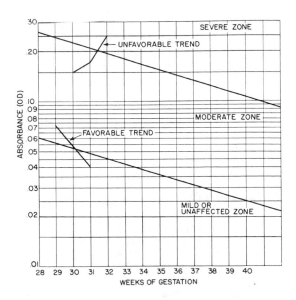

FIGURE 10–1. The Liley graph showing the relationship of duration of pregnancy and net optical density of amniotic fluid at 450 mμ. (From Wenk et al,[15] p. 504, with permission.)

TABLE 10-2. Freda Management Table

Optical Density Difference 450 nm	Grade	Interpretation
0-0.20	1+	Fetus unaffected or mildly affected by hemolysis
0.20-0.35	2+	Fetus definitely affected but not in jeopardy
0.35-0.70	3+	Fetus in distress
0.70 and greater	4+	Impending fetal demise

From: Wenk et al,[15] p. 505, with permission.

It should be noted that substances other than bilirubin may cause abnormal spectrophotometric results. Maternal hemoglobin from a traumatic amniocentesis, methemalbumin, and meconium in amniotic fluid may cause false elevations, as will fetal acidosis. Fetal hemoglobin may be differentiated from maternal hemoglobin by staining and cytological techniques. The presence of methemalbumin indicates marked hemolysis and impending fetal demise.[15] Falsely decreased bilirubin levels may occur if the amniotic fluid sample is exposed to light or if there is dilution by excessive amniotic fluid volume. Other disorders that may cause elevated amniotic fluid bilirubin levels include anencephaly and intestinal obstruction.[16]

TESTS FOR FETAL MATURITY

Tests for fetal maturity are generally performed after the 35th week of pregnancy, when preterm delivery is being considered because of fetal or maternal problems. The lungs are the last of the fetal organs to mature; therefore, the most common complication of early delivery is newborn respiratory distress syndrome (RDS). Tests of amniotic fluid for fetal maturity focus on determining fetal lung maturity and include the lecithin-sphingomyelin (L/S) ratio, as well as measures of other lung surface lipids such as phosphatidyl glycerol and phosphatidyl inositol. If the lungs are found to be mature by these tests, the other body organs also are assumed to be mature.[17,18] Tests of amniotic fluid, which may be used to indicate maturity of other fetal organ systems, include creatinine and bilirubin determinations, as well as examination of fetal cells for type and lipid content.

During the last trimester of pregnancy, fetal lung enzyme systems initiate the production of surfactant by type II pneumocytes, which line the alveoli. Surfactant, a phospholipid mixture, lowers the surface tension in the alveoli and prevents them from collapsing during exhalation. The phospholipid components of surfactant are (1) lecithin (phosphatidyl choline); (2) sphingomyelin; (3) phosphatidyl glycerol (PG); (4) phosphatidyl ethanolamine (PE); (5) phosphatidyl inositol (PI); and phosphatidyl serine (PS). Surfactant appears in amniotic fluid as a result of fetal respiratory movements, which cause it to diffuse from fetal airways.[19]

Lecithin constitutes about 75 percent of surfactant in mature lungs and is responsible for most of the surface activity of surfactant. The saturated form of lecithin, alpha-palmitic beta-myristic lecithin, is seen early in the third trimester; the desaturated form, dipalmitic lecithin (L), begins to appear at approximately 35 weeks' gestation and continues to increase throughout the remainder of the pregnancy. Sphingomyelin, a surfactant component without major surface activity properties, remains fairly constant during pregnancy. The L/S ratio measures the relationship between these two components; if the increasing amount of lecithin over the relatively constant amount of sphingomyelin produces a ratio of 2:1 or more, fetal lung maturity is generally indicated, as long as the pregnancy is uncomplicated and the amniotic fluid sample is not contaminated with blood or meconium.[20]

A more reliable measure of fetal lung maturity is the "lung profile," in which the concentrations of the several lung surface lipids (i.e., PG, PI, PS, and PE) are measured in addition to lecithin and sphingomyelin. Next to lecithin, PG is the second major constituent of surfactant and is believed to aid in maintaining alveolar stability. PG appears in amniotic fluid at about 36 weeks' gestation and indicates secretion of mature surfactant. It has been found that if PG is present in amniotic fluid, RDS in the newborn will not occur. PI is found in amniotic fluid prior to the appearance of PG and indicates immature fetal lungs. PI has a peak concentration at approximately 5 weeks before term and then decreases thereafter. Measurement of PG and PI are most useful since they are unaffected by the presence of blood and meconium, although PG is affected by dilution of the specimen with water and by variations in test performance techniques. In addition to their usefulness in evaluating bloody or meconium stained samples of amniotic fluid, lung profiles aid in determining lung maturity in fetuses of diabetic mothers. In maternal diabetes, the L/S ratio may indicate fetal lung maturity even though PG is not present. If the infant were delivered, RDS would be likely to occur. Measurement of PG in such situations aids in determining if delivery should be attempted.[21,22] The significance of measures of PS and PE in lung profiles has not yet been determined.

A bedside test to estimate fetal lung maturity may be performed when immediate results are needed. The shake test is based on the ability of surfactant to form stable foam, even in the presence of alcohol which impairs foaming of most other biological compounds. In this test, equal amounts of 95 percent ethanol and amniotic fluid are shaken together vigorously for 15 seconds and then allowed to stand undisturbed for 15 minutes. If a complete ring of bubbles is present at the meniscus, the test result is reported as positive, which indicates that sufficient lecithin is available for fetal lung maturity.[23] The sample of amniotic fluid for the shake test also may be diluted with saline to various concentrations in order more accurately to estimate fetal lung maturity. There should be a positive test result even when amniotic fluid has been diluted with two parts of saline.[24]

Other tests of amniotic fluid for fetal maturity include creatinine and bilirubin determinations, and examination of fetal cells for type and lipid content. Creatinine appears in increased amounts in amniotic fluid at about the 36th week of gestation owing to excretion of urine by the fetal kidneys and increased fetal muscle mass. A creatinine concentration of greater than 2.0 mg/dl indicates a fetal age of at least 36 to 37 weeks.[25,26] As noted previously, bilirubin levels decline throughout the last several weeks of pregnancy. Thus, a bilirubin level of less than 0.025 mg/dl at term is considered an indication of fetal maturity. It should be noted, however, that bilirubin levels may not be used to assess fetal maturity in isoimmunized mothers, because levels will be elevated due to hemolytic disease involving the fetus.

During the second and third trimesters, fetal epithelial cells are shed into the amniotic fluid. As the fetus matures, the percentage of cells containing lipids increases. The test is performed by staining the cells with Nile blue stain. Cells containing lipid will appear orange.[27] Although only 1 percent of the cells contain lipid at 34 weeks' gestation, 10 to 50 percent will contain lipid at 38 to 40 weeks.[28] Fetal maturity also may be evaluated by examining the types of cells present. While basal cells are present until about 32 weeks' gestation, cornified cells appear at 36 weeks and are the predominant cell type after 38 weeks.[29]

Clinical Applications Data *(Background Information, p. 399)*

Reference Values

Chromosome analysis	Normal karyotype
Alpha-fetoprotein (AFP)	13–41 μg/ml at 13–14 weeks
	0.2–3.0 μg/ml at term
Acetylcholinesterase	Absent
Bilirubin	<0.075 mg/dl early in pregnancy
	<0.025 mg/dl at term
L/S ratio	<1.6:1 prior to 35 weeks
	>2.0:1 at term
Phosphatidyl glycerol (PG)	Present at approximately 36 weeks
Phosphatidyl inositol (PI)	Peak amounts present 5 weeks prior to term, followed by a decline
Shake test	Positive
Creatinine	1.8–4.0 mg/dl at term

Interfering Factors

■ Failure to promptly deliver samples for chromosomal analysis to the laboratory performing the test, and/or improper incubation of the sample such that cells do not remain alive, will make karyotyping impossible to perform; sample should also be protected from light

■ AFP and acetylcholinesterase may be falsely elevated if the sample is contaminated with fetal blood

■ Bilirubin may be falsely elevated if maternal hemoglobin, methemalbumin, or meconium are present in the sample; fetal acidosis also may lead to falsely elevated bilirubin levels

■ Bilirubin may be falsely decreased if the sample is exposed to light or if amniotic fluid volume is excessive

■ Contamination of the sample with blood or meconium may yield inaccurate L/S ratios

Indications/Purposes for Amniotic Fluid Tests

■ Family or parental history of genetic disorders such as Tay-Sachs disease, mental retardation, chromosome or enzyme anomalies, or inherited hemoglobinopathies

■ Advanced maternal age (chromosomal analysis is routine in mothers aged 35 or older)

■ Prenatal sex determination when the mother is a known carrier of a sex-linked abnormal gene that could be transmitted to male offspring

■ In utero diagnosis of metabolic disorders such as cystic fibrosis, diabetes mellitus, or other errors of lipid, carbohydrate, or amino acid metabolism

■ Suspected neural tube defect as indicated by elevated AFP and acetylcholinesterase levels

■ Known or suspected hemolytic disease involving the fetus as indicated by rising bilirubin levels, especially after the 30th week of gestation

■ Determination of fetal maturity when preterm delivery is being considered, with fetal maturity indicated by L/S ratio of 2:1 or greater, presence of PG, positive shake test, creatinine >2.0 mg/dl, and bilirubin <0.025 mg/dl (nonisoimmunized mother)

Contraindications

■ History of premature labor or incompetent cervix
■ Presence of placenta previa or abruptio placenta

Client Preparation

Client Teaching. Explain to the client:

■ the purpose of the test
■ that it will be done by a physician and will require 20 to 30 minutes
■ the precautions taken to avoid injury to the fetus (i.e., careful palpation, localization of the fetus and placenta by ultrasound, and use of strict aseptic technique)
■ the positioning used for the procedure and the necessity of remaining still during it
■ that the skin will be injected with a local anesthetic at the needle insertion site and that this may cause a stinging sensation
■ that a sensation of pressure may be felt when the needle is inserted for the amniotic fluid sample
■ how to use focusing and controlled breathing for relaxation during the procedure
■ that slight cramping may occur following the procedure
■ that if the test is being done for chromosomal studies, it may be 2 to 4 weeks before results are available

Encourage questions and verbalization of concerns appropriate to the client's age and mental status.
Ensure that a signed consent for the procedure has been obtained.

Physical Preparation

■ If an ultrasound is to be performed immediately prior to the amniocentesis, in order to localize the fetus and placenta, hydrate the client to ensure a full bladder
■ After the ultrasound, have the client empty the bladder to prevent perforation during the amniocentesis (the most common nonamniotic fluid obtained during the procedure is maternal urine[30])
■ Provide a hospital gown
■ Record maternal vital signs and fetal heart rate

The Procedure (Amniocentesis)

The necessary equipment is assembled. This includes an amniocentesis tray with solution for skin preparation, local anesthetic, a 10 or 20 ml syringe, needles of various sizes (including a 22-gauge, 5-inch spinal needle), sterile drapes, and sterile gloves. Special specimen collection tubes (either brown or foil-covered) also are needed.

The client is assisted to a supine position. The head or legs may be raised slightly to promote client comfort and to relax abdominal muscles. If the uterus is large, a pillow or rolled blanket is placed under the client's right side to prevent hypotension due to great vessel compression.

The skin of the lower abdomen is prepared with an antiseptic solution and protected with sterile drapes. The local anesthetic is injected. A 5-inch, 22-gauge spinal needle is inserted, usually at the midline, through the abdominal and uterine walls. The stylet is withdrawn and a plastic syringe of sufficient volume for the sample to be obtained is attached. A sample of at least 10 ml of amniotic fluid is withdrawn and placed in appropriate containers.

When the desired amount of fluid has been removed, the needle is withdrawn and slight pressure applied to the site. If there is no evidence of bleeding or other drainage, a sterile adhesive bandage is applied to the site. The specimens should be sent to the laboratory immediately.

Aftercare

The client is assisted to a position of comfort. If the client is Rh negative, RhoGAM is administered to prevent potential sensitization to fetal blood. The client is reminded to report fever, leaking amniotic fluid, vaginal bleeding, or uterine contractions to her physician. Changes in fetal activity—either an increase or a decrease—also should be reported.

Nursing Observations

Pretest

■ Assess the client's responses to explanations provided (if the client appears unduly anxious about the procedure or unable to cooperate during it, the physician performing the amniocentesis should be so informed)
■ Take and record maternal vital signs and fetal heart sounds and compare with the client's usual baseline
■ Observe for uterine contractions

During the Test

■ Observe the client for diaphoresis, dizziness, and nausea

Post-Test

■ Take and record maternal vital signs and fetal heart sounds every 15 minutes for one half to 1 hour
■ Assess the client for contractions, pain, and vaginal bleeding each time vital signs are checked
■ Observe the puncture site for bleeding or other drainage

REFERENCES

1. Moore, ML: Realities in Childbearing, ed 2. WB Saunders, Philadelphia, 1983, p 762.
2. Wenk, RE, Rosenbaum, JM and Statland, BE: Assessment of Fetal Condition and Amniotic Fluid Analysis. In Henry, JB: Clinical Diagnosis and Management by Laboratory Methods, ed 17. WB Saunders, Philadelphia, 1984, p 502.
3. Strasinger, SK: Urinalysis and Body Fluids. FA Davis, Philadelphia, 1985, p 175.
4. Wenk et al, op cit, p 503.
5. Widmann, FK: Clinical Interpretation of Laboratory Tests, ed 9. FA Davis, Philadelphia, 1983, p 492.
6. Ibid, pp 490–491.
7. Strasinger, op cit, p 176.
8. Wenk et al, op cit, pp 511–512.
9. Widmann, op cit, pp 493–494.
10. Wenk et al, op cit, p 512.
11. Ibid, p 503.
12. Ibid, pp 503–504.
13. Ibid, p 503.
14. Strasinger, op cit, p 177.
15. Wenk et al, op cit, pp 504–505.

16. Fischbach, FT: A Manual of Laboratory Diagnostic Tests, ed. 3. JB Lippincott, Philadelphia, 1988, p 867.
17. Wenk *et al, op cit,* p 506.
18. Strasinger, *op cit,* p 177.
19. Wenk *et al, op cit,* p 506.
20. *Ibid,* pp 506–509.
21. *Ibid,* p 509.
22. Strasinger, *op cit,* pp 177–178.
23. Wenk *et al, op cit,* pp 507–508.
24. Moore, *op cit,* p 430.
25. Strasinger, *op cit,* p 178.
26. Moore, *op cit,* p 430.
27. Pagana, KD and Pagana TJ: Diagnostic Testing and Nursing Implications: A Case Study Approach, ed 2. CV Mosby, St Louis, 1986, p 175.
28. Moore, *op cit,* p 430.
29. *Ibid.*
30. Wenk *et al, op cit,* p 506.

BIBLIOGRAPHY

Corbett, JV: Laboratory Tests and Diagnostic Procedures with Nursing Diagnoses, ed 2. Appleton & Lange, Norwalk, CT, 1987.

Diagnostics, ed 2. Springhouse Corp, Springhouse, PA, 1986.

Jensen, MD, Benson, RC and Bobak, IM: Maternity Care: The Nurse and the Family. CV Mosby, St Louis, 1977.

Kee, JL: Laboratory and Diagnostic Tests with Nursing Implications, ed 2. Appleton & Lange, Norwalk, CT, 1987.

Lamb, JO: Laboratory Tests for Clinical Nursing. Robert J Brady, Bowie, MD, 1984.

Schmeck, H: Fetal defects discovered early by new method. New York Times, Oct 18, 1983.

Skydell, B and Crowder, AS: Diagnostic Procedures. Little, Brown & Co, Boston, 1975.

11

SEMEN ANALYSIS

OVERVIEW OF SEMEN FORMATION AND ANALYSIS

Semen is a fluid that consists of sperm suspended in seminal plasma. It is composed of four main fractions that are contributed by (1) the testis and epididymis, (2) the seminal vesicle, (3) the prostate gland, and (4) the bulbourethral and urethral glands (Fig. 11–1). Sperm, which comprise less than 5 percent of the volume of semen, are produced in the testis and mature in the epididymis. It is thought that the epididymis secretes a number of proteins that are essential to the fertilizing capability of sperm. Most mature sperm are stored in the vas deferens until released by emission and ejaculation. While in the vas deferens, sperm are relatively inactive because of the diminished oxygen supply and acid environment, however, they can survive for up to 1 month in this location.[1,2]

The seminal vesicles, which contribute approximately 60 percent to the volume of semen, are attached to the vas deferens near the base of the urinary bladder. They secrete a viscous, slightly alkaline fluid with high levels of fructose, flavin, potassium, and citric acid. Fructose provides the major nutrient for sperm after emission. (Sperm may survive in the vagina for more than 72 hours after sexual intercourse.[3]) Flavin is responsible for the fluorescence of semen in ultraviolet light, thus allowing for detection of semen on clothing or other fabrics in rape cases. The significance of the high potassium and citric acid levels in seminal fluid has not yet been established. The fluid secreted by the seminal vesicles also contains prostaglandins, which are thought to stimulate muscular contractions in female reproductive organs, and a fibrinogen-like substance which causes semen to coagulate after ejaculation.[4,5]

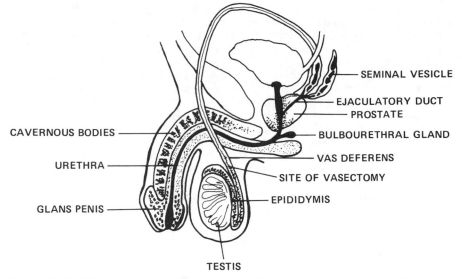

FIGURE 11-1. Diagram of male genitalia. (From Strasinger, SK: Urinalysis and Body Fluids. FA Davis, Philadelphia, 1985, p. 159, with permission.)

The prostate gland, which contributes about 20 percent to the volume of semen, secretes a milky fluid with a pH of 6.5 due largely to its high citric acid content. Prostatic fluid also is high in proteolytic enzymes and acid phosphatase. The proteolytic enzymes are believed to act upon seminal fluid causing coagulation and, subsequently, liquifaction of the ejaculate.[6,7] The bulbourethral and urethral glands secrete a clear, mucus-like fluid that cleanses the urethra and lubricates the end of the penis in preparation for intercourse. This fluid contributes less than 10 to 15 percent to the volume of semen.[8,9]

When ejaculation occurs, the components of semen enter the urethra individually but in rapid succession. Secretion of the bulbourethral and urethral glands occurs first, followed by prostatic secretion and most of the sperm. Note that the first two components contribute only about 40 percent of the total ejaculate. Finally the seminal vesicles empty, contributing the bulk of the fluid. The sequence in which these fluids appear is an important consideration in the method of specimen collection for semen analysis. If, for example, coitus interruptus is used, it is possible that the sperm-rich portion will be missed and that the sample will consist primarily of fluid from the seminal vesicles.[10]

Freshly ejaculated semen is viscous, opaque, and white or grayish-white. It coagulates almost immediately, but within 10 to 30 minutes liquifies to become a translucent fluid that pours in droplets and does not appear clumped or stringy. The pH of semen is slightly alkaline (average 7.7). A pH of less than 7.0 is indicative of a sample consisting mainly of prostatic secretions, and may indicate congenital aplasia of the seminal vesicles. Increased turbidity after liquifaction may indicate the presence of leukocytes and inflammation. Blood in the sample is abnormal. The usual volume of the ejaculate is 2 to 5 ml, although the amount may range from 0.7 to 6.5 ml and still be considered normal. Extending the time between ejaculations does not lead to an increase in volume. Increased volumes of sperm-poor semen are associated with male infertility, while greatly decreased volumes may impair penetration of the cervical mucus by those sperm present.[11,12]

Semen is examined in the laboratory for four main reasons: (1) to investigate infertility, (2) to evaluate the effectiveness of vasectomy, (3) to support or disprove sterility in a paternity suit, and (4) to investigate alleged or suspected rape. For fertility studies, the optimal method of obtaining a specimen is masturbation with collection of the ejaculate in a clean glass or plastic container. Other approaches include obtaining the specimen by coitus interruptus and collection of the sample using a condom. The problems associated with collecting the specimen by coitus interruptus have been noted previously. The use of condoms presents problems because many of them contain spermicides. If used, the condom should be thoroughly washed and dried first.

When rape is alleged or suspected, the specimen may be swabbed from the vagina with a Papanicolaou stick or cotton-tipped applicator or may be obtained by aspiration with a bulb syringe to which a rubber catheter is attached, or with saline lavage. Samples of dried semen on the skin may be obtained by sponging the site with saline moistened gauze. Sections of clothing and other fabric samples containing semen may be soaked in saline for 1 hour. The resulting solution is then subjected to semen analysis.[13,14]

TESTS OF SEMEN

Background Information (Clinical Applications Data, p. 413)

Tests of semen are discussed in relation to those used to determine fertility and those used when rape is suspected.

TESTS FOR FERTILITY

In addition to examining the sample for appearance, viscosity, and pH (see p. 409), fertility tests include assessment of sperm count, sperm motility, and sperm morphology. Other tests include determining the viability of sperm, the presence of fructose in the sample, the presence of antibodies to sperm, and the ability of sperm to penetrate the cervical mucus following coitus.

The sperm count is performed in a manner similar to that used to do blood counts. With the liquified specimen diluted to immobilize the sperm, the number of sperm in a given microscopic area are counted and the result multiplied by a factor of either 100,000 or 1,000,000 to obtain the sperm count. The normal sperm count ranges from 40 to 160 million per milliliter, with counts of 20 to 40 million per milliliter considered borderline normal. For postvasectomy tests, only the sperm count is necessary. It should eventually be negative for sperm on two consecutive monthly examinations.

As sperm must migrate through the cervical mucus and the fallopian tubes, sperm motility is a key indicator of fertility. For this test, the motility of at least 200 sperm is examined microscopically. The percentage of sperm showing progressive forward motion is recorded and should normally be greater than 60 percent within 3 hours of collecting the sample. Those sperm showing progressive motility also may be graded according to the quality of the movement observed (Table 11–1).[15]

Tʜᴇ 11-1. **Grades of Sperm Motility**

Grade I	Minimal forward progression
Grade II	Poor to fair activity
Grade III	Good activity with tail movements
Grade IV	Full activity with tail movements difficult to visualize

From Cannon, DC: Seminal Fluid. In Henry, JB: Clinical Diagnosis and Management by Laboratory Methods, ed 17. WB Saunders, Philadelphia, 1984, p 518, with permission.

Sperm morphology involves microscopic examination of sperm to detect abnormal forms and shapes that may render the sperm incapable of fertilization. The appearance of both the head and the tail of a minimum of 200 sperm is evaluated. Normally, the sperm has an oval head, which measures about 3×5 μm, and a long tapering tail.[16] Abnormal head structures (Fig. 11–2) are associated with failure to penetrate the ovum. Abnormal tail structures are associated with poor sperm motility. The finding of numerous immature sperm (spermatids) is also an abnormal finding, since sperm usually mature in the epididymis. In a normal specimen, fewer than 30 percent abnormal sperm will be found.[17]

If abnormalities in sperm count, motility, or morphology are detected, additional tests may be performed. Tests for sperm viability are indicated when the sperm count is normal but motility markedly decreased. Sperm viability is tested by staining the sample such that dead and living sperm appear different on microscopic examination.[18] If the sperm count is low, the sample may be examined for the presence of fructose. As noted previously (p. 408), the fluid secreted

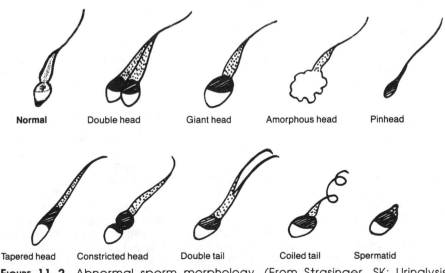

Fɪɢᴜʀᴇ 11–2. Abnormal sperm morphology. (From Strasinger, SK: Urinalysis and Body Fluids. FA Davis, Philadelphia, 1985, p. 161, with permission.)

by the seminal vesicles is high in fructose, a major nutrient for sperm. Thus, presence of fructose in the sample indicates that adequate support medium is available for the sperm and also that the ejaculatory ducts are patent.[19,20]

Both men and women may produce antibodies to sperm. Male antibodies are suspected when semen analysis shows decreased sperm motility with clumping. Female antibodies are suspected when semen analysis is normal and assessment of the female reveals no cause for continuing infertility. The test is performed by mixing sperm with serum from either the male or female and then observing for agglutination or immobilization of the sperm. The quantity of antibodies present may be determined through radioimmunoassay techniques.[21]

Postcoital tests of semen are performed to determine both the quality of cervical mucus and the ability of sperm to penetrate the cervical mucus and still remain active. The test is performed during the ovulatory phase of the menstrual cycle, within 6 to 8 hours of coitus. Normally, at least 10 motile sperm should be present per high-power microscopical field. During the ovulatory phase, cervical mucus should be clear and somewhat watery with a spinnbarkeit of 10 cm. A spinnbarkeit is a measure of tenacity of the cervical mucus and is determined by grasping a portion of the cervical mucus with a forceps and seeing how far it can be drawn before breaking.[22,23]

TESTS FOR THE PRESENCE OF SEMEN

Tests for the presence of semen are performed when rape is alleged or suspected. These tests include examination for sperm, acid phosphatase determination, and detection of blood group substances.

As noted previously (p. 408), the flavin content of semen is responsible for the fluorescence of semen in ultraviolet light. Thus, a preliminary scan of the victim's clothing may help in identifying specific areas that may yield samples for analysis. The presence of sperm in samples obtained from clothing as well as in vaginal secretions may be detected with various staining techniques and microscopic examination. It should be noted, however, that sperm will not be detected if the male has had a vasectomy or is sterile for some other reason.

A more sensitive test to ascertain the presence of semen is the acid phosphatase test, as semen is the only body fluid high in this substance. The acid phosphatase test specifically indicates the presence of prostatic fluid and does not depend on the presence of sperm for a positive result. Vaginal samples as well as clothing stains may be examined. It has been found that acid phosphatase can be detected in semen stains that are several months old.[24]

If the presence of semen is positively determined, testing for the presence of A, B, or H blood group substances may be employed to ascertain if the semen sample is of the same or different blood group as that of the suspect. Inheritance of the H gene is necessary for the normal expression of the ABO genes and the subsequent development of A, B, and H antigens and related blood groups. The H gene is found in over 99 percent of the population. Inheritance of the A gene leads to conversion of nearly all the H antigen on the red cell surface to A antigen sites. Similarly, inheritance of the B gene will lead to conversion of H antigen to B antigen sites. When both the A and B genes are inherited, somewhat more H antigen sites are changed to B than to A. Inheritance of the O gene does not produce such changes in the H structure. Thus, blood group O has the highest level of H antigen. In addition to their presence on red blood cells, A, B, and H antigens may be found on white blood cells and platelets, and in all body secretions—including semen—in 80 percent of the population.[25,26]

Clinical Applications Data *(Background Information, p. 410)*

Reference Values

pH	>7.0 (average 7.7)
Volume	0.7–6.5 ml/ejaculate (usually 1.5–5 ml)
Sperm count	40–160 million/ml (20–40 million/ml = borderline normal)
Sperm motility	>60% within 3 hr of specimen collection
	Quality greater than Grade II (see Table 11–1, p. 411)
Sperm morphology	<30% abnormal sperm
Fructose	Present and/or >150 mg/dl
Sperm antibodies	Negative for male and female antibodies
Postcoital test	At least 10 motile sperm/high-powered microscopical field within 6 to 8 hours of coitus
Acid phosphatase	2500 King-Armstrong units/ml (average)

Interfering Factors

■ Improper specimen collection (e.g., use of condoms containing spermicide; loss of sperm-rich portion of the sample through use of coitus interruptus)
■ Failure to deliver the ejaculated sample to the laboratory within 1 hour
■ Failure to maintain the ejaculated specimen at body temperature until liquifaction occurs (20 to 60 minutes)

Indications/Purposes for Semen Analysis

■ To investigate infertility
■ To evaluate the effectiveness of vasectomy as indicated by two sperm-free samples collected 1 month apart
■ To support or disprove sterility in a paternity suit
■ To investigate alleged or suspected rape

Client Preparation

Male Clients
Client Teaching. Explain to the client:

■ the purpose of the test
■ the various procedures that may be used to obtain the sample
■ the desirability of abstaining from sexual activity for approximately 3 days prior to sample collection, to promote the highest sperm count
■ the importance of transporting the sample promptly to the laboratory, while maintaining it at body temperature, if the sample is collected at home

Encourage questions and verbalization of concerns about the test.

Physical Preparation

■ Provide appropriate specimen collection containers.

Female Clients
Client Teaching. Explain to the client:

■ the purpose of the test
■ that samples will be collected by vaginal examination
■ the positioning on the pelvic examination table
■ that if saline lavage is used to collect the sample, the client may experience a sensation of cold

Encourage questions and verbalization of concerns about the procedure.
The rape victim may need additional support to cope with having a vaginal examination.

Physical Preparation

■ Assist the client to don an examination gown; if rape is suspected, handle the client's clothes carefully because additional specimens may be obtained from them
■ Advise the client to void prior to the procedure; rape victims should not wipe after voiding, so as not to remove possible semen

The Procedure

Ejaculated Sample. The ideal sample is obtained in the laboratory by masturbation and is collected in a glass or plastic specimen container. If the sample is collected at home by masturbation, it must be transported to the laboratory within 1 hour of collection and must be maintained at body temperature.

If the client is unable to produce the specimen by masturbation for either religious or psychological reasons, the specimen may be obtained during the sexual act through the use of condoms or coitus interruptus. If a condom is used, it must be washed and dried thoroughly before use to rid it of possible spermicides. If coitus interruptus is used, the client must be informed of the potential for loss of the sperm-rich portion of the sample (see p. 409).

If none of the aforementioned approaches is acceptable to the client, a final alternative is to obtain postcoital samples from the cervical canal and vagina of his partner.

Cervical/Vaginal Samples. The necessary equipment is assembled. This includes vaginal speculums, Papanicolaou sticks, cotton-tipped applicators, gloves, saline and syringes for lavage (if necessary), slides, and small jars containing 95 percent ethanol.

The client is assisted to the lithotomy position on the pelvic examination table. A vaginal speculum is inserted and the specimen obtained by direct smear, aspiration, or saline lavage. The specimens are labeled and sent immediately to the laboratory.

Samples From Skin and Clothing. Samples of dried semen on the skin may be obtained by sponging the site with saline moistened gauze. Sections of clothing and other fabric samples containing semen may be soaked in saline for 1 hour. The resulting solution is then subjected to semen analysis.

Aftercare and Nursing Observations

There is no specific aftercare unless postejaculatory or postcoital cleansing is desired. The rape victim may be given a spermicidal douche in addition to the prescribed medication for prevention of pregnancy.

The nurse should assess the client's understanding of all explanations provided and should be sensitive to possible feelings of embarrassment on the part of the client.

REFERENCES

1. Cannon, DC: Seminal Fluid. In Henry, JB: Clinical Diagnosis and Management by Laboratory Methods, ed 17. WB Saunders, Philadelphia, 1984, p 516.
2. Strasinger, SK: Urinalysis and Body Fluids. FA Davis, Philadelphia, 1985, p 158.
3. Diagnostics, ed 2. Springhouse Corp, Springhouse, PA, 1986, p 701.
4. Cannon, *op cit*, p 516.
5. Hole, JW: Human Anatomy and Physiology, ed 4. Wm C Brown, Dubuque, IA, 1987, p 815.
6. Strasinger, *op cit*, pp 158–159.
7. Cannon, *op cit*, pp 516–518.
8. Hole, *op cit*, p 815.
9. Cannon, *op cit*, p 517.
10. *Ibid.*
11. *Ibid.*
12. Strasinger, *op cit*, p 159.
13. Diagnostics, *op cit*, p 701.
14. Cannon, *op cit*, p 521.
15. Cannon, *op cit*, p 518.
16. Strasinger, *op cit*, p 161.
17. *Ibid.*
18. *Ibid*, p 162.
19. *Ibid.*
20. Widmann, FK: Clinical Interpretation of Laboratory Tests, ed 9. FA Davis, Philadelphia, 1983, p 472.
21. Strasinger, *op cit*, p 162.
22. Cannon, *op cit*, pp 519–520.
23. Diagnostics, *op cit*, pp 700, 703.
24. Cannon, *op cit*, p 521.
25. *Ibid.*
26. Pittiglio, DH: Modern Blood Banking and Transfusion Practices. FA Davis, Philadelphia, 1983, pp 94–96.

BIBLIOGRAPHY

Kee, JL: Laboratory and Diagnostic Tests with Nursing Implications, ed 2. Appleton & Lange, Norwalk, CT, 1987.

Lamb, JO: Laboratory Tests for Clinical Nursing. Robert J Brady, Bowie, MD, 1984.

Luckmann, J and Sorensen, KC: Medical-Surgical Nursing: A Psychophysiologic Approach, ed 3. WB Saunders, Philadelphia, 1987.

Michaels, D: Diagnostic Procedures: The Patient and the Health Care Team. John Wiley & Sons, New York, 1983.

Wallach, J: Interpretation of Diagnostic Tests: A Handbook Synopsis of Laboratory Medicine, ed 4. Little, Brown & Co., Boston, 1986.

Widmann, FK: Pathobiology: How Diseases Happen. Little, Brown & Co, Boston, 1978.

12

ANALYSIS OF GASTRIC AND DUODENAL SECRETIONS

------------------------------ **OVERVIEW OF GASTRIC AND**
DUODENAL SECRETIONS ------------------------------

The stomach secretes 1,500 to 3,000 ml of gastric juice each day in response to ingestion of food; the sight, smell, or thought of food; and excessive stress, alcohol, and caffeine. Normally, stomach secretions aid in preparing ingested food for absorption in the small intestine, initiate the digestion of proteins, and promote absorption of vitamin B_{12}.

The chief cells of the stomach secrete digestive enzymes. The major enzyme secreted is pepsinogen, which is converted to pepsin in the presence of hydrochloric acid. Hydrochloric acid is secreted by the parietal cells of the stomach in a highly concentrated form with a pH of approximately 0.8. Pepsin, which functions in the beginning digestion of proteins, is most active in an acidic environment. It functions optimally at a pH of 2, and a pH of not greater than 5.[1] In addition to hydrochloric acid, the parietal cells secrete intrinsic factor, which

416

aids in the absorption of vitamin B_{12}. The goblet cells and mucous glands of the stomach secrete a viscous alkaline material that protects the stomach lining from damage by the acidic gastric juices.[2] Gastric juices also contain other substances such as electrolytes (sodium, potassium, chloride, and bicarbonate) and other enzymes such as gastric lipase, urease, lysozyme, and carbonic anhydrase.[3]

Gastric juices are produced continuously, although amounts vary in relation to food intake and other factors that stimulate or inhibit gastric secretion. The production of gastric juices is normally lowest early in the morning. Gastric secretion is mediated by the autonomic nervous system via the vagus nerve. When an individual ingests food—or thinks of, sees, or smells food—parasympathetic impulses travel via the vagus nerve to the stomach and stimulate the G cells of the stomach to secrete the hormone gastrin. Gastrin then stimulates the various cells in the stomach to increase their secretions.[4] In addition to distention of the stomach with food, exposure of the gastric mucosa to substances called secretagogues also stimulates the secretion of gastrin. Examples of such substances are alcohol, caffeine, meat extracts, and spices.

Because parasympathetic impulses increase gastric secretions, sympathetic nervous system activity will inhibit them. Gastric secretion, for example, is inhibited when food enters the small intestine. This inhibition is thought to be due to sympathetic impulses that are triggered when acidic gastric contents come into contact with the upper part of the small intestine. These sympathetic impulses ultimately inhibit those of the vagus nerve. Hormones secreted by the small intestine also inhibit gastric secretion. These include enterogastrone, secretin, and cholecystokinin-pancreozymin (CCK-PZ).

In addition to the normal neural and humoral mechanisms involved in gastric secretion, numerous other substances, including many drugs, may stimulate or inhibit gastric secretion. Substances that stimulate gastric secretion include histamine, nicotine, adrenocorticotropic steroids, insulin, and parasympathetic agents such as acetylcholine, reserpine, and pilocarpine. Substances that inhibit gastric secretion include belladonna alkaloids (e.g., atropine), anticholinergic drugs (e.g., probanthine), and histamine receptor antagonists (e.g., cimetidine, ranitidine). Aspirin causes changes in the gastric mucosa and decreases the secretion of mucus by the stomach, resulting in insufficient protection of the stomach lining from gastric juices.[5]

In the small intestine, digestion and absorption of nutrients is completed. This is accomplished by a combination of intestinal juices, pancreatic juices, and bile. As with the stomach, intestinal secretions consist of enzymes, hormones, and mucus. Intestinal enzymes include peptidases, sucrase, maltase, lactase, intestinal lipase, intestinal amylase, and nucleases which break down ingested proteins, carbohydrates, and fats so that they may be absorbed from the small intestine into the blood. In addition, enterokinase is secreted. This enzyme activates trypsin, which is a peptidase secreted by the pancreas. Other pancreatic enzymes include chymotrypsin, carboxypeptidase, pancreatic amylase, pancreatic lipase, and nuclease.

Normally, 1,200 to 1,500 ml of duodenal juices are secreted each day. Digestive juices are clear, have a high bicarbonate content, and range in pH from 8 to 8.5. As noted previously, hormones secreted by the small intestine include secretin and cholecystokinin-pancreozymin. When acidic gastric contents enter the duodenum, the resultant decrease in pH stimulates the mucosal cells of the small intestine to produce secretin. Secretin stimulates secretion of pancreatic juices which have a high bicarbonate content. Cholecystokinin-pancreozymin also stimulates the pancreas to release its juices, especially enzymes, although the source of the stimulation in this case is thought to be from the presence of polypeptides or fatty acids in the small intestine.[6]

Tests of gastric and intestinal secretions include analysis of contents and tests of normal function (e.g., tests that stimulate gastric and duodenal secretions). Most of these tests involve inserting a nasogastric or intestinal tube and may be quite uncomfortable for the client. Newer nonlaboratory procedures are beginning to replace tests of gastric and intestinal secretions, as they are more accurate, less time-consuming, and less uncomfortable for the client. These newer procedures include endoscopy, various radiological techniques, measurement of hydrogen ion concentration (pH) via electrodes, radioimmunoassay of serum gastrin levels, cytological examination of gastric contents for malignant cells, and serum analysis of intrinsic factor, anti-intrinsic factor antibodies, and antiparietal cell antibodies.[7,8] Many of these tests are not widely used at this time; only those tests in more common use will be discussed in this chapter.

TESTS OF GASTRIC SECRETIONS

Background Information

ANALYSIS OF GASTRIC CONTENTS (CLINICAL APPLICATIONS DATA, p. 421)

Gastric fluid analysis has two major components: (1) macroscopic analysis and (2) microscopic analysis. Macroscopic analysis includes examining the specimen for overall physical and chemical characteristics such as color, presence of mucus and blood, and pH determination. Microscopic analysis involves examining the specimen for organisms such as bacteria and parasites. Cytological examination for abnormal (i.e., malignant) exfoliated cells also may be done, although special techniques must be used so that the cells are not destroyed prior to analysis.

Specimens for gastric analysis are normally collected in the morning after the client has been fasting for 12 hours. Approximately 20 to 100 ml of gastric fluid should be present in the stomach at that time. If digestion is normal, and if the client has observed fasting instructions, no food particles should be present.[9]

Macroscopic Analysis

Color. Gastric juice is normally a translucent, pale gray, slightly viscous fluid. If the gastric aspirate is yellow to green in color, the presence of bile is indicated. This may be due to reflux of bile from excessive gagging when the nasogastric tube was inserted for the test or it may indicate an obstruction in the small intestine distal to the ampulla of Vater, the site where bile is secreted into the small intestine.[10] Pink, red, or brownish gastric secretions indicate the presence of blood (see further on).

Mucus. Mucus is normally present in gastric secretions and derives mainly from the mucus secreted by the gastric glands. The mucus content is responsible for the viscosity of gastric secretions. Saliva also may contribute to the mucus content, but it is frothy and tends to float on top of the sample. In tests of gastric secretions, clients are instructed to expectorate saliva during the test so as not to contaminate the sample. If mucus from the respiratory tract is present, it tends to be more tenacious than gastric secretions and sometimes contains dust particles. Small amounts of mucus from duodenal reflux also may be present in the sample.[11]

Blood. Blood is not normally present in gastric secretions. Small particles or streaks of fresh blood may be present owing to trauma during nasogastric intubation. Larger amounts of blood or "coffee ground" material indicates bleeding of a greater magnitude and is usually due to some type of gastric lesion (e.g., ulcer, gastritis, carcinoma). Blood swallowed from the mouth, nasopharynx, or lungs also may be present in the sample. Whether overt blood appears in the sample or not, the specimen should always be tested for blood.[12]

pH. The pH of gastric secretions is usually less than 2.0 and is not normally greater than 6.0, if gastric secretion is normal. Lack of normal gastric acidity is seen in pernicious anemia, gastric carcinoma, aplastic or hypochromic anemia, and with immune-related disorders of the thyroid, stomach, and connective tissue. Elevated pH in gastric juice also supports ruling out peptic ulcer disease as a diagnostic.[13] In addition to peptic ulcer disease, low pH levels are seen in Zollinger-Ellison syndrome (non–beta cell adenomas of the pancreas that produce excessive gastrin).

Microscopic Analysis

Red Blood Cells. As noted earlier, the presence of a few red blood cells may be due to the trauma of gastric intubation. Larger numbers, however, may indicate serious disorders and require additional diagnostic follow-up.

White Blood Cells. Normally, a few white blood cells are present in gastric juices. Elevated numbers may indicate inflammation of the gastric mucosa, mouth, paranasal sinuses, or respiratory tract. White blood cells found in gastric aspirates also may be due to inflammation of the duodenum, pancreas, or biliary tract, although this is a less common finding.[14]

Epithelial Cells. A few epithelial cells are normally present because of sloughing from mucosal surfaces. Clumps of cells may be due to dislodgment during intubation. Gastritis also may lead to the finding of increased epithelial cells in gastric fluid.

Bacteria and Yeasts. Because of the highly acidic environment of the stomach, bacteria are not normally found in gastric contents. In most cases, those bacteria (and yeasts) that are cultured from gastric fluid are normal flora of the mouth or respiratory tract. Increased numbers of bacteria may be found in gastric contents that have an abnormally high pH. Excessive numbers of yeasts are associated with retention of gastric contents owing to some type of blockage (e.g., pyloric obstruction).[15] Cultures for mycobacterium tuberculosis are done in individuals who are suspected of having pulmonary tuberculosis but who are unable to expectorate sputum effectively for analysis. Gastric samples for cytology are best collected through procedures designed to cause cells to exfoliate (i.e., exfoliative cytology). In addition to gastric aspiration, samples may be obtained by gastroscopy and use of balloons and brushes. The best method is said to be gastric lavage with a solution containing chymotrypsin.[16]

Parasites. Parasites may be found in gastric fluid, mainly resulting from reflux of duodenal contents. These include *Giardia lamblia*, trophozoites or cysts, strongyloidis larvae, and hookworm ova.

TESTS OF GASTRIC ACIDITY (CLINICAL APPLICATIONS DATA, p. 423)

Tests of gastric acidity are used to determine the presence and/or amount of hydrochloric acid in the stomach and to diagnose disorders associated with altered secretion of gastric acids. Three main types of tests are used to evaluate gastric acidity: (1) basal gastric acidity test, (2) gastric acid stimulation tests, and (3) tubeless gastric analysis test. The basal gastric acidity test usually is performed with tests of gastric acid stimulation.

Basal Gastric Acidity Test

This test is used to determine if there is elevated gastric acidity, which is seen in Zollinger-Ellison syndrome and peptic ulcer disease. The test involves inserting a nasogastric tube and collecting a 1-hour sample of gastric secretions, usually at four 15-minute intervals. The sample is examined for volume, pH, and total acid secretion in each specimen as well as in the total sample. Total acid secretion is expressed as basal acid output (BAO) in mEq/hour. The BAO is somewhat lower in the elderly and in women and varies directly with body weight.[17]

Gastric Acid Stimulation Tests

Gastric acid stimulation tests are performed to determine the response to substances that are administered to induce increased gastric acid secretion. Elevated acid output is associated with peptic ulcer disease and Zollinger-Ellison syndrome. Decreased acid output is usually associated with pernicious anemia and gastric carcinoma; however, it may also be seen in a variety of other disorders, including hypochromic anemia, nutritional megaloblastic anemia, steatorrhea, rheumatoid arthritis, and myxedema.

Substances used to induce gastric secretion in these tests include histamine, Histalog, and pentagastrin, with the latter being the drug of choice. Histamine is a substance that occurs naturally in the body and is implicated in various allergic and inflammatory responses. It also has the effect of stimulating gastric acid secretion. Unfortunately, when used for gastric acid stimulation tests, histamine produces numerous unpleasant side effects such as flushing, bradycardia, headache, nasal stuffiness, lacrimation, and alterations in blood pressure.[18] Histalog is an analog of histamine that also produces increased gastric acid secretion but more slowly. It has minimal side effects, but requires a longer testing period when used for gastric acid stimulation tests. Pentagastrin is a synthetic compound that induces gastric secretion as rapidly as histamine, but without major side effects. For these reasons, it is the current drug of choice for gastric acid stimulation tests.

Gastric acid stimulation tests are performed by first determining the basal acidity and then evaluating the response to the drug administered. Studies in which pentagastrin or histamine are used require sampling of gastric secretions for 1 hour following administration of the drug. Tests in which Histalog is used require sampling for 2 hours after the drug is administered.

As with basal gastric acidity tests, samples obtained from gastric acid stimulation tests are examined for volume, pH, and amount of acid secreted. First, basal acid output (BAO) is determined. Maximal acid output (MAO) is also determined by adding the total milliequivalents of acid secreted in all samples after injection of the gastric acid stimulant.[19] Peak acid output (PAO) also may be determined by adding the greatest acid output in two consecutive 15-minute samples. Finally, BAO and MAO are compared as a ratio, which normally ranges from 0.3 to 0.6. That is, the maximal output should be one and a half to three times the basal output.[20]

Hollander Insulin Test. This test is used to evaluate the effectiveness of vagotomy (i.e., severing vagal nerve connections to the stomach) as a treatment for persistent peptic ulcer disease, and involves stimulation of the vagus nerve through insulin-induced hypoglycemia. Hypoglycemia is normally a potent stimulator of gastric secretions and causes impulses to be transmitted via the vagus nerve. If the vagus nerve has been severed, however, the normal physiological response will not occur.

This tests involves performing a 2-hour basal secretion test and then injecting the client with regular insulin (usually 15 to 20 units). Gastric contents are then sampled every 15 minutes for 2 hours. Measurements performed on the samples are the same as those used for other gastric acid stimulation tests.

This test is not used very frequently, as it may be dangerous for the client (i.e., a blood sugar of less than 45 to 50 mg/dl is needed to provoke gastric secretion). In addition, data from the test do not always provide a clear distinction between normal and abnormal results, false-positive and false-negative results are common, and the results do not correlate strongly with recurrent ulcer disease.

Tubeless Gastric Analysis Test (Diagnex Blue Test)

Tubeless gastric analysis is used to determine the absence or presence of hydrochloric acid in the stomach by measuring excretion of dye in urine. The advantage of the test is that intubation is not required. The disadvantage is that exact measures of gastric acid and pH are not possible.

The test is performed by administering caffeine in tablet form to stimulate gastric secretion and then orally administering a dye (i.e., Diagnex blue). The dye is bound to a resin and is released in the stomach only if the pH is below 3.5. The dye is then absorbed in the small intestine and excreted in the urine, where it produces a blueish-green coloration. Appearance of the dye in the urine indicates that sufficient hydrochloric acid was present to induce release of the dye.

Because other more accurate tests are now available to evaluate gastric acidity and response to gastric stimulation, this test is no longer used in clinical practice.

Clinical Applications Data

ANALYSIS OF GASTRIC CONTENTS (BACKGROUND INFORMATION, p. 418)
Reference Values

Macroscopic Analysis	
Volume (fasting)	20–100 ml
Color	Pale gray, translucent
Mucus	Present such that the sample is slightly viscous
Blood	Negative
pH	<2.0 (never >6.0)

Microscopic Analysis	
Red blood cells	Negative to a few
White blood cells	Negative to a few
Epithelial	Few
Bacteria	Absent to few
Yeasts	Absent to few
Parasites	Absent
Abnormal Cells	Absent

Interfering Factors

■ Failure to follow dietary restrictions such that food particles are present
■ Exposure to the sight, smell, or thought of food immediately prior to the test

- Ingestion of drugs that may alter gastric secretions (e.g., alcohol, histamine, nicotine, adrenocorticotropic steroids, insulin, parasympathetic agents, belladonna alkaloids, anticholinergic drugs, histamine receptor antagonists, aspirin)
- Contamination of the sample with saliva and respiratory secretions, which should be expectorated rather than swallowed during the procedure
- Failure to send the samples to the laboratory promptly for analysis of cells, which may disintegrate in gastric juices

Indications/Purposes for Analysis of Gastric Contents

- Suspected peptic ulcer disease, as indicated by low to normal pH and (possibly) the presence of blood
- Suspected Zollinger-Ellison syndrome, as indicated by low to normal pH
- Suspected gastric carcinoma, as indicated by lack of normal gastric acidity, blood (possibly), and abnormal cells on cytological examination
- Suspected pernicious anemia as indicated by lack of normal gastric acidity
- Suspected pulmonary tuberculosis, as indicated by positive cultures for mycobacterium tuberculosis
- Suspected parasitic infestation of the gastrointestinal tract

Client Preparation

Client Teaching. Explain to the client:

- the purpose of the test (*note:* gastric analysis is often performed as a component of specific tests for gastric acidity)
- that fasting for 12 hours prior to the test is necessary, although water may be permitted up to 8 hours before the test
- that smoking is not permitted for 8 hours prior to the test
- that certain medications may be withheld, upon the physician's order, for up to 24 hours prior to the test
- that a stomach tube will be passed through the nose or mouth into the stomach
- that the client will be asked to swallow periodically when the tube is passed, as this facilitates its passage
- that the tube may cause a sensation of burning or irritation as it is passed and that gagging may occur when the tubing touches the back of the throat
- that saliva and respiratory secretions should be expectorated rather than swallowed during the test
- that a sample of stomach juices will be removed via the tube
- that the tube will be removed upon completion of the test

Encourage questions and verbalization of concerns appropriate to the client's age and mental status.

Physical Preparation

- Ensure to the extent possible that dietary, smoking, and medication restrictions are followed
- Provide the client with a hospital gown

The Procedure

The equipment needed is assembled. This includes a nasogastric tube, lubricant, gloves, a 50 ml syringe adapted for use with nasogastric tubes, saline, and specimen containers with appropriate labels. Tissues and an emesis basin also should be available for expectoration of secretions by the client.

With the client seated comfortably, the nasogastric tube is passed into the stomach and the syringe is attached. All gastric contents are aspirated, placed in a container, and labeled. If a specimen for tubercle bacilli is to be obtained, gastric washings with saline may be performed to obtain the sample. This is accomplished by irrigating the nasogastric tube with saline and withdrawing the contents.

When all needed samples are obtained, the nasogastric tube is removed. The samples should be sent to the laboratory immediately.

Aftercare

The client is assisted to a position of comfort. Mouth and nose care is provided. Any foods and medications withheld for the test are resumed. Lozenges may be used to alleviate sore throat due to irritation by the tube.

Nursing Observations

Pretest

■ Assess the client's response to explanations provided; if the client is extremely anxious, the individual performing the test should be so informed

During the Test

■ Note the presence of food, blood, tissue, or bile in the sample; also, note the odor of the specimen—fecal odor and greenish-brown color may indicate bowel obstruction

Post-Test

■ Assess the client's comfort level
■ Assess the client's ability to resume normal food and fluid intake

TESTS OF GASTRIC ACIDITY (BACKGROUND INFORMATION, p. 419)
Reference Values

Volume	20–100 ml (usually 30–60 ml)
Basal acid output (BAO)	2–6 mEq/hr (values may be slightly lower in women and the elderly; values vary directly with body weight)
Maximal acid output (MAO) (after stimulation tests)	16–26 mEq/hr or at least 1½–3 times the BAO
BAO/MAO ratio	0.3–0.6 (usually <0.4)

Interfering Factors

■ Failure to follow dietary restrictions resulting in stimulation of gastric secretions
■ Exposure to the sight, smell, or thought of food immediately prior to and during the test
■ Ingestion of drugs that may alter gastric secretions (e.g., alcohol, histamine, nicotine, adrenocorticotropic steroids, insulin, parasympathetic agents, belladonna alkaloids, anticholinergic drugs, and histamine receptor antagonists) unless administered as part of the testing procedure

■ Dilution of the samples with saliva and respiratory secretions, which should be expectorated during the test

Indications/Purposes for Gastric Stimulation Tests

■ Suspected duodenal ulcer as indicated by elevated BAO (5 to 7 mEq/hr), and MAO (greater than 40 mEq/hr) (individuals with peptic ulcer disease who have stomach ulcers may have low to normal BAO and MAO)
■ Suspected Zollinger-Ellison syndrome as indicated by elevated BAO, normal or elevated MAO (elevated MAO after gastric stimulation is frequently not seen in these individuals since gastric acid output is already at maximum levels), and high BAO/MAO ratio
■ Suspected pernicious anemia as indicated by decreased or absent gastric acid output with BAO, MAO, and BAO/MAO ratio frequently at 0
■ Suspected gastric carcinoma as indicated by decreased BAO (e.g., 1.0 mEq/hr), decreased MAO (e.g., 4.0 mEq/hr), and decreased BAO/MAO ratio (e.g., 0.25)
■ Evaluation of effectiveness of vagotomy in the treatment of peptic ulcer disease as indicated by absence of response to gastric stimulation with insulin (Hollander insulin test)

Client Preparation

Client preparation is essentially the same as that for analysis of gastric contents (see p. 422). For gastric stimulation tests using pentagastrin, Histalog, and histamine, the client should be informed that a medication will be injected that increases stomach secretions and that the test will require 2 to 3 hours for completion. The client should be advised to report unusual symptoms such as flushing, headache, nasal stuffiness, dizziness, faintness and nausea.

For the insulin test, the client should be informed that insulin will be injected intravenously to lower the blood sugar, and should be reassured that glucose will be available for administration if necessary. The client should also be advised that it may be necessary to insert an intermittent venous access device (e.g., heparin lock). The client should be informed that it takes approximately 4 hours to complete this test.

Depending upon the institution, signed consents may be required for gastric acid stimulation tests because they involve injection of drugs.

The Procedure

Equipment needed for the tests discussed subsequently is essentially the same as for analysis of gastric secretions (see p. 422). In some institutions, the serial gastric aspirates are obtained by connecting the nasogastric tube to a suction device. Manual aspiration of gastric contents is, however, the preferred approach. For the Hollander insulin test, equipment to insert an intermittent venous access device (i.e., heparin lock) will be needed, as well as a syringe of 50 percent glucose.

Basal Gastric Acidity Test. A nasogastric tube is inserted and the stomach contents aspirated. The tube is clamped. After 15 minutes, the tube is opened and the gastric contents aspirated. This procedure is continued until a total of four samples have been obtained. Each sample is labeled with the time and sequence of collection. The samples should be transported promptly to the laboratory.

Gastric Acid Stimulation Tests. A basal gastric acidity test is performed; then the gastric stimulant (pentagastrin, Histalog, or histamine) is injected subcutaneously. For pentagastrin and histamine tests, gastric samples are obtained at 15-minute intervals for 1 hour after injection of the drug; for Histalog, the samples are obtained at 15-minute intervals for 2 hours after drug injection. If side effects of the drugs become severe, epinephrine or ephedrine may be administered. These drugs antagonize the effects of histamine, except for those on gastric secretions.[21]

Hollander Insulin Test. A 2-hour basal gastric acidity test is performed. A baseline blood sugar level is then measured. An intermittent venous access device (i.e., heparin lock) may also be inserted for administration of insulin and for glucose, if extreme hypoglycemia should occur. This device also may be used to obtain blood sugar samples during the test. Regular insulin is then administered in a dosage of 15 to 20 units or 0.2 units/kg body weight. Gastric aspirates are then obtained every 15 minutes for 2 hours. Blood glucose determinations also are done at 30, 60, and 90 minutes after injection of the insulin.

A syringe of 50 percent glucose should be available for administration if extreme hypoglycemia occurs. Sweetened orange juice or milk also may be administered orally if necessary. Note that a blood sugar level of 45 to 50 mg/dl is needed to provoke gastric secretions.

All specimens are labeled with the time and sequence of collection. The nasogastric tube and venous access device are removed upon completion of the test.

Aftercare

Aftercare is essentially the same as that for a routine gastric analysis (see p. 423). Foods and medications withheld for the test are resumed and client comfort is promoted.

Nursing Observations

Nursing observations are essentially the same as those for a routine gastric analysis. For gastric stimulation tests, the client's blood pressure and pulse may be monitored before, during, and after the test. The client also should be assessed for side effects of the drugs administered to induce gastric secretion. For the Hollander insulin test, the client is monitored for signs of hypoglycemia and is encouraged to resume usual dietary intake as soon after the test is completed as possible.

TESTS OF DUODENAL SECRETIONS

Background Information

ANALYSIS OF DUODENAL CONTENTS (CLINICAL APPLICATIONS DATA, p. 427)

Duodenal fluid analysis is used mainly to evaluate clients with chronic pancreatitis or suspected carcinoma of the pancreas. It also may be used in evaluating infants suspected of having cystic fibrosis or with diarrhea or steatorrhea of unknown etiology.[22]

Duodenal fluid samples are more difficult and time-consuming to obtain than are gastric samples. Duodenal samples are obtained by inserting a double-lumen tube. One lumen opens into the stomach and drains gastric secretions so that they do not interfere with duodenal fluid analysis. The end of the tube is positioned near the ampulla of Vater, so that the second lumen of the tube actually drains duodenal and pancreatic fluids. Correct tube placement must be confirmed by fluoroscopic radiological procedures. It should be noted that duodenal samples may be obtained during endoscopic procedures.

Specimens for duodenal analysis are usually collected in the morning, after the client has been fasting for 12 hours. Approximately 20 ml of duodenal fluid should be obtained at that time. If digestion is normal, and if the client has observed fasting instructions, no food particles should be present.

Macroscopic Analysis

Color. Duodenal secretions are normally pearly gray, translucent, and moderately viscous. Yellow or green coloration indicates that bile is present, but this finding is generally of no major clinical significance. Pink, red, or brownish secretions may indicate the presence of blood (see further on). If food particles are present, it may indicate either failure to follow dietary restrictions, intestinal obstruction, or duodenal diverticulum.[23]

Blood. Blood is not normally present in duodenal secretions. Small particles or streaks of fresh blood may be present due to the trauma of intubation. Larger amounts of blood suggest pancreatic carcinoma.

pH. The pH of duodenal fluid normally ranges from 8.0 to 8.5. Increased pH is associated with chronic pancreatitis.

Bicarbonate. Bicarbonate may be measured as part of a routine analysis but is more likely to be done as part of stimulation tests. Decreased bicarbonate levels are seen in chronic pancreatitis.

Microscopic Analysis

Red Blood Cells. As previously noted, the finding of red blood cells may indicate intubation trauma or carcinoma of the pancreas.

White Blood Cells and Epithelial Cells. Normally a few white blood cells and epithelial cells are present in duodenal aspirates. Larger amounts are associated with inflammation of the duodenum, bile ducts, or pancreas.

Bacteria. Bacteria are not normally present in duodenal secretions owing to the effects of gastric acid. Samples for routine analysis are rarely cultured for bacteria.

Parasites. Parasites are rarely seen in duodenal secretions. When present, they usually consist of the following: (1) larvae of *Strongyloides stercoralis;* (2) cysts or trophozoites of *Giardia lamblia* or *Entamoeba histolytica;* and (3) ova of *Necator, Ancylostoma,* or *Ascaris.*[24]

DUODENAL STIMULATION TESTS (CLINICAL APPLICATIONS DATA, p. 429)

Duodenal stimulation tests involve administering substances that stimulate pancreatic secretion and then measuring the pancreatic substances as they appear in duodenal aspirates. Two such tests are performed: (1) secretin test and (2) cholecystokinin-pancreozymin test.

Secretin Test

Secretin is a hormone normally secreted by the small intestine (see p. 417). It acts to stimulate the pancreas to secrete increased volumes of pancreatic juices with high bicarbonate content. In this test, secretin is administered intravenously (1 clinical unit per kg body weight), and three duodenal samples are aspirated at 20-minute intervals. A decreased response to secretin is seen in any disorder characterized by chronic inflammation and scarring of the pancreas (e.g., chronic pancreatitis). This test also may aid in diagnosing carcinoma of the pancreas, as bicarbonate values in this disorder are higher than in chronic pancreatitis after stimulation with secretin. Deficiency in pancreatic secretion is associated also with cystic fibrosis. The main use of this test, however, is to monitor declining pancreatic function in individuals with chronic pancreatitis.[25]

Cholecystokinin-Pancreozymin Test

Cholecystokinin-pancreozymin is a hormone normally secreted by the small intestine. It acts to stimulate the pancreas to secrete increased amounts of pancreatic enzymes. This test, which is sometimes performed after the secretin test, involves administration of cholecystokinin-pancreozymin and then aspirating duodenal secretions. The aspirated samples are then assayed for the pancreatic enzyme amylase, lipase, or trypsin, with amylase the enzyme most commonly measured. The results of this test generally parallel those of the secretin test; that is, if overall pancreatic function is decreased, enzyme production also will be decreased.

Clinical Applications Data

ANALYSIS OF DUODENAL CONTENTS (BACKGROUND INFORMATION, p. 425)
Reference Values

Macroscopic Analysis	
Volume (fasting)	20 ml
Color	Pearly gray, translucent
Blood	Negative
pH	8.0–8.5
Bicarbonate	145 mEq/l
Microscopic Analysis	
Red blood cells	Negative
White blood cells	Few
Epithelial cells	Few
Bacteria	Negative
Parasites	Negative

Interfering Factors

■ Failure to follow dietary restrictions, resulting in the presence of food particles in the aspirate
■ Improper tube placement, resulting in aspiration of gastric secretions

Indications for Analysis of Duodenal Contents

■ Suspected carcinoma of the pancreas as indicated by decreased volume, the presence of blood (possibly), and normal bicarbonate
■ Known or suspected chronic pancreatitis as indicated by decreased volume, pH, and bicarbonate

■ Suspected cystic fibrosis as indicated by decreased volume, pH, and bicarbonate
■ Suspected infestation with parasites, especially *Giardia lamblia*

Client Preparation

Client Teaching. Explain to the client:

■ the purpose of the test (*note:* analysis of duodenal contents is often performed as a component of duodenal stimulation tests)
■ that fasting from foods and fluids for 12 hours prior to the test is necessary
■ that smoking is not permitted for 8 to 12 hours prior to the test
■ that a tube will be passed through the mouth or nose into the small intestine
■ that various positions may need to be assumed (e.g., sitting, lying on side or back) while the tube is passed (see under Procedure, below)
■ that the client may be asked to swallow or deep breathe periodically as the tube is passed
■ that a mild sedative may be administered prior to insertion of the tube
■ that the tube may cause a sensation of burning as it is passed and that gagging may occur when the tube touches the back of the throat
■ that tube placement will be checked by an x-ray examination
■ that a sample of juices from the small intestine will be removed from the tube by using a suction apparatus
■ that the tube is removed upon completion of the test

Encourage questions and verbalization of concerns appropriate to the client's age and mental status.
A signed consent may be required for this test, depending upon the institution.

Physical Preparation

■ Ensure to the extent possible that dietary and smoking restrictions are followed
■ Provide the client with a hospital gown

The Procedure

The equipment needed is assembled. This includes a double-lumen intestinal tube to aspirate duodenal contents, lubricant, gloves, a 20 or 50 ml syringe adapted for use with the intestinal tube, and specimen containers. Tissues and an emesis basin also should be available for client use. A mechanical suction device for removing gastric secretions continuously during the test will be needed, as will a suction device for removing duodenal secretions.

With the client seated comfortably, the double lumen tube is passed into the upper part of the stomach. The client is then positioned on the left side and the tube passed into the lower part of the stomach. The client is then assisted to a sitting position and asked to lean forward from the waist as far as possible. He or she also is instructed to take several deep breaths at this time, which should move the tip of the tube into the portion of the stomach near the pyloric sphincter. The client is then assisted to lie on the right side; this position, along with normal peristalsis, should move the tube into the duodenum. The client is then assisted to a back-lying position and the tube advanced another 10 to 15 cm. Approximately 15 minutes are required to pass the tube in this manner. Under fluoroscopic visualization, the tube is positioned so that the tip is in the middle of the third portion of the duodenum, distal to the ampulla of Vater.[26] When proper location of the tube is ascertained, the tube is secured to the client's face with tape.

The gastric lumen of the tube is connected to a suction device throughout the procedure. Duodenal secretions are collected by mechanical suction for 20 minutes and then sent to the laboratory for analysis. The gastric aspirate is discarded. If tests of duodenal stimulation are to be performed, they will be done prior to removal of the intestinal tube.

Aftercare

The client is assisted to a comfortable position. Mouth and nose care is provided. Any foods withheld for the test are resumed. Lozenges may be used to alleviate sore throat due to irritation by the tube. If the client received a sedative prior to the test, appropriate care for a sedated individual should be implemented.

Nursing Observations

Pretest

■ Assess the client's response to explanations provided; if the client is extremely anxious, the individual performing the test should be so informed and an order for a preprocedure sedative should be obtained
■ Assess the client's degree of mobility, as the client will need to assume various positions (sitting, side-lying, back-lying) while the tube is passed; if the client's mobility is impaired, the individual performing the test should be so informed so that sufficient assistance is available for client positioning

During the Test

■ Note the presence of food or blood in the specimen
■ Note the client's response to the procedure

Post-Test

■ Assess the client's comfort level
■ Assess the client's degree of sedation and take appropriate safety measures
■ Assess the client's ability to resume normal food and fluid intake

DUODENAL STIMULATION TESTS (BACKGROUND INFORMATION, p. 426)
Reference Values

Volume	2–4 ml/kg body weight
Bicarbonate	90–130 mEq/l
Pancreatic amylase	6.6–35.2 U/kg body weight

Interfering Factors

■ Failure to follow dietary restrictions, resulting in stimulation of pancreatic secretion by food particles
■ Improper tube placement, resulting in aspiration of gastric secretions

Indications/Purposes for Duodenal Stimulation Tests

■ Monitoring the progression of chronic pancreatitis with worsening disease indicated by decreased volume, decreased bicarbonate, and decreased enzyme secretion

■ Suspected cancer of the pancreas as indicated by decreased volume, normal bicarbonate, and decreased enzyme secretion

Client Preparation

Client preparation is the same as that for routine analysis of duodenal contents (see p. 428). The client should be informed that a medication will be administered that stimulates pancreatic secretion. Intradermal skin tests to determine sensitivity to secretin or to cholecystokinin-pancreozymin, or to both, may be performed prior to the test. Since secretin is administered intravenously, an intermittent venous access device (i.e., heparin lock) may be inserted for the test.

The Procedure

The procedure begins with aspiration of baseline (fasting) duodenal secretions (see p. 428). For the secretin test, secretin is administered intravenously in the amount of one clinical unit per kg body weight. Three samples of duodenal aspirate are then obtained at 20-minute intervals. For the cholecystokinin-pancreozymin test, the hormone is administered and samples for pancreatic enzymes (usually amylase) are withdrawn.

Aftercare and Nursing Observations

Aftercare and nursing observations are essentially the same as those for routine analysis of duodenal fluids (see p. 429). In addition, the client should be observed for allergic reactions to the hormones even though skin tests may have been negative.

REFERENCES

1. Bullock, BL and Rosendahl, PP: Pathophysiology: Adaptations and Alterations in Function. Little, Brown, & Co, Boston, 1984, p 489.
2. Hole, JW: Human Anatomy and Physiology, ed 4. Wm C Brown, Dubuque, IA, 1987, p 506.
3. Bullock and Rosendahl, *op cit*, p 488.
4. Hole, *op cit*, p 507.
5. Bullock and Rosendahl, *op cit*, p 490.
6. Widmann, FK: Clinical Interpretation of Laboratory Tests, ed 9. FA Davis, Philadelphia, 1983, pp 577–578.
7. Strasinger, SK: Urinalysis and Body Fluids. FA Davis, Philadelphia, 1985, p 187.
8. Cannon, DC: Examination of Gastric and Duodenal Contents. In Henry, JB: Clinical Diagnosis and Management by Laboratory Methods, ed 17. WB Saunders, Philadelphia, 1984, p 558.
9. Cannon, *op cit*, p 554.
10. *Ibid.*
11. *Ibid.*
12. *Ibid.*
13. Widmann, *op cit*, p 576.
14. Cannon, *op cit*, p 554.
15. *Ibid*, pp 554–555.
16. *Ibid*, p 558.
17. Widmann, *op cit*, p 575.
18. Cannon, *op cit*, p 556.

19. *Ibid*, p 553.
20. Widmann, *op cit*, p 575.
21. Bergensen, BS: Pharmacology in Nursing, ed 14. CV Mosby, 1979, p 700.
22. Cannon, *op cit*, p 561.
23. *Ibid*, pp 559–560.
24. *Ibid*, p 560.
25. Widmann, *op cit*, p 578.
26. Cannon, *op cit*, p 559.

BIBLIOGRAPHY

Beare, PG, Rahr, VA and Ronshausen, CA: Nursing Implications of Diagnostic Tests, ed 2. JB Lippincott, Philadelphia, 1985.
Braunstein, H: Outlines of Pathology. CV Mosby, St Louis, 1982.
Byrne, CJ, Saxton, DF, Pelikan, PK and Nugent, PM: Laboratory Tests: Implications for Nursing Care. Addison-Wesley, Menlo Park, CA, 1986.
Diagnostics, ed 2. Springhouse Corporation, Springhouse, PA, 1986.
Fischbach, FT: A Manual of Laboratory Diagnostic Tests, ed 3. JB Lippincott, Philadelphia, 1988.
Guyton, AC: Textbook of Medical Physiology, ed 6. WB Saunders, Philadelphia, 1981.
Kee, JL: Laboratory and Diagnostic Tests With Nursing Implications, ed 2. Appleton & Lange, Norwalk, CT, 1987.
Lamb, JO: Laboratory Tests for Clinical Nursing. Robert J Brady, Bowie, MD, 1984.
Luckmann, J and Sorensen, KC: Medical-Surgical Nursing: A Psychophysiologic Approach, ed 3. WB Saunders, Philadelphia, 1987.
Malseed, R: Drug Therapy and Nursing Considerations. JB Lippincott, Philadelphia, 1983.
Michaels, D: Diagnostic Procedures: the Patient and the Health Care Team. John Wiley & Sons, New York, 1983.
Pagana, KD and Pagana, TJ: Diagnostic Testing and Nursing Implications: A Case Study Approach, ed 2. CV Mosby, St Louis, 1986.
Skydell, B and Crowder, AS: Diagnostic Procedures. Little, Brown, & Co, Boston, 1975.
Tilkian, SM, Conover, MB and Tilkian, AG: Clinical Implications of Laboratory Tests, ed 4. CV Mosby, St Louis, 1987.
Widmann, FK: Pathobiology: How Diseases Happen. Little, Brown & Co, Boston, 1978.
Williams, SR: Nutrition and Diet Therapy, ed 4. CV Mosby, St Louis, 1981.

13

FECAL ANALYSIS

COMPOSITION AND CHARACTERISTICS OF FECES

Feces consist mainly of cellulose and other undigested foodstuffs, bacteria, and water (as much as 70 percent). Other substances normally found in stools include epithelial cells shed from the gastrointestinal tract, small amounts of fats, bile pigments in the form of urobilin (see Fig. 6–1, p. 300), gastrointestinal and pancreatic secretions (see Chapter 12), and electrolytes.[1,2] The average adult excretes 100 to 300 g of fecal material per day, the residue of approximately 10 liters of liquid material that enters the intestinal tract each day.[3]

Feces are normally brown because of bacterial degradation of bile pigments to stercobilin. The characteristic odor of feces is due to bacterial action on proteins and other residues that produces substances such as indole, skatole, phenol, hydrogen, sulfide, and ammonia.[4] The normal consistency of feces is described as "plastic;" that is, stools should not normally be liquid, mushy, or hard.[5] The shape and caliber of normal stools is the same as that of the distal colon.

Alterations in color, odor, consistency, and/or shape may indicate the presence of disease. Although these characteristics are not always specifically studied in the laboratory, the nurse may observe them when providing care. Feces that are abnormal in terms of gross characteristics require additional diagnostic follow-up. Table 13–1 depicts normal and abnormal characteristics that may be observed and possible causes of alterations.

Laboratory analysis of feces includes microscopic examinations, chemical tests for specific substances, and microbiological tests. It should be noted that

TABLE 13-1. Normal and Abnormal Gross Characteristics of Feces

Characteristic	Normal	Alterations	Possible Causes of Alterations
Volume	100–300 g	Large volume, malodorous, floating	Malabsorption of fats or protein
Odor	Pungent		Cystic fibrosis, pancreatitis, postgastrectomy syndrome, bile duct obstruction, primary small bowel disease
Shape/Caliber	Shape and caliber of the distal colon	Large caliber	Dilatation of the colon
		Small, ribbon-like	Decreased elasticity of the colon
			Partial bowel obstruction
Color	Brown	Red	Lower GI tract bleeding
			Red beet ingestion
			BSP dye, pyridium compounds
		Black	Upper GI tract bleeding
			Charcoal, licorice, iron, or bismuth ingestion
		Dark brown	Hemolytic anemia
			Diet high in meat
			Prolonged exposure of the sample to air
		Gray	Chocolate and cocoa ingestion
		Gray, silvery	Steatorrhea
		Pasty, gray-white	Barium ingestion
			Bile duct obstruction
		Very pale gray	Diet high in milk products
		Green, yellow-green	Ingestion of spinach, other greens, laxatives of vegetable origin, indomethacin
			Rapid transit time through the intestine preventing oxidation of bile pigments
		Green-black	Meconium, infant
		Green-yellow (watery)	Transitional stool, infant
		Yellow, pasty	Breastfed infant
		Yellow-brown	Cow's milk–fed infant
Consistency	Plastic	Small, round, hard masses	Habitual constipation
		Mucoid, watery but without blood	Irritable bowel syndrome, diffuse superficial bowel inflammation, villous adenoma
		Mucoid, bloody	Inflammatory bowel syndrome, carcinoma, typhoid, Shigella, ameba
		Sticky, tarry, black	Upper GI tract bleeding
		Voluminous, watery, little-formed material	Osmotic catharsis
			Noninvasive infections (cholera toxigenic, E. coli, staphylococcal food poisoning)
		Loose, purulent or with necrotic tissue	Diverticulitis, abscess, necrotic tumor, parasites
Mucus	Absent	Present	Colitis, bacillary dysentary, diverticulitis, carcinoma

Adapted from Widmann, FK: Clinical Interpretation of Laboratory Tests, ed 9. FA Davis, Philadelphia, 1983, pp 553–554.

laboratory analysis of feces is performed much less frequently than studies of blood, urine, and other body fluids. One reason for this is that clients and health care providers dislike collecting stool specimens. Furthermore, fecal samples cannot usually be collected on demand the way blood samples can, with the possible exception of small samples obtained during rectal examination which may be sufficient for screening tests (e.g., occult blood). Despite these disadvantages, analysis of fecal material aids in diagnosing gastrointestinal and other disorders.[6]

TESTS OF FECES

Background Information

MICROSCOPIC ANALYSIS OF FECES (CLINICAL APPLICATIONS DATA, p. 440)

Microscopic analysis of stool specimens includes examining the sample for leukocytes, epithelial cells, qualitative fat, meat fibers, and parasites. These tests may be performed singly, in combination with other tests, or as routine screening tests.

Leukocytes

Examination of feces for leukocytes, especially neutrophils and monocytes, is usually performed in the initial evaluation of diarrhea of unknown etiology. The presence or absence of leukocytes can provide important diagnostic clues faster than awaiting the results of stool cultures. Leukocytes are seen in disorders that affect the intestinal wall such as ulcerative colitis and certain bacterial infections (e.g., *Salmonella, Shigella, Yersinia,* and invasive *Escherichia coli*). Leukocytes also are occasionally seen in antibiotic-related colitis. It should be noted that as few as three leukocytes per high-power field (HPF) may indicate a disorder involving the intestinal wall. Leukocytes are absent in infections with organisms that cause diarrhea by toxins rather than by intestinal wall damage. Examples of such organisms are viruses, toxigenic bacteria (e.g., *Staphylococcus,* noninvasive *E. coli, Clostridium perfringens, Vibrio cholerae*), and parasites (e.g., *Giardia, Entamoeba*). Leukocytes also may be absent in inflammatory processes deep within the intestinal wall.[7,8]

Epithelial Cells

Normally small to moderate numbers of epithelial cells are present in feces. Large numbers of epithelial cells (or large amounts of mucus), however, indicate that the intestinal mucosa is irritated.[9]

Qualitative Fat

Fats are found in the feces primarily in the forms of triglycerides (neutral fats), fatty acids, and fatty acid salts. Their presence is determined through various staining techniques prior to microscopic examination. Through these methods, the number of fat droplets and their size can be determined, and the type of fat present can be identified. The finding of more than 60 fat droplets per HPF usually indicates steatorrhea, which simply means excess fat in the stool. The size of the droplet also must be considered in arriving at a diagnosis. The fat droplets in steatorrhea are usually larger than normal.

Excess fat in the stool is usually due to either malabsorption syndromes or deficiency in pancreatic enzymes. Microscopic examination for fecal fat may aid in differentiating between these two disorders. An increase in triglycerides generally indicates a deficiency of pancreatic enzymes which normally break down triglycerides to fatty acids. In contrast, individuals with malabsorption syndromes usually have normal amounts of triglycerides in their stools but excessive fatty acids, as these clients are unable to absorb the fats once they are broken down.[10] Other causes of excessive fecal fat include surgical resection or fistulas of the intestines and recent intake of excessive amounts of dietary fats. False-negative results may occur in individuals with malabsorption problems who restrict their fat intake due to anorexia.

Microscopic tests for fecal fats are essentially qualitative in nature. The test simply indicates if there is excessive fat present, and if so, the nature of that fat. The definitive test for evaluating steatorrhea is quantitative analysis for fecal fat. This is accomplished through a 72-hour stool collection while the client is on a diet containing 100 g of fat per day (see p. 436).[11]

Meat Fibers

Microscopic examination of stool specimens for meat fibers aids in evaluating the efficiency of digestion. If protein digestion is adequate, meat fibers will not be found. If they are present, inadequate proteolysis is indicated. The finding of meat fibers in feces usually correlates positively with the finding of steatorrhea.[12] Individuals who have difficulty digesting proteins also have difficulty digesting fats.

Parasites

Microscopic tests for parasites augment observation of gross characteristics of stools; that is, certain types of parasites (e.g., tapeworm segments) may be apparent in stool samples without the aid of a microscope.[13] Microscopic analysis for parasites is usually indicated in individuals with intestinal disorders of unknown etiology, history of possible exposure to parasites, or eosinophilia of unknown cause that could be due to parasitic infestation.

Parasites commonly found in stools include roundworms (e.g., *Ascaris lumbricoides*), tapeworms (e.g., *Diphyllobothrium latum, Taenia saginata*), hookworms (e.g., *Necator americanus*), ameba (e.g., *Entamoeba histolytica*), and protozoa (e.g., *Giardia lamblia*).[14] In collecting specimens for parasites, it is important that the sample be transported immediately to the laboratory. The best samples are considered to be those that contain blood and mucus because they are also most likely to contain parasites.

TESTS FOR SPECIFIC SUBSTANCES IN FECES (CLINICAL APPLICATIONS DATA, p. 442)

Fecal samples can be chemically analyzed for a variety of substances including occult (hidden) blood, qualitative fats, trypsin, urobilinogen, and bile. In addition, estimates of carbohydrate utilization can be made.

Occult Blood

The most frequently performed test of feces is chemical screening for occult (hidden) blood. The purpose of the test is to detect pathological lesions (e.g., carcinoma) before they produce symptoms and while the condition is still amenable to treatment. Indeed, such testing is widely used in mass screening programs for colorectal cancer, with 75 percent of such cancers detected while still localized.[15]

A number of easy-to-use test kits for detection of occult blood are available. Prior to such kits, the traditional method was to expose the sample to a sequence of solutions that included glacial acetic acid, gum guaiac solution, and hydrogen peroxide. A blue color indicated a positive test result. The test kits use these same principles, with some using paper impregnated with guaiac. For these reasons, analysis of feces for occult blood is sometimes still referred to as a "stool for guaiac."

One of the main problems of testing stools for occult blood is the number of false-positive results that occur. A diet high in meat, for example, may cause stools to test positive for blood, as will diets high in certain vegetables (i.e., horseradish and turnips) and in bananas. In addition, bleeding from the gums or nasal passages may produce positive results for occult blood in stools. Therapy with many drugs may lead to positive results due to direct or indirect drug effects on the gastrointestinal tract. These include aspirin (as little as one 300 mg tablet per day), iron preparations, anticoagulants, adrenocorticosteroids, colchicine, and phenylbutazone. In contrast, ascorbic acid may lead to false-negative results.

Numerous pathological conditions may cause bleeding into the intestinal tract. Table 13–2 details these disorders, including severity of bleeding and other clinical features.

Sometimes bleeding appears so obvious that one may be tempted not to confirm visual observations with appropriate testing. Stools that are grossly red or black are usually assumed to contain blood. Such assumptions, however, must always be confirmed, as certain foods and medications also may impart these colors to stools (see Table 13–1, p. 433). If blood is present in sufficient quantity, the color of the stool reflects the source of the bleeding and/or the length of time the blood was in the gastrointestinal tract. Black stools, for example, are associated with upper GI bleeding when the hemoglobin has come in contact with gastric acid and has been converted to acid hematin. In such cases, stools may remain black for as long as 5 days after the initial bleeding occurred. If, however, upper GI bleeding is massive and the volume increases GI motility (e.g., as occurs in bleeding from esophageal varices), stools may be red or maroon and of somewhat liquid consistency. Generally, though, bright red stools are associated with lower GI bleeding from hemorrhoids, ulcerative colitis, and carcinomas.[16]

For occult blood studies, samples are obtained on rectal examination or portions of bowel movements may be used. It is recommended that the client follow a meat-free, high-bulk diet for 3 days prior to testing and that drugs that may alter test results be withheld. In practice, however, these restrictions frequently are not applied.

Quantitative Fats

As noted previously (p. 435), the definitive test for excessive fecal fat is the 72-hour quantitative measure, with the amount of fat present expressed as a percentage of solid material. Because fat output may vary on a day-to-day basis, the 3-day collection is believed to be the most reliable approach. In adults, a controlled fat diet of 100 g per day also is followed during the collection. In infants and children, for whom such a diet could not be used, results of the collection are based on the estimated intake of dietary fat. Thus, it is important to know what foods were ingested during the test period.[17]

Quantitative fat studies are generally indicated when pancreatic insufficiency or malabsorption syndromes are suspected. They may also be used to

TABLE 13-2. Conditions Associated With Gastrointestinal Bleeding

Condition	Usual Age of Occurrence	Severity	Other Features
Upper GI Tract			
Peptic ulcer (gastric or duodenal)	Any, including young children	Variable, from occult to life-threatening	Pain, typical history often absent
Erosive gastritis	Usually adults over age 25	Usually mild; may be very severe	Aspirin, alcohol use often predispose Severe uremia, chronic liver disease predispose
Atrophic gastritis	Adults over age 25	Usually mild	Associated with pernicious anemia, autoantibodies, decreased gastric acidity
Esophageal varices	Adults; children with portal hypertension	Massive, sudden	Common in alcoholic liver disease Cirrhosis or portal hypertension always present
Mallory-Weiss tears at gastroesophageal junction	Any, but usually older adults	Variable depending on depth, location of tear	Common in alcohol abusers
Hiatus hernia, esophagitis	Progressively increasing incidence over age 40	Usually mild	Persistent painless bleeding a common cause of iron deficiency anemia in elderly
Small and Large Bowel			
Meckel's diverticulum	Commonest in children and young adults	Moderate; stools red or maroon	Caused by peptic ulceration of ectopic gastric mucosa
Polyps	Any age	Usually mild; often intermittent	Diarrhea, mucus in stools sometimes accompany
Infectious diarrheas	Any age	Usually mild or moderate	Ameba, *Shigella*, *Clostridium difficile*
Inflammatory bowel disease (Crohn's disease, ulcerative colitis)	Adolescents, adults under age 60	Usually mild, but may be massive	Diarrhea, pain, weight loss more common in Crohn's disease than in ulcerative colitis Bleeding more prominent in ulcerative colitis

TABLE 13-2—*Continued*

Condition	Usual Age of Occurrence	Severity	Other Features
Diverticular disease	Progressively increasing incidence over age 40	Usually mild, frequently occult	Often asymptomatic, unless inflammation or abscess develops
Vascular malformations	Older adults	Usually mild; may be life-threatening in ~15%	Bleeding often recurrent Often misdiagnosed as peptic ulcer or diverticular disease
Carcinoma	Older adults	Variable, from occult to moderate	Common cause of iron deficiency anemia in older persons Red blood more common with distally located tumors
Rectum and Anus Hemorrhoids	Older adults	Usually mild; blood is bright red	May be painless or symptomatic Often associated with constipation
Anorectal fissure	Any age	Usually mild; blood is bright red	Nearly always painful Crohn's disease, anal intercourse may predispose

From Widmann, FK: Clinical Interpretation of Laboratory Tests, ed 9. FA Davis, Philadelphia, 1983, pp 558–559, with permission.

monitor the effectiveness of treatment for such disorders. Severe liver disease and biliary tract disease also may cause excessive fat to be present in stools. Such disorders, however, usually lead to jaundice and blood chemistry abnormalities. Thus, fecal fat analysis does not contribute much additional diagnostic data.[18] Fecal fat also may be elevated if there is increased GI motility or alterations in normal bacterial flora of the intestines.

Trypsin

Trypsin is an enzyme secreted by the pancreas. It is normally not present in stools, except in children under the age of 2. If it is absent from the stools of children under 2, pancreatic deficiency is indicated. It should be noted that trypsin may not be detected if the child is constipated, owing to the prolonged action of normal intestinal bacteria on the enzyme.[19]

Carbohydrate Utilization

Individuals with various disorders related to malabsorption (e.g., celiac disease, tropical sprue, disorders involving the small intestine) may have difficulty with carbohydrate absorption as well as fat absorption. Thus, a thorough investigation of the finding of steatorrhea (excess fat in the stool) includes evaluation of carbohydrate metabolism. Such an evaluation includes performing oral and intravenous glucose tolerance tests (see Chapter 5) and comparing the results. Persons with carbohydrate malabsorption have normal results on intravenous glucose tolerance tests, but not on oral glucose tolerance tests.[20]

If carbohydrates cannot be absorbed normally, excessive amounts will appear in the stool. This is tested by placing a Clinitest tablet (Ames Company, Elkhart, Indiana) in a portion of stool which has been emulsified with water. It should be noted that Clinitest tablets are one of the methods used to detect excess sugar in urine. When performed on fecal samples, a positive Clinitest result indicates carbohydrate malabsorption.[21] This test is easily performed and may be used as a screening test to detect metabolic and intestinal disorders.

Urobilinogen

Urobilinogen is produced from bilirubin, a breakdown product of red blood cells, and normally appears in urine (see Chapter 6) and feces. In individuals with liver and biliary tract disorders, bilirubin metabolism may be impaired with decreased amounts appearing in the feces. Low levels also may be seen in certain anemias when red cell production is low, as less than normal amounts of bilirubin are produced due to deficient quantities of circulating red blood cells. In contrast, elevated fecal urobilinogen levels may be seen in disorders characterized by excessive red cell destruction (e.g., various hemolytic anemias).

Because blood and urine samples for products of bilirubin metabolism are more easily obtained than stool samples, this test is rarely used. Factors that may lead to falsely decreased values include antibiotic therapy and exposure of the sample to light.[22]

Bile

Bile should not be present in feces of adults, as it is broken down in the intestines during normal digestion; however, tests for bile may be normally positive in children. Bile may appear in the stools of adults if there is rapid transit through the gastrointestinal tract (e.g., diarrhea). It may also be found in clients with hemolytic anemias that produce jaundice.[23]

MICROBIOLOGICAL TESTS OF FECES (CLINICAL APPLICATIONS DATA, p. 444)

Stool Cultures

Certain bacteria are normally found in feces (i.e., the "normal flora" of the bowel). The presence of pathological types of bacteria may, however, produce diarrhea and other signs of systemic infection. Thus, most stool cultures are done to evaluate diarrhea of unknown etiology, in order to identify possible causative bacteria. Bacteria produce diarrhea in three main ways: (1) the organisms invade the intestinal wall, damaging tissue; (2) the organisms produce toxins within the intestine that alter gastrointestinal motility; and (3) toxins produced by bacteria are ingested (e.g., via foods) and produce diarrhea, although the organisms themselves are not detected in feces.[24] Table 13–3 lists the organ-

---

TABLE 13–3. **Mechanisms of Bacterial Diarrhea**

Organisms Damage Tissue Directly
Typhoid *(Salmonella typhi)*
Other salmonellas
Some shigellas
Staphylococcal pseudomembranous colitis
E. coli in infants ("enteropathogenic" species)
Yersinia species
Campylobacter fetus

Intraluminal Multiplication Causes Accumulation of Toxin, Which Causes Diarrhea
Cholera *(Vibrio cholerae)*
Travelers' diarrhea *(Escherichia coli)*
Pseudomembranous colitis *(Clostridium difficile)*
Some shigellas
Other *Vibrio* organisms
Clostridium perfringens

Preformed Toxin Ingested; Organisms Absent From Feces
Staphylococcal food poisoning
Clostridium botulinum

From Widmann, FK: Clinical Interpretation of Laboratory Tests, ed 9. FA Davis, Philadelphia, 1983, pp 355, with permission.

---

isms associated with these three main mechanisms. The primary purpose of stool cultures is to identify organisms that cause damage to intestinal tissue.

Samples for stool cultures may be obtained either by rectal swab or by collecting a sample of a bowel movement. It is important that such samples are not exposed to air or room temperature more than necessary, as this may damage bacteria so that they cannot be grown in culture. Thus, samples obtained by rectal swab must be placed in preservative, while those obtained from bowel movements must be placed in tightly sealed containers. The samples should be received in the laboratory within 1 hour of collection.

Clinical Applications Data

MICROSCOPIC ANALYSIS OF FECES (BACKGROUND INFORMATION, p. 434)
Reference Values

Leukocytes	Negative
Epithelial cells	Few to moderate
Fat (qualitative)	<60 normal-sized droplets/HPF
Triglycerides (neutral fats)	1–5%
Fatty acids	5–15%
Meat fibers	Negative
Parasites	Negative

Interfering Factors

■ A diet too high or too low in fat may alter results of qualitative tests for fats
■ Failure to send fresh stool specimens immediately to the laboratory, avoiding excessive exposure to room temperature and air, may damage any parasites present such that they cannot be identified microscopically
■ Contamination of the sample with urine or toilet bowl water
■ Use of laxatives for several days prior to the tests
■ Presence of barium in the stool following x-ray procedures
■ Antibiotic therapy

Indications/Purposes for Microscopic Analysis of Feces

■ Abnormal appearance of stools (see Table 13–1, p. 433)
■ Diarrhea of unknown etiology
  □ Diarrhea due to disorders involving the intestinal wall (e.g., ulcerative colitis and bacterial infection with *Salmonella*, *Shigella*, *Yersinia*, and invasive *E. coli*) is associated with the presence of leukocytes in the sample
  □ Diarrhea due to organisms that cause diarrhea by toxin rather than by intestinal wall damage (e.g., viruses, *Staphylococcus*, noninvasive *E. coli*, *Clostridium perfringens*, *Vibrio cholerae*, *Giardia*, *Entamoeba*) is associated with absence of leukocytes in the sample
■ Suspected inflammatory bowel disorder as indicated by large numbers of epithelial cells
■ Suspected pancreatitis as indicated by excessive fecal fat (steatorrhea) with elevated triglycerides (neutral fats)
■ Suspected malabsorption syndromes as indicated by steatorrhea, normal triglycerides, and elevated fecal fatty acids
■ Suspected alteration in protein digestion as indicated by the presence of meat fibers
■ Suspected infestation with intestinal parasites
■ Eosinophilia of unknown etiology, with suspicion of parasitic infestation

Client Preparation

Client Teaching. Explain to the client:

■ the purpose of the test
■ the importance of following a normal diet for several days prior to the collection, or notifying the physician if this cannot be done
■ the importance of not taking laxatives for several days prior to the collection, or notifying the physician if this avoidance is not possible
■ the method for collecting a sample of a bowel movement (see under Procedure)
■ how to transfer the sample from the specimen pan to the sample container (e.g., use of tongue blades, obtaining the sample from the midportion of the stool, including any portion of the stool with visible blood, mucus, pus, or parasites such as tapeworms)
■ the importance of not contaminating the specimen with urine or water
■ the importance of delivering the sample to the laboratory within 30 to 60 minutes of collection; if this is not possible, the sample may be refrigerated (*exception:* Samples for parasites may not be refrigerated and must be received in the laboratory while still warm)
■ the importance of placing the sample in a tightly covered container

Encourage questions and verbalization of concerns appropriate to the client's age and mental status.

Physical Preparation

■ Ensure to the extent possible that the client has followed a relatively normal diet and has not used laxatives for several days prior to testing
■ Provide a specimen collection container (e.g., plastic "hat" device, which is placed under the toilet seat), gloves, and tongue blades
■ Provide the specimen container in which the sample is to be sent to the laboratory

The Procedure

The sample is collected in either a plastic "hat" type receptacle, which is placed under the toilet seat, or in a bedpan. It is important that the "hat" or bedpan be clean and dry, and that the sample not be contaminated with urine or water. Gloves are worn and two clean tongue blades are used to transfer the mid-portion of the sample to a clean, dry plastic container with a tightly fitting lid. Any visible blood, mucus, pus, or parasites should be included in the sample. The container should be covered tightly as soon as the sample is obtained.

The tongue blades should be double-wrapped in paper towels and may be inserted into one of the gloves when they are removed. The collection container (e.g., plastic "hat" or bedpan) should be thoroughly cleansed or disposed of, preferably in a large plastic bag. Hands should be washed thoroughly.

In infants and young children, samples may be obtained from diapers, provided that contact with urine is avoided. Another approach is to insert a small-diameter (e.g., ¼ inch) glass tube into the infant's rectum while the child is held on the parent's lap. In the majority of cases, a core of feces will be obtained that can then be pushed out into a specimen container.[25]

The sample should be sent, properly labeled, to the laboratory within 30 to 60 minutes. If this is not possible, the sample may be refrigerated, except for samples for parasites, which must be sent to the laboratory while still warm.

Aftercare

There is no specific aftercare following collection of a stool sample.

Nursing Observations

If the client is to collect the sample independently, assess his or her ability to do so. If assisting with sample collection, observe and record the gross characteristics of the specimen (see Table 13–1, p. 433).

TESTS FOR SPECIFIC SUBSTANCES IN FECES (BACKGROUND INFORMATION, p. 435)
Reference Values

Occult Blood	Negative (0.5–2 ml/day)
	5–7% of dietary intake
Quantitative fat (72-hour collection)	<5 g/24 hr
	10–25% of dry fecal matter
Neutral fat	1–5% of dry fecal matter
Fatty Acids	5–15% of dry fecal matter
Trypsin	Positive (2+–4+)

Carbohydrates (Clinitest)	Negative
Urobilinogen	
Random sample	Negative
24-hour collection	40–200 mg/24 hr
	80–280 Ehrlich units/24 hr
Bile	
Child	Positive
Adult	Negative

Interfering Factors

- Ingestion of a diet high in meat, certain vegetables (e.g., horseradish and turnips), and bananas may cause false-positive results in tests for occult blood
- Therapy with numerous medications may lead to positive results in tests for occult blood due to direct or indirect drug effects; examples of such drugs are aspirin, anticoagulants, adrenocorticosteroids, iron preparations, colchicine, and phenylbutazone
- Ingestion of ascorbic acid may lead to false-negative results in tests for occult blood
- A diet too high or too low in fats, or failure to follow the prescribed diet (100 g of fat per day) may alter results of quantitative fat tests
- Constipation may lead to false-negative results in tests for fecal trypsin in children
- Ingestion of antibiotics and exposure of the fecal sample to light may produce false-negative results in tests for fecal urobilinogen

Indications/Purposes for Tests for Specific Substances in Feces

Occult Blood

- Known or suspected disorder associated with gastrointestinal bleeding (see Table 13–2, p. 437)
- Therapy with drugs that may lead to gastrointestinal bleeding (e.g., aspirin, anticoagulants)

Quantitative Fats

- Suspected intestinal malabsorption or pancreatic insufficiency as indicated by elevated fat levels (see p. 441)
- Monitoring effectiveness of therapy for intestinal malabsorption or pancreatic insufficiency

Trypsin

- Suspected pancreatic insufficiency in very young children as indicated by negative or decreased results

Carbohydrate Utilization (Clinitest)

- Suspected malabsorption syndromes as indicated by positive results

Urobilinogen

- Suspected anemias characterized by decreased red blood cell production as indicated by decreased levels
- Suspected liver and biliary tract disorders as indicated by decreased levels
- Suspected hemolytic anemias as indicated by increased levels

Bile

■ Suspected hemolytic anemias, which lead to excessive levels

Client Preparation

Client preparation is essentially the same as that for microscopic analysis of feces (see p. 441). For tests for occult blood, the client should eat a high-bulk, low-meat diet for 3 days prior to testing. Medications that may alter test results (e.g., aspirin) also may be withheld for 3 or more days prior to the test, although this should be confirmed with the person ordering the study.

For qualitative fat studies, the client should follow a diet containing 100 g of fat for 3 days prior to testing as well as during the test. Alcohol, antacids, laxatives, and antibiotics also may be withheld. The client should be provided with a large container (usually a gallon paint can) and should be instructed to refrigerate the sample.

If the test is for urobilinogen, the client should not be taking antibiotics and should be supplied with a light-protected container.

The Procedure

The procedure is essentially the same as that described on p. 442. Fecal specimens for analysis of specific substances are usually obtained on random samples, although the test for quantitative fats requires a 72-hour collection. Such a study is usually begun early in the morning of a given day, and is then continued for 3 consecutive days. The sample is maintained in a large, refrigerated container (usually a gallon paint can). Fecal studies for urobilinogen may be done on a 24-hour basis.

When random samples are used, the tests are often repeated on a serial basis. This is especially true of studies for occult blood. When this approach is used, it is desirable to obtain the samples on 3 different days.

Aftercare and Nursing Observations

Aftercare and nursing observations are essentially the same as those described on p. 442. If dietary or medication regimens were modified for the test, they may be resumed upon completion of the study.

MICROBIOLOGICAL TESTS OF FECES (BACKGROUND INFORMATION, p. 439)
Reference Values

Stool culture	Normal flora

Interfering Factors

■ Therapy with antibiotics may decrease the type and amount of bacteria present
■ Excessive exposure of the sample to air or room temperature may damage bacteria so that they will not grow in culture
■ Failure to transport the sample to the laboratory within 1 hour of collection

Indications/Purposes for Stool Cultures

■ Diarrhea of unknown etiology that may be due to bacteria that damage intestinal tissue (see Table 13–3, p. 440)

Client Preparation

Client preparation is essentially the same as that for other tests of feces. If the sample is to be obtained by rectal swab, explain to the client how this will be done.

The Procedure

If the sample is to be obtained by rectal swab, a clean or sterile swab and preservative will be needed. Prepackaged sterile swabs with cylinders containing preservative are commercially available for obtaining various types of samples for culture (e.g., wound drainage, throat secretions). The swab is inserted into the rectum (*without* the use of a lubricant) past the anal sphincter. It is rotated gently and then withdrawn.[26]

For samples of portions of bowel movements, the procedure is the same as that described on p. 442. The sample should be placed in a clean, dry container. As certain nonpathological bacteria are normally present in feces, it is not necessary for the container to be sterile.

All samples should be protected from air and sent to the laboratory within 1 hour of collection. Samples should not be refrigerated.

Aftercare and Nursing Observations

There are no specific aftercare or nursing observations related to obtaining samples for stool culture, other than to observe the gross characteristics of the specimen. If the client is to collect the sample independently, assess his or her ability to do so.

REFERENCES

1. Hole, JW: Human Anatomy and Physiology, ed 4. Wm C Brown, Dubuque, IA, 1987, pp 527–528.
2. Strasinger, SK: Urinalysis and Body Fluids. FA Davis, Philadelphia, 1985, p 195.
3. Widmann, FK: Clinical Interpretation of Laboratory Tests, ed 9. FA Davis, Philadelphia, 1983, p 551.
4. Hole, *op cit*, p 528.
5. Widmann, *op cit*, p 552.
6. *Ibid*, p 551.
7. Strasinger, *op cit*, p 196.
8. Kao, YS and Scheer, WD: Malabsorption, Diarrhea, and Examination of Feces. In Henry, JB: Clinical Diagnosis and Management by Laboratory Methods, ed 17. WB Saunders, Philadelphia, 1984, pp 564–565.
9. Widmann, *op cit*, p 560.
10. Strasinger, *op cit*, pp 196–197.
11. Kao and Scheer, *op cit*, p 564.
12. *Ibid*, p 569.
13. Widmann, *op cit*, p 557.
14. Diagnostics, ed 2. Springhouse Corp, Springhouse, PA, 1986, p 526.
15. Strasinger, *op cit*, p 197.

16. Widmann, *op cit*, pp 554–557.
17. Kao and Scheer, *op cit*, p 564.
18. Widmann, *op cit*, p 561.
19. Fischbach, FT: A Manual of Laboratory Diagnostic Tests, ed 3. JB Lippincott, Philadelphia, 1988, p 212.
20. Widmann, *op cit*, pp 561–562.
21. Strasinger, *op cit*, p 199.
22. Diagnostics, *op cit*, p 808.
23. Fischbach, *op cit*, p 212.
24. Widmann, *op cit*, p 354.
25. Kao and Scheer, *op cit*, p 568.
26. Diagnostics, *op cit*, p 509.

BIBLIOGRAPHY

Beare, PG, Rahr, VA and Ronshausen, CA: Nursing Implications of Diagnostic Tests, ed 2. JB Lippincott, Philadelphia, 1985.
Byrne, CJ, Saxton, DF, Pelikan, PK and Nugent, PM: Laboratory Tests: Implications For Nursing Care. Addison-Wesley, Menlo Park, CA, 1986.
Jacob, SW, Francone, CA and Lossow, WJ. Structure and Function in Man, ed 5. WB Saunders, Philadelphia, 1982.
Kee, JL: Laboratory and Diagnostic Tests With Nursing Implications, ed 2. Appleton & Lange, Norwalk, CT, 1987.
Lamb, JO: Laboratory Tests For Clinical Nursing. Robert J Brady, Bowie, MD, 1984.
Luckmann, J and Sorenson, KC: Medical-Surgical Nursing: A Psychophysiologic Approach, ed 3. WB Saunders, Philadelphia, 1987.
Pagana, KD and Pagana, TJ: Diagnostic Testing and Nursing Implications: A Case Study Approach, ed 2. CV Mosby, St Louis, 1986.
Porth, C: Pathophysiology: Concepts of Altered Health States, ed 2. JB Lippincott, 1986.
Tilkian, SM, Conover, MB and Tilkian, AG: Clinical Implications of Laboratory Tests, ed 4. CV Mosby, St Louis, 1987.
Wallach, J: Interpretation of Diagnostic Tests: A Hardbook Synopsis of Laboratory Medicine, ed 4. Little, Brown & Co., Boston, 1986.
Widmann, FK: Pathobiology: How Diseases Happen. Little, Brown & Co, Boston, 1978.

ANALYSIS OF CELLS AND TISSUES

TESTS COVERED

OVERVIEW OF CYTOLOGICAL AND HISTOLOGICAL METHODS

The various cells and tissues of the body may be analyzed through cytological and histological methods. Cytology refers to the study of the structure, function, and pathology of cells. Histology deals with the study of the structure, function and pathology of tissues. Both methods are used primarily in the detection of cancer.

Cytological methods are used mainly as screening procedures to detect precancerous or malignant cells. The laboratory techniques used were developed by Papanicolaou, who identified characteristics that allowed for differentiation of normal from neoplastic cells. This differentiation is based on changes that occur in the relationships between the cytoplasm and the nucleus of the cells.[1] In performing cytological examinations, slides with cells are stained with various substances and are then examined microscopically. Malignant cells, for example, may show large, darkly stained irregular nuclei.[2]

The most common site examined through cytological methods is the uterine cervix (i.e., the "Pap smear"). Cells from the respiratory tract also are frequently examined. Samples of such cells may be obtained through sputum specimens (see Chapter 7), bronchial brushings or washings obtained during bronchoscopic examinations, or from postbronchoscopy sputum specimens. Various body fluids also may be examined for abnormal cells. These include urine (see Chapter 6); cerebrospinal fluid (see Chapter 8); and pleural, peritoneal, pericardial, and synovial effusions (see Chapter 9).

The method of reporting results of cytological examinations varies somewhat with the laboratory. Papanicolaou developed a numerical classification system for the various types of cells found on cytological examination. Owing to problems with overlapping classes and variation in laboratory interpretation, narrative descriptions of the cells present are now more likely to be used.[3]

It should be noted that cellular changes that mimic neoplastic changes may occur in response to inflammatory processes. Thus, the cytologist should be provided with information about the client so that accurate interpretation of the cells types present may be made.[4]

In addition to its use in cancer detection, cytological study may provide other types of diagnostic information. By examining cells obtained from the oral cavity, female sexual chromosomes (Barr bodies) may be identified. Various Papanicolaou stains may elicit cell types associated with viral or fungal infections. Analysis of cells from effusions also may demonstrate cell types associated with collagen vascular diseases such as systemic lupus erythematosus and rheumatoid arthritis. The nature of the cells present in vaginal smears may indicate the client's estrogen levels.[5]

Histological methods are used primarily to confirm the diagnosis of cancer when screening tests are positive for abnormal cells. Histological techniques involve obtaining samples of tissue by biopsy and examining them microscopically. Such an evaluation involves examining the structure of the tissues and may also include cytological study of the cells through the use of various staining techniques. Electron microscopy methods also have been used.[6]

If the tissue sample is that of a tumor, it is examined in relation to anatomical size, position, and extent of the tumor. Whether or not malignant cells have invaded blood or lymphatic channels also is assessed.[7] Sections of tissue obtained at surgery may be frozen (i.e., "frozen sections") and analyzed during the surgical procedure to determine if more extensive surgery is needed, thus avoiding the client's being subjected to a second procedure.

In addition to samples obtained during surgery, biopsies of tissues may be performed by local excision, needle aspiration, or with special instruments such as tissue punches and curettes. Tissue samples also may be obtained during various endoscopic procedures. Common sites for biopsies are the skin, mucous membranes, serous membranes (e.g., pleura), synovial membranes lining joints, various organs (e.g., liver, kidney, lung), glands (e.g., thyroid, prostate), lymph nodes, bone, muscle, and female reproductive tissues. Bone marrow biopsies also are performed (see Chapter 1).

TESTS OF CELLS AND TISSUES

Background Information

PAPANICOLAOU SMEAR (PAP SMEAR) (CLINICAL APPLICATIONS DATA, p. 452)

The Pap smear is used primarily in the early detection of cervical cancer. Malignant cells from such cancers slough readily and can be detected with cytological methods. In addition to cancer detection, Pap smears may be used to assess estrogen levels and response to estrogen therapy. Inflammatory changes and infections due to viruses and fungi also may be detected with Pap smears.

Results of Pap smears are reported in various ways depending upon the laboratory's preference. The traditional method for reporting results is shown here:

Class I	Normal cells
Class II	Atypical cells, but not malignant
Class III	Atypical cells, suspicious of malignancy
Class IV	Atypical cells, suggestive of malignancy
Class V	Cancer cells present, conclusive for malignancy

Abnormal results of Pap smears should be followed by either repeat Pap smears or cervical biopsies. It is recommended that women between the ages of 20 and 40 have a Pap smear at least every 3 years. Women over 40 should have a Pap smear every year. More frequent examinations may be performed in women who are at high risk for developing cervical cancer (e.g., positive family history).

SKIN BIOPSY (CLINICAL APPLICATIONS DATA, p. 454)

Skin biopsies are performed to detect malignancies and are indicated when there are skin lesions of suspicious appearance or when skin lesions change in size, color, or texture. Skin biopsies may be performed with a biopsy punch or by scraping or excising the lesion using a scalpel.

BONE BIOPSY (CLINICAL APPLICATIONS DATA, p. 455)

A bone biopsy consists of removing a plug of bone with a special serrated needle, or surgical excision of a sample of bone for examination prior to further surgery for bone disease. If performed by surgical excision (i.e., "open" biopsy), the preparation and procedure are the same as that for any orthopedic surgical procedure requiring general anesthesia. Bone biopsies are generally indicated when x-ray examination shows evidence of a lesion involving bone.

BREAST BIOPSY (CLINICAL APPLICATIONS DATA, p. 456)

Breast lesions can be localized by palpation, mammography, or ultrasound, but the nature of the lesion can be confirmed only by biopsy. The tissue sample may be obtained by needle aspiration or by open incision. Many physicians perform only open biopsies, excising the entire lesion rather than aspirating only a small sample of it.

CERVICAL PUNCH BIOPSY (CLINICAL APPLICATIONS DATA, p. 458)

Punch biopsy of the uterine cervix may be performed during a routine pelvic examination, if abnormal areas are noted, or it may be indicated by abnormal results of a Pap smear (see p. 448) or a positive Schiller test. The Schiller test involves applying iodine solution to the cervix. Normal tissues stain dark brown, but abnormal tissues fail to pick up the color. Both the Schiller test and punch biopsy of the cervix are performed using a colposcope, a specialized binocular microscope that allows direct visualization of the cervix. Punch biopsy results may indicate the need for the more extensive cone biopsy of the cervix. This operative procedure involves excision of cervical tissue and requires general anesthesia.

BIOPSY OF THE BLADDER AND/OR URETER (CLINICAL APPLICATIONS DATA, p. 459)

Biopsies of the bladder and ureter are usually performed during cystoscopical examinations of the bladder. Such biopsies are indicated if a bladder tumor is visualized radiologically, if there are persistent symptoms following excision of bladder polyps or tumors, and if there is evidence of hydroureter without kidney stones. The purpose of the test is to differentiate between benign and malignant lesions or to monitor recurrent lesions for malignant changes.

RENAL BIOPSY (KIDNEY BIOPSY) (CLINICAL APPLICATIONS DATA, p. 461)

Renal biopsy involves obtaining a sample of kidney tissue for histological and cytological evaluation. The test may be performed by percutaneous needle biopsy (closed biopsy) or through surgical incision (open biopsy). Lesions of the kidney may be localized by renal CAT scan or ultrasound. In addition to identified lesions, other indications for renal biopsy include hematuria, proteinuria and/or casts in the urine of unknown etiology, nephrotic syndrome, acute or rapidly progressing renal failure of unknown etiology, systemic lupus erythematosus with urinary abnormalities, suspected renal cysts, and monitoring transplanted kidneys.

Renal biopsy, especially when performed by the percutaneous method, is not without its attendant risks. Bleeding within the kidney, damage to renal tissue, and infection may occur. Therefore, this procedure is performed only when absolutely necessary to obtain data not otherwise available through blood, urine, and noninvasive radiological tests.

CHORIONIC VILLUS BIOPSY (CVB) (CLINICAL APPLICATIONS DATA, p. 464)

Chorionic villus biopsies are used to detect fetal abnormalities due to various genetic disorders. The advantage of CVB over amniocentesis (see Chapter 10) is that CVB can be performed as early as the eighth week of pregnancy, thus permitting earlier decisions to retain or terminate the pregnancy.

Chorionic villi are finger-like projections that cover the embryo and anchor it to the uterine lining prior to development of the placenta. Since chorionic villi are of embryonic origin, samples of them provide information about the developing baby. Chorionic villi samples are best obtained between the eighth and tenth weeks of pregnancy. After 10 weeks of pregnancy, the villi are overgrown with maternal cells.

CVB can be used to detect hundreds, and potentially even thousands, of genetic defects. It cannot, however, be used to detect neural tube defects such as spina bifida. For the latter, amniocentesis is still the test of choice.

CVB is performed in a manner similar to an amniocentesis, although entry into the amniotic sac is not necessary. The test carries with it the risks of damage to the chorionic membrane, bleeding, and possible spontaneous abortion even as late as 18 to 20 weeks of pregnancy. The number of spontaneous abortions attributed to CVB is estimated to be as low as 2 percent.[8]

In addition to CVB's advantage of being performed earlier than amniocentesis, results are also available more quickly—many times within 48 hours of the study.

Tissue samples obtained via CVB are cultured in Petri dishes and are then examined microscopically. The cells grown in culture are assessed for chromosomal abnormalities.

It should be noted that the developing embryo and chorion may be localized prior to or during the procedure by ultrasound or endoscopic tests.

LIVER BIOPSY (CLINICAL APPLICATIONS DATA, p. 465)

Liver biopsy involves obtaining a sample of hepatic tissue for histological and cytological evaluation. The test may be performed by percutaneous needle biopsy (closed biopsy) or through surgical incision (open biopsy). This test is indicated when liver disease is suspected, but is not evidenced by less invasive procedures such as ultrasounds and CAT scans.

Liver biopsy, especially when performed by the percutaneous method, is not without its attendant risks: bleeding within the liver, damage to hepatic tissue, and infection may occur. Therefore, this procedure is performed only when absolutely necessary.

MUSCLE BIOPSY (CLINICAL APPLICATIONS DATA, p. 468)

A muscle biopsy consists of obtaining a sample of tissue, usually from the deltoid or gastrocnemius muscle, for histological study. Muscle biopsies are indicated when there is a family history of Duchenne's muscular dystrophy, when fungal or parasitic infestation of muscle is suspected, and in various neuromuscular disorders to differentiate neuropathy from myopathy.

LYMPH NODE BIOPSY (CLINICAL APPLICATIONS DATA, p. 469)

Lymph node biopsies are performed when there is persistent enlargement of lymph nodes and/or signs and symptoms of systemic disease that may indicate malignant or infectious processes. The lymph nodes most commonly biopsied are the cervical, axillary, and inguinal nodes. Cervical lymph nodes drain the scalp and face; axillary lymph nodes drain the arms, breasts, and upper chest; and inguinal nodes drain the legs, external genitalia, and lower abdominal wall.

Lymph node biopsies may be performed by needle aspiration or by surgical excision. The latter approach is preferred for deeper nodes and when a larger or more complete sample of the node is required.

INTESTINAL BIOPSY (SMALL INTESTINE) (CLINICAL APPLICATIONS DATA, p. 470)

Biopsies of the small intestine are generally performed during endoscopic procedures. During these tests, samples of intestinal tissue may be obtained via the endoscope, if abnormal lesions are visualized. The main purpose of the test is to differentiate between benign and malignant lesions of the small intestine. Other purposes include differentiating among the various small intestinal disorders such as lactose intolerance, enzyme deficiencies, sprue, and parasitic and other infections.

LUNG BIOPSY (CLINICAL APPLICATIONS DATA, p. 473)

Lung biopsy is the removal of a sample of lung tissue for cytological and histological study. The sample may be obtained through "closed" methods such as insertion of a needle through the chest wall and fiberoptic bronchoscopy, or by "open" biopsy, which entails a thoracotomy and general anesthesia.

Lung biopsies are indicated when there is diffuse pulmonary disease of unknown etiology; when malignancy, infection, or parasitic infestation is suspected; and when other less invasive tests such as chest x-ray examinations, CAT scans, and sputum analyses are inconclusive.

Complications of lung biopsies (especially needle biopsies) include bleeding into lung tissue, pneumothorax, hemothorax, and infection. Thus, this test should be performed with caution and only when necessary to obtain diagnostic information not otherwise available through less invasive procedures.

PLEURAL BIOPSY (CLINICAL APPLICATIONS DATA, p. 475)

Pleural biopsy is the removal of a sample of pleural tissue for cytological and histological study. It is usually performed by needle biopsy and may be done as part of a thoracentesis (see Chapter 9). Open biopsy, requiring a thoracotomy using general anesthesia, also may be performed.

Pleural biopsies may be performed when there is evidence of a pleural effusion of unknown etiology; when a tumor is suspected (to differentiate between benign and malignant disease); and to diagnose suspected infection, fibrosis, and collagen vascular disease involving the pleura.

Complications of pleural biopsies (especially needle biopsies) include bleeding into lung tissue, pneumothorax, hemothorax, and infection. Thus, this test should be performed with caution and only when necessary to obtain diagnostic information not otherwise available through less invasive procedures.

PROSTATE GLAND BIOPSY (CLINICAL APPLICATIONS DATA, p. 477)

Prostate gland biopsy involves the removal of a sample of prostatic tissue for histological and cytological examination. This test is indicated when there is enlargement of the prostate gland of unknown etiology or when cancer of the prostate gland is suspected.

Several approaches to obtaining the sample are possible: transurethral, transrectal, and perineal. Possible complications include bleeding and infection at the biopsy site, although these are not frequent problems.

THYROID GLAND BIOPSY (CLINICAL APPLICATIONS DATA, p. 478)

Thyroid gland biopsy involves the removal of a sample of thyroid tissue for histological and cytological examination. This test is indicated when thyroid nodules are demonstrated or when there are symptoms of thyroiditis or hyperthyroidism to determine the cause.

Thyroid tissue samples may be obtained by needle aspiration (closed biopsy) or surgical incision (open biopsy). Needle biopsies require local anesthesia, whereas open biopsies are performed in a manner similar to that used for a thyroidectomy.

Clinical Applications Data

PAPANICOLAOU SMEAR (PAP SMEAR) (BACKGROUND INFORMATION, p. 448)
Reference Values

No abnormal cells (class I Pap smear).

Interfering Factors

- Douching within 24 hours of the test, which may wash away cells that would have been obtained on sampling
- Use of lubricating jelly on the vaginal speculum, which may alter the sample
- Improper specimen collection (samples for cancer screening are obtained

from the posterior vaginal fornix and from the cervix; samples for hormonal evaluation are obtained from the vagina)
■ Improper preservation of the specimen upon collection
■ Collection of the sample during menstruation, as blood in the sample may impair identification of abnormal cells

Indications/Purposes for a Pap Smear

■ Routine screening for cervical cancer
■ Evaluation of estrogen levels and response to therapy with estrogen
■ Identification of inflammatory tissue changes
■ Detection of viral and fungal vaginal infections

Client Preparation

Client Teaching. Explain to the client:

■ the purpose of the test
■ that the test should not be performed when the client is menstruating
■ that the client should not douche for at least 24 hours prior to the test
■ that all clothing below the waist will need to be removed, except for the shoes, which may be kept on (if the Pap smear is to be performed along with a breast examination, it may be necessary to remove all clothing and to don an examination gown)
■ that the examination will be performed with the client positioned on a gynecological examination table
■ that a metal or plastic vaginal speculum will be inserted in order to visualize the cervix
■ that slight discomfort may be experienced when the speculum is inserted
■ that relaxation and controlled breathing aid in reducing discomfort during the examination
■ that samples of vaginal and cervical cells will be obtained with a small wooden spatula or with a cotton-topped applicator
■ that the examiner may perform a bimanual examination involving the vagina, rectum, and pelvic cavity as part of the examination
■ that a breast examination also may be performed as part of the gynecological evaluation
■ that the entire procedure should take approximately 15 minutes

Encourage questions and verbalizations of concerns by the client.
Obtain a brief gynecological history that includes the date of the last menstrual period, frequency of periods, duration of periods, type of menstrual flow, date of last Pap smear, and use of birth control pills or other medications containing hormones.

Physical Preparation

■ Assist the client to disrobe and provide an examination gown if necessary; if breast examination is to be performed, the gown should be donned so that it opens in the front
■ Ensure that the client voids immediately prior to the examination

The Procedure

The equipment needed is assembled. This includes a vaginal speculum, gloves, wooden spatulas or cotton-tipped applicators, slides, preservative or spray fixative, marking pens for labeling the samples, and lubricant if a bimanual examination is to be performed after the Pap smear has been obtained.

The client is positioned on the examination table. The feet should not be placed in the stirrups until immediately before the Pap smear is to be obtained. When the feet have been positioned, the client should be instructed to allow her legs to ''drop'' to each side and to attempt to relax as much as possible. The client's legs should be draped to avoid excessive and unnecessary exposure and chilling.

The speculum may be dipped or rinsed in water to aid in insertion but should not be lubricated. With the speculum positioned, vaginal and cervical samples are obtained and placed on slides. The slides should be fixed with spray or placed in preservative immediately.

The speculum is removed. If a bimanual pelvic examination is to be performed, it will be done at this time. In contrast, a breast examination is usually performed prior to obtaining the Pap smear.

Aftercare and Nursing Observations

The client is assisted to remove her legs from the stirrups and is allowed to rest for a few minutes in a supine position. Excess lubricant or secretions should be cleansed from the perineal area. The client may wish to do this herself. If cervical bleeding occurs, the client should be provided with a perineal pad. The client should be assisted to dress, if necessary.

The client should be informed when results of the test will be available and when she should have her next Pap smear.

SKIN BIOPSY (BACKGROUND INFORMATION, p. 449)

Reference Values

No abnormal cells or tissue present.

Indications/Purposes for Skin Biopsy

- Evaluation of skin lesions that are suspected of being malignant
- Diagnosis of keratoses, warts, moles, keloids, fibromas, cysts, or inflammatory lesions

Client Preparation

Client Teaching. Explain to the client:

- the purpose of the test
- that foods and fluids are not restricted for the procedure
- that the test involves removing a small skin sample or portion of a skin lesion
- that the test will be performed by a physician
- that it may be necessary to shave the site prior to the biopsy
- that a local anesthetic will be either sprayed onto or injected at the biopsy site to prevent pain
- that one or two sutures may be necessary to close the biopsy site, depending on its extent
- that a dressing or Bandaid will be applied to the site following the procedure

Encourage questions and verbalization of concerns appropriate to the client's age and mental status.
Ensure that a signed consent has been obtained.

Physical Preparation

- If the area to be biopsied is hirsute, it may be necessary to shave it prior to the biopsy

■ Depending on the biopsy site, the client may need to be assisted to disrobe and be provided with a hospital gown

The Procedure

The equipment needed is assembled. This includes sterile drapes (depending on the site and the extent of the lesion), materials for cleansing the skin, equipment for obtaining the sample, local anesthetic, a jar with formalin to preserve the specimen, suture or other material to close the biopsy site, sterile gloves, and dressings or Bandaids.

The client is assisted to a position of comfort and the area to be biopsied is adequately supported and exposed. The area is then cleansed with antiseptic solution. A local anesthetic is applied by either topical spray or needle infiltration. Depending on the size of the lesion to be biopsied, the area may be draped with sterile drapes.

If the sample is to be obtained by curettage, the surface of the lesion is scraped with a curette until adequate tissue samples are obtained. The scrapings are placed on a microscope slide and preserved with an appropriate fixative. The sample is sent to the laboratory immediately. If bleeding occurs, a Bandaid is applied to the site.

If the sample is to be obtained by shaving or excision, a scalpel is used to remove the portion of the lesion that protrudes above the epidermis. Bleeding is controlled with digital pressure. A sterile dressing or Bandaid is applied to the site. The sample is placed in an appropriate fixative (usually in formalin) and sent to the laboratory immediately.

If the sample is to be obtained by punch biopsy, a small round "cookie cutter" punch, 4 to 6 mm in diameter, is rotated into the skin to the desired depth. The cylinder of skin is pulled upward with a forceps and separated at its base with a pointed scalpel or scissors. The site may then be closed using sutures or other material, and a sterile dressing is applied. The specimen is placed in an appropriate fixative and sent to the laboratory immediately.

Aftercare and Nursing Observations

The client may be allowed to rest for a few minutes following the procedure. The dressing or Bandaid should be assessed for excessive bleeding. The client should be instructed in care and observation of the site. If sutures were used, the client should have a follow-up appointment for suture removal.

BONE BIOPSY (BACKGROUND INFORMATION, p. 449)

Reference Values

No abnormal cells or tissue present.

Indications/Purposes for Bone Biopsy

■ Radiographical evidence of a bone lesion
■ Differentiation of benign from malignant bone lesions
■ Identification of the source of a metastatic lesion involving bone

Client Preparation

Client Teaching. Explain to the client:

■ the purpose of the test
■ the method that will be used to obtain the sample (needle biopsy or surgical excision)

- that the procedure will be performed by a physician
- that foods and fluids are usually not restricted prior to a needle biopsy but are restricted prior to an open biopsy
- that special skin preparation may be required (e.g., shave, orthopedic skin prep), especially for an open biopsy
- the type of anesthetic to be administered (local infiltration for needle biopsies, general anesthesia for open biopsies)
- that, if a needle biopsy is to be performed, momentary discomfort may be experienced when the periosteum is penetrated
- that a dressing will be applied to the site
- that analgesics may be administered following the procedure to alleviate any discomfort

Encourage questions and verbalization of concerns about the procedure. Ensure that a signed consent has been obtained.

Physical Preparation

- For an open biopsy, the physical preparation is the same as that for any surgical procedure requiring general anesthesia. A shave and/or orthopedic skin prep may be required prior to the procedure.
- For a needle biopsy, a shave and orthopedic skin prep may be required. The client should be assisted to disrobe as necessary and should be provided with a hospital gown.

The Procedure

For an open biopsy, the samples are obtained through surgical excision during the operative procedure.

For a needle biopsy, the client is assisted to a position of comfort, and the biopsy site is supported and exposed. The skin is cleansed with an antiseptic solution, injected with local anesthetic and draped with sterile drapes. A small incision is made and the biopsy needle is inserted to obtain a plug of bone. The sample is placed in formalin and sent to the laboratory immediately. The incision may be closed with sutures or other material and a sterile dressing applied.

Aftercare and Nursing Observations

Following an open biopsy, the client is cared for and observed in the same manner as anyone who has had surgery using general anesthesia.

For a needle biopsy, the client is allowed to rest for several minutes following the procedure. The client's response to the procedure is monitored.

For both approaches, the dressing is observed for excessive bleeding. The client should be instructed on care and observation of the site. If sutures were used, follow-up arrangements for suture removal should be made.

The client also should be assessed for level of discomfort following the procedure, and prescribed analgesics should be administered accordingly.

BREAST BIOPSY (BACKGROUND INFORMATION, p. 449)

Reference Values

No abnormal cells or tissue present.

Indications/Purposes for Breast Biopsy

■ Evidence of a breast lesion by palpation, mammography, or ultrasound
■ Observable breast changes such as "peau d'orange" skin changes, scaly skin of nipple or areola, drainage from nipple, and ulceration of skin
■ Differentiation of benign from malignant breast lesions

Client Preparation

Client Teaching. Explain to the client:

■ the purpose of the test
■ that the procedure will be performed by a physician
■ the method that will be used to obtain the sample (needle biopsy or surgical excision)
■ that foods and fluids are not usually restricted prior to a needle biopsy, but are restricted prior to an open biopsy
■ the type of anesthetic to be administered (local infiltration for a needle biopsy, general anesthesia for an open biopsy)
■ that a dressing will be applied to the site
■ that analgesics may be administered following the procedure to alleviate any discomfort

Encourage questions and verbalization of concerns about the procedure.
Ensure that a signed consent for the procedure has been obtained.

Physical Preparation

■ For an open biopsy, the physical preparation is the same as that for any surgical procedure requiring general anesthesia
■ For a needle biopsy, the client should disrobe from the waist up and be provided with a hospital gown with the opening in the front

The Procedure

For an open biopsy, the sample is obtained through surgical excision during the operative procedure.

For a needle biopsy, the client is assisted to a supine position, and the area to be biopsied is exposed. The skin is cleansed with an antiseptic, injected with local anesthetic, and draped with sterile drapes. A needle (either a Vim-Silverman biopsy needle or an 18-gauge needle) is inserted into the mass. A plug of tissue or bolus of fluid is aspirated via a syringe connected to the needle. The tissue is placed in a specimen container with normal saline; fluid is gently expelled into a green-topped (heparinized) blood collection tube. The samples should be sent to the laboratory immediately. A sterile dressing is applied to the biopsy site.

Aftercare and Nursing Observations

Following an open biopsy, the client is cared for and observed in the same manner as with anyone who has had surgery using general anesthesia.

For a needle biopsy, the client is allowed to rest for several minutes following the procedure. The client's response to the procedure is monitored.

For both approaches, the dressing is observed for excessive bleeding or drainage. The client should be instructed on care and observation of the biopsy site. If sutures were used, follow-up arrangements for suture removal should be made.

The client also should be assessed for level of discomfort following the procedure, and prescribed analgesics should be administered accordingly.

CERVICAL PUNCH BIOPSY (BACKGROUND INFORMATION, p. 449)
Reference Values

No abnormal cells or tissue present.

Indications/Purposes for Cervical Punch Biopsy

- Abnormal Pap smear
- Schiller test positive for abnormal cells or tissue (see p. 449)
- Appearance of abnormal cells or tissue (e.g., ulceration, leukoplakia, polyps) on colposcopic examination
- Differentiation of benign from malignant cells or tissue

Contraindications

- Acute pelvic inflammatory disease
- Cervicitis
- Bleeding disorder

Client Preparation

Client Teaching. Explain to the client:

- the purpose of the test
- that the test should not be performed when the client is menstruating and is best performed approximately 1 week after her period has ended
- that all clothing below the waist will need to be removed, except for the shoes, which may be kept on
- that the procedure will be performed with the client positioned on a gynecological examination table
- that a metal or plastic vaginal speculum will be inserted to visualize the cervix
- that slight discomfort may be experienced when the speculum is inserted
- that relaxation and controlled breathing aid in reducing discomfort during the examination
- that the cervix may be swabbed with iodine in order to aid in identification of abnormal cells (if the client is allergic to iodine, this should be noted prior to the test)
- that a microscope-like device will be used to more clearly visualize the cervix, but that it is not inserted into the vagina
- that a small sample of cervical tissue will be obtained with forceps
- that mild discomfort may be experienced when the sample is removed as well as after the test
- that the entire procedure should take approximately 15 minutes
- that a small amount of cervical bleeding may occur after the procedure
- that a gray-green vaginal discharge may persist for a few days to a few weeks following the procedure
- that strenuous exercise should be avoided for 8 to 24 hours following the procedure
- that douching and intercourse should be avoided for approximately 2 weeks after the procedure or as directed by the physician

Encourage questions and verbalization of concerns about the procedure. Ensure that a signed consent has been obtained.

Physical Preparation

■ Assist the client to disrobe from the waist down and provide an examination gown if necessary
■ Ensure that the client voids immediately prior to the procedure

The Procedure

The client is positioned on the examination table. The legs are draped and the external genitalia cleansed with an antiseptic solution. The vaginal speculum is inserted using water as a lubricant if a Pap smear is to be performed prior to the biopsy (see p. 452).

For the biopsy, the cervix is swabbed with 3 percent acetic acid to remove mucus and improve the contrast between tissue types. If a Schiller test is to be performed, the cervix is swabbed with iodine solution to aid in identification of abnormal cells. The colposcope is inserted through the speculum and is focused on the cervix. If an area is identified as abnormal, the biopsy forceps are inserted through the speculum or colposcope, and tissue samples are obtained. The samples are placed in specimen containers with formalin solution. The containers should be labeled with the source of the samples.

Bleeding, which is not uncommon following a cervical punch biopsy, may be controlled by cautery, suturing or by applying silver nitrate or ferric subsulfate to the site. If bleeding persists, a tampon may be inserted by the physician following removal of the speculum.

Aftercare and Nursing Observations

Excess lubricant, solutions, or secretions are cleansed from the perineal area. The client is assisted to remove her legs from the stirrups and is allowed to rest for a few minutes in a supine position. The client is then assisted to dress, if necessary.

If a vaginal tampon was inserted, the client should be informed as to when it may be removed (usually in 8 to 24 hours). After this, pads should be worn if there is bleeding or drainage. The client should be told to report excessive vaginal bleeding.

The client should be reminded that a gray-green vaginal discharge may persist for a few days to a few weeks after the procedure, that strenuous exercise should be avoided for 8 to 24 hours, and that douching and intercourse should be avoided for 2 weeks or as otherwise directed by the physician.[9]

BIOPSY OF BLADDER AND/OR URETER (BACKGROUND INFORMATION, p. 450)

Reference Values

No abnormal cells or tissue present.

Indications/Purposes for Biopsy of Bladder and/or Ureter

■ Differentiation between benign and malignant lesions involving the bladder and/or ureter, especially if there is evidence of a bladder tumor on radiological examination or if hydroureter is present without stones
■ Monitoring recurrent lesions of the bladder or ureter for malignant changes

Contraindications

■ Acute cystitis
■ Bleeding disorders

Client Preparation

Client Teaching. Explain to the client:

■ the purpose of the test
■ that it will be performed by a urologist during a cystoscopic examination of the bladder
■ that a sedative may be administered prior to the procedure to promote relaxation
■ the type of anesthetic to be administered (local or general anesthesia may be used)
■ that, if general anesthesia is to be used, foods and fluids are withheld for 8 hours prior to the procedure
■ that, if local anesthesia is to be used, only clear liquids may be taken for 8 hours prior to the test
■ that the test will be performed with the client positioned on a special urological table and that the legs will be elevated in stirrups
■ that after he or she is positioned on the table the legs will be draped and the external genitalia will be cleansed with antiseptic solution
■ that a special microscope-like instrument will be inserted into the urethra in order to visualize the bladder
■ that, if local anesthesia is used, a sensation of pressure or of having to void, or both sensations, may be experienced
■ that a small amount of tissue will be removed from the bladder and/or ureter with a special brush or forceps inserted through the cystoscope
■ that after tissue removal and inspection of the bladder and urethra, the cystoscope will be removed
■ that vital signs and urinary output will be monitored closely following the test
■ that burning or discomfort on urination may be experienced for the first few voidings after the test
■ that urine may be blood-tinged for the first and second voidings after the test

Encourage questions and verbalization of concerns about the procedure.
Ensure that a signed consent has been obtained.

Physical Preparation

■ Assist the client to disrobe from at least the waist down, and provide a hospital gown if necessary
■ Ensure to the extent possible that dietary or fluid restrictions, or both, are followed prior to the test
■ If general anesthesia is to be used, the physical preparation is the same as that for any surgical procedure requiring general anesthesia
■ If local anesthesia is to be used, the client's vital signs are checked, and the premedication is administered if ordered

The Procedure

The client is positioned on the examination table and the legs are placed in the stirrups and draped. If general anesthesia is to be used, it is administered prior to positioning on the table. The external genitalia are cleansed with antiseptic solution. If a local anesthetic is to be used, it is instilled into the urethra and retained for 5 to 10 minutes. A penile clamp may be used for male clients to aid in retention of the anesthetic.

The cystoscope alone may be used for the examination, or a urethroscope may be used to examine the urethra prior to cystoscopy. The urethroscope has a sheath that may be left in place and the cystoscope inserted through it, thus avoiding multiple instrumentations. After the cystoscope is inserted, the bladder is irrigated and then inspected. Urine samples may be obtained prior to bladder irrigation.

The area of the bladder to be biopsied is identified and tissues are removed by cytology brush or biopsy forceps. If a tumor is found, and if it is small and localized, it may be excised. Bleeding may be controlled using electrocautery. If ureteral samples are needed, small catheters may be inserted into them via the cystoscope. Specimens obtained for biopsy are placed in appropriate containers and sent to the laboratory immediately.

Upon completion of cystoscopy and collection of tissue samples, the cystoscope is withdrawn. The client's legs are removed from the stirrups and the supine position is assumed.

Aftercare and Nursing Observations

If general anesthesia was used, the client is cared for in the same manner as anyone who has had such anesthesia.

For local anesthesia, the client is allowed to rest in the supine position for several minutes before being assisted from the table. Vital signs may be taken and compared with baseline readings.

Special attention must be paid to resumption of normal voiding patterns. Time and amount of voidings and the appearance of the urine should be monitored for at least 24 hours following the procedure. The urine may be blood-tinged for the first and second voidings but is usually clear by the third voiding. The client also should be assessed for bladder distention; incomplete emptying of the bladder; suprapubic or flank pain; chills; and fever. If bladder spasms occur, analgesics may be administered. Warm sitz or hip baths may also alleviate discomfort. Prophylactic antibiotics also may be ordered.

Foods and fluids withheld prior to the test are resumed. Unless medically contraindicated, a fluid intake of 3,000 ml within 24 hours after the test is desirable.

Clients who have the procedure performed as an outpatient should be instructed on how to monitor urinary output and on the necessity of reporting symptoms such as pain, chills, and fever immediately.

RENAL BIOPSY (KIDNEY BIOPSY) (BACKGROUND INFORMATION, p. 450)

Reference Values

No abnormal cells or tissue present.

Indications/Purposes for Renal Biopsy

■ Determination of the nature of lesions of the kidney identified by renal CAT scan or ultrasound (e.g., benign versus malignant lesions)
■ Hematuria, proteinuria, and/or casts in the urine of unknown etiology to determine the nature of the renal disorder
■ Monitoring the progression of nephrotic syndrome
■ Acute or rapidly progressing renal failure of unknown etiology

- Systemic lupus erythematosus with urinary abnormalities to determine the extent of renal involvement
- Suspected renal cysts to confirm the diagnosis
- Monitoring the function of a transplanted kidney

Contraindications

- Bleeding disorders
- Advanced renal disease with uremia
- Severe, uncontrolled hypertension
- Solitary kidney (except transplanted kidney)
- Gross obesity and severe spinal deformity (contraindicates percutaneous needle biopsy)
- Inability of the client to cooperate during the procedure (contraindicates percutaneous needle biopsy)

Nursing Alert

- Renal biopsy, especially when performed by the percutaneous method, may result in bleeding within the kidney, damage to renal tissue, and infection
- Prior to the procedure the client's hematological status and blood clotting ability must be assessed; therefore, a complete blood count (CBC), platelet level, prothrombin time, partial thromboplastin time, clotting time, and bleeding time should be performed prior to the test (in addition, a type and cross-match for 2 units of blood may be ordered)
- Following the procedure, the client's vital signs, amount of urine output, characteristics of urine output, and comfort level must be monitored closely for early detection of possible complications

---

Client Preparation

Client Teaching. Explain to the client:

- the purpose of the test
- that the procedure will be performed by a physician
- the method that will be used to obtain the sample (percutaneous [closed] biopsy or surgical [open] biopsy)
- the type of anesthesia to be administered (local infiltration for needle biopsies, general anesthesia for open biopsies)
- that foods and fluids are withheld for 6 to 8 hours prior to the procedure
- that a sedative may be administered prior to the procedure
- that, if a needle biopsy is performed, it will be necessary to remain motionless and breathe as instructed during certain portions of the procedure
- that, if a needle biopsy is performed, a pressure dressing will be applied to the site
- that, following a needle biopsy, the client will need to lie on the biopsied side for at least 30 minutes, with a pillow or sandbag under the site to prevent bleeding
- that bed rest is required for 24 hours after the procedure
- that vital signs and urinary output will be monitored closely for at least 24 hours following the test
- that, unless medically contraindicated, the client should have a fluid intake

of approximately 3 quarts (3,000 ml) for at least the first 24 hours following the test
■ that strenuous activity, sports, and heavy lifting should be avoided for at least 2 weeks following the test
■ that any discomfort, especially in the area of the kidneys, shoulders, or abdomen, should be reported immediately

Encourage questions and verbalization of concerns about the procedure.
If the client appears unduly anxious or unable to cooperate with a percutaneous needle biopsy (including assuming the prone position for the test), the physician performing the procedure should be so informed.
Ensure that a signed consent for the procedure has been obtained.

Physical Preparation

■ If the skin at the biopsy site is unusually hirsute, it may be necessary to shave the site prior to the procedure
■ Ensure to the extent possible that dietary and fluid restrictions are followed prior to the test
■ If an open biopsy is to be performed, the physical preparation is the same as that for any surgical procedure requiring general anesthesia
■ For a percutaneous needle biopsy, the client's vital signs are taken and compared with baseline levels; the client should void immediately prior to the procedure and be provided with a hospital gown (the premedication, if ordered, is administered 30 to 60 minutes prior to the procedure)

The Procedure

For an open biopsy, the samples are collected during the operative procedure.

For a percutaneous needle biopsy, the client is assisted to the prone position. A sandbag may be placed beneath the abdomen to aid in moving the kidneys to the posterior and in maintaining the desired position. The biopsy site is exposed, cleansed with antiseptic, and draped with sterile drapes. The skin and subcutaneous tissues are then infiltrated with a local anesthetic.

To facilitate downward movement and subsequent immobilization of the kidneys the client is instructed to take a deep breath and hold it as the biopsy needle (usually a Vim-Silverman needle) is inserted. As the needle enters the kidney, the client is instructed to exhale. The needle is then rotated to obtain a plug of tissue. The needle is then withdrawn and manual pressure is applied to the site for 5 to 20 minutes. If there is no evidence of bleeding, a pressure dressing is applied. The tissue sample is placed in a container with buffered saline and sent immediately to the laboratory.

Aftercare

Following an open biopsy, the client is cared for in the same manner as anyone who has had surgery requiring general anesthesia.

For a percutaneous biopsy, the client is positioned on the biopsied side with a small pillow or sandbag under the biopsy site for at least 30 minutes. Complete bed rest is maintained for 24 hours after the test. Siderails on the bed should be up, especially if the client received a sedative prior to the procedure. Foods and fluids withheld prior to the test may be resumed. Unless medically contraindicated, the client should be assisted to take in 3,000 ml of fluid during the first 24 hours following the procedure. Because of activity restrictions, the client will need assistance with eating and elimination. A urine specimen for culture and sensitivity may be collected 24 hours after the test.

Nursing Observations

Pretest

■ Assess the client's response to explanations provided
■ Take and record vital signs and compare with the client's baseline readings

During the Test

■ Monitor the client's response to the procedure (percutaneous biopsy)

Post-Test

■ Take and record vital signs as for a postoperative client whether the biopsy was performed by open or closed technique (i.e., every 15 minutes times four, every 30 minutes times four, every hour times four, and then every 4 hours for 24 hours)
■ Assess the biopsy site for bleeding, hematoma formation, and inflammation each time vital signs are taken
■ Assess the client's comfort level and report immediately any complaints of perirenal, shoulder, or abdominal pain
■ Monitor time and amount of each voiding
■ Assess each voiding for the presence of blood; this may involve using "dipsticks" to detect microscopic blood; report immediately any grossly bloody urine

CHORIONIC VILLUS BIOPSY (CVB) (BACKGROUND INFORMATION, p. 450)

Reference Values

No chromosomal abnormalities detected.

Indications/Purposes for Chorionic Villus Biopsy

■ Family history of genetic disorders (e.g., chromosomal abnormalities, enzyme deficiencies, sickle cell anemia or other hemoglobinopathies, Tay-Sachs disease)
■ Maternal age over 35 to screen for disorders such as Down's syndrome
■ Prenatal sex determination when the woman is a known carrier of a sex-linked disorder such as hemophilia
■ Need for early decision to terminate or maintain pregnancy when fetal abnormality is suspected

Contraindications

■ History of incompetent cervix

Client Preparation

Client Teaching. Explain to the client:

■ the purpose of the study
■ that it will be performed by a physician and will require approximately 15 minutes
■ the precautions taken to avoid injury to the fetus (e.g., localization of the embryo by ultrasound)
■ that all clothing below the waist will need to be removed, except for the shoes, which may be kept on
■ that the procedure will be performed with the client positioned on a gynecological examination table

- that a metal or plastic vaginal speculum will be inserted in order to visualize the cervix
- that slight discomfort may be experienced when the speculum is inserted
- that relaxation and controlled breathing aid in reducing discomfort during the examination
- that a small catheter will be inserted through the cervix to a site between the wall of the uterus and the developing embryo
- that a small amount of tissue will be removed by gentle suction
- that the suction catheter and speculum will then be removed

Encourage questions and verbalization of concerns about the procedure, the pregnancy, or both.

Ensure that a signed consent has been obtained.

Physical Preparation

- Assist the client to disrobe from the waist down and provide an examination gown if necessary
- Ensure that the client voids immediately prior to the procedure
- Take and record vital signs and compare with baseline readings

The Procedure

The client is positioned on the examination table. The legs are draped and the external genitalia may be cleansed with an antiseptic solution. The vaginal speculum is then inserted. For the biopsy, a suction catheter is inserted via the speculum through the cervical os to the biopsy site. The catheter is then connected to a 20 ml syringe, and approximately 10 ml of suction is applied. The suction is maintained as the catheter is withdrawn to avoid introducing cervical secretions into the uterus. The outside of the catheter is wiped to remove maternal secretions and the tissue sample is flushed onto Petri dishes with an appropriate culture medium. The samples are labeled and sent to the laboratory immediately.

Aftercare and Nursing Observations

Excess lubricant and secretions are cleansed from the perineum. The client is then assisted to remove her legs from the stirrups and is allowed to rest for a few minutes in the supine position. Vital signs may be taken at this time. The client is then assisted to dress.

The client should be instructed to report immediately any abdominal cramping or vaginal bleeding.

LIVER BIOPSY (BACKGROUND INFORMATION, p. 451)

Reference Values

No abnormal cells or tissue present.

Indications/Purposes for Liver Biopsy

- Suspected disease of the liver parenchyma (e.g., cirrhosis, malignancy, hemachromatosis, sarcoidosis, hepatitis, amyloidosis) to determine nature of the pathological problem
- Hepatomegaly (enlarged liver) or jaundice of unknown etiology
- Persistently elevated liver enzymes of unknown etiology

Contraindications

- Bleeding disorders
- Suspected vascular tumor of the liver
- Ascites, which may obscure location of the liver for percutaneous biopsy
- Subdiaphragmatic or right hemothoracic infection
- Infection involving the biliary tract
- Inability of the client to cooperate during the procedure (contraindicates percutaneous needle biopsy)

Nursing Alert

- Liver biopsy, especially when performed by the percutaneous route, may result in bleeding within the liver, damage to hepatic tissue, and infection
- Clients with liver disease frequently have impaired blood coagulation and are especially at risk for bleeding during or after this procedure
- Prior to the procedure the client's hematological status and blood clotting ability must be assessed; therefore, a complete blood count (CBC), platelet level, prothrombin time, partial thromboplastin time, clotting time, and bleeding time should be performed prior to the study
- Following the test, the client's vital signs must be monitored closely; in addition, the client's comfort level must be assessed: complaints of right shoulder or pleuritic chest pain should be reported immediately (respiratory distress due to bleeding within the liver or inadvertent pneumothorax also may occur)

Client Preparation

Client Teaching. Explain to the client:

- the purpose of the test
- that it will be performed by a physician
- the method that will be used to obtain the sample (percutaneous [closed] biopsy or surgical [open] biopsy)
- the type of anesthesia to be administered (local infiltration for needle biopsies, general anesthesia for open biopsies)
- that foods and fluids are withheld for 6 to 8 hours prior to the procedure
- that, if a needle biopsy is performed, it will be necessary to remain motionless and breathe as instructed during certain portions of the procedure
- that, if a needle biopsy is performed, the client may experience slight discomfort in the area of the right shoulder when the biopsy needle is introduced
- that, if a needle biopsy is performed, a pressure dressing will be applied to the site
- that following a needle biopsy, the client will need to lie on the right side with a rolled towel or small pillow under the site to create pressure and prevent bleeding, and that this position will need to be maintained for at least 2 hours
- that bed rest is required for 24 hours after the procedure
- that vital signs will be monitored closely for at least 24 hours following the test
- that any unusual or persistent discomfort or any difficulty breathing should be reported immediately

Encourage questions and verbalization of concerns about the procedure.
If the client appears unduly anxious or unable to cooperate with a percutaneous
needle biopsy, the physician performing the procedure should be so informed.
Ensure that a signed consent for the procedure has been obtained.

Physical Preparation

- If the skin at the biopsy site is unusually hirsute, it may be necessary to shave the site prior to the procedure
- Ensure to the extent possible that dietary restrictions are followed
- If an open biopsy is to be performed, the physical preparation is the same as that for any surgical procedure requiring general anesthesia
- For a percutaneous needle biopsy, the client's vital signs are taken and compared with baseline readings; the client should void immediately prior to the procedure and be provided with a hospital gown

The Procedure

For an open biopsy, the samples are collected during the operative procedure.

For a percutaneous needle biopsy, the client is assisted to the supine or left lateral position with the right hand under the head. The biopsy site is exposed, cleansed with antiseptic, and draped with sterile drapes. The skin and subcutaneous tissues are then infiltrated with a local anesthetic. The syringe is attached to the biopsy needle. The client is then instructed to take a deep breath, exhale forcefully, and hold his or her breath. The biopsy needle is then inserted, rotated to obtain a core of liver tissue, and quickly removed. It is important that the client remain motionless during biopsy needle insertion. After the needle is removed, the client may resume normal breathing. A pressure dressing is applied to the site. The sample is expelled from the needle into a container with formalin solution and sent to the laboratory immediately.

Aftercare

Following an open biopsy, the client is cared for in the same manner as anyone who has had surgery requiring general anesthesia.

For a percutaneous biopsy, the client is positioned on the right side with a rolled towel or small pillow under the biopsy site to create pressure and prevent bleeding. This position is maintained for at least 2 hours. Complete bed rest is maintained for 24 hours after the test. Foods and fluids withheld for the test may be resumed. Because of activity restrictions, the client will need assistance with eating and elimination. If ordered, administer analgesics for postbiopsy discomfort.

Nursing Observations

Pretest

- Assess the client's response to explanations provided
- Take and record vital signs and compare with the client's usual baseline readings

During the Test

- Monitor the client's response to the procedure (percutaneous needle biopsy)

Post-Test

■ Take and record vital signs as for a postoperative client, whether the biopsy was performed by open or closed technique (i.e., every 15 minutes times four, every 30 minutes times four, every hour times four, and then every 4 hours for 24 hours)
■ Assess the biopsy site for bleeding, hematoma formation, bile leakage, and inflammation each time vital signs are taken
■ Assess the client's comfort level and report immediately pleuritic pain, persistent right shoulder pain, or abdominal pain
■ Assess the client's respiratory status and immediately report any signs or symptoms of respiratory distress

MUSCLE BIOPSY (BACKGROUND INFORMATION, p. 451)

Reference Values

No abnormal cells or tissue present.

Indications/Purposes for Muscle Biopsy

■ Family history of Duchenne's muscular dystrophy
■ Diagnosis of suspected fungal or parasitic infestation of muscle
■ Neuromuscular disorders of unknown etiology to differentiate between neuropathy and myopathy

Interfering Factors

■ Electromyography, if performed prior to muscle biopsy, may produce residual inflammation leading to false-positive biopsy findings

Client Preparation

Client Teaching. Explain to the client:

■ the purpose of the test
■ that it will be performed by a physician and will take approximately 15 minutes
■ the site from which the sample will be obtained (usually the deltoid or gastrocnemius muscle)
■ that it may be necessary to shave the biopsy site prior to the study
■ that the procedure involves making a small incision over the muscle and removing a small bit of muscle tissue with a biopsy forceps
■ that a local anesthetic will be injected at the biopsy site to alleviate discomfort
■ that suture or other material may be necessary to close the biopsy site
■ that a dressing will be applied to the biopsy site
■ that the muscle will be tender to touch and movement for several days following the procedure

Encourage questions and verbalization of concerns about the procedure.
Ensure that a signed consent has been obtained.

Physical Preparation

■ If the area to be biopsied is hirsute, it may be necessary to shave it prior to the biopsy
■ Depending on the biopsy site, the client may need to be assisted to partially disrobe and be provided with a hospital gown

The Procedure

The client is assisted to the necessary position (supine for deltoid biopsy, prone for gastrocnemius biopsy). The biopsy site is exposed, cleansed with antiseptic, and draped with sterile drapes. The skin and subcutaneous tissues are then infiltrated with a local anesthetic. A small incision is made over the muscle with a scalpel, and a bit of muscle tissue is then grasped with a forceps and excised. The sample is placed in normal saline and sent to the laboratory immediately. The incision is closed with sutures or other material and a sterile dressing is applied.

Aftercare and Nursing Observations

The client is assisted to a position of comfort and allowed to rest for a few minutes. The dressing should be assessed for excessive bleeding. The client should be instructed in care and observation of the biopsy site. The client should have a follow-up appointment for removal of sutures or for evaluation of healing of the biopsy site, or for both purposes.

LYMPH NODE BIOPSY (BACKGROUND INFORMATION, p. 451)

Reference Values

No abnormal cells or tissue present.

Indications/Purposes for Lymph Node Biopsy

- Persistent enlargement of one or more lymph nodes of unknown etiology, especially if accompanied by signs of systemic illness such as weight loss, fever, night sweats, cough, edema, and pain
- Differentiation between benign (e.g., sarcoidosis) and malignant (e.g., lymphomas, leukemias) disorders that may lead to enlarged lymph nodes
- Suspected fungal or parasitic infections involving the lymph nodes
- Staging of metastatic carcinomas, with the stage indicated by the extent of lymph node involvement

Client Preparation

Client Teaching. Explain to the client:

- the purpose of the test
- the method that will be used to obtain the sample (needle biopsy or surgical excision)
- that foods and fluids are usually not restricted prior to a needle biopsy but are restricted prior to an excisional biopsy
- that the procedure will be performed by a physician
- the type of anesthesia to be administered (local infiltration for needle biopsies, general anesthesia for excisional biopsies if deeper nodes are to be removed)
- that, if an excisional biopsy is performed, sutures or other material may be used to close the biopsy site
- that a dressing will be applied to the biopsy site
- that analgesics may be administered following the procedure to alleviate any discomfort

Encourage questions and verbalization of concerns about the procedure.
Ensure that a signed consent has been obtained.

Physical Preparation

■ If the skin at the biopsy site is unusually hirsute, it may be necessary to shave the site prior to the procedure
■ Ensure to the extent possible that dietary restrictions are followed
■ Take and record vital signs and compare with baseline readings
■ Provide a hospital gown

The Procedure

The site to be biopsied is exposed, cleansed with antiseptic, and draped with sterile drapes. If done under local anesthesia, the skin and subcutaneous tissues are so infiltrated.

For surgical excision of the node, a small incision is made over the node. The lymph node is then grasped with forceps and placed in normal saline solution. The biopsy site is closed with sutures or other materials and a sterile dressing is applied.

For a needle biopsy, the lymph node is grasped with the fingers, and a needle with syringe attached is inserted directly into the node. A specimen is then aspirated and is placed in a container with normal saline solution. Pressure is applied to the site. If there is no bleeding, a sterile dressing is applied.

All specimens are sent to the laboratory immediately.

Aftercare and Nursing Observations

If general anesthesia was administered, care and observation of the client are the same as for anyone who has had a surgical procedure using general anesthesia.

If local anesthetic was used, the client is assisted to a position of comfort and allowed to rest for a few minutes. Vital signs are taken and recorded.

For both approaches, the dressing is observed for excessive bleeding or drainage. The client should be instructed on care and observation of the biopsy site. If sutures were used, follow-up arrangements should be made for suture removal.

The client should also be assessed for level of discomfort following the procedure, and prescribed analgesics should be administered accordingly. Any foods or fluids withheld prior to the procedure should be resumed.

INTESTINAL BIOPSY (SMALL INTESTINE) (BACKGROUND INFORMATION, p. 451)

Reference Values

No abnormal cells or tissue present.

Indications/Purposes for Biopsy of the Small Intestine

■ Suspected malignant or premalignant tissue change on endoscopic visualization
■ Differentiation between benign and malignant disorders involving the small intestine
■ Diagnosis of various intestinal disorders such as lactose intolerance, enzyme deficiencies, sprue, and parasitic infestations

Interfering Factors

■ Barium swallow within the preceding 48 hours

Contraindications

■ Aneurysm of the aortic arch
■ Inability of the client to cooperate during the procedure
■ Bleeding disorders

Client Preparation

Client Teaching. Explain to the client:

■ the purpose of the test
■ that it will be performed during an endoscopic examination of the stomach and small intestine
■ that foods and fluids are withheld for 6 to 8 hours prior to the procedure
■ that a sedative may be administered prior to the procedure to promote relaxation
■ that full or partial dentures should be removed prior to the procedure
■ that the test may be performed with the client in a sitting or semireclined position
■ that a flexible, microscope-like instrument will be inserted through the mouth and passed into the stomach and small intestine
■ that the throat will be sprayed with a local anesthetic to make passage of the tube less uncomfortable
■ that this anesthetic will have a bitter taste, may create a sensation of warmth and may impair swallowing
■ that a device may be inserted into the mouth to protect the teeth and prevent biting the endoscope
■ that saliva will be removed by suctioning during the procedure (similar to dental suctioning)
■ that after the tube is inserted, the client may be assisted to a side-lying position
■ that air may be injected into the stomach during the test to aid in visualization and that this may cause a sensation of fullness or bloating
■ that the procedure may take from 45 minutes to an hour
■ that after the stomach and intestine have been visualized and tissue samples obtained, the endoscope and mouth device will be removed
■ that vital signs will be monitored closely following the procedure
■ that the client will not be permitted to eat or drink until the local anesthetic has worn off
■ that activity may be restricted until the premedication has worn off
■ that the client should report immediately any chest pain or upper abdominal pain, pain on swallowing, difficulty breathing, and expectoration of blood

Encourage questions and verbalization of concerns about the procedure.
Ensure that a signed consent for the procedure has been obtained.

Physical Preparation

■ Ensure to the extent possible that dietary and fluid restrictions are followed prior to the test
■ Remove full or partial dentures; if the client has any permanent crowns on the teeth (i.e., "caps"), the physician performing the test should be so informed
■ Assist the client to disrobe, and provide a hospital gown
■ Have the client void
■ Take and record vital signs and compare with baseline values
■ Administer premedication if ordered (this may consist of an analgesic or tran-

quilizer to reduce discomfort and promote relaxation, as well as atropine to reduce secretions)

The Procedure

With the client seated in a semireclined position, a local anesthetic is sprayed into the throat and may also be swabbed in the mouth. A protective guard is inserted to cover the teeth. A bite block also may be inserted to maintain adequate opening of the mouth without client effort.

The endoscope is passed through the mouth, and the client is assisted to the left lateral position. The dental suction device is inserted to drain saliva. The esophagus may be examined and then the scope is advanced into the stomach. Gastric lavage may be performed to clear the stomach of residual. After the stomach is examined, the scope is advanced into the duodenum. Air may be injected through the endoscope to aid in visualizing structures. A cytology brush or biopsy forceps is introduced through the endoscope to obtain tissue samples. Specimens are placed in appropriate containers and are sent to the laboratory immediately. The dental suction device is removed, the endoscope is withdrawn, and the tooth guard and bite block are removed.

Aftercare

The client is assisted to a position of comfort and allowed to rest for a few minutes. Vital signs are checked. The client may then be transported to a recovery area for additional monitoring. A side-lying position may be maintained for 1 to 2 hours to prevent aspiration of secretions. Appropriate safety precautions for the sedated client are taken. If the procedure is performed on an out-patient basis, transportation should be arranged because driving is contraindicated by the premedication.

The client should be reminded not to eat or drink until the local anesthetic has worn off and normal swallowing ability has returned. The client also should be reminded to report immediately any chest or upper abdominal pain, pain on swallowing, difficulty breathing, and expectoration of blood.

Nursing Observations

Pretest

■ Assess the client's response to explanations provided
■ Take and record vital signs and compare with the client's baseline readings

During the Test

■ Monitor the client's response to the procedure

Post-Test

■ Take and record vital signs; additional readings may be required until vital signs are stable
■ Assess and record breath sounds and characteristics of respirations
■ Assess the client's ability to swallow
■ Assess the client's recovery from the premedication
■ Assess the client's comfort level and report immediately any complaints of chest pain, epigastric pain, periumbilical pain, and pain on swallowing
■ Assess the client's ability to resume usual food and fluid intake

LUNG BIOPSY (BACKGROUND INFORMATION, p. 451)

Reference Values

No abnormal cells or tissue present.

Indications/Purposes for Lung Biopsy

- Determination of the cause of diffuse pulmonary disease of unknown etiology
- Diagnosis of suspected malignancy, infection, or parasitic infestation
- Inconclusive results of less invasive tests such as chest x-ray examiniations, CAT scans, and sputum analyses

Contraindications

- Bleeding disorders
- Hyperinflation of the lung
- Cor pulmonale
- Inability of the client to cooperate with the procedure (contraindicates needle biopsies and bronchoscopies done under local anesthesia)

Nursing Alert

- Lung biopsies may result in bleeding into lung tissue, pneumothorax, hemothorax, and infection
- Prior to the procedure the client's hematological status and blood clotting ability must be assessed; therefore, a complete blood count (CBC), platelet level, prothrombin time, partial thromboplastin time, clotting time, and bleeding time should be performed
- Following the procedure the client's vital signs, lung sounds, and comfort level are monitored closely for early detection of possible complications

---

Client Preparation

Client Teaching. Explain to the client:

- the purpose of the test
- that the procedure will be performed by a physician
- the method that will be used to obtain the sample (needle biopsy, bronchoscopy, or thoracotomy)
- the type of anesthesia to be administered (local anesthesia for needle biopsies, topical or general anesthesia for bronchoscopy, general anesthesia for thoracotomy)
- that foods and fluids are withheld for 6 to 8 hours prior to the procedure, especially if bronchoscopy is to be performed or general anesthesia is to be used
- that a sedative may be administered prior to the procedure
- that if the specimen is to be obtained by bronchoscopy or thoracotomy, full or partial dentures should be removed prior to the procedure
- that, if a needle biopsy is to be performed, the client should remain as still as possible and refrain from coughing after the biopsy needle is inserted
- that, if a bronchoscopy is to be performed, a microscope-like instrument will be inserted through the mouth and passed into the trachea ("windpipe")

■ that, if a thoracotomy is to be performed, a chest incision will be made and a chest tube will be inserted before the incision is closed
■ that, following the procedure, vital signs and respiratory status will be monitored closely
■ that, following the procedure, the client should report immediately any difficulty breathing or other discomforts
■ that sputum samples may be collected following bronchoscopy
■ the type of activity restrictions that may be necessary following the procedure

Encourage questions and verbalization of concerns about the procedure. Ensure that a signed consent has been obtained.

Physical Preparation

■ Ensure to the extent possible that dietary and fluid restrictions are followed prior to the procedure
■ For bronchoscopy or thoracotomy, remove full or partial dentures; if the client has any permanent crowns on the teeth (i.e., "caps"), the physician performing the procedure should be so informed
■ Assist the client to disrobe and provide a hospital gown
■ Have the client void
■ Take and record vital signs and compare with baseline readings
■ Administer premedication as ordered

The Procedure

For a needle biopsy, the client is assisted to a sitting position with arms supported on a pillow on an overbed table. The needle insertion site is cleansed with an antiseptic solution, infiltrated with a local anesthetic, and draped with sterile drapes. The client is reminded to remain as still as possible and to avoid coughing during the procedure. The needle is inserted through the posterior chest wall into the selected intercostal space. A small incision may be made prior to needle insertion. After insertion, the needle is rotated to obtain the sample and is then withdrawn. Pressure is applied to the biopsy site. If there is no bleeding, a pressure dressing is applied. The sample is placed in formalin solution and sent to the laboratory immediately. If cultures are desired, the sample may be divided into two portions, with the part for culture placed in a sterile container.

For a bronchoscopy, the client initially is positioned in relation to the type of anesthesia to be used. If general anesthesia is to be administered, the client is placed in the supine position and anesthetized. The neck is hyperextended and the bronchoscope introduced through the mouth. If local anesthesia is used, the client is seated and the tongue and oropharynx are sprayed and swabbed with anesthetic. The client is then assisted to a supine or side-lying position and the bronchoscope is introduced through the mouth. Additional anesthetic is applied through the scope as it approaches the vocal cords and the carina, eliminating reflexes in these sensitive areas. After inspection through the bronchoscope, the samples are collected by bronchial brush or biopsy forceps. Specimens are placed in appropriate containers and sent to the laboratory immediately.

Open biopsies are performed in the operating room under general anesthesia. A thoracotomy is performed to obtain the sample, and a chest tube is inserted following the procedure.

Aftercare and Nursing Observations

Following a needle biopsy or bronchoscopy using local or topical anesthesia, the client is usually positioned in semi-Fowler's position to permit maximum ventilation, and is allowed to rest for a few minutes. Vital signs are checked and compared with baseline levels. Vital signs may be repeated at 15- to 30-minute intervals for 1 to 2 hours or until stable.

If a needle biopsy was performed, the biopsy site is assessed for bleeding each time vital signs are taken. Breath sounds also are assessed, and the client is observed for any signs of respiratory distress. The client's comfort level also is evaluated. Foods and fluids withheld for the procedure are resumed if assessment data indicates that the client is stable.

If a bronchoscopy was performed using local anesthesia, vital signs are monitored and the client is observed for signs of laryngospasm, bronchospasm, and laryngeal edema as indicated by wheezing, stridor, absence of air movement at the mouth or nares, anxiety, and cyanosis. Breath sounds are carefully assessed, as is the client's comfort level. Gargles or lozenges may be prescribed for throat discomfort. Foods and fluids may be resumed after the local anesthetic has worn off and if assessment data indicated client stability.

For an open biopsy, care and observation are the same as those for anyone who has had a thoracotomy under general anesthesia.

PLEURAL BIOPSY (BACKGROUND INFORMATION, p. 452)

Reference Values

No abnormal cells or tissue present.

Indications/Purposes for Pleural Biopsy

■ Evidence of pleural effusion of unknown etiology
■ Suspected tumor involving the pleura
■ Differentiation between benign and malignant disorders involving the pleura
■ Determination of the cause of infection involving the pleura (i.e., viral, fungal, bacterial, and parasitic infections)
■ Diagnosis of fibrosis or collagen vascular disease involving the pleura

Contraindications

■ Bleeding disorders
■ Inability of the client to cooperate with the procedure (contraindicates needle biopsies)

Nursing Alert

■ Plueral biopsies may result in bleeding into lung tissue, pneumothorax, hemothorax, and infection
■ Prior to the procedure the client's hematological status and blood clotting ability must be assessed; therefore, a complete blood count (CBC), platelet level, prothrombin time, partial thromboplastin time, clotting time, and bleeding time should be performed
■ Following the procedure the client's vital signs, lung sounds, and comfort level are monitored closely for early detection of possible complications

---

Client Preparation

Client Teaching. Explain to the client:

- the purpose of the test
- that the procedure will be performed by a physician
- the method that will be used to obtain the sample (needle biopsy or open biopsy via thoracotomy)
- the type of anesthesia to be administered (local anesthesia for needle biopsy, general anesthesia for open biopsy)
- that foods and fluids are generally not withheld prior to a needle biopsy but are restricted for 6 to 8 hours prior to an open biopsy
- that a sedative may be administered prior to the procedure
- that, if a thoracotomy is to be performed, full or partial dentures should be removed prior to the procedure
- that, if a needle biopsy is to be performed, the client should remain as still as possible and refrain from coughing after the biopsy needle is inserted
- that, if a thoracotomy is performed, a chest incision will be made, and that a chest tube will be inserted before the incision is closed
- that, following the procedure, vital signs and respiratory status will be monitored closely
- that, following the procedure, the client should report immediately any difficulty breathing or other discomforts
- the type of activity restrictions that may be necessary following the procedure

Encourage questions and verbalization of concerns about the procedure.
Ensure that a signed consent has been obtained.

Physical Preparation

- Ensure to the extent possible that any dietary and fluid restrictions are followed prior to the procedure
- For thoracotomy, remove full or partial dentures
- Assist the client to disrobe and provide a hospital gown
- Have the client void
- Take and record vital signs and compare with baseline readings
- Administer premedication if ordered

The Procedure

For a needle biopsy, the client is assisted to a sitting position with arms supported on a pillow on an overbed table. The needle insertion site is cleansed with an antiseptic solution, infiltrated with a local anesthetic, and draped with sterile drapes. The client is reminded to remain as still as possible and to avoid coughing during the procedure. The needle is inserted through the posterior chest wall into the selected intercostal space, rotated to obtain the sample, and then withdrawn. Pressure is applied to the biopsy site. If there is no bleeding, a pressure dressing is applied. The sample is placed in formalin solution and sent to the laboratory immediately.

Open biopsies are performed in the operating room under general anesthesia. A thoracotomy is performed to obtain the sample, and a chest tube is inserted following the procedure.

Aftercare and Nursing Observations

Following a needle biopsy, the client is usually positioned in semi-Fowler's position to permit maximum ventilation. Vital signs are checked and compared with baseline levels. Vital signs may be repeated at 15- to 30-minute intervals for 1 to 2 hours or until stable. The biopsy site is assessed for bleeding each time vital signs are taken. Breath sounds also are assessed, and the client is observed for any signs of respiratory distress. The client's comfort level also is evaluated. Foods and fluids withheld prior to the procedure are resumed if assessment data indicate that the client is stable.

For an open biopsy, care and observation are the same as those for anyone who has had a thoracotomy under general anesthesia.

PROSTATE GLAND BIOPSY (BACKGROUND INFORMATION, p. 452)
Reference Values

No abnormal cells or tissue present.

Indications/Purposes for Prostate Gland Biopsy

■ Prostatic hypertrophy of unknown etiology
■ Suspected cancer of the prostate gland

Contraindications

■ Bleeding disorders

Client Preparation

Client Teaching. Explain to the client:

■ the purpose of the test
■ that it will be performed by a physician
■ that foods and fluids are usually not restricted prior to the test
■ that a sedative may be administered to promote relaxation
■ the method that will be used to obtain the sample
■ the type of positioning that may be used for the test (see under Procedure)
■ that a local anesthetic will be administered to prevent pain, but that the client may feel a "pinching" or "pulling" sensation during the procedure
■ the importance of remaining still during the procedure
■ that an antibiotic may be administered to prevent infection
■ that vital signs and urinary output will be monitored closely following the procedure
■ that, following the procedure, any rectal pain or bleeding, blood in the urine, or fever should be reported immediately
■ any special site care necessary (e.g., a dressing is applied when the perineal approach is used)

Encourage questions and verbalization of concerns about the procedure.
Ensure that a signed consent has been obtained.

Physical Preparation

■ Administer enemas, if ordered—if the perineal or transurethral approach is to be used, one enema is usually ordered; if the transrectal approach is to be used, saline enemas until clear may be ordered
■ Assist the client to disrobe and provide a hospital gown
■ Have the client void
■ Take and record vital signs and compare with baseline readings
■ Administer premedication if ordered

The Procedure

For the transurethral approach, the client is positioned on a urological examination table as for a cystoscopy (see p. 460). The external genitalia are cleansed with antiseptic solution, and a local anesthetic is instilled into the urethra. The endoscope is then inserted. The prostate gland is visualized and the tissue for biopsy removed with a cutting loop. The sample is placed in formalin solution and sent to the laboratory immediately. The disadvantage of this approach is that malignant nodules or tissue may not be included in the sample, even though the endoscope is under direct visual guidance.

For the transrectal approach, the client is assisted to the Sims' position and a rectal examination is performed to locate potentially malignant nodules. A biopsy needle guide is then passed along the examining finger and the stylet removed. The biopsy needle is inserted through the needle guide and rotated to obtain a core of tissue. The needle is then withdrawn and the sample placed in formalin solution. The disadvantage of this appraoch is the perforation of the rectum and the creation of a tract through which cells from the nodule may be seeded. Possible complications include infection, hemorrhage, and perforation of the bladder.

For the perineal approach, the client is assisted to the position desired by the physician. This is usually the jack-knife position or the lithotomy position, both achieved by using a special examination or operative type table. The client is draped appropriately with the perineum exposed. The perineum is cleansed with an antiseptic solution and infiltrated with a local anesthetic. A small incision is made and either a biopsy needle or a biopsy punch inserted. Samples are taken from several locations and placed in formalin solution. Digital pressure is applied to the site. If there is no bleeding, a sterile dressing is applied.

Aftercare and Nursing Observation

The client is assisted to a position of comfort and allowed to rest for a few minutes. Vital signs are taken and compared with baseline readings, and may be repeated every 4 hours for 24 hours. If the perineal approach was used, the biopsy site should be observed for bleeding or other drainage. If the transurethral approach was used, the client should be monitored for resumption of usual voiding patterns. The appearance of the urine should also be observed. If the client received a sedative prior to the procedure, appropriate safety precautions for the sedated client should be taken.

The client should be reminded to report immediately any rectal pain or bleeding, blood in the urine, or fever. If the perineal approach was used, site care should be reviewed with him.

THYROID GLAND BIOPSY (BACKGROUND INFORMATION, p. .452)

Reference Values

No abnormal cells or tissue present.

Indications/Purposes for Thyroid Gland Biopsy

■ Abnormal thyroid scan
■ Enlargement of the thyroid gland of unknown etiology
■ Signs and symptoms of thyroiditis or hyperthyroidism
■ Presence of thyroid nodules of unknown etiology to differentiate between benign and malignant nodules
■ Differentiation between thyroid cysts and solid tumors

■ Differentiation between inflammatory thyroid diseases (Hashimoto's thyroid-itis versus granulomatous thyroiditis)
■ Confirmation of the diagnoses of hyperthyroidism and nontoxic nodular goiter

Contraindications

■ Bleeding disorders

Client Preparation

Client Teaching. Explain to the client:

■ the purpose of the test
■ that the procedure will be performed by a physician
■ the method that will be used to obtain the sample (needle biopsy or open biopsy)
■ the type of anesthesia to be administered (local anesthesia for needle biopsy, general anesthesia for open biopsy)
■ that foods and fluids are generally not withheld prior to a needle biopsy but are restricted for 6 to 8 hours prior to an open biopsy
■ that a sedative may be administered prior to the procedure
■ that, if a needle biopsy is to be performed, the client will be positioned on an examining table with a pillow, sandbag, or folded blanket under the shoulders to make the thyroid gland more accessible
■ that, if a needle biopsy is to be performed, the client should remain as still as possible and should refrain from swallowing as the local anesthetic is injected
■ that, if an open biopsy is to be performed, an incision will be made at the front of the neck
■ that, following the procedure, vital signs and respiratory status will be monitored carefully
■ that, the client may have a sore throat following the procedure

Encourage questions and verbalization of concerns about the procedure.
Ensure that a signed consent has been obtained.

Physical Preparation

For a needle biopsy, the client is assisted to the supine position and a small pillow, sandbag, or folded blanket is placed under the shoulders, the skin is cleansed with an antiseptic solution, injected with a local anesthetic, and draped with sterile drapes. The client is reminded not to swallow as the local anesthetic is injected. The biopsy needle is inserted, the specimen obtained, and the needle withdrawn. Pressure is applied to the biopsy site. If there is no bleeding, a pressure dressing is applied to the site. The sample is placed in formalin solution and sent to the laboratory immediately.

For an open biopsy, the sample is obtained through surgical excision during the operative procedure.

Aftercare and Nursing Observations

Following a needle biopsy, the client is allowed to rest for a few minutes following the procedure. Vital signs are checked and compared with baseline readings. Vital signs may be repeated every 15 minutes for 1 hour, every hour for 4 hours, and then every 4 hours for 24 hours. The biopsy site is assessed for bleeding each time the vital signs are taken. The client also is evaluated for dyspnea, hoarseness, and difficulty swallowing. Comfort level is monitored, and analgesics may be administered for throat discomfort.

For an open biopsy, care and observation are essentially the same as those for a client who has had a thyroidectomy.

REFERENCES

1. Halsted, JA and Halsted, CH: The Laboratory in Clinical Medicine: Interpretation and Application, ed 2. WB Saunders, Philadelphia, 1981, 138.
2. *Ibid*, p 139.
3. *Ibid*, p 138.
4. *Ibid*.
5. *Ibid*, pp 138–139.
6. *Ibid* pp 140–141.
7. *Ibid*, pp 141.
8. Packer, B: Early prenatal testing—a chorionic villus update. *Mothers Today*, May/Jun 1987, p 12.
9. Diagnostics, ed 2. Springhouse Corp, Springhouse, PA, 1986, p 493.

BIBLIOGRAPHY

Braunstein, H: Outlines of Pathology. CV Mosby, St Louis, 1982.
Jacob, SW, Francone, CA and Lossow, WJ: Structure and Function in Man, ed 5. WB Saunders, Philadelphia, 1982.
Levine, DZ: Care of the Renal Patient. WB Saunders, Philadelphia, 1983.
Nealon, TF: Fundamental Skills in Surgery, ed 2. WB Saunders, Philadelphia, 1971.
Parrish, JA: Dermatology and Skin Care. McGraw-Hill, New York, 1975.
Price, SA and Wilson, LM: Pathophysiology: Clinical Concepts of Disease Processes, ed 3. McGraw-Hill, New York, 1986.
Widmann, FK: Clinical Interpretation of Laboratory Tests, ed 9. FA Davis, Philadelphia, 1983.
Widmann, FK: Pathobiology: How Diseases Happen. Little, Brown & Co, Boston, 1978.

OBTAINING PERIPHERAL BLOOD SPECIMENS

INTRODUCTION

Most of the hematology tests, as well as numerous other laboratory tests, require venous blood. Microsamples of capillary blood may be obtained, if necessary, from the fingertips or earlobes of older children and adults, and from the heels of infants. Capillary punctures also may be used instead of venipunctures if the client has poor veins or a limited number of usable veins, and when the client is extremely apprehensive about having a venipuncture. When the amount of blood needed is greater than 1.5 ml, however, a venipuncture must be done.

Blood samples also may be obtained from vascular access devices such as heparin locks, triple lumen subclavian catheters, and arterial lines. Such procedures avoid the necessity of repeated skin punctures but must be performed with strict aseptic technique to avoid contamination of the indwelling device and possible septicemia. A "discard sample" of 3 to 5 ml is obtained prior to withdrawing samples for testing, to avoid altered results due to drugs and intravascular infusions.

Nursing Alert

According to the most recent guidelines from the Centers for Disease Control, gloves should always be worn when obtaining and handling blood samples.

CLIENT PREPARATION

Client preparation is essentially the same for all sites and for all studies. *Client Teaching.* Explain to the client:

■ the purpose of the test
■ the procedure, including the site from which the blood sample is likely to be obtained
■ that momentary discomfort may be experienced when the skin is pierced
■ food, fluids, and/or drugs to be withheld prior to the test

For children, a doll may be used as the "patient" for demonstration purposes. A laboratory technician's equipment basket may hold the child's attention during the actual procedure.

For all clients, encourage questions and verbalization of concerns about the procedure.

Physical Preparation

■ The skin is assessed for lesions, edema, and temperature, as the site selected should be warm and free of lesions or edema: application of warm compresses for 3 minutes will dilate capillaries if the skin feels cool or looks pale or cyanotic
■ For venipunctures, the condition of the veins should be noted, and the use of tortuous, sclerotic veins or those in which phlebitis has previously occurred should be avoided, as should the use of an extremity with an intravenous site or heparin lock; if the extremity must be used, obtain the sample from a site distal to the IV or heparin lock (extremities with functioning hemodialysis access sites should not be used, nor should the arm on the affected side following mastectomy be used)
■ The skin is prepared by cleansing with an antiseptic such as povidone-iodine (Betadine) or 70% alcohol, and is allowed to airdry or is dried with sterile gauze (drying prevents dilution of the sample with antiseptic); for the immunosuppressed patient, povidone-iodine should be used, followed by a 70% alcohol pad taped over the site for 10 minutes—the site should be allowed to air-dry or be dried with sterile gauze prior to the venipuncture

THE PROCEDURE

Capillary Punctures (Fingertip, Earlobe, Heel)

The equipment needed is assembled: sterile lancet, skin disinfectant, gauze pads or cotton balls, collection device, bandage, and materials to label the sample. The client is placed in a position of comfort and safety, either sitting or lying down. If an extremity is to be used, it is supported on the bed or a table. A small pillow or rolled towel or blanket may be used to improve positioning of the extremity or to promote comfort.

The site is selected and the skin prepared as described previously. The area to be used is grasped firmly. The skin is punctured with the sterile lancet using a quick, firm motion to a depth of approximately 2 millimeters. With one wipe, the first drip of blood is removed. If flow is poor, the site should not be squeezed, as this may produce more tissue fluid than blood. A hand or foot may be held in the dependent position to improve blood flow.

The sample is collected in microhematocrit tubes or pipettes and evacuated into a container holding the proper reagent. For smears, a drop of blood is placed on a clean microscope slide and spread gently with the edge of another slide.

The sample is labeled with the patient's name and other required identifying information and is sent promptly to the laboratory.

Venipunctures

The equipment needed is assembled: tourniquet; skin disinfectant; gauze pads or cotton balls; syringe and needle or vacuumized tube, holder, and needle; bandage; and materials to label the specimen. A 20-gauge needle is usually used to prevent damage to blood cells. Needles with smaller lumens may be used depending on the age of the client, the size of the vein, and the size of the vacuumized tube. Soft rubber tubing, approximately 1-inch wide, may be used for the tourniquet; however, a rubber tourniquet of the same width with a Velcro closure is prefereable.

The vacuumized tubes used in collecting samples of venous blood come in various sizes appropriate to the age of the client or the type of laboratory analysis equipment, and may or may not contain an anticoagulant. The color of the rubber stopper used to seal the tube indicates the presence and type of anticoagulant (Table A-1). Care must be taken to ensure that the correct tube is used for the test to be performed.

A syringe and needle may be used to obtain a venous blood sample if it is felt that the vacuumized tube system will collapse the vein before the volume of blood needed is obtained. In such instances, the sample must be transferred promptly to the appropriate blood tube. To accomplish this, the needle is removed from the syringe and the rubber stopper from the tube, and blood is allowed to flow gently down the inside of the tube. Another approach is to insert the needle into the rubber stopper of the vacuumized tube, allowing the vacuum to draw the blood into the tube. This may be done safely, without hemolysis of blood cells, if the needle used is 21 gauge or larger. Most authorities recommend changing the needle before injecting the rubber stopper. If the sample is for a blood culture, the rubber stopper is cleansed with povidone-iodine before the needle is inserted.

The client is placed in a position of comfort and safety, either sitting or lying down. The extremity to be used is supported on the bed or a table. A small pillow or rolled towel or blanket may be used to improve positioning of the extremity or to promote comfort.

The tourniquet is applied 1 to 1½ inches above the site to be used. Tourniquets should be applied tightly enough to cause the veins to enlarge but should never occlude arterial circulation. They should not be kept in place for more than 1 minute prior to the venipuncture or for more than 2 to 3 minutes for the entire procedure. If a vein in the arm is to be used, the client is asked to open and close the hand a few times and then to clench the fist. If the puncture cannot be made within 1 minute, the tourniquet is removed and then reapplied when the puncture site is definitely located. This prevents hemoconcentration, which may alter test results.

The skin is cleansed as described previously (see under Physical Preparation). If the vein is palpated after the skin is prepared, the site is recleansed.

The needle cover is removed and the needle inserted into the vein approximately ½ inch below the point where the needle is expected to enter the vein itself. When the needle is smaller than the vein, it is inserted bevel up at a 15- to 45-degree angle through the skin. When the needle is larger than the vein, it is inserted bevel down and almost parallel to the skin. This allows the skin to

TABLE A-1. **Types of Vacuumized Tubes Used for Blood Tests**

Color of Stopper	Substance in Tube	Action of Substance	Tests Used/Not Used for
Red, Pink	None	—	Used for tests in which *serum* is required (e.g., many chemistry and serology tests). *Serum* is plasma that has been withdrawn from the body and in which the fibrinogen has been used up during normal coagulation of the sample. Not used for tests requiring whole, uncoagulated blood.
Lavender, Purple	Ethylenediamine-tetraacetic acid (EDTA)	Blocks coagulation by binding calcium. Causes minimal distortion of the size and shape of blood cells. Prevents platelet aggregation.	Used mainly for hematology tests.
Light Blue	Sodium citrate	Blocks coagulation by binding calcium. May result in dilution of the specimen due to volume needed to anticoagulate the sample.	Most frequently used in coagulation studies. Not used for cell counts or chemistry studies.
Green (Navy Blue, Tan)	Sodium heparin	Prevents coagulation by blocking the action of thrombin. Does not alter blood cell size. May cause a bluish background when blood smears are stained.	Used for red cell osmotic fragility studies. May also be used for selected chemistry and toxicology studies. Not used for coagulation studies.
Gray	Sodium fluoride and potassium oxalate	Blocks coagulation by binding calcium. Blocks action of enzymes in red blood cells which break down glucose and alcohol. May also inactivate cardiac and liver enzymes.	Used primarily for blood glucose and alcohol testing. Not used for blood glucose tests if the laboratory uses an enzyme testing procedure for determining blood glucose levels. Not used for studies of cardiac and liver enzymes.

TABLE A–1—*Continued*

Color of Stopper	Substance in Tube	Action of Substance	Tests Used/Not Used for
Black	Sodium oxalate	Blocks coagulation by binding calcium. May distort blood cells. May result in dilution of the specimen due to the volume needed to anticoagulate the sample.	Used for coagulation studies. Not used for blood smears, cell counts, or chemistry tests.
Yellow	Sodium polyanethole-sulfonate (SPS)	Blocks coagulation. Inactivates white blood cells and antibiotics.	Used primarily for blood cultures. (Blood sample must be added to blood culture bottle containing additional SPS within 1 hour of obtaining sample.)

be punctured first, then the vein, and is a useful approach for entering difficult veins.

If the vacuumized tube system is used, the tube is pushed into the holder until the rubber stopper is punctured and blood flows into the tube. If more than one tube of blood is required, the filled tube is removed from the holder and another inserted until the desired number of samples is obtained. The sequence for obtaining multiple samples using different types of tubes is as follows: (1) blood culture tubes (the rubber stopper must be cleansed before inserting into the holder to prevent contamination of the sample); (2) tubes with no additives; (3) tubes for coagulation studies; and (4) tubes with additives (see Table A–1).

If a syringe is used, pull back on the plunger until the desired amount of blood is obtained. The sample is then transferred into the desired blood tubes as described previously (see p. 483).

The tourniquet is released and the client is instructed to unclench the fist. The needle is removed and pressure is immediately applied to the puncture site with a gauze pad or cottonball. Pressure should be maintained for 3 minutes to prevent hematoma formation. If the puncture site is on the dorsum of the hand, the hand is elevated while pressure is applied. Pressure is maintained until bleeding has stopped.

The sample is labeled with the client's name and other required identifying information and sent promptly to the laboratory.

AFTERCARE

- After bleeding has stopped, apply an adhesive bandage
- Application of an adhesive bandage on the finger of a child under 6 years of age is not recommended, as the child may swallow the bandage and choke on it

NURSING OBSERVATIONS

Pretest

■ Assess the client's understanding of explanations provided
■ Assess the client's degree of anxiety about the procedure
■ Inspect the skin for puncture sites to be used (see p. 482)

During the Test

■ Note the client's responses to the procedure

Post-Test

■ Check the venipuncture site in 5 minutes to be sure a hematoma is not forming
■ If the client is immunosuppressed, check the puncture site every 8 hours for signs of infection and watch for signs of septicemia such as fever, chills, petechiae, and inflamed joints

APPENDIX II

OBTAINING VARIOUS TYPES OF URINE SPECIMENS

One of the main reasons for invalid results of urine tests is improper specimen collection and maintenance. Thus, the nurse must know how the specimens are collected and how to instruct clients on specimen collection. The various types of specimens are discussed here.

RANDOM SPECIMENS

Random specimens are urine samples that are collected at any time of day in clean containers. Usually 15 to 60 ml of urine are sufficient for tests performed on random samples. Random samples are used for routine screening tests to detect obvious abnormalities. The client is instructed to void directly into the urine container or to void in some other type of clean container, after which the sample is transferred to another type of laboratory container. If the sample is collected by the client at home, it must be transported to the laboratory within 2 hours, or test results may be inaccurate.

FIRST MORNING SPECIMENS

First morning specimens are collected upon arising in the morning, when urine is most concentrated. Such samples are ideal for screening purposes, as substances may be detectable in them that are not found in more dilute samples. In addition to routine screening tests, first morning samples are desirable for pregnancy tests and tests for orthostatic proteinuria.

487

DOUBLE-VOIDED SPECIMENS

Double-voided specimens are used when testing urine for sugar and acetone. The purpose of this approach is to ensure that the urine tested is fresh so that it serves as a valid indicator of current blood glucose and ketone levels. The client is instructed to empty the bladder and, if possible, to drink a glass of water. Approximately one half hour later, the client voids again. The second sample is then tested. Some individuals advocate testing the first sample as well, in case the client cannot void a second time. The validity of results on the first sample may, however, be questionable. The double-voided specimen is particularly critical for the first urine sample of the day because urine that has accumulated in the bladder overnight is not a valid indicator of current status.

CLEAN-CATCH MIDSTREAM SPECIMENS

Clean-catch midstream specimens are used to avoid contamination of the sample with urethral cells, microorganisms, and mucus. The procedure is as follows. The client is provided with a clean-catch kit containing materials for cleansing the meatus and a sterile specimen container. The male client should cleanse the urinary meatus with the agent provided (or with soap and water), void a few milliliters of urine into the toilet or urinal, and then void directly into the specimen container. Women should cleanse the labia minora and meatal orifice carefully, working from front to back, and then manually keep the labia separated while voiding a few milliliters into the toilet or bedpan. With the labia still separated, the client should then void directly into the collection container. If menstruating, or if a heavy vaginal discharge is present, the woman should insert a clean vaginal tampon before beginning the cleansing process. Care must be taken by all clients to avoid touching the inside of the urine container and lid.

Clean-catch midstream urine specimens are used primarily for microbiological and cytological analysis of urine. Some individuals also advocate using this method for specimens for routine urinalysis, especially in women, since the sample is less likely to be contaminated with substances that alter results of routine screening tests.

CATHETERIZED SPECIMENS

Urine specimens may be obtained from one-time "straight" catheterizations or from indwelling Foley catheters. "Straight" catheterization is indicated when the client is unable to void for a random or clean-catch specimen without excessively contaminating the sample. It is also used for samples for microbiological and cytological studies.

Indwelling catheters may be placed for a variety of reasons. In some cases, they may be inserted when serial urine specimens are needed at exact time intervals. In other cases, the catheter is already in place and must be used for urine sampling.

When obtaining a sample from an indwelling catheter, be sure that the drainage tube is empty; then clamp the tube distal to the specimen collection port. The sample is obtained with a needle (25- to 21-gauge) and a 3 to 5 ml (larger if a greater amount is needed) syringe after the tubing has been clamped for approximately 15 minutes. The specimen port is cleansed with an antiseptic swab (e.g., alcohol sponge) and the sample aspirated. The sample is then placed in a sterile container or rubber-stoppered test tube and sent promptly to the laboratory. Bedside screening tests (e.g., for glucose and ketones) may be performed by instilling the sample directly from the syringe to the reagent strip. Care must be taken to be sure that the catheter is unclamped after the sample is obtained.

TWENTY-FOUR HOUR (TIMED) SPECIMENS

Twenty-four hour specimens allow for quantification of substances in urine. Methods of preserving the accumulating sample vary among laboratories, and therefore, the laboratory should be consulted for advice regarding the use of a preservative or the need for refrigeration, or both. It is critical that all urine excreted during the 24-hour period be collected.

When a 24-hour specimen is required, it is desirable to begin it in the morning, usually sometime between 6 and 8 A.M. First the client voids and discards the specimen. The time that the discard sample is obtained is the time that the collection begins. All urine voided thereafter is collected. The next day, at the same time the specimen collection was begun, the client is instructed to void again. This final voiding is added to the sample, and the collection ends. The dates and times of specimen collection should be noted on the laboratory slip. In the hospital setting, it is helpful if a reminder to collect all urine is posted in or near the client's bathroom so that neither the client nor hospital personnel inadvertently discard any portion of the specimen. The client should be instructed not to place toilet paper in the specimen container (devices that fit into toilet seats are often used). Individuals who use a bedpan should be instructed not to void into a pan containing feces.

Sometimes it is necessary to insert a Foley catheter for 24-hour urine collections. This is especially true if the client is unable to participate in specimen collection. Other times, a Foley catheter may already be in place. When a 24-hour urine collection is to be obtained via an indwelling catheter, the collection should begin by changing the tubing and drainage bag so that a clean, fresh system is in use. If a preservative is required, it can be obtained from the laboratory and placed directly into the drainage bag. Others advocate using a container with preservative and emptying the drainage bag contents into it at frequent intervals (e.g., every 2 hours). If refrigeration of the specimen is necessary, the drainage bag is placed in a basin filled with ice. The ice supply will need to be renewed frequently to ensure that the specimen is properly chilled. If the urine must be protected from light, the drainage bag may be covered with dark plastic or aluminum foil. If the drainage tubing is positioned correctly for continuous drainage, it need not be covered.

When the collection is completed, the sample should be transported promptly to the laboratory.

Some urine tests require 2-hour samples. A 2-hour sample is collected in the same manner as a 24-hour sample, with the exact starting and stopping times noted.

SUPRAPUBIC ASPIRATION

Suprapubic aspiration involves inserting a needle directly into the bladder to obtain a urine sample. Since the bladder is normally sterile, this method allows for collection of samples that are free of extraneous contamination. In this procedure, the skin over the suprapubic area is cleansed with antiseptic and draped with sterile drapes. A local anesthetic may then be injected. The needle is inserted and the sample is removed, after which a sterile dressing is applied. The site is observed for inflammation and abnormal drainage. Suprapubic aspiration may be used for samples for microbiological and cytological analysis. It may also be used to obtain samples in infants and young children.

PEDIATRIC SAMPLES

Pediatric samples are usually collected by attaching clear plastic bags with adhesive to the genital area of both girls and boys.

GENERAL INDEX

A "T" following a page number indicates a table. An "F" following a page number indicates a figure. For your convenience, a special index listing all of the tests covered in the book appears on p. xiii, at the front of the book.

Index of Tests Covered appears on p. xiii, at the front of the book.

Index of Tests Covered appears on p. xiii, at the front of the book.

Index of Tests Covered appears on p. xiii, at the front of the book.

Index of Tests Covered appears on p. xiii, at the front of the book.

Index of Tests Covered appears on p. xiii, at the front of the book.

Index of Tests Covered appears on p. xiii, at the front of the book.

Index of Tests Covered appears on p. xiii, at the front of the book.

Index of Tests Covered appears on p. xiii, at the front of the book.

Index of Tests Covered appears on p. xiii, at the front of the book.

Index of Tests Covered appears on p. xiii, at the front of the book.

Index of Tests Covered appears on p. xiii, at the front of the book.

Index of Tests Covered appears on p. xiii, at the front of the book.

Index of Tests Covered appears on p. xiii, at the front of the book.

Index of Tests Covered appears on p. xiii, at the front of the book.

Index of Tests Covered appears on p. xiii, at the front of the book.

Index of Tests Covered appears on p. xiii, at the front of the book.

Index of Tests Covered appears on p. xiii, at the front of the book.

Index of Tests Covered appears on p. xiii, at the front of the book.

Neisseria meningitidis, 366
Nephrogenic diabetes insipidus, 214
Nephrotic syndrome
  laboratory correlations in, 308T
  proteinuria in, 295
Nephrotoxic drugs, serum creatinine and, 157
Neural tube defects, amniotic fluid tests for, 400, 400T
Neurogenic diabetes insipidus, 214
Neurohypophysis, 208
Neuromuscular disorders, aldolase and, 200
Neurosyphilis, serological tests for, 366–367
  clinical applications data for, 372
Neutrophils, 20T, 41
  altered levels of, causes of, 42T
  peritoneal fluid, 390
  synovial fluid, 381, 382T, 393
Newborn
  hemolytic disease of, 400–402, 401F, 402T
  physiological jaundice of, 175
Nicotine, toxicity of, 286T
Nifedipine, blood levels of, 284T
Nigrosin, cryptococcal infections and, 366
Nitrite, urinary, 301–302
Nitrogenous compounds, 149–152. *See also specific substance*
Nonesterified fatty acids (NEFA), 161
Nonimmune transformation tests, 87, 93
Norepinephrine
  serum, 219, 221–222, 246–248
  urinary, 328–329, 339
Norpace (disopyramide), blood levels of, 283T
5'-Nucleotidase, 181
  clinical applications data for, 192
Null cells, 83
  reference values for, 91
Nutrition. *See* Diet; Parenteral nutrition

O antigen test, 106T, 109
O₂ saturation, 273–276
Occult blood, fecal, 435–436, 437T–438T, 442–444
OCT. *See* Ornithinecarbamoyl transferase
OGTT. *See* Oral glucose tolerance test
17-OHCS. *See* 17-Hydroxycorticoids
25-(OH)D₃, 278, 280–281
Oligohydramnios, 399
Open biopsy. *See* Biopsy; *specific type, e.g.,* Bone biopsy
Oral glucose tolerance test (OGTT), 135
  aftercare with, 141
  client preparation for, 140
  factors interfering with, 139

indications for, 139–140
  nursing alert for, 140
  nursing observations with, 141
  procedure for, 140–141
  reference values for, 139
Organophosphorus insecticides, toxicity of, 286T
Orinase (tolbutamide), 136, 143–145
Ornithinecarbamoyl transferase (OCT), 182
  aftercare with, 196
  client preparation for, 196
  factors interfering with, 195
  indications for, 195
  nursing observations with, 196
  procedure for, 196
  reference values for, 195
Orthostatic proteinuria, 295
Osmolality
  plasma, 314
  serum, 265
  urine, 314. *See also* Concentration tests
Osmotic fragility, 31, 31T
  clinical applications data for, 38
Oval fat bodies, 303
Ovaries, hormones secreted by. *See also* Estrogen(s); Progesterone
  serum, 222–223
  urinary, 329–330
Oxalate, urinary, 332
Oxalic acid, toxicity of, 286T
Oxidant drugs, G-6-PD and, 32
Oxygen saturation, 273–276

P. *See* Phosphorus
Packed red cell volume. *See* Hematocrit
PAH (para-aminohippuric acid), 312
Pain, liver biopsy followed by, 466
Pancreas
  amylase and
    duodenal stimulation tests and, 429
    serum, 183, 196
    urinary, 325
  duodenal fluid analysis and, 425–426
  serum lipase and, 184, 197
Pancreatic hormones, 225–226. *See also specific hormone, e.g.,* Insulin
Pancreatic secretion, duodenal stimulation tests and, 426–427
Pancreatitis, pleural effusion and, 388
Papanicolaou smear (Pap smear), 448–449
  aftercare with, 454
  client preparation for, 453
  factors interfering with, 452–453
  indications for, 453
  procedure for, 453–454
  reference values for, 452

Index of Tests Covered appears on p. xiii, at the front of the book.

Index of Tests Covered appears on p. xiii, at the front of the book.

Index of Tests Covered appears on p. xiii, at the front of the book.

Index of Tests Covered appears on p. xiii, at the front of the book.

Index of Tests Covered appears on p. xiii, at the front of the book.

Index of Tests Covered appears on p. xiii, at the front of the book.

Index of Tests Covered appears on p. xiii, at the front of the book.

Syndrome of inappropriate antidiuretic
hormone secretion (SIADH), 214–
215
Syneresis, 51
Synovial fluid, 376, 377
Synovial fluid analysis, 380–384
aftercare with, 395
client preparation for, 394–395
crystals in, 382–383, 383T
factors interfering with, 393
indications for, 393–394
nursing observations with, 395–396
procedure for, 395
reference values for, 393
white blood cells and inclusions in,
382T
Synovial lining cell, 382T
Synovial membranes, 375–376
Syphilis, central nervous system and,
366–367, 372
Syphilis tests, 111–114, 112T
Syrup of ipecac, toxicity of, 285T
Systemic lupus erythematosus (SLE)
FTA-ABS test and, 111
synovial fluid analysis and, 394

T₃. *See* Triiodothyronine
T₄. *See* Thyroxine
"T₇," 216
Talcum crystals, 381–382
Tamm-Horsfall protein, 304
Tapeworms, 435
Tartaric acid, prostatic acid phosphatase
and, 184
TBG. *See* Thyroxine-binding globulin
TCT. *See* Thrombin clotting time
Tegretol (carbamazepine), blood levels of,
283T
Template method, bleeding time and, 62
Testosterone, 223
aftercare with, 251
client preparation for, 251
factors interfering with, 250
hCG and, 213
indications for, 250–251
nursing observations with, 251
procedure for, 251
reference values for, 250
Thalassemias, 28, 29, 30F
Thallium salts, toxicity of, 286T
Theophylline, blood levels of, 283T
Thiamine, urinary, 346
Thirst, antidiuretic hormone and, 214
Thoracentesis, 376
procedure for, 389
Thrombin, 51, 53

Thrombin clotting time (TCT, plasma
thrombin time), 68
clinical applications data for, 75
Thrombocytes. *See* Platelet *entries*
Thrombocytopenia, 54
causes of, 56T
Thrombocytosis, causes of, 56T
Thrombopoietin, 54
Thymocytes, monoclonal antibodies and,
87
Thymus, cellular immunity and, 83–84
Thyrocalcitonin. *See* Calcitonin
Thyroglobulin, 215
Thyroid gland biopsy, 452
aftercare with, 479–480
client preparation for, 479
contraindications to, 479
indications for, 478–479
nursing observations with, 479–480
procedure for, 479
Thyroid hormones, 215–218. *See also*
specific hormone, e.g.,
Triiodothyronine (T₃)
Thyroid screen, 216
Thyroid-stimulating hormone (TSH), 211
aftercare with, 233
client preparation for, 233
factors interfering with, 233
indications for, 233
nursing observations with, 233
procedure for, 233
prolactin and, 210
reference values for, 232
Thyroid-stimulating hormone (TSH)
stimulation test, 211–212
aftercare with, 234
client preparation for, 234
indications for, 233–234
nursing observations with, 234
procedure for, 234
reference values for, 233
Thyroid-stimulating immunoglobulins
(TSI, TSIg), 218
clinical applications data for, 242
Thyrotoxicosis
thyroxine in, 216
triiodothyronine in, 217
Thyrotropin. *See* Thyroid-stimulating
hormone
Thyrotropin-releasing hormone (TRH),
211
TSH stimulation test and, 211–212
Thyroxine (T₄), 215–216
aftercare with, 239
blood glucose and, 132T
client preparation for, 239
factors interfering with, 238

Index of Tests Covered appears on p. xiii, at the front of the book.

Index of Tests Covered appears on p. xiii, at the front of the book.

Index of Tests Covered appears on p. xiii, at the front of the book.

Index of Tests covered appears on p. xiii, at the front of the book.